voices of

THE WOMEN'S HEALTH MOVEMENT

VOLUME TWO

voices of

THE WOMEN'S HEALTH MOVEMENT

VOLUME TWO

BARBARA SEAMAN

with LAURA ELDRIDGE

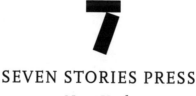

SEVEN STORIES PRESS

New York

Seven Stories Press
140 Watts Street
New York, NY 10013
www.sevenstories.com

College professors may order examination copies of Seven Stories Press titles for a free six-month trial period. To order, visit http://www.sevenstories.com/textbook or send a fax on school letterhead to (212) 226-1411.

Book design by Jon Gilbert

Library of Congress Cataloging-in-Publication Data

Voices of the women's health movement / edited by Barbara Seaman ; with Laura Eldridge.
    p. cm.
Includes bibliographical references and index.
ISBN 978-1-60980-444-2 (v. 1) -- ISBN 978-1-60980-446-6 (v. 2)
  1. Women--Health and hygiene. 2. Women--Health and hygiene--History. I. Seaman, Barbara. II. Eldridge, Laura.
[DNLM: 1. Women's Health--United States--Collected Works. 2. Feminism--United States--Collected Works. 3. Feminism--history--United States--Collected Works. 4. History, 19th Century--United States--Collected Works. 5. History, 20th Century--United States--Collected Works. 6. Women's Health--history--United States--Collected Works. 7. Women's Rights--United States--Collected Works. 8. Women's Rights--history--United States--Collected Works. WA 309]
  RA564.85.V65 2012
  362.1082--dc22
                        2010016341

Printed in the United States of America

9 8 7 6 5 4 3 2 1

Contents

Acknowledgments xv

Introduction
    by Barbara Seaman with Laura Eldridge..1

CHAPTER 12: SEX

Parlor Massages
    by Leora Tanenbaum 6

The Sexual Revolution Wasn't Our War
    by Anselma Dell'Olio 9

The Liberated Orgasm
    by Barbara Seaman 13

The Sexuality Questionnaire
    by Shere Hite...19

Shere Hite Debunks Freud's Vaginal Orgasm
    by Sarah J. Shey 23

A New View of Women's Sexual Problems
    by The Working Group on a New View of Women's Sexual Problems 27

Boys, Girls, Men, and Women: Variables of Experience
    by Rebecca Plante 30

Sex is Not a Natural Act
    by Leonore Tiefer...34

The Rise of Viagra: How the Little Blue Pill Changed Sex in America
    by Meika Loe...38

Slut! Growing Up Female With a Bad Reputation
    by Leora Tanenbaum 42

"Tell Me More, Tell Me More": Young Women's Locker Room Talk as a
    Boomer-Feminist Legacy
    by Paula Kamen..45

CHAPTER 13: SELF-HELP GYNECOLOGY

Self-Help Gynecology
    edited by Kofi Taha...48

Carol Downer's History-Bearing: Brushes with the Law
    by Gena Corea 56

Empowering the Pelvic Exam
    by Lila A. Wallis...57

Self-Helpless Gynecology
    by Caedmon Magboo Cahill..59

The Bridal Shower: We Haven't Come a Long Way, Baby
    by Betty Dodson 60

CHAPTER 14: MIND AND BODY: PSYCHOLOGY AND WOMEN

Psychology Constructs the Female
    by Naomi Weisstein..66

Demeter Revisited
    by Phyllis Chesler 70

Dominants
    by Jean Baker Miller..75

Mental Patients' Political Action Committee
    by Ellen Frankfort...77

An Interview with Jules Masserman
    Kathryn Watterson 78

Lineal Victims
    by Phyllis L. Fine..83

Airless Spaces
    by Shulamith Firestone..84

Catfight
    by Leora Tanenbaum 85

Women and Madness: a Feminist Diagnosis
    by Phyllis Chesler 92

Maud
    by Nell Casey 98

Addiction by Prescription: Women and the Problem of Tranquilizers
    by Andrea Tone..100

Women and Drug Addiction
    by Stephen R. Kandall...104

Silver Hills
    by Erica Warren 106

CHAPTER 15: RAPE AND VIOLENCE AGAINST WOMEN

Against Our Will: Men, Women, and Rape
    by Susan Brownmiller..116

Rape Doesn't End with a Kiss
    by Pauline Bart 118

Rape in Great Art
    by Audrey Flack 122

Working to End Sexual Violence on College Campuses
    by Helen Lowery and Nicole Levitz 128

Trauma and Recovery
    by Judith Herman...130

How to Befriend a Battered Woman
    by Barbara Seaman and Leslye E. Orloff 139

Fifty Ways Not to Leave an Abusive Spouse
    by Elaine Weiss 145

Out of Control
by Norma Fox Mazer 147

Our Guys
by Bernard Lefkowitz 150

The Campaign to Free Charline
by Jennifer Gonnerman 152

Surviving Intimate Terrorism
by Hedda Nussbaum 155

CHAPTER 16: WOMEN IN SPORTS

Women in Motion
by Lucinda Franks 160

The Athletic Triad: A Dangerous Triangle
by Lila A. Wallis 163

Patsy Mink on Title IX
interview by Tania Ketenjian 164

Why Feminists Are in Such Good Shape
by Amelia Richards 165

CHAPTER 17: BODY IMAGE

Fat Is a Feminist Issue
by Susie Orbach..168

Such a Pretty Face: Being Fat in America
by Marcia Millman 171

The Beauty Myth
by Naomi Wolf 175

Sacrificing Ourselves for Love
by Jane Wegscheider Hyman and Esther R. Rome 176

CHAPTER 18: BODY PARTS

FACE

Aging (balm for a 27th birthday)
by Erica Jong 179

The No-Nonsense Approach to Cleaning Your Face
by Deborah Chase 180

Susan Brownmiller on Appearance and Makeup
by Carrie Carmichael 183

HAIR

Body Hair: The Last Frontier
by Harriet Lyons and Rebecca Rosenblatt 185

All Hair the Conquering Heroine
by Lois Gould 186

Femininity
by Susan Brownmiller and Carrie Carmichael 188

Memoirs of a (Sorta) Ex-Shaver
by Carolyn Mackler 189

Browbeating
by Hagar Scher 192

Dreading It . . . Or How I Learned to Stop Fighting My Hair and
Love My Nappy Roots
by Veronica Chambers 193

BREASTS

The Anatomy of Your Breasts
by Marvin S. Eiger and Sally Wendkos Olds 195

The Bra Story
by Lori Barer 198

Breast Reduction
by Marta Drury 201

VAGINA

Breakthrough Against Female Genital Mutilation
by Noy Thrupkaew 201

CHAPTER 19: SEXUALLY TRANSMITTED INFECTIONS

Charity Girl
    by Michael Lowenthal...208

Sexually Transmitted Diseases on College Campuses
    by Lori Barer 211

A Circle of Women
    by Tara Greenway 212

And for Breast-feeding, Too, the Band Played On
    by Edith White 214

Midlife and Older Women Living with HIV/AIDS
    by Jane P. Fowler 217

Breaking the Walls of Silence: AIDS and Women in a Maximum State Prison
    by AIDS Counseling and Education Program,
    Bedford Hills Correctional Facility 219

Women's Health Care in Prison
    by Cassandra Shaylor...220

CHAPTER 20: CHRONIC ILLNESS

The Oral History of Rose Kushner
    interview by Anne S. Kasper..224

Dr. Susan Love
    interview by Tania Ketenjian...225

Stolen Conflicts: A Feminist Revisioning
    by Sharon Batt 230

Fighting the "War" on Breast Cancer: How a Metaphor Has Shaped the
    Debate on Early Detection and Treatment
    by Barron H. Lerner 234

Anne S. Kasper
    interview by Tania Ketenjian...236

Women's Hearts at Risk
    by Charlotte Libov...239

The Myth of Osteoporosis
 by Gillian Sanson...243

CHAPTER 21: INFORMED CONSENT, CONFLICT OF INTEREST, AND PHARMACEUTICAL COMPANIES

The Amazing Story of DES
 by Barbara Seaman and Gideon Seaman......................................249

It's Only Once Around the Merry-Go-Round
 by Margot Adler..256

How Do You Know It's True?
 by Victor Cohn...257

Diana Petitti, MD
 interview by Tania Ketenjian...261

A Different Prescription
 by Anne Rochon Ford 265

Should Prescription Drugs Be Advertised?
 by Michael Castleman and Maryann Napoli 271

The American Cancer Society: The World's Wealthiest "Nonprofit" Institution
 by Sam Epstein...272

CHAPTER 22: END OF LIFE ISSUES

Out of Pain and Anger
 by Marilyn Webb 276

Good Mourning, America
 by Amy Pagnozzi 281

Dying into Grace: Mother and Daughter . . . a Dance of Healing
 by Artemis March..284

CHAPTER 23: WOMEN'S HEALTH, MOVING FORWARD

Changing Concepts of Women's Health: Advocating for Change
 by Julia Scott..293

The Whole Woman
    by Germaine Greer...296

Women's Health and Government Regulation: 1950–1980
    by Suzanne White Junod..303

Map of the Women's Health Movement
    by Sheryl Burt Ruzek...308

Cindy Pearson
    interview by Tania Ketenjian..315

On Young Feminism
    by Sunny Daly...321

Our Bodies, Our Voices, Our Choices
    by the National Black Women's Health Project...322

Patsy Mink on Health Issues for Asian Women
    interview by Tania Ketenjian..341

Charon Asetoyer
    interview by Tania Ketenjian..344

In Conclusion, In Memoriam, In Hope 347

About the Contributors...351

About the Editors 366

Index..367

Contents of Volume One...382

To My Daughter, Elana Felicia
—Barbara

To My Grandmothers, Grace, Ellen, and Ray
—Laura

Acknowledgments

FIRST AND FOREMOST, thanks to our agent, Valerie Borchardt, who is generous and patient with her time and good advice, and also to Anne and Georges Borchardt.

Many thanks to our editor, Theresa Noll, whose talent and calm never cease to amaze us—this book bears evidence of her vision and hard work in every section. Our gratitude goes also to Amy Scholder, who helped us to imagine what the book might look like and saw our plans realized. Our deepest admiration and thanks to Dan Simon, who we have been fortunate to know and work with for many years.

Barbara thanks her co-founders of the National Women's Health Network: Alice Wolfson, Belita Cowan, Phylis Chesler, PhD, and Mary Howell, MD. Also to Cindy Pearson, Olivia Cousins, PhD, and Amy Allina who carried on our goals. We are grateful to Phil Corfman, MD, and Richard Crout, MD (who stood up for informed consent in women's health care), Judy Norsigian (OBOS), Pat Cody and Sybil Shainwald (on behalf of DES families), Maryann Napoli (Center for Medical Consumers), Susan Wood, PhD (formerly of the FDA), and Nancy Krieger, PhD.

We are grateful also to Andrea Tone, Leonore Tiefer, Shere Hite, Gloria Steinem, Congresswoman Carolyn Maloney, Minna Elias, Sheryl Burt Ruzek, Barbara Brenner, Barbara Ehrenreich, Alice Yaker, Suzanne Parisian, MD, Byllye Avery, Susan Love, MD, David Michaels, PhD, Devra Lee Davis, PhD, Carolyn Westhoff, MD, Elizabeth Siegel Watkins, PhD, Pat Cody, Gordon Guyatt, MD, Bruce Stadel, Diane Meier, MD, Ben Loehnen, Jennifer Baumgardner, Nikki Scheuer, Sheila and Donald Bandman, Judge Emily Jane Goodman, Daniel Simon, Thomas Hartman, E. Neil Schachter, Debra Chase, Tara Parker Pope, Senator Ron Wyden, Nora Coffey, Warren Bell, MD, Alan Cassels, Wendy Armstrong, Colleen Fuller, Anne Rochon-Ford, Leora Tanenbaum, Abby Lippman, PhD, Harriet Rosenberg, PhD, Amy Richards, Pam Martens, Ariel Olive, Ann Fuller, Barbara Mintzes, Aubrey Blumsohn, MD, Frances C. Whittelsey, K-K Seaman, Ronnie Eldridge, Mavra Stark, Joan Michel, and Linda K. Nathan.

To our top-notch assistants: Sara Germain was relentless in helping us contact authors and choose selections. Megan Buckley, Helen Lowery, Reed Eldridge, and Seven Stories' Daniella Gitlin were all helpful at crucial moments. Thanks to Kim Chung, who against all odds kept our computers running, and Maria Tylutki, who made sure everything else around the office was organized and as efficient as possible. And as always we are grateful to Agata Rumprecht-Behrens, who knows where things are better than either of us and who helps with whatever project we are working on despite her own busy schedule.

ADDITIONAL ACKNOWLEDGMENTS FROM BARBARA:

My deepest gratitude to Dr. Susan Love, Dr. Neil Schachter, Deborah Chase, and Dr. Diane Meier.

I am grateful to Ruth Gruber, my stepmother; my sisters, Elaine Rosner Jeria and Jeri Drucker, and Jeri's husband Ernest Drucker, PhD; my children, Noah, Shira, and Elana; my sons-in-law, Urs Bamert and Timothy Walsh; my cousins, Amelia Rosner and Richard Hyfler; and Jesse Drucker, Nell Casey, and Henry Jeria.

All my love to my grandchildren, Sophia Bamert, Idalia Bamert, Liam Walsh, and Ezekiel Walsh.

ADDITIONAL ACKNOWLEDGMENTS FROM LAURA:

I would like to thank Irene Xanthoudakis, Rebecca Kraut, Lauren Porsch, Molly Barry, Rachel Fisher, Rumela Mitra, Helen Lowery, April Timko, Nicole Richman, Stephanie Kirk, Chi-Hyun Kim, Susan Masry, Rob Tennant, Rabbi Sari Laufer, Leonore Tiefer, Danie Greenwell, Alisa Kraut, Brian Cooke, Chris Rugen, Kim Jordan, Jenny Tomczak, Caroline Cruz, Amy Troy, Melissa Barrett, Jennifer Smith-Garvin, Karla Wiehagen, Anne Taylor, Kate Jefferson, Chad and Sonya Cooper, Miriam Silberstein, and Katie Walker.

Much, much love goes to my brothers, David, Reed, and Peter, my dearest friends, and to my grandfather Paul Eldridge, Sr.

My gratitude to the Seaman family, who have supported me through the years, and given me the chance to love and grieve my dear friend properly. They are like a second family and I am blessed to have them in my life.

Many thanks to Sheldon, Beth, Marnie, Zachary and Josh Weinberg, and to the entire Weinberg/Josell/Alperin family.

My parents Paul and Susan Eldridge are my best examples of how to lead meaningful, ethical lives. They have given me big shoes to fill and helped me as best they could to be up to the task. My son, Levi Jacob, has blessed and challenged me in countless ways. Jeremy Weinberg has been an unending source of love, patience and support. His kindness, intelligence, and humor are the great pleasures of my life, and I am truly fortunate to have him as my partner in everything I undertake.

Introduction

WHEN ELIZABETH CADY STANTON decided to re-set her son's collarbone in the mid-nineteenth century she wasn't trying to be radical, she was trying to be a good mother. She wasn't trying to empower female healing and reject the mostly male medical establishment. She was trying to respond to the unalleviated pain of a cherished love one.

In addition to her tireless writing and activism, Stanton was a mother of five children. Never daunted, Stanton moved her writing desk into the nursery and worked in between spending time with her brood. When her eldest son Daniel was born with a dislocated collarbone, the Stantons tried to get him the best medical care. Repeated doctors' visits resulted in bandaging and treatments that actually made the problem worse. When a nurse helping Daniel refused to respond to the fact that his hand was turning blue from the bandages, saying, "I shall never interfere with the doctor," Stanton sprang into action. She replaced the doctor only to be disappointed a second time. She wasn't about to be fooled a third time, and, to the nurse's shock, took off her son's bandages and with arnica (a homeopathic remedy) and gentle pressure re-dressed her son's bones. She concluded, "I learned another lesson in self-reliance. I trusted neither men nor books absolutely after this . . . but continued to use my 'mother's instinct,' if 'reason' is too dignified a term to apply to a woman's thoughts."

Her decisiveness goes to the heart of women's health activism. It is almost always born of personal experience, often a social injustice acted out on the body. It is inherently and un-self-consciously radical. Throughout human history—and more recently the nineteenth and twentieth centuries, we have witnessed brilliant and courageous examples of women taking control of their bodies and health choices. These experiences have often led to a greater sense of autonomy and equality. In many ways, it is an original rebellion.

In these days as we debate the basic right of human beings to have medical care, it is an often-made point that one of the simplest ways to control a citizenry is through access to health services. Women have known this for a long time, and the process of coming to understand and reject this system of control often helps them to see themselves as independent agents in a larger sense.

In the nineteenth century, medical services were consolidated by doctors taken with new and changing medical technologies. As physicians and scientists pioneered surgeries, pharmaceuticals, and new mental health practices, they pushed out traditional (often female) providers, including midwives and makers of alternative medicines. Because these doctors were almost entirely male, they treated distinctively female body parts and health issues as disease. Male bodies were healthy and female ones were pathological. Nineteenth- and early twentieth-century ideas of the hysterical woman appall our twenty-first century sensibilities, but they haven't entirely gone away. The way that menopause has been treated as a disease state is evidence that while there is now a different language used to misinterpret and medicate women's bodies, the tendency persists.

When Elizabeth Cady Stanton and the other first-wave feminists abandoned the recommendations of physicians, they were creating a model of resistance that lived on in small pockets of activism throughout the twentieth century and then was taken up again in major ways in the 1970s. I was lucky enough to be a part of that movement.

When we talk about the "women's health movement," we are, of course, talking about many movements. We can look to the work of women who writer Susan Brownmiller has termed our "heroic antecedents," daring women in past centuries who stood up against a culture that discouraged open speech about health problems, or who provided alternative care when none was available. We can speak specifically about the second-wave women's movement in the 1970s and look at the foundational writings that have changed the landscape of women's health. And we can listen to the voices of young activists who help us to understand the new issues we face today.

So many of my friends recall sitting in rooms where secrets were shared among women. Typically any shameful feelings we may have had lifted as we learned that our private experiences often turned out to be universal.

I remember the voices: "Yes, I had an illegal abortion." "Yes, I was raped." "Yes, my neighbor (brother, father, uncle, priest, doctor, therapist, teacher) hassled me sexually." "Yes, I faked orgasms." "Yes, every birth control method I've ever used was a disaster." "Yes, my gynecologist makes me feel uncomfortable, but I can't admit it, he's so esteemed. His pelvic exams are so rough it hurts." "Yes, I took a drug that made me very sick, but my doctor told me to keep taking it."

Women talked, listened, and spread the word. We went back to our communities, started our own women's groups, consciousness-raising groups, and know-your-body courses. By 1975, there were nearly 2,000 official women's self-help projects scattered around the United States and countless unofficial ones.

Do women talk less to each other now than they did then? The very possibility is troubling.

If I have a single hope for this book it is that the women who read it be inspired to talk among themselves about health, since women who talk to each other about health will go on to talk to each other about anything and everything.

At the turn of the millennium, a Barnard College senior asked Judy Norsigian of *Our Bodies, Ourselves* what she hopes to see when the continuously updated volume celebrates its fiftieth anniversary in the year 2020. Norsigian answered, "The creation of a health and a medical care system that is far more responsive to women's needs and accessible to all women regardless of age, income, sexual preference, race, etc. . . . And using technology in the most appropriate way—that is science-based, not profit-based . . ." People need to be in control of their own health. But in order for that to be possible, they must have information from a trustworthy source.

I asked Cindy Pearson, executive director of the National Women's Health Network, what she thinks about patients taking their health into their own hands. "Thirty years ago," Pearson said, "if anyone talked about a bad experience they had with the health care system . . . the response would usually be 'You need a better doctor. . . .'" Today, in part through the hard-won battles of consumer advocates, AIDS activists, and the feminist health movement, among others, that isn't the only answer. Pearson continues, "People talked about finding a good doctor but then realized good doctors aren't the answer, informed patients are the answer."

We believe that within the yin and yang of these two thoughtful responses there is to be found the right approach: good science combined with leadership from the patients' points of view. What makes a good doctor these days isn't always easy to say. But if there is one quality we should all be looking for in our doctors, it is the willingness to listen seriously to their patients.

CHAPTER 12

Sex

SEXUALITY HAS ALWAYS BEEN a feminist battleground. It has been an issue around which we have organized and come together and at other times it has torn us apart. From activism around the access and safety of birth control to writings about sexual pleasure and bedroom equality and of course notorious debates about pornography, women's health writers have a lot to say and a lot to teach us.

Few issues are at once so private and so public, and elicit such strong feelings on all sides. You could feel the whole world shake a little in the mid-1970s when the beautiful and brilliant Shere Hite published her paradigm-changing *Hite Report on Female Sexuality*. Building on earlier works by women's health movement writers, as well as thousands of questionnaires that the young graduate student published in her apartment and distributed everywhere she could, the book revealed the extent of women's dissatisfaction with the sexual status quo and posed serious critiques of the classic Masters and Johnson model of sexuality. Hite rejected the still-perpetuated idea that most women could climax from heterosexual intercourse, further dismantling the idea that women who failed to do so were frigid. That Hite struck a nerve with both women and men was evident in the intense media scrutiny that followed Hite in the decades after the original *Hite Report*. After the publication of *Women and Love: A Cultural Revolution in Progress*, Hite was so abused and criticized that she fled America for Europe, where she lives today.

If feminists thought the ideas of the frigid woman died with the twentieth century, they were mistaken. In the late 1990s, a little blue pill called Viagra became an unprecedented success and changed the relationship between drugs and the bedroom. An intense search began for a female version, a sexual aid that could be marketed to women. Along with the chemical search for compounds that would work in the body, another quest was underway: pharmaceutical companies began looking for women who could be diagnosed with "female sexual dysfunction" (FSD). Conferences at esteemed medical schools backed by drug company dollars began turning out terrifying statistics suggesting that the *majority* of women might have this disease, and strived to develop "treatment alternatives."

From this dark moment for women's health, so dominated by pharmaceutical greed, ersatz science, and sexism, rose one of the most original and powerful voices in women's health activism today. Leonore Tiefer is a New York–based psychologist and sexologist. A lifelong feminist, Tiefer's critique of the new FSD fervor led to the establishment of the grass roots group A New View of Women's Sexual Problems. Far from being only a medical problem, Tiefer and the New View argued, most female sexual problems were also psychological and social. By reducing the complexities of sexuality to a tiny pill, scientists were ignoring histories of physical abuse, social stigmas on sexual expression, and decades of people living with fear, pain, and guilt about their sexual practice. Voices like the New View helped contribute to the successful blocking of FDA approval for a testosterone patch for sexual dysfunction, and continues to advocate for women as the frantic search for female Viagra rolls along.

In addition to providing important analytical tools for women interested in resisting the medicalization of sex, the New View provided an outlet for older and younger activists to work together. Many women in the group were still in their twenties when they became active.

Parlor Massages

LEORA TANENBAUM

Leora Tanenbaum, adapted from "Parlor Massages," a review of Rachel P. Maines, *The Technology of Orgasm: "Hysteria," the Vibrator, and Women's Sexual Satisfaction*, Baltimore: Johns Hopkins University Press, 1999, published in *The Women's Review of Books*, April 1999. Reprinted by permission.

A bizarre episode in the history of physician "manipulation" of female sexuality has been accidentally discovered by Rachel Maines in The Technology of Orgasm, *here reviewed by Leora Tanenbaum.*

Many people equate sex with heterosexual intercourse. So widespread is the idea that oral sex, for instance, "doesn't count" as sex that teenagers who engage in it exclusively identify themselves as virgins. Indeed, in the "Sex in America" national survey of a few years ago, in which over 3,000 Americans were queried about their sexual practices, 95 percent said that they had had vaginal intercourse the last time they had had sex. Eighty percent said that they had had vaginal intercourse every single time they'd had sex within the past year. Despite the opportunity for variety, coitus is far and away the most popular heterosexual act.

Which is too bad. We females know all too well that intercourse is not necessarily—how shall I put this?—the most satisfying sexual act. As Shere Hite revealed in her *Hite Report* on female sexuality back in 1976, the majority of women simply do not experience orgasm through penetration alone. It is obvious that intercourse benefits men far more than women: For the heterosexual man, coitus nearly always leads to orgasm, regardless of whether he pays any extra-coital attention to his partner's pleasure.

So where is a sexually frustrated heterosexual woman to turn to relieve her frustration? The answer: the vibrator. Easy, quick, and practically guaranteed effective, the vibrator, as many of us know, is far more efficient than manual masturbation.

The vibrator has been around far longer than you might think. In *The Technology of Orgasm*, historian Rachel Maines traces the evolution of this sex aid back to the 1880s. She also finds that the precursor to the vibrator—midwife- or physician-assisted genital massage—dates all the way back to Hippocrates. For millennia, genital massage was a medically sanctioned procedure, designed to help supposedly ill or deviant women diagnosed with "hysteria." Maines uses the vibrator as a tool (so to speak) to expose Western medicine's long-standing preference for coitus and mistrust of women who are not sexually satisfied through penetration alone. In this original, witty, thoroughly researched, and eye-opening book (complete with photographs and drawings of old-fashioned vibrators), Maines skewers male-centered beliefs about female sexual satisfaction as well as the whole concept of "hysteria."

How Maines found her topic is almost as fascinating as vibrator history itself. She started out, she explains, doing graduate research on needlework history, which meant combing through turn-of-the-century women's magazines such as *Modern Priscilla* and *Woman's Home Companion*. But her attention kept wandering to the sides of the pages, which contained vibrator advertisements. At first Maines reacted to "their turgid prose" by assuming that "I simply had a dirty mind." Surely masturbation was not the purpose of these electrical appliances. (One, White Cross, was named after an 1880s British Episcopalian sexual purity organization to suggest virtue and chastity, she notes.) But her curiosity was piqued, and she investigated this sideline interest at the Bakken Library and Museum of Electricity in Life, in Minneapolis, which houses eleven turn-of-the-century vibrators (listed in their catalogue as "musculo-skeletal relaxation devices"). Encouraged by the museum staff, Maines dropped her textile history research to pursue the origins of this "capital-labor substitution innovation."

Beginning in the fifth century BCE, a woman was diagnosed with hysteria if she exhibited any or all of the following: anxiety, sleeplessness, irritability, nervousness, muscle spasms, sensations of heaviness in the abdomen, or "a tendency to cause trouble for others." Hysteria was believed to result from sexual deprivation. But "sex" meant "marital coitus"; any woman who did not reach orgasm through coitus, then, was potentially diseased. In the late nineteenth century, as many as three-quarters of the American female population were diagnosed with hysteria; it is one of the most frequently diagnosed diseases in history.

Maines observes that "hysteria"—a Greek word meaning "that which proceeds from the uterus"— essentially pathologizes all women, since "this purported disease . . . displayed a symptomatology consistent with the normal functioning of female sexuality." The American Psychiatric Association only officially eliminated hysteria from its canon of diseases in 1952.

The standard treatment for hysteria was genital massage to orgasm, conducted either by the physician himself or by a midwife. Masturbation was forbidden, since it was believed to cause disorders and diseases (in men as well as women). In the first century CE, Galen noted that genital massage therapy resulted in the release of a fluid from the vagina, after which the patient was cured of her symptoms (at least temporarily). Soranus instructed physicians who practiced genital massage to "moisten these parts freely with sweet oil, keeping it up for some time." In the Middle Ages and Renaissance, physicians began to turn over the task of genital massage to midwives. Maines quotes from a 1653 medical compendium in which the author advises: "We think it necessary to ask a midwife to assist, so that she can massage the genitalia with one finger inside, using oil of lilies, musk root, crocus, or [something] similar. And in this way the afflicted woman can be aroused to the paroxysm."

The amazing thing is that no one seemed to notice that the paroxysm was in fact an orgasm. Since no penetration occurred, physicians did not recognize the treatment as being sexual in nature, nor did they realize that their patients derived sexual gratification from their "hysterical paroxysm." Maines does point out that occasionally, one or two physicians would publicly express concern about "whether to draw this harmful fluid out of the uterus by exciting and rubbing the private parts," but they seem to have been vastly outnumbered by their massage-happy colleagues.

In nineteenth-century Europe and the United States, it was widely believed that women were satisfied with intercourse regardless of whether they experienced what we now define as an orgasm, or even that "normal" women possessed no sexual desire at all. Either way, the sexual nature of genital massage was camouflaged, "since in the first case no penetration (and therefore nothing sexual) was occurring during the treatment and in the second case sexual pleasure on the part of the patient was theoretically impossible."

Lest you suppose that physicians performed genital massage for their own titillation, Maines is quick to point out that they did not enjoy the treatment. "On the contrary," she writes, "this male elite sought every opportunity to substitute other devices for their fingers, such as the attentions of a husband, the hands of a midwife, or the business end of some tireless and impersonal mechanism. . . . Like many husbands, doctors were reluctant to inconvenience themselves in performing what was, after all, a routine chore." Indeed, Maines titles her chapter detailing the history of medical genital massage "The Job Nobody Wanted."

The electromechanical vibrator was invented in the 1880s by a British physician: the first reliable treatment for hysteria. (Hydrotherapy, a precursor to the vibrator—the use of pumped water aimed at the pelvis—had been popular for "female disorders" during the previous hundred years, but the appliances were inordinately expensive.) The vibrator was eagerly embraced by doctors, who could now significantly increase the number of patients they could treat, and the income they could generate. (Women diagnosed with hysteria formed a particularly lucrative market: their "disease" was not deadly, and they required regular treatment.) By 1900, there were over a dozen vibrators available to physicians. The "Cadillac of vibrators," the 125-pound Chattanooga, cost $200 plus freight charges in 1904.

By 1905, many models were portable, allowing their use on house calls. Soon after, manufacturers began to bypass doctors altogether and targeted their wares directly to women's magazines such as *McClure's, Needlecraft*, and *Hearst's*. They were marketed as a health and relaxation aid, promising women that "all the pleasures of youth . . . will

throb within you." In 1918 the Sears, Roebuck, and Company Electrical Goods catalog offered six vibrator models, ranging in price from $5.95 to a deluxe model with numerous vibrators at $28.75.

In the 1920s, the vibrator fell out of use. The camouflage disappeared, revealing the sexual purpose of the device: Freud and others had correctly identified the clitoral orgasm as a sexual climax (though Freud mistakenly differentiated it from the so-called vaginal orgasm). Vibrators began to appear in erotic films. No longer was it possible to pretend that a vibrator-assisted masturbatory session at the local doctor's office was just another hum-drum treatment for a chronic disease. The vibrator only resurfaced in the 1960s as a sex aid. Today, you can purchase a vibrator quite easily: You can visit a women's sex store like Good Vibrations in San Francisco and Eve's Garden in New York City, or you can stop by your local electrical appliance store and pick one up, now sold (again) as a massage relaxation aid.

The Technology of Orgasm is a fun read. But it's frightening how many of the old attitudes about female sexuality continue to thrive. As recently as 1965, one medical authority said that he did not like to recommend clitoral stimulation to his patients because "most men . . . feel that the need to bring a woman to climax through clitoral stimulation is a burden." Maines observes that even today, heterosexual women are made to feel guilt if they cannot reach orgasm through penetration alone. Many men, eager to preserve their own hassle-free pleasure or worried that they may be sexually inadequate, or both, scoff when presented with the mechanical facts of female sexuality.

The male preference for penetration is so strong that Maines has been unable to carve an academic career in the area of female sexuality, despite her obvious research and analytic talents. In 1986, after she published her first article on vibrators, she lost her teaching job at Clarkson University, in part because the school feared that alumni would stop giving money if they discovered her line of research. She also tells us that after one early presentation of her findings, a male tenured professor told her that he was not convinced by her arguments, since "the sexual experience of women using vibrators and their predecessors was 'not the real thing.'"

Maines retails this reaction to illustrate that many men can't even fathom male-female sexual relations without penetration. But the comment is revealing in another way as well. Perhaps the professor intended to suggest that an act should not be classified as "sex" if those involved do not think of it as such. And he would have had a point. When a midwife genitally massaged a female patient as part of her workday routine, should that act be identified as a lesbian sexual experience? I would say no. Likewise, when a male physician masturbated a patient for medical reasons, the two could hardly be said to be engaging in sex, either.

As Maines so deftly shows, "sex" means different things to different people. Harm is done, however, when female sexual needs go unrecognized because of a narrow, male-oriented definition of "sex." So let's penetrate, if you will, the myth of penetrative sex and broaden women's sexual experiences.

The Sexual Revolution Wasn't Our War

ANSELMA DELL'OLIO

Anselma Dell'Olio, "The Sexual Revolution Wasn't Our War," *Ms.*, Spring 1972. Reprinted by permission.

The women's liberation movement caught men off guard. They thought women had *already* been liberated by the sexual revolution.

According to most men, a liberated woman was one who put out sexually at the drop of a suggestive comment, who didn't demand marriage, and who "took care of herself" in terms of contraceptives. As far as men were concerned, that's all the liberation any woman needed. The bonus of bralessness and economically independent women simply fueled the misconception that the women's liberation movement was in some way a continuation of the sexual revolution, also known as the more-free-sex-for-us revolution.

In truth, women had been liberated only from the right to say no to sexual intercourse with men. Kinsey in the fifties, and Masters and Johnson in the sixties, contributed scientific ammunition for the sexual revolution which freed women from Victorian morality. This gift relieved us of centuries of moral and social pressure which had dictated that no *nice* woman would ever "go all the way" with a man until marriage.

But it destroyed the sanctuary of maidenhood, pressuring us to give our bodies without respite from late adolescence to old age, or until our desirability as sex objects waned. For the first time, we were shorn of all protection (patronizing as it may have been, and selective in terms of class privilege) and openly exhorted to prostitute ourselves in the name of the new morality.

We have come to see that the so-called sexual revolution is merely a link in the chain of abuse laid on women throughout patriarchal history. While purporting to restructure the unequal basis for sexual relationships between men and women, our munificent male liberators were in fact continuing their control of female sexuality.

With the advent of the new feminism, women finally began to ask, "What's in it for us?" And the answer is simple: We've been sold out. The sexual revolution was a battle fought by men for the greater good of mankind. Womankind was left holding the double standard. We're supposed to give, but what do we get? Kinsey's *Sexual Behavior in the Human Female* offered a priceless handbook for the revolution in its finding that (1) women could and did enjoy sex after all, (2) there is no such thing as a frigid woman, only inept men, (3) virginity in women was no longer considered important or particularly desirable by most men, and (4) women and men were now equals in bed and equally free to screw their bottoms off for the sheer fun of it.

What the popularizers of Kinsey's findings neglected to emphasize would have provided the seeds for a *real* revolution in the bedroom. We still remained ignorant about the difference between orgasm and ejaculation, about the speed-of-response differential between male and female orgasm, about the fallacy of the vaginal-clitoral orgasm dichotomy, about women's multiorgasmic nature, and so on. Because of this deliberate or unconscious *excising* of Kinsey, and later Masters and Johnson, we have managed to survive into the seventies with the double standard intact, alive and well in the minds of average American males. And many females as well.

The new freedom of the sexual revolution was at best a failure, at worst a hoax—because it never caused significant changes in the social attitudes and behavior of men to correspond with this new morality being forced upon women. There has been no real revolution in the bedroom. For this crucial reason, the sexual revolution and the women's movement are polar opposites in philosophy, principles, goals, and spirit.

The real point is that there are not many women—liberated, unliberated, feminist, or otherwise—who are sleeping around for the sheer pleasure of it. The Achilles' heel of the sexual revolution is persistent male ignorance of the female orgasm.

Now, if there was anything that a sexual revolution should have been able to accomplish, especially with the data made available by Kinsey as early as 1953, it should have been more pleasure for women during intercourse. Yet nineteen years later, the majority of women have to put up with relatively infrequent orgasms during sexual—at least heterosexual—encounters.

Of course, before Freud, the question of orgasm was moot because women weren't supposed to enjoy sex at all. Decent women submitted to it with clenched teeth. With Freud, female orgasm was rediscovered, and the high incidence of female frigidity was declared to be an emotional and psychological problem of "sexually immature" women. Vexed by the fact that women could reach orgasm freely and quickly through masturbation, but less frequently during standard intercourse, Freud thought there must be two kinds of female orgasm: clitoral and vaginal. The clitoral orgasm, which worked for most women, but was difficult in the standard male-gratifying positions, was defined as "adolescent." The vaginal orgasm was declared to be the only true, mature, womanly orgasm. It could only be achieved during intercourse through vaginal penetration by the penis. Since overwhelming numbers of women weren't experiencing the "mature" orgasm, Freud concluded that women, recognizing their inferiority to men, were loath to accept their femininity. For this dreadful condition he prescribed psychiatric assistance.

Over the decades psychiatrists have treated scores of us with little success, trying to get us to surrender to our destinies by transferring our orgasms from clitoris to vagina. Generations of women, including the present one, grew up masturbating in secret (men talked about masturbating long before women did), and faking orgasm during intercourse.

Kinsey and Masters and Johnson should have changed all that. Neither study produced a shred of evidence in defense of the double-orgasm theory. As a result of their extensive experiments, Masters and Johnson advanced three important conclusions:

1. The dichotomy of vaginal and clitoral orgasm is entirely false. Anatomically, all orgasms are centered in the clitoris, whether they result from direct manual pressure applied to the clitoris, indirect pressure resulting from the thrusting of the penis during intercourse, or generalized sexual stimulation of other erogenous zones, such as the breasts.

2. Women are naturally multiorgasmic. That is, if a woman is immediately stimulated following orgasm, she is likely to experience several orgasms in rapid succession. This is not an exceptional occurrence, but one of which most women are capable. In all of their students, Masters and Johnson

found no incidence of a totally or clinically frigid woman.

3. While women's orgasms do not vary in kind, they vary in intensity. The most intense orgasms experienced by the research subjects were by masturbatory manual stimulation by the partner. The least intense orgasms were experienced during intercourse.

These findings were surely cataclysmic and should have been liberating, at least to the degree that they served to destroy established myths. Yet five years after publication, they still have had little or no impact on men's minds or women's lives.

Many women are still not having orgasms and still, as noted earlier, not sleeping around for pleasure—an unchanging fact despite the sexual revolution. In the meantime, men *are* pursuing sex for just that reason.

If pleasure is rarely the reward, women's continued willingness to have intercourse doesn't make sense. Why, then, are we doing it?

The truth is we are often pressured into it, and not only by the litany of the sexual revolution. It may be the need for affection and attention. Or the desire to please; the need for approval. It's no news to any of us that men can have intercourse with women they are totally disinterested in as human beings. For many women, sex fails to bring physical satisfaction, and depersonalized sex denies women even the side benefits of communication and approval.

What the sexual revolution should have taught us is that *need* shouldn't be confused with *love*; that men and women can neither give nor receive love until we stop confusing it with a need for security and approval. The women's movement is trying to teach that lesson. Love is not getting high on fantasies of romance, the perfect lover, absolute happiness, and sexual ecstasy. Love is based on two-way communication and respect, and that only exists between equals.

When feminists are critical of romance, there is often a panicked reaction: "But you can't possibly want to get rid of love?"

No, we don't want to negate the emotion. We want a better definition. We want to get rid of the sick and hoary old illusions that women have pursued relentlessly at the price of our humanity. What is called love now is so clearly exploitative and unsatisfactory that it should make us suspicious that men want to preserve it at all costs. What is called love now is vital to the oppression of women.

Men have poured their creative energies into work; we have poured ours into love, and an unequal social and sexual relationship was the inevitable result. And because this was the situation the sexual revolution failed to correct, feminists are moving into an area they have won by default.

The problems are enormous. Whenever we manage to combat our sense of insecurity long enough to go out and actually do something, our attitude is betrayed by our conditioned belief that women's work is dispensable, our contributions secondary. When the man in our life complains about our absorption in work, we are apologetic. We turn somersaults to accomplish it at odd hours rather than claim our time as our own and risk his disapproval, anger, or complete rejection. Often, we apologize for our work even before a man has time to object—so thorough is our conditioning. And men most often accept our sacrifice as their due. The *droit du seigneur* of the sexual revolution.

Therefore, a sexually liberated woman without a feminist consciousness is nothing more than a new variety of prostitute for the sexual revolution. If we don't sell ourselves for money in the street or security in the suburbs, we sell ourselves in exchange for some measure of approval and (we hope) lasting affection.

Feminism was reborn in part to protest and correct the fact that, although women are no longer burdened by an old-fashioned morality (which is good), we are now saddled with the entire range of emotional and physical consequences of sexual availability (which is bad).

That old form of censure—every woman a virgin or else—was simply one side of the coin.

The ancient epithet of "promiscuous" was always the other, and the coin has now been turned over. Promiscuity has lost none of its old sting. It has only acquired a whole new negative connotation with the aid and comfort of psychology, psycho-analysis, and psychiatry. Practitioners in these fields have taken to accusing the sexually active woman of "emotional" frigidity, inability to relate, nymphomania, etc. So even the apparent gain for women is illusory. If we are no longer expected to be virgins physically, we are still expected to be "practicing" virgins—mentally pure, and only "in love" with one man.

There are many women who have decided to challenge the hypocrisy of the sexual revolution by refusing to tolerate this double-standard non-sense and becoming at least as sexually liberated as men are. They soon find out that, emotional problems aside (and they are not insignificant), the physical obstacles are close to insurmountable. The physical price a woman stands to pay for sexual nonchalance is staggering. A woman's chances of getting pregnant are still good (meaning bad), and those chances get better (meaning worse) as the frequency of, and number of partners for, intercourse increases.

The pill is hazardous, and other forms of con-traception are a drag, a distraction, and a nuisance, not to mention being failure-prone. Tampering with women's vastly more complex reproductive system is all right with men, but vasectomy, still the most practical, inexpensive method of birth control which can be performed in minutes in the doctor's office, is not; at least, not with most men. The virility-fertility connection is sacrosanct. And there you have the clearest evidence of why feminists view the sexual revolution as one more male ego trip. What kind of sexual revolution is it when, in the year 1971, the possibility of a practical male contraceptive still goes largely unresearched and unpublicized?

It's now clear that the dice are loaded and the women's movement is the one force that can make the game honest. The rising chorus of laments

about a growing incidence of male impotence probably means that our feeble attempts to correct the situation are going in the right direction. It can't hurt for men to begin to experience a small dose of the medicine women have had to swallow for a century.

The sexual politics imbedded in the culture shows itself clearly through the language bias. When men don't function sexually, they are called "impotent," *without power.* When women don't, they are called "frigid," *icy cold.* The active-passive dichotomy is apparent. Men know a good thing when they have it, and they go to whatever lengths are necessary to protect their potency. If a woman is a threat to that potency, then her ego must be crushed. Notice that we never hear about females being "castrated" when our egos are destroyed and our potency denied. Such melodramatic sym-bolism is reserved for men. In fact, a woman's loss—her frigidity, her inability to derive pleasure from sex—is frequently described by men as "cas-trating." Frigidity is our fault, and male impotency is our fault too!

Perhaps the best evidence of the phoniness of the sexual revolution is the prevailing eighteenth-century attitude toward masturbation. For men, it is a fact of life. Locker rooms and little boys' habits have made it so. But for women, autoeroti-cism is a newly discovered secret. In view of the fact that there are women who still fake orgasm, women who feel embarrassed to request their own satisfaction in intercourse, or women who flatly tell a partner, "I don't come, so don't wait for me," it's about time we perfected the art of mas-turbation. Not as a substitute for intercourse, but as one means to pleasure and to the understanding of our own bodies.

These subjects remain difficult to discuss in plain language, and so the women's movement has rushed in where the sexual revolution feared to tread. And none too soon. As Susan Lydon says in *Sisterhood Is Powerful,* "Appearances notwith-standing, the age-old taboos against conversation about personal sexual experience haven't yet been broken down." This reluctance on the part of most people to discuss the issues openly and honestly has allowed the creation of many myths about sexual supermen and superwomen. Men who are inadequate lovers squirm out of their plight by claiming that a previous girlfriend was a real sexpot who had fourteen vaginal orgasms in five minutes, so what's wrong with *you* anyway? Men strangle us with our sisters' lies. The next time you're tempted to fake orgasm, just think of the harm you may be doing to the next woman, if not to yourself.

A man with some respect for himself and you will not be turned off by your honesty. You may be the first woman who ever talked to him straight, and he may welcome the opportunity to clear up doubts of his own. And if he is turned off, you are well rid of him. As long as you allow yourself to be victimized, rest assured you *will* be—again and again. If female sexuality has been such a mystery to women for so long, think how mysterious it must be to men.

Men are severely troubled by women picking lovers with an awareness of self-interest. We are still ridiculed for wanting, after all this time, to reclaim our true sexuality. We are accused of *demanding* orgasms like spoiled children demanding sweets before dinner. Men are never accused of the same. For them, orgasms are regarded as necessary to health.

As often as we repeat the following story, it never seems to be enough: According to Ovid, Tiresias, the blind prophet of Thebes who had been both a man and a woman, was asked to mediate in a dispute between Jove and Juno as to which sex got more pleasure from lovemaking. Tiresias unhesitatingly answered that women did. Two thousand years and several sexual revolutions later, we still believe the opposite to be true.

Ideally, of course, we shouldn't have to *demand,* but we are going to have to start becoming more vocal and insisting on a sexual bill of rights if the situation is ever to change. Otherwise we will end up abandoning the idea of men as sexual partners or accepting our own mutilated sexuality. It's a radical truism that power is never relinquished, it must be taken—and potency is a synonym of power.

The Liberated Orgasm

BARBARA SEAMAN

Barbara Seaman, excerpt from "The Liberated Orgasm," *Free and Female,* as it appeared in *Ms.*, August 1972. Reprinted by permission.

Years ago, Margaret Mead suggested that "the human female's capacity for orgasm is to be viewed . . . as a potentiality that may or may not be developed by a given culture."

We don't need to be anthropologists to realize that our Western culture has not only failed to develop that potentiality, but it has stifled and repressed it.

As a result, we women have been afraid to think for ourselves about our own sexual tastes and pleasures. We have tried to model our own preferences after the prevailing views of normality. We have been shy about telling our lovers what we want. We have feared it would be unwomanly to do other than let the male take the lead, however ineptly.

The modern sex manuals are filled with misinformation—for instance, the standard advice to men that they should flail away at the sensitive clitoris. But even when their suggestions are applicable to some women in some moods, they are rarely applicable to all women in all moods, and they foster a certain technical rigidity that is antithetical to really good sex.

Female sexuality is so easily bruised and buried in the myths and medical models of the prevailing culture that the self-awareness needed for liberation will be difficult to achieve unless women explore their own true sexual feelings and needs.

We know that all orgasms are similar on a motor level, and that all orgasms are different on a sensory level.

We know also that there is no ideal or norm,

except in our own imaginations. The truth is that the liberated orgasm is an orgasm *you* like, under any circumstances *you* find comfortable. (The only qualification is that liberated persons don't exploit each other—that's just for masters and slaves.)

In the spring of 1971, my research assistant Carol Milano and I completed an informal but we think rather enlightening sex survey of 103 women. They were career women or students: models of the new woman who enjoys more than average sexual awareness and freedom.

In our survey, all but six regularly achieved some sort of orgasm with relative ease. This is substantially higher than the figure for women in general in our society, especially when you consider that perhaps one-third of the women in our survey were under twenty-five. (From the Kinsey report and more recent investigations, we know that while the majority of women do achieve orgasms sooner or later, for many it is later. It often takes years or even decades for adult women to achieve sexual satisfaction.)

[Some in our survey] could not comment on the clitoral versus the vaginal orgasm at all; to them, the whole debate seemed meaningless. These women simply did not experience their orgasms in one place more than the other. But with this group left out, there were the two extremes of women who stated a preference for, or more frequent experience of, one type or the other. Regardless of the actual physiology of the event, they *felt* most of their orgasms in either the vagina or the clitoris.

Women are so varied in their sexuality that even those who seem alike are different. Let us contrast two, whom I shall call Marie and Antoinette.

Both women are sexually informed and active, and both have given considerable thought to their sexual needs. To achieve orgasms, both require direct clitoral stimulation.

They are not militant clitorists, for neither doubts that some women obtain orgasms via vagi-

nal stimulation, but it doesn't work for them. Marie says, "I know that lots of girls do *not* need as much direct stimulation as I do—but I think this is because they have larger and better placed clitorises." Antoinette says, "I don't think anyone really knows what percentage of women have orgasms during intercourse. It would seem to depend on individual anatomy and placement of the clitoris."

Although clitorises are highly variable in size as well as placement, Masters and Johnson say that in eleven years of research they found no evidence to support the belief that differences in clitoral anatomy can influence sexual response. This, however, must be viewed as a highly tentative finding since they were unable to observe any clitorises during orgasms. Masters and Johnson think that in certain women the thrusting penis does not exercise the traction on the labia and clitoral hood that it does for others. So perhaps idiosyncracies of the vagina, rather than the clitoris, better explain the anatomical need for direct stimulation. Direct clitoral stimulation can be obtained in sexual intercourse, provided the woman is on top or the couple is side by side, and the pubic bones of the man and woman are touching.

What, in the experience of Marie and Antoinette, is the most common lovemaking error that men make?

Marie: "Not enough direct manipulation of the clitoris."

Antoinette: "Many men don't realize that the clitoris is the source of orgasms."

Analysts are undoubtedly telling us the truth when they report that they have "converted" thousands of women to vaginally experienced orgasms. The point is merely that, for some women at least, the strong desire to notice vaginal sensations makes these more noticeable. If Masters and Johnson are correct, all orgasms are essentially the same and quite sensibly involve all the pertinent parts God gave us.

But if all orgasms are the same, why do women not recognize the fact? Are we hopelessly stupid or recalcitrant?

Or are we complex human organisms whose responses are as varied and individual as we are ourselves? Some women noted a difference in their response to vaginal stimulation after childbirth. Several other women noted that they first experienced "vaginal" orgasm—that is, orgasm without direct clitoral stimulation—during intercourse with men who could either sustain vaginal thrusting for an exceptionally long period of time (compared to other lovers) or who had organs that seemed exceptionally large and "filling." One woman also noted a difference in male "sex rhythms": "With some of my lovers I need my clitoris fondled to reach orgasm, and with others I don't."

Several of the women who need direct clitoral stimulation gave what appeared to be very sound anatomical explanations of their preference. Here is one example: "Before the birth of my son, who weighed over nine pounds and had an inordinately large head, I used to reach orgasm without needing to have my clitoris massaged. I don't believe that my vagina was repaired properly after childbirth. I think it must have gotten stretched out of shape because my same husband, with the same penis (and to whom I feel closer than ever), cannot bring me to orgasm so easily by his thrusting alone. I enjoy sex more than ever. My desire, if anything, has increased. But something is different about me, and if my understanding of Masters and Johnson is correct, I believe that the difference is that my vagina was slightly damaged, so that my husband's thrusting no longer provides as much traction on my clitoris."

So, allowing for the probability that there are anatomical differences that may have a strong bearing, what were the other differences between "vaginal" and "clitoral" women?

From [our] evidence, there were more women in the vaginal group whose early experience with men had been favorable and who had not had to struggle to learn to enjoy sex. These women, perhaps because they were more "trusting" or perhaps,

more simply, because their earliest lovers were better controlled and had stimulated them vaginally for long enough periods to bring them to orgasm by that route, had somehow learned to experience "feeling" in their vaginas and to let themselves come to orgasms through vaginal stimulation alone.

The "clitoral" types generally had been exposed to more selfish or fumbling lovers, particularly in their early experiences. Some, of course, had themselves insisted on the practice of merely "petting to climax" in order to preserve a token virginity during their premarital years.

Outside or in, clitoral or vaginal, we are in no way as standardized as Hugh Hefner's airbrushed and siliconed playmates. For example, while fourteen women in our survey complained that their lovers did not engage in enough physical foreplay, and eight others complained that their lovers did not engage in enough verbal foreplay, pillow talk, or conversation, two respondents took the opposite position. They like to get down to the main business of sex more swiftly than their lovers. One observed: "I find foreplay detrimental." The second woman asks wryly: "I have very little interest in foreplay. Is that an inhibition or a total lack of it?"

Or consider the question of the handsome stranger, an alleged apparition in the dreams of younger females. Most of the women in my survey did not like sex with strangers. Over and over they emphasized the importance (to them) of warmth, intimacy, trust, tenderness.

Some women even deem it best to withdraw entirely from men. A prominent feminist confided: "I think it's wonderful that women have discovered masturbation, because it will enable us to keep apart from men as long as necessary. When you have work to do, you can't allow yourself to be diverted by sexual relationships. Masturbation is what male revolutionaries have always used to relieve themselves. Some of the women I know are so pathetic. They run around looking for a man, any man at all."

But what precisely is the female orgasm (which may or may not be developed by a given culture) and where does it take place? A women knows when she's had one (if she doubts it, she hasn't), but since her orgasm is not punctuated by the sure sign of ejaculation, men have felt free to develop lunatic theories about it, and women have not learned to trust their own bodies.

A woman's external sex organs consist of labia majora, or outer lips; labia minora, or inner lips; and the highly eroticized clitoris, the only organ known to man or woman whose sole purpose is to receive and transmit sexual pleasure. The hood of the clitoris is attached to the labia minora, which are directly affected by penile thrusting. Thus, intercourse causes the labia to exert traction on the clitoral hood, producing rhythmic friction between it and the clitoris itself.

Masters and Johnson have proved—or believe they have proved; their work has not yet been replicated—that virtually all feminine orgasms, however vaginal some of them may seem, do include indirect clitoral stimulation, the labia minora being the agent of mediation. Some Freudian analysts have long maintained that vaginal orgasms are entirely distinct from clitoral orgasms and are, indeed, the hallmark of a sexually mature woman. If clitoral stimulation, whether direct or transmitted through the labia, occurs in all orgasms, then distinguishing them is invalid. So is the complicated mystique attached to the distinction. Vaginal women have been said to be mature, feminine, loving, and happy, while clitoral women have had all the opposite traits attributed to them.

However, if I read Masters and Johnson correctly, they are saying that clitoral stimulation may occur in orgasm, but orgasm does not chiefly occur in the clitoris.

To the contrary, orgasm, which is a total body response, is always marked by vaginal contractions. No specific physiologic response in the clitoris has yet been recorded.

Let us review the physiology of the female sex cycle:

STAGE 1: EXCITEMENT. Within ten to thirty seconds after erotic stimulation starts, the vaginal lining is moistened with a lubricating fluid. Nipples become erect, and the breasts begin to swell, increasing in size by one-fifth to one-quarter in women who have not nursed a baby. (Breasts that have been suckled do not enlarge as much.) Other changes start to occur in the clitoris, labia, and vagina as vasocongestion (the engorgement of vessels and organs with blood) and muscular tension start to build. Late in the excitement phase, some women may start to develop a measles-like rash, or sex flush, across their bodies. (Seventy-five percent of the women evaluated by Masters and Johnson showed this response on some occasions.)

STAGE 2: PLATEAU. The tissue surrounding the outer third of the vagina engorges and swells, creating an "orgasmic platform." The deeper portion of the vagina balloons out to form a cavity. The uterus enlarges. The swelling of the outer third of the vagina reduces its diameter, allowing it to grip the penis better. The clitoris retracts, and it becomes harder to locate.

Just prior to the orgasmic phase, the labia minora undergo a marked color change called the sex skin reaction. In the woman who has not had children, the labia minora turn pink or bright red. In the mother, they turn bright red or deep wine (presumably because she has a greater number of varicosities). This coloration remains throughout orgasm, but disappears ten to fifteen seconds afterward. When a woman develops sex skin, she is almost certain to go on to orgasm. Women who are aroused to plateau levels but not brought to orgasm experience a prolonged and sometimes uncomfortable ebbing away of vasocongestion and muscular tension.

STAGE 3: ORGASM. The typical orgasm lasts only ten or fifteen seconds, if that long. Changes occur throughout the body. Muscles of the abdomen, buttocks, neck, arms, and legs may contract; pulse and breathing are more rapid; and blood pressure climbs. The woman experiences a series of rhythmic contractions in the outer third of the vagina and the tissues surrounding it and in the uterus. These contractions, each taking about four-fifths of a second, serve to discharge the accumulated vaso-congestion and tension that have been brought on by sexual stimulation. A mild orgasm usually involves three to five contractions; an intense one, as many as fifteen.

From time to time a woman may experience what some Samoan Islanders call the "knockout" orgasm, and what Masters and Johnson term the "status orgasmus." Masters and Johnson suspect, but are not certain, that the woman is probably having rapidly connected multiple orgasms, over a time period of sixty seconds or so.

In prolonged intercourse a woman may have three, four, or five separate orgasms, and in a few primitive cultures, where men have good control of themselves, multiple female orgasms are apparently the norm. Some masturbating women can have up to fifty successive orgasms according to clinical observation.

Multiple orgasms are most apt to occur when intercourse is prolonged. Thus, while the much vaunted "mutual orgasm" has some very nice features, it also has some drawbacks from the woman's point of view. Or to put it another way, there is no need for a woman to hold back deliberately, for if the male can maintain effective thrusting for a long enough period, the woman will have several preliminary orgasms and, quite possibly, another when he reaches his.

Women who don't have multiple orgasms may fear that they are missing something, but women who do have them often report that these are not their most pleasurable experiences. "If I've had a great orgasm, I can't bear to go on," one such woman explained.

This mysterious thing called orgasmic intensity is measured, principally, in the number of contractions. Masters and Johnson maintain that females have the most intense orgasms when they are free to please themselves only— "without the distraction of a partner." But they do qualify it. "A woman might tell me that she had a delightful experience with the machine," Dr. Masters com-mented at the New York Academy of Medicine in 1968, "but the next night with her husband might have been even better, in her opinion, although we registered fewer orgasmic contractions."

STAGE 4: RESOLUTION. Blood vessels emptied and muscular tensions relieved, the various parts and organs return to their normal condition, some rapidly and some slowly. One woman in three develops a film of perspiration across her body.

According to Masters and Johnson, the clitoris contributes crucially to the buildup of sexual tensions, but orgasm itself is more correctly described as centering in the vagina. Tensions established, it is vaginal contractions that bring relief by emptying engorged organs and vessels. Masters and Johnson call these vaginal contractions "the visible manifestations of female orgasmic experience."

Yet, even for those lucky women who can fantasize to orgasm, the clitoris serves as receptor and transformer of sexual stimuli, while vaginal contractions punctuate the orgasm itself.

However, it is important to note that some women who do not possess a clitoris seem to be capable of orgasm. Dr. Michael Daly, a Philadelphia gynecologist, reports that he has studied in depth two patients in whom the total clitoris was removed because of cancer. Both continued to have orgasms, and both said that their sexual responsiveness after surgery was as great as it was before.

There also are established cases of women in whom an artificial vagina had to be created, because they were born without one. These women also are capable of reaching orgasm.

Apparently, it is lucky for us that most of our sex tissue is internal and can be stimulated by an almost infinite variety of methods.

It is clearly false to say "vaginal orgasm is a myth." But does the vagina contribute to sexual arousal? Or (as some sex researchers, most notably Kinsey, and some women have thought) does it have no feeling?

Yes, it does. Vaginal sensations are believed to be proprioceptive, which means that they are sensations resulting from a stimulus within our own bodies, not imposed from outside.

Close your eyes; extend an arm and bend it. If you can describe the position of your arm, if you know whether it is bent or straight, you are receiving and using proprioceptive information. Ordinarily, we do not pay much conscious attention to our proprioceptive intelligence, but without it we would not even be able to walk.

The vagina is most apt to develop proprioceptive abilities during states of sexual arousal and distention. In unaroused states, as, for example, when a gynecologist inserts a speculum, it may be quite unresponsive.

Obviously, there is a crucial distinction between motor experience (what's happening) and sensory experience (what we're aware of). Masters and Johnson do not always draw this distinction as sharply as many psychologists (and women) might wish.

Some orgasms seem to be experienced vaginally or deep in the vagina, while others seem to be in the clitoris. Some orgasms occur while direct clitoral stimulation is taking place, while others occur only with vaginal stimulation. The experts who have been discussing this have never even defined the terms "vaginal" and "clitoral" orgasm, and women could hardly be sure whether a clitoral orgasm meant an orgasm that was induced by clitoral stimulation, an orgasm that seemed to be experienced in the clitoris, or both.

The same woman may, at different times, experience orgasms in different locations or from different types of stimulation. Women know this, but as a rule men appear to have difficulty comprehending it. In 1968, Drs. Jules Glenn and Eugene Kaplan accused psychoanalysts of assuming, incorrectly, that clitorally stimulated orgasms are necessarily experienced clitorally. They said that their patients have reported a great variation in the location of the experienced orgasm. Occasionally, sites other than the vagina and clitoris (the abdomen, the anus) seem to be the focus of feeling. The area in which the orgasm is experienced need not be the area of stimulation, and there is great variation in the area

or areas where orgasm is felt. The terms "vaginal orgasm" and "clitoral orgasm," according to Glenn and Kaplan have been "widely used but ill-defined."

The charge of technical rigidity is frequently leveled against not only writers of certain types of sex manuals, but also sex researchers, such as Kinsey, and Masters and Johnson.

There is a great deal that can be said against Masters and Johnson, and some of it has been said very well and very publicly. Among the many eloquent critics, Yale psychologist Kenneth Keniston has observed that Masters and Johnson are, although unintentionally, "helping to perpetuate rather than to remedy some of the more prevalent ills of our time—the confusion of human sexuality with the physiology of sexual excitement, naiveté with regard to the psychological meaning of the sexual act, and an inability to confront the ethical implications of sex." He also points out how little has been told of actual laboratory procedures and adds, "Masters and Johnson repeatedly reduce human sexuality to physical responses."

Dr. Natalie Shainess considers the Masters and Johnson view one in which "sex seems little more than a stimulus-response reflex cycle, devoid of intrapsychic or interpersonal meaning. . . . What is the attitude toward sex in a researcher who says, 'Masturbating women concentrate on their own sexual demand without the distraction of a coital partner'? Distraction! Is that the meaning of a partner in sex?"

But with all this, the fact remains that Masters and Johnson have recorded some sexual response cycles in women, and have done it in a way that helps clarify many issues for us. It is probably too much to ask that they be humanitarians and love advisers, as well as intrepid researchers.

Some of the anatomical details are interesting and useful to know, certainly for gynecologists and perhaps for women. And yet the interest we express in their work is, above all, a testament to the abysmal limits put on us by our own timidity.

Certain marriage counselors have long maintained that a loving wife is content merely to satisfy her husband, for instance, and that it need be of no consequence if she fails to achieve satisfaction. We have Masters and Johnson to thank for convincing them that sexual frustration can even give a woman cramps and headache. But how sad it is that we had to wait for sex researchers to demonstrate it. Didn't we know it all the time?

If there is going to be a breakthrough in human sexuality—and I think that such a breakthrough may be in the wind—it is going to occur because women will start taking charge of their own sex lives. It is going to occur because women will stop believing that sex is for men and that men (their fathers, their doctors, their lovers and husbands, their popes and kings and scientists) are the authorities. We need only study a little anthropology or history to understand that sexuality is incredibly plastic and easily repressed.

Women must discover and express their own sexuality, without shame or inhibition. And instead of following sex manuals or trusting the locker-room sexpertise of their fellows, men must learn to seek and receive signals from the women they love.

The Sexuality Questionnaire

SHERE HITE

Shere Hite, ed., excerpt from *Sexual Honesty: By Women for Women*, New York: Warner Books, 1974. Reprinted by permission.

INTRODUCTION

This book is a forum for our public discussion with each other of the nature of our sexuality, the first in a series intended for the reexamination and redefinition of our sexuality. We have never before attempted as a group to define or discover what the physical nature of our sexuality might be, and have in fact more or less just accepted the role which society handed to us. Never before have we tried to determine what feelings might lie buried beneath the layers and layers of myth we live by, or buried beneath the weight of the many "authoritative" books written by male "experts" who presume to tell us how we feel. It is time we made up our own minds, ended the ban on talking about sex, and came to terms with our own personal lives and how we intend to live them.

Most of the extant works on female sexuality contain distortions related to not knowing what female sexuality is about. The most damaging of this literature, often written by male doctors, is nothing more than the reiteration of "marriage manual" techniques for improving our "responsiveness," with some worn-out platitudes thrown in to "liberate" us from our "hang-ups." The most helpful of this literature has been the more scientific clinical studies, which, while in themselves valid and necessary, have also unfortunately been interpreted through the perspectives of unexamined preconceptions about our sexuality. There has rarely been any acknowledgment that female sexuality might have a nature of its own, which would involve more than merely being the logical counterpart of male sexuality. Actually, no one really knows much about the subject yet because women are just beginning to think about it. Therefore, even though some of these clinical efforts have been helpful, it is time women themselves spoke out and began to define their own sexuality.

What exactly is meant by "defining our own sexuality"? Perhaps we have become so submerged in our culture's idea of what we are supposed to be, that we have lost touch with what we really feel, and how to express it. So our first step, for which the questionnaires were designed, should be to try to get back in touch with our more instinctive feelings, and even perhaps to discover feelings never before articulated or consciously felt. Not only are we out of touch with ourselves, but we are also out of touch with each other, and with each other's feelings about sex, since no channels exist for communication on this subject. If we were lucky, our mothers or friends shared their experiences with us, but all too often this was not the case. Perhaps this lack of real information made us wonder if we were somehow "different" from other women. Furthermore, although the kind of material presented here is always part of the scientific investigation of sexuality, access to primary data is something the public is not ordinarily trusted with, and so even this possible channel of communication was closed off. With this book we have, perhaps for the first time, a means of sharing our feelings about sex and getting acquainted on a broad scale, a forum for discovering common experiences and needs, and for beginning the redefinition of who we are. Of course this book does not pretend to represent any kind of final definition of our sexuality, nor is it a statistical sample of all the replies received. It merely represents forty-five out of the over 2,000 replies received to the questionnaires to date. Neither will this book be the end of our newly opened dialogue, but rather a beginning, as it will be followed by the publication of more of these answers, and eventually by the complete analysis of all the answers received. Therefore it is vitally important that you also participate in this discussion by sending in your own answers to the questions, and thus adding your own feelings to this redefinition.

The ultimate intention of this research is to formulate a critique of our current cultural definitions of sex, based on what we have all said. This book, to be published in 1975, perhaps together with some concluding original replies, will not be statistically oriented in that it will not attempt to correlate such things as age and background with attitude and "performance." Rather, it will attempt to answer the questions which formed the basis for this study, namely:

1. Insofar as we can possibly know them, what are the "instinctive" (natural, not socially conditioned) physical expressions of our sexuality?
2. How do these compare with the basic physical activities we usually engage in?
3. What changes, based on the findings of (1)

and (2), might we want to make in our sexual definitions and in our actual physical relations? What would be the implications of these changes for our present cultural definitions of sexuality, for the institutions related to them, and for men's perceptions of their own sexuality?

It does, even now, seem fairly clear that this reawakening of our sensitivity to what is instinctive and natural to us will be part of larger changes which involve not only such things as bedroom habits, but which will also have profound and far-reaching effects on all of our social relations.

SEXUALITY QUESTIONNAIRE II, JANUARY 1973

1. Is having sex important to you? What part does it play in your life?

2. Do you have orgasms? When do you usually have them? During masturbation? Intercourse? Clitoral stimulation? Other sexual activity? How often?

3. Is having orgasms important to you? Do you like them? Do they ever bore you? Would you enjoy sex just as much without ever having them? Does having good sex have anything to do with having orgasms?

4. If you almost never or never have orgasms, are you interested in having them? Why or why not? If you are interested, what do you think would contribute to your having them? Did you ever have them?

5. Could you describe what an orgasm feels like to you? Where do you feel it, and how does your body feel during orgasm?

6. Is having orgasms somewhat of a concentrated effort? Do you feel one has to learn how to have orgasms?

7. Is one orgasm sexually satisfying to you? If not, how many? How many orgasms are you capable of? How many do you usually want? During masturbation? During clitoral stimulation with a

partner? During intercourse?

8. Please give a graphic description or drawing of how your body could best be stimulated to orgasm.

9. Do you enjoy arousal? For its own sake—that is, as an extended state of heightened sensitivity not necessarily leading to orgasm? What does it feel like?

10. Do you like to remain in a state of arousal for indefinite or long periods of time? Or do you prefer to have arousal and orgasm in a relatively short period of time?

11. Do you ever go for long periods without sex? (Does this include masturbation or do you have no sex at all?) Does it bother you or do you like it?

12. How often do you desire sex? Do you actively seek it? Is the time of the month important? Do you experience an increase in sexual desire at certain times of the month?

13. Do you enjoy masturbation? Physically? Psychologically? How often? Does it lead to orgasm usually, sometimes, rarely, or never? Is it more intense with someone or alone? How many orgasms do you usually have?

14. What do you think is the importance of masturbation? Did you ever see anyone else masturbating? Can you imagine women you admire masturbating?

15. How do you masturbate? What is the sequence of physical events which occur? Please give a detailed description. For example, what do you use for stimulation—your fingers or hand or a vibrator, etc.? What kinds of motions do you make—circular, patting, up and down, etc.? Do you use two hands, or if not, what do you do with the other hand(s)? Where do you touch yourself? Does it matter if your legs are together or apart? Do you move very much? .

16. What positions and movements are best for stimulating yourself clitorally with a partner? Do you have orgasms this way usually, sometimes, rarely, or never? Please explain ways you and your partner(s) practice clitoral stimulation. Can you think of other ways?

17. What other sexual play do you enjoy? Is it important for reaching orgasm? How important is kissing (mouth stimulation), breast stimulation, caressing of hips and thighs, general body touching, etc.?

18. Do you like vaginal penetration/intercourse? Physically? Psychologically? Why? Does it lead to orgasm usually, sometimes, rarely, or never? How long does it take? Do you ever have any physical discomfort? Do you usually have adequate lubrication? Do you ever have a decrease in vaginal-genital feeling the longer intercourse continues?

19. What kinds of movements do you find most stimulating during penetration—soft, hard, pressure to the back or front or neither, with complete or partial penetration, etc.? Which positions do you find stimulating? Does the size and shape of penis or penetrating "object" matter to you?

20. Do you have intercourse during your period? Oral sex?

21. Is it easier for you to have an orgasm when intercourse is not in progress? In other words, do you have orgasms more easily by clitoral stimulation than intercourse? Are the orgasms different? How?

22. Do you enjoy cunnilingus? Do you have orgasms during cunnilingus usually, sometimes, never, or rarely? Do you have them during oral/clitoral or oral/vaginal contact or both? Explain what you like or dislike about it.

23. Do you use a vibrator to have orgasms? What kind of vibrator is it? On which body area(s) do you use it? Do you use it during masturbation or sexual play or intercourse or other times?

24. Do you enjoy rectal contact? What kind? Rectal penetration?

25. What do you think about during sex? Do you fantasize? What about?

26. Does pornography stimulate you? What kinds? Which actions?

27. What do you think of sado-masochism? Of domination-submission? What do you think is their significance?

28. Do you prefer to do things to others or to have things done to you, or neither?

29. Which would cause you to become more excited—physical teasing, direct genital stimulation, or psychological "foreplay"?

30. Who sets the pace and style of sex—you or your partner? Who decides when it's over? What happens if your partner usually wants to have sex more often than you do? What happens if you want to have sex more often than your partner?

31. Do you usually have sex with the people you want to have sex with? Who usually initiates sex or a sexual advance—you or the other person?

32. Describe how most men and women have had sex with you (if there are any patterns, etc.).

33. Do most of your partners seem to be well informed about your sexual desires and your body? Are they sensitive to the stimulation you want? If not, do you ask for it or act yourself to get it? Is this embarrassing?

34. Do you feel guilty about taking time for yourself in sexual play which may not be specifically stimulating to your partner? Which activities are you including in your answer?

35. Are you shy about having orgasms with a partner? With only new partners or with everyone? Why?

36. Do you think your vagina and genital area are ugly or beautiful? Do you feel that they smell good?

37. Do you ever find it necessary to masturbate to achieve orgasm after "making love"?

38. How long does sex usually last?

39. Do you ever fake orgasms? During which sexual activities? How often? Under what conditions?

40. What would you like to try that you never have? What would you like to do more often? What changes would you like to make in the usual "bedroom" scene?

41. What were your best sex experiences?

42. How old were you when you had your first sexual experiences? With yourself? With another person? What were they? How old were you when you had your first orgasm? During what activity? At what age did you first look carefully at your vagina and genitals?

43. What is it about sex that gives you the greatest pleasure? Displeasure?

44. What can you imagine you would like to do to another person's body? How would you like to relate physically to other bodies?

45. Do you enjoy touching? Whom do you touch—men, women, friends, relatives, children, yourself, animals, pets, etc.? Does this have anything to do with sex?

46. How important are physical affection and touching for their own sakes (not leading to sex)? Do you do as much of them as you would like? Do you ever have sex with someone mainly to touch and be touched and be close to them? How often?

47. Do you ever touch someone for purposes of sensual arousal but not "real" sex? Please explain. (If desired, refer to question 9).

48. Is there is a difference between sex and touching? If so, what is that difference?

49. In the best of all possible worlds, what would sexuality be like?

50. Do you think your age and background make any difference as far as your sex life is concerned? What is your age and background—education, upbringing, occupation, race, economic status, etc.?

51. Do you usually prefer sex with men, women, either, yourself, or not at all? Which have you had experience with and how much?

52. What do you think of the "sexual revolution"?

53. How does or did contraception affect your sexual life? Which methods have you used? Did you ever take birth control pills?

54. Do you feel that having sex is in any way political?

55. Have you read Masters and Johnson's recent scientific studies or sexuality? Kinsey's? Others? What did you think of them?

56. Please add anything you would like to say that was not mentioned in this questionnaire.

57. How did you like the questionnaire?

Shere Hite Debunks Freud's Vaginal Orgasm

SARAH J. SHEY

Sarah J. Shey, excerpts from *Women as Revolutionary Agents of Change: The Hite Reports and Beyond [WRAC]*, Madison: University of Wisconsin Press, 1993. Reprinted by permission.

With the publication of *The Hite Report on Female Sexuality* in 1976, Shere Hite killed Freud's notion of the superiority of the vaginal orgasm. Drs. William Masters and Virginia Johnson, Dr. Mary Jane Sherfey, Ann Koedt, Barbara Seaman, and, to some extent, even Dr. Alfred Kinsey had all challenged the "mature" orgasm that Freud popularized, but Hite's documentation—going beyond the handful of subjects Freud used to construct theories of women and distributing an essay questionnaire to 3,500 women on their sexuality—proved to be the psychoanalyst's undoing.

Naomi Weisstein, scientist and author of *How Psychology Constructs the Female*, notes the astounding impact the Hite reports had when they were first published.

> Hite . . . became involved with the feminist movement, and, taking seriously the idea that the personal is the political, undertook a major effort to find out what really happens in women's sexual lives.
>
> From 1972 to 1976 she distributed a lengthy essay questionnaire to women all over the country; in 1976, on publication of the findings from the responses of 3,500 women, she explained her goals: "The purpose of this project is to let women define their own sexuality—instead of doctors or other (usually male) authorities. Women are the real experts on their own sexuality; they know how they feel and what they experience, without needing anyone to tell them. . . . In this study, for the first time, women themselves speak out about how they feel about sex, how they define their own sexuality, and what sexuality means to them." Hite's background in social and cultural history helped her to provide a cultural framework for this discussion, to see female sexuality for what it is, rather than how it fits into the prevalent patriarchal ideology.

Hite's basic finding was that 70 percent of women do not have orgasms from intercourse, but do have them from more direct clitoral stimulation. This testimony from thousands of women blew the lid off the question of female orgasm. . . .

Hite's documentation with such a large sample of exactly how women do have orgasms easily—during self-stimulation—and that they do not usually have orgasms during simple intercourse without additional stimulation, as well as her declaration that there was nothing "wrong" with this,

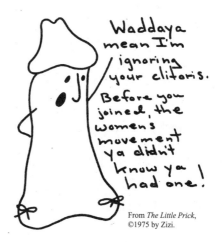

From *The Little Prick*,
©1975 by Zizi.

that if the majority of women said this, it must be "normal" for women—no matter what "professional sexologists" said—was, after an initial period of shock among some in the sex research community, accepted widely, and eventually Hite received the distinguished service award from the American Association of Sex Educators, Counselors and Therapists.[1]

Hite herself enumerated the varied contributions of *The Hite Report on Female Sexuality* during a speech delivered to Harvard Forum in 1976, and again to the University of Pennsylvania in 1977.

The Hite Report on Female Sexuality is so long that very often it is understood on one level only. However, in reality there are three important levels on which to understand it. First, to hear women's voices on this subject is an historic breakthrough. Can you believe that, before this, we had almost no recorded descriptions of how orgasm feels to women, only how it feels to men? The second contribution of *The Hite Report on Female Sexuality* is that it provides a new cultural and historical framework for the definition of physical relations as we know it, i.e., "sex." And finally, [it] provides many new findings for sex research, especially relating to how women achieve orgasm.

Perhaps one of the most widely publicized of those findings, and deservedly so, is that intercourse/coitus itself does not automatically lead to orgasm for most women. For centuries, women have been described as having "problems" with sex. However, it is now becoming clear that is not women who have a problem with sex, but the society that has a problem with its definition of sex, a definition that hurts both women and men, but a definition we can change.[2]

It becomes useful, at this point, to look at some of the findings in *The Hite Report on Female Sexu-*

ality, which would eventually become the first in a trilogy based on Hite's sex research.

1. MOST WOMEN DO NOT ORGASM AS A RESULT OF INTERCOURSE PER SE. The overwhelming majority of women require specific clitoral contact for orgasm. Women know how to orgasm whenever they want, easily and pleasurably, and women who masturbate can orgasm easily and regularly. Women are free to use this knowledge during sex with others. It is no more difficult for a woman to orgasm than for a man; women are not "dysfunctional" or slow to arouse—it is our definition of sex that makes women "dysfunctional."

In her latest book, *Women as Revolutionary Agents of Change*, Hite concludes that her earlier findings were essentially valid.

> "If you don't have orgasms during intercourse, you're hung up." The influence of these psychiatric theories on women has been strong and pervasive. Whether or not a woman has been in analysis, she has heard these unfounded and anti-woman theories endlessly repeated—from women's magazines, popular psychologists, and men during sex. Everyone—of all classes, backgrounds, and ages—knows a woman should orgasm during intercourse. If she doesn't, she knows she has only herself and her own hang-ups to blame.
>
> "I see my failure to have orgasms during intercourse as my failure largely, i.e., I've had plenty of men who (1) were adept, (2) lasted a long time, (3) were eager for my orgasm to occur, but none of them were successful. I guess I have a fear of childbearing, a fear of responsibility—I don't know."
>
> There was a lot of psychic jargon in the women's answers. The women may have been in therapy, but it's just as easy to pick up these terms from numerous articles by therapists and others in the women's magazines, and also from male "experts" with

whom you may have "sex."

The idea that if we would "just relax and let go" during intercourse we would automatically have an orgasm is, of course, based on the fallacious idea that orgasm comes to us automatically by the thrusting penis, and all we have to do is to give ourselves over to what our bodies will naturally and automatically do—that is, orgasm. As one woman put it, "It's our fault that we can't be as natural as they are." . . .

Insisting that women should have orgasms during intercourse, from intercourse, is to force women to adapt their bodies to inadequate stimulation, and the difficulty of doing this and the frequent failure that is built into the attempt breeds recurring feelings of insecurity and anger. As Ann Koedt put it in *The Myth of the Vaginal Orgasm*:

"Perhaps one of the most infuriating and damaging results of this whole charade has been that women who were perfectly healthy sexually were taught that they were not. So in addition to being sexually deprived, these women were told to blame themselves when they deserved no blame. Looking for a cure to a problem that has none can lead a woman on an endless path of self-hatred and insecurity. For she is told by her analyst that not even in her one role allowed in male society—the role of a woman—is she successful. She is put on the defensive, with phony data as evidence that she better try to be even more feminine, think more feminine, and reject her envy of men. That is: Shuffle even harder, baby."

Finally, there are two myths about female sexuality that should be specifically cleared up here.

First, supposedly women are less interested in sex and orgasms than men, and more interested in "feelings," less apt to initiate sex, and generally have to be "talked

into it." But the reason for this, when it is true, is obvious: women often don't expect to, can't be sure to, have orgasms.

"I suspect that my tendency to lose interest in sex is related to my having suppressed the desire for orgasms, when it became clear it wasn't that easy and would 'ruin' the whole thing for him."

The other myth involves the mystique of female orgasm, and specifically the idea that women take longer to orgasm than men, mainly because we are more "psychologically delicate" than men, and our orgasm is more dependent on feelings. In fact, women do not take longer to orgasm than men. The majority of the women in Kinsey's study masturbated to orgasm within four minutes, similar to the women in this study. It is, obviously, only during inadequate or secondary, insufficient stimulation like intercourse that we take "longer" and need prolonged "foreplay."[3]

2. DEFINING SEX AS "FOREPLAY" FOLLOWED BY INTERCOURSE TO MALE ORGASM IS A SEXIST DEFINITION OF SEX, WITH A CULTURAL, RATHER THAN A BIOLOGICAL, BASE. Historically, Hite wrote, this definition is only 3,000 years old. She reiterated this point in *Women as Revolutionary Agents of Change*:

There need not be a sharp distinction between sexual touching and friendship. Just as women described "arousal" as one of the best parts of sex, and just as they described closeness as the most pleasurable aspect of intercourse, so intense physical intimacy can be one of the most satisfying activities possible—in and of itself.[4]

3. MEN MAKE THEIR OWN ORGASMS DURING SEX, AND WOMEN SHOULD BE ABLE TO ALSO. Men should not be in charge of both their own and women's orgasms.

During "sex" as our society defines it both people know what to expect and how to make it possible for the man to orgasm. The whole thing is prearranged, prea-greed. . . . But we can change this pattern, and redefine our sexual relations with others. On one level, we can take control over our own orgasms. We know how to have orgasms in masturbation. How strange it is, when you think about it, that we don't use this knowledge during so much of sex we have with men. . . . A man controls his own orgasm . . . [and] is not considered "selfish" or "infantile" because there is an ideology to back it up.

However, women, do not usually, are not supposed to, control their own stimu-lation:

"I have never tried to stimulate myself clitorally with a partner—I have always been afraid to."

"It seems too aggressive when I act to get the stimulation I want." . . .

There is no reason why making your own orgasms should not be as beautiful or as deeply shared as any other form of sex with another person—perhaps even more so. The taboo against touching yourself says essentially that you should not use your own body for your own pleasure, that your body is not your own to enjoy. . . . Controlling your own stimulation symbol-izes owning your own body, and is a very important step toward freedom.[5]

4. AGE IS NOT A FACTOR IN FEMALE SEXUALITY. "Older women are *not* less sexual than younger women—and they are often more sexual," she wrote. "Young women and girls are not less sexual than adults, but are often misinformed about the nature of their sexuality. . . . Girls are still being kept from finding out about, exploring, and dis-covering their won sexuality—and called 'bad girls' when they try. At puberty, girls are given information about their reproductive organs and menstruation, but rarely told about the clitoris!"

Ultimately, Hite wrote, the sexual revolution did not "free" women, but was, in many ways, a step backward for women:

The "sexual revolution" of the 1960s was a response to long-term social changes that affected the structure of the family and women's role in it. (Contrary to popular opinion, the birth control pill was more a technological response to these same social changes than their cause.) Up until the second half of this century, and throughout most periods of history, a high birth rate has been considered of primary importance by both individuals and society. . . .

The change in the women's role was double-edged. In traditional terms, insofar as having many children had become less important, women's status declined. That is, since women had traditionally been seen almost completely in terms of their childbearing role, they themselves as a class became less important and less re-spected when that role was no longer so important. At the same time, it was said that, now that women were "free" from their old role, they could be "sexually free like men," etc. . . . However, as with the slaves after emancipation, becoming in-dependent was easier said than done. In fact, women did not have equal opportu-nities for education or employment, and so they were stuck in their traditional role of being dependent on men. In spite of the so-called sexual revolution, women (feeling how peripheral, decorative, and expendable they had become to the over-all scheme of things) became more sub-missive to men than ever. This was even more true outside of marriage than inside, since marriage did offer some forms of protection in traditional terms. This in-creased submissiveness and insecurity was reflected in the child-like, baby-doll fashions of the 1960s—short little-girl dresses, long straight (blond) hair, big innocent (blue) eyes, and of course always looking as young and pretty as possible. . . . This situation eventually led to the women's movement of the late 1960s and 1970s, which was now trying to implement some of the positive potentials of the change in women's role, to make women truly independent and free.[6]

Drawing from Hite's findings, Weisstein explored the traditional definition of sex and its lasting ramifications on women:

> If women had been compelled to hide how they could easily reach orgasm during masturbation, then the definition of sex, it follows, is sexist and culturally linked. . . . *The Hite Report on Female Sexuality* linked the definition of sex as we know it to a particular society and historical cultural tradition, saying sex as we know it is created by our social system; it is a social institution.[7]

Looking back, Hite says that she intended "not to create one new definition (i.e., redefinition) of sexuality, but to allow for many—hence, 'undefining.'" *The Hite Report on Female Sexuality* allowed women to voice their opinions en masse on a subject that had been misconstrued for thousands of years. Women spoke—and women and men are listening. The revelatory undefining of sex is taking place.

NOTES

1. Shere Hite, *Women as Revolutionary Agents of Change: The Hite Reports and Beyond* (Madison, WI: University of Wisconsin Press, 1993), 1–3.
2. Ibid., 28–29.
3. Ibid., 45–46.
4. Ibid., 33.
5. Ibid., 61–62.
6. Ibid., 89–90.
7. Ibid., 3–4.

A New View of Women's Sexual Problems

THE WORKING GROUP ON A NEW VIEW OF WOMEN'S SEXUAL PROBLEMS

The Working Group on a New View of Women's Sexual Problems, excerpt from *The New View of Women's Sexual Problems Manifesto*, 2008. Reprinted by permission.

INTRODUCTION: BEYOND THE MEDICAL MODEL OF SEXUALITY

In recent years, publicity about new treatments for men's erection problems has focused attention on women's sexuality and provoked a competitive commercial hunt for "the female Viagra." But women's sexual problems differ from men's in basic ways which are not being examined or addressed. We believe that a fundamental barrier to understanding women's sexuality is the medical classification scheme in current use, developed by the American Psychiatric Association (APA) for its *Diagnostic and Statistical Manual of Disorders* (DSM) in 1980, and revised in 1987 and 1994. It divides (both men's and) women's sexual problems into four categories of sexual "dysfunction": sexual desire disorders, sexual arousal disorders, orgasmic disorders, and sexual pain disorders. These "dysfunctions" are disturbances in an assumed universal physiological sexual response pattern ("normal function") originally described by Masters and Johnson in the 1960s. This universal pattern begins, in theory, with sexual drive, and proceeds sequentially through the stages of desire, arousal, and orgasm.

In recent decades, the shortcomings of the framework, as it applies to women, have been amply documented. The three most serious distortions produced by a framework that reduces sexual problems to disorders of physiological function, comparable to breathing or digestive disorders, are:

1) A false notion of sexual equivalency between men and women. Because the early researchers emphasized similarities in men's and women's physiological responses during sexual activities,

they concluded that sexual disorders must also be similar. Few investigators asked women to describe their experiences from their own points of view. When such studies were done, it became apparent that women and men differ in many crucial ways. Women's accounts do not fit neatly into the Masters and Johnson model; for example, women generally do not separate "desire" from "arousal," women care less about physical than subjective arousal, and women's sexual complaints frequently focus on "difficulties" that are absent from the DSM.

Furthermore, an emphasis on genital and physiological similarities between men and women ignores the implications of inequalities related to gender, social class, ethnicity, sexual orientation, etc. Social, political, and economic conditions, including widespread sexual violence, limit women's access to sexual health, pleasure, and satisfaction in many parts of the world. Women's social environments thus can prevent the expression of biological capacities, a reality entirely ignored by the strictly physiological framing of sexual dysfunctions.

2) The erasure of the relational context of sexuality. The American Psychiatric Association's DSM approach bypasses relational aspects of women's sexuality, which often lie at the root of sexual satisfactions and problems—e.g., desires for intimacy, wishes to please a partner, or, in some cases, wishes to avoid offending, losing, or angering a partner. The DSM takes an exclusively individual approach to sex, and assumes that if the sexual parts work, there is no problem; and if the parts don't work, there is a problem. But many women do not define their sexual difficulties this way. The DSM's reduction of "normal sexual function" to physiology implies, incorrectly, that one can measure and treat genital and physical difficulties without regard to the relationship in which sex occurs.

3) The leveling of differences among women. All women are not the same, and their sexual needs, satisfactions, and problems do not fit neatly into categories of desire, arousal, orgasm, or pain. Women differ in their values, approaches to sexuality, social and cultural backgrounds, and current situations, and these differences cannot be smoothed over into an identical notion of "dysfunction"—or an identical, one-size-fits-all treatment. Because there are no magic bullets for the sociocultural, political, psychological, social, or relational bases of women's sexual problems, pharmaceutical companies are supporting research and public relations programs focused on fixing the body, especially the genitals. The infusion of industry funding into sex research and the incessant media publicity about "breakthrough" treatments have put physical problems in the spotlight and isolated them from broader contexts. Factors that are far more often sources of women's sexual complaints—relational and cultural conflicts, for example, or sexual ignorance or fear—are downplayed and dismissed. Lumped into the catchall category of "psychogenic causes," such factors go unstudied and unaddressed. Women with these problems are being excluded from clinical trials on new drugs, and yet, if current marketing patterns with men are indicative, such drugs will be aggressively advertised for all women's sexual dissatisfactions.

A corrective approach is desperately needed. We propose a new and more useful classification of women's sexual problems, one that gives appropriate priority to individual distress and inhibition arising within a broader framework of cultural and relational factors. We challenge the cultural assumptions embedded in the DSM and the reductionist research and marketing program of the pharmaceutical industry. We call for research and services driven not by commercial interests, but by women's own needs and sexual realities.

SEXUAL HEALTH AND SEXUAL RIGHTS: INTERNATIONAL VIEWS

To move away from the DSM's genital and mechanical blueprint of women's sexual problems, we turned for guidance to international documents. In 1974, the World Health Organization held a unique conference on the training needs for sexual health workers. The report noted: "A growing body of knowledge indicates that problems in human sexuality are more pervasive and more important to the well-being and health of individuals in many cultures than has previously been recognized." The report emphasized the importance of taking a positive approach to human sexuality and the enhancement of relationships. It offered a broad definition of "sexual health" as "the integration of the somatic, emotional, intellectual, and social aspects of sexual being."

In 1999, the World Association of Sexology, meeting in Hong Kong, adopted a Declaration of Sexual Rights. "In order to assure that human beings and societies develop healthy sexuality," the Declaration stated, "the following sexual rights must be recognized, promoted, respected, and defended":

➤ The right to sexual freedom, excluding all forms of sexual coercion, exploitation, and abuse
➤ The right to sexual autonomy and safety of the sexual body
➤ The right to sexual pleasure, which is a source of physical, psychological, intellectual, and spiritual well-being
➤ The right to sexual information . . . generated through unencumbered yet scientifically ethical inquiry
➤ The right to comprehensive sexuality education
➤ The right to sexual health care, which should be available for prevention and treatment of all sexual concerns, problems, and disorders

WOMEN'S SEXUAL PROBLEMS: A NEW CLASSIFICATION

Sexual problems, which The Working Group on a New View of Women's Sexual Problems defines as discontent or dissatisfaction with any emotional, physical, or relational aspects of sexual experience, may arise in one or more of the following interrelated aspects of women's sexual lives.

I. SEXUAL PROBLEMS DUE TO SOCIOCULTURAL,

POLITICAL, OR ECONOMIC FACTORS

A. Ignorance and anxiety due to inadequate sex education, lack of access to health services, or other social constraints.

    1. Lack of vocabulary to describe subjective or physical experience.

    2. Lack of information about human sexual biology and life-stage changes.

    3. Lack of information about how gender roles influence men's and women's sexual expectations, beliefs, and behaviors.

    4. Inadequate access to information and services for contraception and abortion, STD prevention and treatment, sexual trauma, and domestic violence.

B. Sexual avoidance or distress due to perceived inability to meet cultural norms regarding correct or ideal sexuality, including:

    1. Anxiety or shame about one's body, sexual attractiveness, or sexual responses.

    2. Confusion or shame about one's sexual orientation or identity, or about sexual fantasies and desires.

C. Inhibitions due to conflict between the sexual norms of one's subculture or culture of origin and those of the dominant culture.

D. Lack of interest, fatigue, or lack of time due to family and work obligations.

II. SEXUAL PROBLEMS RELATING TO PARTNER AND RELATIONSHIP

A. Inhibition, avoidance, or distress arising from betrayal, dislike, or fear of partner, partner's abuse or couple's unequal power, or arising from partner's negative patterns of communication.

B. Discrepancies in desire for sexual activity or in preferences for various sexual activities.

C. Ignorance or inhibition about communicating preferences or initiating, pacing, or shaping sexual activities.

D. Loss of sexual interest and reciprocity as a result of conflicts over commonplace issues such as money, schedules, or relatives, or resulting from traumatic experiences, e.g., infertility or the death of a child.

E. Inhibitions in arousal or spontaneity due to partner's health status or sexual problems.

III. SEXUAL PROBLEMS DUE TO PSYCHOLOGICAL FACTORS

A. Sexual aversion, mistrust, or inhibition of sexual pleasures due to:

1. Past experiences of physical, sexual, or emotional abuse.

2. General personality problems with attachment, rejection, cooperation, or entitlement.

3. Depression or anxiety.

4. Sexual inhibition due to fear of sexual acts or of their possible consequences, e.g., pain during intercourse, pregnancy, sexually transmitted disease, loss of partner, loss of reputation.

IV. SEXUAL PROBLEMS DUE TO MEDICAL FACTORS

Pain or lack of physical response during sexual activity despite a supportive and safe interpersonal situation, adequate sexual knowledge, and positive sexual attitudes. Such problems can arise from:

A. Numerous local or systemic medical conditions affecting neurological, neurovascular, circulatory, endocrine, or other systems of the body.

B. Pregnancy, sexually transmitted diseases, or other sex-related conditions.

C. Side effects of many drugs, medications, or medical treatments.

D. Iatrogenic conditions.

Boys, Girls, Men, and Women: Variables of Experience

REBECCA PLANTE

Rebecca Plante, excerpt from *Sexualities in Context*, Colorado: Westview Press, 2006. Reprinted by permission.

THE REALITY OF INTERSEXUALITY

"'Intersex' is a general term used for a variety of conditions in which a person is born with a reproductive or sexual anatomy that doesn't seem to fit the typical definitions of female or male." For example, a person might be born appearing to be female on the outside, but having mostly male-typical anatomy on the inside. Or a person may be born with genitals that seem to be in-between the usual male and female types—for example, a girl may be born with a noticeably large clitoris, or lacking a vaginal opening, or a boy may be born with a notably small penis, or with a scrotum that is divided so that it has formed more like labia. Or a person may be born with mosaic genetics, so that some of her cells have XX chromosomes and some of them have XY.

Though we speak of intersex as an inborn condition, intersex anatomy doesn't always show up at birth. Sometimes a person isn't found to have intersex anatomy until she or he reaches the age of puberty, or finds himself [to be] an infertile adult, or dies of old age and is autopsied. Some people live and die with intersex anatomy without anyone (including themselves) ever knowing.[1]

The Intersex Society of North America (ISNA) was founded in 1993 by Cheryl Chase. Chase and many others have spent the last twelve years working "to end shame, secrecy, and unwanted genital surgeries for people born with an anatomy that someone decided is not standard for male or female" (www.isna.org). There is a range of circumstances in which a person may be defined, usually by medical professionals, as "intersex." Klinefelter and Turner syndromes are only two of a handful of sex variations, which include congenital adrenal hyperplasia (CAH), androgen insensitivity syndrome, and hypospadias. There are estimates that about one in every two thousand individuals has an intersexed condition.

SEX VARIATIONS

A few of the many intersex conditions have physiological or biological aspects that represent what ISNA calls "real medical emergencies," calling for immediate intervention at the time of birth; one of these is congenital adrenal hyperplasia. The other conditions do not require parents and medical professionals to make quick or hasty decisions. CAH creates problems in the adrenal glands, small structures that sit atop the kidneys and are responsible for releasing cortisone, a hormone that helps the body deal with stress. CAH inhibits the production of cortisone and wreaks havoc on the ability to monitor salt levels. Because the adrenals add various hormones to the bloodstream, a "broken genetic recipe" (www.isna.org) can lead to high levels of virilizing hormones, creating larger than average clitoral structures and labia that look like a scrotum (in XX individuals). That "broken recipe" is implicated in virilizing effects that continue into puberty, such as thick body hair, receding hairline, deep voice, and so on.

Androgen insensitivity syndrome (AIS) is a condition where individuals "are chromosomally and gonadally male (that is, XY with testicles), but lack a key androgen receptor that facilitates the ability, fetally and onward, to respond to androgens (male hormones) produced in normal amounts by the testes."[2] So the individual would have no internal "female" organs while also having no epididymis, vas deferens, and seminal vesicles, all of which are responsible for delivering semen from the testes. Babies with AIS will have genitalia that look "female," undescended (internal) testes, and a vagina but no uterus, fallopian tubes, or ovaries. Sometimes AIS is not discovered until puberty, when the girl does not menstruate and may not develop *secondary sexual characteristics,* such as pubic and underarm hair.

Remember that "'Intersex' is a general term used for a variety of conditions in which a person is born with a reproductive or sexual anatomy that doesn't seem to fit the typical definitions of female or male."[3]

Hypospadias is one such condition and may contribute most to the one in two thousand estimate cited earlier. It relates to the position of the urethral opening on the penis, which is usually at the top of the penis. Hypospadias can result in an opening that is anywhere along the penis, thus creating "nonstandard" genitalia. This is not a medical emergency in most circumstances; the most extreme instances may involve a missing urethra (which causes urine to leave the bladder behind the penis).

In and of themselves, genitalia that do not look like the standard "male" and "female" bits of skin are not life-threatening. Yet virtually all intersex conditions have been treated this way, until recently. Activist and educational groups like ISNA, Bodies Like Ours, and Survivor Project have been created by people diagnosed with intersex conditions. Not all intersexuality awareness groups have the same aims—two organizations focusing on CAH and AIS are oriented for parents (and medical professionals), while Survivor Project and Intersex Initiative Portland are more explicitly aimed at activism. But their broader goals are similar: to draw attention to the involuntary surgeries (intersex genital mutilation), stigmatizing and arbitrary judgments, and narrowness of binary models.

Physicians and scientists, themselves members of a culture with a dualistic gender system, have played a large role in the modern development of intersexuality. Sociologist Sharon Preves, who interviewed thirty-seven intersex individuals in North America, describes what happens when an infant is born: ". . . a common method of handling an ambiguous birth includes telling the parent(s) that their child's genitals are not yet 'fully developed' before quickly whisking the infant away for myriad medical diagnostic procedures with which to ascertain the infant's 'most appropriate' gender assignment."[4] This treatment perpetuates the myth that there is something *medically* wrong with the child, when it is really more of a *social* emergency.[5] In an examination of the medical aspects of intersexuality, psychologist Suzanne Kessler reviewed the literature describing operative and diagnostic techniques, interviewed physicians, and concluded that doctors respond according to societal conceptualizations of "normal" sex and gender.

"Normal" and "medically acceptable" is a clitoris between 0 and 0.9 centimeters, or three-eights of an inch.[6] But to be considered a penis, the organ must be between 2.4 and 4.5 centimeters. (Penile size standards for infants were published in the 1960s, and clitoral standards were published in the late 1980s.) Without even knowing the metric system, one can still see that there is a gap between 0.9 centimeters and 2.5 centimeters. The marks on the ruler in this gap therefore represent something "unacceptable," a limbo that has traditionally been addressed by involuntary surgeries (what some call intersex genital mutilation) to shorten the clitoral structure. The surgeries often leave the clitoris scarred and with diminished or absent sensation. But medical thinking has been informed by cultural viewpoints that privilege the penis. Many infants are assigned the sex "female" if physicians do not believe that the "micropenis" has the potential to grow more at puberty. Kessler's research made medical logic clear: if an intersex boy would be ostracized in a locker room or public restroom due to the size of his phallus, then the boy should be assigned "female" at birth and undergo "clitoral" reduction.

Medical professionals, as members of the broader culture, react in accord with their socialization into that culture. So the construction of sex as binary and opposite informs physicians' responses, along with our belief that *anatomy is destiny*. This underlies the fear that a clitoris of an unexpected length is unacceptable for a baby assigned female. It underlies the assessment that a penis of an unexpected (smaller) length is unacceptable and must be turned into a clitoris for a baby reassigned to female. How do any of us know what "normal" is, especially when we are discussing genitalia? "Anatomy is destiny" is an expression of our positivist belief that the body tells the truth about who we are—that "true sex" can be ascertained via genitalia. The belief that one body has or

should have only one sex in it ("one-body-one-sex") is another way to maintain the binary gender and sexuality status quo.[7] When intersex children are assigned sexes and genders as youth, the physicians' criteria for "success" include ultimately being able to have penile-vaginal intercourse.

One intersex condition, Mayer-Rokitansky-Kuster-Hauser (MRKH) syndrome, involves congenital absence of the vagina combined with, often, internal primary sexual characteristics (e.g., fallopian tubes, cervix, and/or uterus). The vulva, clitoris, and chromosomes are not affected by MRKH, but there may be kidney abnormalities, skeletal problems, and hearing problems. Given that physicians emphasize normalization and heterosexuality in obliterating intersex bodies (via phallic/clitoral reductions, removal of testes, and so on), it is not surprising that doctors' main response to MRKH is to create a vagina:

My life completely changed when I was thirteen and sent home from camp with abdominal pain. When I was examined they discovered an imperforate hymen prohibiting the flow of menstrual fluid. I had my first surgery then, to open my hymen so I could bleed. But they found that nothing was there. I had no vagina, just a dimple, and they could detect no uterus. I had secondary sex characteristics, body hair and breasts, so they guessed I had ovaries but no one knew where. The medical profession has known about MRKH since 1838, but I was diagnosed with "congenital absence of vagina" because that's what they cared about. My abdominal pain was quickly forgotten. I was suddenly and shamefully different. Puberty was over for me. I went from selling Girl Scout Cookies to correcting my sexual dysfunction in one afternoon.

My doctors talked to my parents about vaginal reconstruction so I could have a normal sex life with my husband. What husband? And why couldn't he adjust as he would for any other "birth defect"? My parents did the right thing. They took me down the only path available, the path of "corrective" surgery. But I was staggering from the loss of my fertility, the dream of having children. I received sympathy and even pity about that, but the most pressing concern was to create my vagina ASAP.[8]

Medical interventions are not benign and often are wholly unnecessary from the standpoint of physical health.[9] The problem with the sex assignment process and "intersex genital mutilation" is that medical professionals have failed to see the human effects of these interventions. Persistent feelings of shame and bodily alienation can combine with feelings of disfigurement and invasion (due to multiple surgeries), inhibition, pain, and the sense of bearing a huge, incomplete secret. The development of healthy self-concept is often hampered by profound sociocultural stigmatization of people born with genitalia that do not conform to expected norms.

Max Beck, assigned female at birth and named Judy, writes about the effects of forced surgeries, secrecy, and silence:

> I grew into a rough-and-tumble tomboy, a precocious, insecure, tree-climbing dress-hating show-off with a Prince Valiant haircut and razor-sharp wit who was constantly being called "little boy" and "young man."
>
> I quickly came to understand that the tomboy—the gender identity with which I had escaped childhood—was less acceptable in adolescence. Yearly visits to endocrinologists and pediatric urologists, lots of genital poking and prodding, and my mother's unspoken guilt and shame had all served to distance me considerably from my body: I was a walking head. In retrospect, it seems odd that a tomboy should have been so removed from her body. But instead of a daily, muddy, physical celebration of life, my tomboyishness was marked by a reckless disregard for the body and a strong desire to be annihilated. So I reached ado-

lescence with no physical sense of self, and no desire to make that connection. All around me, my peers and former playmates were dating, fooling around, giving and getting hickeys, while I, whose puberty came in pill form, watched aghast from the sidelines.

> What *was* I? The doctors and surgeons assured me I was a girl, that I just wasn't yet "finished." I don't think they gave a thought to what that statement would mean to me and my developing gender identity, my developing sense of self. The doctors who told me I was an "unfinished girl" were so focused on the lie—so invested in selling me "girl"—that I doubt they ever considered the effect a word like "unfinished" would have on me. I knew I was incomplete. I could see that compared to—well, compared to everyone!—I was numb from the neck down. When would I be finished? The "finishing" the doctors talked about occurred during my teen years—hormone replacement therapy and a vaginoplasty. Still, the only thing that felt complete was my isolation. Now the numbness below my neck was real—a maze of unfeeling scar tissue. I wandered through that labyrinth for another ten years, with a gender identity and desires born of those medical procedures. I began to experience myself as a sort of sexual Frankenstein's monster.[10]

Beck's experiences highlight how intersexuality has been perceived as a social emergency, the lie of "girlhood" superseding individual needs, feelings, and happiness.

Writer Jim Costich, an "intersexed activist," clarifies the essential problem with surgical interventions:

> Forced gender assignment and/or surgical procedures and hormone therapy have never made males or females out of the intersexed. It has only made intersexed people who have been made to look something like males and females. Not all of us were

surgically altered. I wasn't. We are all working toward a day when none of us are surgically altered without our informed, mature desire and choice. No child should be mutilated to mollify the gender issues of others.[11]

Intersexuality represents an excellent opportunity for critical thinking. It requires us to explore what it really means to talk about two sexes, and to conceptualize them in the taken-for-granted way, as *opposite* sexes. We must consider how physicians and scientists, as part of the powerful social institution of medicine, have arbitrarily made decisions about what "male" and "female" mean. If we were not as set on promulgating the idea that there are two and only two sexes that are linked directly to the development of two and only two genders, we might have a society that could handle gray areas better. When we persist in seeing biological sex and gender as examples of binary opposites, we perpetuate narrow limitations on individual expression and deny the realities and experiences of many people.

I introduce the concept of intersex here as a way to further the process of critical thinking and to explore social constructionism. The reality of intersexuality forces us to reinterpret what biological sex and social gender are, and to examine the broader social process underlying our definitions of sex and gender. Most importantly, consider what it means to make intersex people's experiences invisible.

NOTES

1. www.isna.org.
2. Sharon E. Preves, *Intersex and Identity: The Contested Self* (New Brunswick, NJ: Rutgers University Press, 2003), 28.
3. www.isna.org.
4. Preves, *Intersex and Identity*, 54.
5. Suzanne Kessler, *Lessons from the Intersexed* (New Brunswick, NJ: Rutgers University Press, 1998).
6. Ibid., citing physicians Meyers-Seifer and Charest.
7. Alice Dreger, *Hermaphrodites and the Medical Invention of Sex* (Cambridge, MA: Harvard University Press, 1998).
8. Esther (Marguerite) Morris, "The Missing Vagina Monologues," *Sojourner: The Women's Forum* 26, no. 7 (March 2001).
9. Kessler, 1998.
10. Max Beck, "My Life As an Intersexual," NOVA Online: Sex Unknown, PBS, October 2001, http://www.pbs.org/wgbh/nova/gender/beck.html.
11. Jim Costich, *An Intersex Primer* (self-published, 2003).

Sex Is Not a Natural Act

LEONORE TIEFER

Leonore Tiefer, excerpt from *Sex Is Not a Natural Act*, Colorado: Westview Press, 2004. © 1995 by Leonore Tiefer. Reprinted by permission.

BECOMING AN ACTIVIST

I have discovered that I have the soul of an activist, a person committed to social change and the amelioration of social problems. The eldest child of leftist Jewish New Yorkers, it should have been obvious that I would grow up expecting to be involved in the struggle against injustice and oppression. The locale of struggle, the particular issues, these would depend on the social and personal vicissitudes of my life and times, but my background inescapably oriented me toward involvement in progressive issues.

I was on the University of California campus at Berkeley from 1963 to 1969 throughout the Free Speech Movement and the various antiwar campaigns, and I must tell you that *then* I didn't lift a finger. I felt agitated a lot; I went to rallies; I watched. I wanted to get involved. But I was frightened and alienated by mass events, no one I knew was involved, and I really didn't understand the politics. Despite my background, political reality really only began for me when the women's movement came along in the 1970s. I became an activist in Fort Collins, Colorado, where I had gone to teach psychology at Colorado State University after getting my PhD from Berkeley in 1969.

As I look back, I realize that these were the questions that concerned me in the early 1970s: How do you maintain your commitment when it becomes clear that the struggle will not soon be over? How do you deal with disappointment and victory? How do you choose which issues to engage? How do you balance the mixed feelings that come with coalitions? How do you deal with the social marginalization of activism? Especially marginalizing was the fact that it seemed that very few people in my profession were active in political change movements and my colleagues often criticized my activities.

For years my feminist activism was separate from my "career" as a sexology researcher and teacher. Although I spent endless hours working for equal access to sports facilities for women students, founding town and campus feminist organizations, advocating gender equity in faculty salaries and promotions, developing a course in the psychology of women, and writing letters to newspapers protesting sexism in news stories and advertisements, I was at the same time publishing my research on prenatal hormones and mating behavior in the golden hamster and the rat and going to conferences listening to other papers on prenatal hormones and mating behavior in the golden hamster and the rat. And in the 1970s, although I noticed the sexist behavior of colleagues at these conferences, and I noticed the paucity of women scientists, I did not see the sexism in the paradigm or in the methods. And I did not see the racism at all.

Beginning with a publication in 1978 (just forget everything before then—for example, my first publication, in 1969, entitled "Mating Behavior of Male *Rattus norvegicus* in a Multiple-Female Exhaustion Test"!), I gradually became aware of how sex research is shaped by social and political values. The single most helpful factor in raising my consciousness about my profession was reading the growing literature in women's, ethnic, and gay and lesbian studies.

In 1982 I joined a biweekly seminar at the New York Institute for the Humanities called "Sex, Gender, and Consumer Culture." It was full of politically active New York journalists and humanities professors trained to look at meaning and to disdain universals. The seminar had no other psychologists

or health-domain types at all. Here were people who relished the links they made between intellectual theories and political context, the complete opposite of the "neutral, objective" stance I had been taught in my profession. Although I admit I was often over my head in that seminar, and for years I couldn't figure out how understanding Picasso in Barcelona or turn-of-the-century French postcards could help me understand sexuality in people's lives today, I gradually underwent a sea change in my perception of how sexual lives are shaped by sociohistorical context.

I began to blend politics with my profession when I volunteered to give a talk on "Changing Conceptions of Sex Roles: Impact on Sex Research" for my graduate school mentor Frank Beach's sixty-fifth birthday celebration in 1976. The theme of the celebration was "Sex Research: Where Are We Now, Where Are We Going?" I volunteered for two reasons: First, I was under the spell of the women's movement, which said, "Speak out!" Since I had been giving countless speeches in Fort Collins about equal pay and equal athletics and equal graduate admissions, I guess I thought I could somehow easily segue into a speech on equal sexology.

Second, I was having a sabbatical year at Bellevue Hospital in New York to learn about human sexuality. At Colorado State I had been assigned the task of teaching human sexuality because I knew a lot about the sexuality of hamsters and rats, and I had learned pretty fast that a background in comparative psychology was not an adequate preparation for teaching human sexuality. New York has more bookstores than Fort Collins, and I was doing a lot of reading that year. I was terrifically excited by one book I read—the first-ever collection of essays on feminist social science. The editorial introduction began:

> Everyone knows the story about the Emperor and his fine clothes. Although the townspeople persuaded themselves that the Emperor was elegantly costumed, a child, possessing an unspoiled vision, showed the citizenry that the Emperor was really naked.

The story instructs us about one of our basic sociological premises: that reality is subject to social definition. The story also reminds us that collective delusions *can be undone* by introducing fresh perspectives. Movements of social liberation are like the story in this respect: *they make it possible for people to see the world in an enlarged perspective . . .* In the last decade no social movement has had a more startling or consequential impact on the way people see and act in the world than the women's movement.[1]

In retrospect, I realize now that part of my motivation at Beach's sixty-fifth birthday party in giving a very provocative paper about feminism and sex research was anger—I wanted to show that the emperor birthday boy and all his buddies were naked, that is, intellectually. In this way, I now realize, I intended to get intellectual revenge for the sexist prejudice I had suffered during my years of graduate training. In addition, as any good clinician will point out, at the very same time I was attempting to win, through some sort of tour de force presentation, the intellectual recognition and approval denied to me by those sexist practices.

The paper criticized biological determinism and genital preoccupations in sex research, exposed the stereotyped assumptions about males and females that limited research designs, and called for more qualitative and subjective elements in sex research. Although my ability to make those arguments was pretty thin in 1976, it surprises me how well the general points have stood the test of time.

The paper was received with quite a lot of anger. People felt it was inappropriate to a birthday celebration to criticize the assumptions guiding the past fifty years of work of the guest of honor, and, of course, now I can see that they were right. Personal motives frequently incite social justice actions, and it neither justifies nor dismisses those actions to acknowledge the motives. People often look for motives of maladjustment in the work of social activists, and indeed, activists *are* malad-

justed, "creatively maladjusted," as Martin Luther King Jr. said. Indeed, if activists weren't maladjusted, they would be adjusted—adjusted to the status quo—and that is the whole point. But there is a time and a place for everything, even social justice, although it's hard sometimes in the heat of the struggle to understand that.

After the party and ceremonies, as I was preparing the chapter based on my talk for publication in the celebration volume, I received several letters from male colleagues suggesting I tone down the feminism. One colleague wrote: "Do you think you can modify your chapter to meet these criticisms? You obviously had something on your mind and you got it said . . . But, I'm not sure that putting all your thoughts and speculations in the 'permanent record' is a good idea for you [or] for the point of view you champion."[2] I opted not to change much of the speech for the published version[3] and in 1979 I received a Distinguished Publication Award from the Association for Women in Psychology for my chapter.

These two extremes have characterized reactions to my work ever since, up to 1993. Until now, my sexologist colleagues have persistently told me that although I had some interesting observations, basically I was too strident, too political, too angry, and too repetitious. In contrast, feminist audiences persistently embraced me, encouraged me, and thanked me for bringing a message about sexuality that they found illuminating and liberating. In all honesty, it's hard to say which reaction has been the greater source of motivation. After all, I am the daughter of a Communist whose passion in life was playing the stock market. I'm used to having my feet in very different camps, to having a fragmented identity, to reading disparate literatures always looking for syntheses. I have kept going to sexological meetings, and I have kept going to feminist meetings.

A MIDLIFE CRISIS?

In 1991, I published a record seven papers, most of which were based on speeches I had been invited to give. Two things seemed to have happened. First, I found that I suddenly had a lot to say, and second, to my astonishment, I found that people in my field wanted to hear me. Why?

I had a lot to say partly because ethnic, gay and lesbian, and women's studies had provided fascinating material that I thought could be relevant to sexology and the study of human sexuality. I was particularly taken with the efforts of feminist writers to show how science constructs nature, rather than discovers it, and in particular how animal research is used to construct images of "human nature" that may not be in women's best interests.[4] The new *Journal of the History of Sexuality*, dominated by gay, lesbian, and feminist scholars, has been making available dozens of fascinating examples of the varying construction of sexualities in the past. And ethnic minority intellectuals have been exposing the limitations of many academic concepts and categories that are blind to factors of race and class.[5]

I also had a lot to say because I could tell a narrative of social construction, the story of the medicalization of male sexuality, from the inside.[6] This narrative gave my years of criticism of sexology's biological reductionism, phallocentrism, stereotyped gender assumptions, and context-stripped research a credibility that overcame, for the moment, the stigma of being an ideologue.

Also, sexologists have wanted to hear my kind of ideas recently because it's become so obvious that sex research is inexorably political. AIDS, abortion, pornography, homosexual rights, and child sexual abuse claims and counterclaims have put sex and sex research continually on the front page. Time has caught up with me in a funny way.

It seems quite possible, however, that my time in the sun may be brief. A recent analysis argues that the radical critique of science, as found over the past twenty-five years in *Science for the People*, has given birth and given way to professionalized sociological treatments of scientific knowledge in a newly reputable subspecialty in sociology.[7] Even if many of my suggestions for transformation and re-

form are heeded, a similar fate may befall sexology if it continues to privilege its own survival rather than the improvement of people's sexual understanding and sexual lives. The transformation of sexology into a tool to fight oppression and injustice is still only a dim possibility far out on the horizon.

But, popular or not, I expect to continue to look for opportunities to move the struggle forward. Let me conclude by describing two I have recently taken. This past year I was able to participate in the National Institutes of Health (NIH) Consensus Development Conference on Impotence. This conference marked the first time the NIH chose a topic in sexuality.[8] *Impotence*, I believe, is a term essential to maintaining phallocentrism in sexology and therefore a term I agitate against whenever I can. Discussion of impotence converts problems of the penis into problems of the man, converts problems with sexual performance into weakness and lack of masculine control. Thus, a field devoted to the diagnosis and treatment of impotence supports the quest for phallic perfection—a quest that ignores women and women's sexual interests—recruiting enormous economic resources for this purpose.

I was invited to speak at the NIH conference about ethnic and cultural influences on impotence, an important topic, but one about which there is no research. Instead, I insisted on discussing nomenclature and partner issues, topics that weren't even on the schedule. I was determined to bring women into this "all boys' toys" situation. And I did make a difference, albeit a small one, in the final report of the NIH consensus panel. Activism extends not only to such participation but also to telling the story of the consensus conference, as I have at several meetings this year, to show how the social constructions of sexuality and gender actually proceed daily in minute ways.

CONCLUSION

What can I abstract from this odyssey of an activist who happens to be a sexologist? It's important to view whatever subject you are interested in from many perspectives by reading, joining interdisciplinary seminars, and participating in out-of-venue activities. It's important to understand political reality and to see how the subject you are interested in fits into politics. Professions exist to perpetuate themselves, and any good they do must be effortfully worked into their mission. You need another place to stand in addition to just being a competent professional. If you are committed to social betterment, you must take action; analysis alone is insufficient. Unfortunately, it's never clear that a particular moment is the right one or that a particular action will make a difference, so you will have to take action without certain knowledge of its impact. Since challenging the status quo is likely to make you unpopular, make sure you have a political base of some sort to provide moral support when the going gets rough.

I said I would mention two opportunities I've recently taken to move the struggle forward. The second one is to put these ideas into speeches such as these. Is this again the manifestation of maladjusted motives? I feel that any venue is the right one to say that feminism is a struggle to eradicate the ideology of domination—the cultural basis of group oppression[9] and to remind anyone within the sound of my voice to extend their feminist thinking to contend with racism as well as sexism.

We live in a time of intensely competing sexual discourses, and sexuality is one of the arenas for struggle against oppression and injustice. There is really no way to be apolitical as a sexologist—every action supports some interests and opposes others. My message is a call for you to choose your work with intentionality and to incorporate race and class analyses into your research and clinical efforts.

NOTES

1. Marcia Millman and Rosabeth Kanter, eds., *Another Voice: Feminist Perspectives on Social Life and Social Science* (London: Octagon press, 1975), vii.
2. Leonore Tiefer, "Feminism and Sex Research: Ten Years' Reminiscences and Appraisal," in Joan C. Chrisler and Doris Howard, eds., *New Directions in Feminist Psychology: Practice, Theory, and Research* (New York: Springer Publishing Company, 1992).
3. Leonore Tiefer, "The Context and Consequences of Contemporary Sex Research: A Feminist Analysis," in W. McGill, D. Dewsbury, and B. Sachs, eds., *Sex and Behavior: Status and Prospectus* (New York: Plenum Press, 1978).
4. See Donna Haraway, *Simians, Cyborgs, and Women: The Reinvention of Nature* (London: Routledge, 1991).
5. See bell hooks, *Feminist Theory from Margin to Center* (Boston: South End Press, 1984); and bell hooks, *Talking Back: Thinking Feminist, Thinking Black* (Boston: South End Press, 1989).
6. Leonore Tiefer, "In Pursuit of the Perfect Penis: The Medicalization of Male Sexuality," *American Behavioral Scientist* 29, 579–599.
7. Brian Martin, "The Critique of Science Becomes Academic," *Science, Technology, and Human Values* 18, no. 2 (Spring 2003): 247–259.
8. Leonore Tiefer, "Nomenclature and Partner Issues," paper presented at National Institutes of Health Consensus Development Conference on Impotence, Bethesda, MD.
9. hooks, *Feminist Theory from Margin to Center*, 25.

The Rise of Viagra: How the Little Blue Pill Changed Sex in America

MEIKA LOE

Meika Loe, excerpt from *The Rise of Viagra*, New York: New York University Press, 2006. Reprinted by permission.

THE SEARCH FOR THE FEMALE VIAGRA

Immediately after Viagra's "blockbuster" debut, many wondered if the little blue pill would work for women. Journalists and comedians reported that middle-aged wives of Viagra users were now asking, "Where is my magic pill?" Countless newspapers and magazines ran stories introducing Viagra for men, followed with the question, " Will it work for women too?" Amid this curiosity, hundreds of women nationwide volunteered for Viagra clinical trials. *The Journal of the American Medical Association* (*JAMA*) shockingly reported, "sexual dysfunction is more prevalent in women (43 percent) than in men (31 percent)." Many pharmaceutical companies, including Pfizer, rushed to cash in on the female market, setting up new research and clinical trials.

In many ways, the rise of female sexual dysfunction (FSD) is similar to that of erectile dysfunction (ED). FSD can be understood as a social phenomenon that continues to be defined, used, and critiqued by a host of experts who have stakes in this medical category, including basic scientists, gynecologists, urologists, psychologists, marketers, and feminists. The key similarity is that FSD is a *medical* diagnosis, signaling that both the problem and the treatment must be focused on the woman's body. FSD, like ED, is a case of what I would call "diagnostic expansion," whereby an older diagnosis, frigidity, gets broadened to include a wider spectrum of sexual problems and concerns. However, unlike the case of ED, defining and treating sexual problems in women is proving to be slow paced, complicated, and controversial.

Will women truly benefit from the search for the female Viagra? Will they benefit from their inclusion in sexual science, and the increased popular and medical attention paid to women's sexual arousal, desire, orgasm, and pain? How could they not, right? The answers are not as simple and perhaps not as optimistic as they first may seem. As many scholars have shown, women have historically been manhandled, quite literally, by Western medicine. History shows that women's bodies, seen as deviant and abnormal by men in power, have long been subjects of medical surveillance and control. "Hysteria," "nymphomania," and "frigidity" were widely used in the modern era to label primarily middle- and upper-class women as "sick." Women have often been used as medical guinea pigs, test subjects for early harmful and even fatal medical treatments such as abortions, birth control pills, fertility drugs (thalidomide), breast cancer treatments (tamoxifen), and hormone replacement. Women (and men) of color have been and continue to be med-

ical test subjects, many times without their knowledge and at great risk to their health. Today, every aspect of a woman's life cycle has been medicalized—from birth to menstruation to childbirth to menopause to death—revealing a growing dependence on medicine that some say is risky and excessive. On the other hand, some would argue that such medical solutions have empowered and enabled women in important ways, for example, in the areas of reproductive control, pain relief, and depression management. Given women's complex historical relationship to medicine, this excerpt explores how medical experts have recently attempted to make sense of women's sexual problems in the Viagra era.

THE RISE OF FSD

The Boston Forum is a perfect site for tracking the rise of FSD. The 1999 Boston Forum meeting was the first large-scale FSD-themed conference of its kind, organized by urologist and ED researcher Irwin Goldstein. By the time of Viagra's debut, Dr. Goldstein was also a major figure in the classification and commercialization of FSD, having researched and written widely about new medical categories of sexual dysfunction for both men and women. Around the time when Pfizer's Viagra was approved by the FDA and released to the public, Goldstein and other Pfizer-funded physicians penned a variety of scientific articles and granted a large number of interviews claiming that 30 to 50 percent of men and women in America have "organic sexual dysfunction." By 1999, Goldstein had published so widely in medical and urological journals such as the *Urology Times*, the *New England Journal of Medicine*, and *JAMA* that he was anointed "FSD" expert by countless mainstream publications, including *Time*, *Playboy*, and *Fortune*.

In 1999 Goldstein began convening a so-called multidisciplinary group of about five hundred practitioners, clinicians, scientists, and pharmaceutical representatives who congregate in Boston annually, near the site of Boston University's medical school and sexual dysfunction clinics, to learn and share "the latest" in FSD. These meetings are the most influential scientific conferences concerning the overall understanding of FSD and have had a great deal of sway over how the scientific and medical community has come to regard women's sexual problems. I attended these four-day Boston meetings for three consecutive years, from 1999 to 2001, eager to understand how women's sexuality and sexual problems were being understood by the "experts." In many ways, what happened at these meetings explains why the search for the female Viagra is still mired in confusion.

While I refer to the meetings as the Boston Forums, it is important to point out that the name has changed slightly every year. What hasn't changed over the years is the subtitle of these gatherings, which is highlighted on the annual conference program: "New Perspectives in the Management of Female Sexual Dysfunction." This subtitle reveals the "management," or treatment-oriented objectives of the meeting, which may or may not require some basic understanding of "sexual function." As Goldstein told me, after the introduction of Viagra, "We work backwards, we expect a treatment for things." This emphasis on treatment-based science is made even more obvious if one acknowledges the role of the pharmaceutical industry in subsidizing the meetings as well as the research. As I will argue, their "pharmaceutical agenda"—that is, their need to find drug treatments for problems—inevitably fuels the construction of women's sexual issues as medical problems.

THE PLAYERS

Understanding how these meetings operate requires recognizing the four overlapping groups of "players" that make the Boston Forum what it is. The four groups include "experts" on FSD, marketers, critics, and journalists. Importantly, the "experts," or so-called Boston Forum grandmasters, are the primary FSD visionaries. They attend various medical meetings, publish in the medical journals, and are the "experts" appearing in or being quoted by the popular media. As in the case of ED, however, many of them have close ties to the pharmaceutical industry as consultants, investigators, and/or stockholders. Because of the recent influx of funding, some have even been able to make a career out of sexual medicine, as in the case with the members of Goldstein's Boston University group. For these experts, "grandmastering" and publishing are the activities that characterize their knowledge production and enable them to reach large audiences.

Marketers are those affiliated with the pharmaceutical industry. Because the Boston Forums are pharmaceutical-industry-sponsored events, companies such as Pfizer, Eli Lilly, Shering-Plough, Solvay Pharmaceuticals, and others provide the funding for the meetings (in the form of educational grants). Most are eager to support research in this area and promote their products at this venue, both in the display area and at the podium, where one can find numerous presentations by industry-affiliated researchers. Thus there is a crucial overlap between the "experts" and the marketers. Since grandmasters are not required to disclose their relationships with pharmaceutical companies during conference presentations, the industry presence and the overlap between marketers and experts is rather covert. For example, I was not aware of this overlap until at one point in the 1999 conference, when an FDA presenter asked who in the audience was *not* an "industry person" and about half of the people in the room kept their hands down—a clear sign that participation in the meeting was linked to industry goals. This close relationship between science and corporate interests raises important questions regarding the nature of and motivation for the scientific claims of FSD.

Critics—specifically a feminist group of health advocates, academics, and therapists called The Working Group on a New View of Women's Sexual Problems—were also in attendance at the meeting, using the annual Boston conference as a site to voice concerns about the ongoing medicalization of women's bodies, the privatization of medicine, and the oversimplification of medical models. This group of critics is actively challenging the conventional scientific wisdom circulating at these meetings. The Working Group is also reminding participants and experts of what feminists have written about for decades—that women's sexuality is as much about politics as it is about biology. They disperse leaflets, speak in smaller venues, and hold press conferences in an attempt to challenge the biological model of sexuality that most participants seem to take for granted. And though I am calling them critics, they may also be experts in their own disciplines. Their leader, clinical psychologist Leonore Tiefer, is both an insider and an outsider at medical meetings, or both a noted expert in psychology and a critic of medical and pharmaceutical industries. Tiefer has been one of the few clinicians to actively express serious concerns at the Boston Forum about the social implications of the medicalization of sexuality for women and men, medical science, and society at large. As you will see, at times during the Boston meetings, the chasm between the experts and the critics is wide, and at other times, concerned experts may literally become critics, revealing another fascinating overlap.

Finally, the annual Boston meeting attracts significant media attention as journalists from the *Boston Globe*, the *Chicago Tribune*, *60 Minutes*, and other regional and national outlets attend. Journalists depend on the above players to report on conference activities, and they also create their own framing of FSD. Typically, in an attempt to get "both sides of the story," the media may incorporate both medical claims, like those of Irwin Goldstein and his Boston research group, and feminist counterclaims, like those of Leonore Tiefer and her Working Group, thus cementing "the sides" and the stakes of each group of players.

EXPERT-OWNERSHIP

Perhaps the most fascinating occurrence at the Boston Forum, at least to me, is the ongoing competition among sexuality experts to understand and, as social-problems theorist Joseph Gusfield would say, to "own" women's sexual problems. Each year, definitions of women's sexual problems are up for debate. Thus, the stakes are high, especially when one is backed by a powerful corporation vying for control of the market in women's sexual problems.

Experts subsidized by pharmacological corporations are called "affiliated experts." Which female sexual dysfunction experts are "affiliated" is difficult to determine because, as noted above, disclosure is not always obvious during presentations at the Boston Forum. In 2000, disclosure statements that came with the conference program revealed that affiliated experts come from many disciplines, especially urology, basic science, and psychiatry, and all employ the scientific method to locate women's sexual problems in the body as medical problems worth treating. Overall, about half (53 percent) of those giving a presentation disclosed a research or consulting relationship with one or more drug companies. More importantly, 88 percent of those giving high-profile, lengthy grandmaster presentations disclosed such links. The most visible and vocal affiliated expert at the Boston Forum meetings is Irwin Goldstein.

In contrast, the group I will call "critical experts" do not accept pharmaceutical funding and actively promote counterclaims at the Boston Forum. In other words, while these professionals acknowledge women's sexual problems, they place the blame for these problems outside of the body, in social and cultural arenas. They make up a tiny minority of FSD experts at the Boston Forum, and, as noted before, their most vocal proponent is Leonore Tiefer.

In between these two extremes are the "semi-affiliated experts" who receive limited pharmaceutical funding (usually acting as temporary consultants rather than investigators) and actively promote sympathetic counterclaims at the Boston Forum. In other words, they express concern with medical definitions or measures but still embrace medical models. They are the minority of FSD experts, primarily those trained in psychology or sex therapy.

Finally, I call those who are not associated with pharmaceutical funding or counterclaims the "neutral experts." Generally, these experts occupy less marketable research areas, such as the area of sexual pain disorders, or are government-affiliated researchers. I am most interested in the first three groups of experts, whose positioning in relation to medical and pharmacological arenas affects the form and content of the claims they make.

One urologist made reference to these expert groups and their competing models for understanding women's sexual problems in his description of the "scene" at the Boston conference:

> I'm not really into the scene. I just have fun watching . . . I mean, there are such disparate groups there. You have the psychologists, the psychiatrists, the sex therapists, and the gynecologists, and then the urologists. The urologists are the most scientific—they see a clinical problem that they want to fix. As urologists, we embrace the scientific method. But the others, I can't figure out what they are doing there. I just can't figure it out. They don't embrace the scientific method at all, and they are singing "Kumbayah" and holding hands. It is just fascinating. I mean, I see it as a problem, FSD, like chest pain. It is a medical problem.

This quotation highlights three things: the dominant role that urologists play as claim-makers at the Boston Forum, the chasm between urological and psychological approaches to constructing claims, and the struggle over defining women's sexual problems as medical or nonmedical.

Slut! Growing Up Female with a Bad Reputation

LEORA TANENBAUM

Leora Tanenbaum, excerpt from *Slut! Growing Up Female with a Bad Reputation,* New York: Seven Stories Press, 1999. Reprinted by permission.

When news broke that Monica Lewinsky had allegedly had consensual sexual relations with President Clinton, I was astounded by the torrent of nasty remarks, headlines, and public opinion polls picking apart her body, hair, psychological state, and sexuality. *New York* magazine reported that as an adolescent, Lewinsky had spent two summers at weight-loss camp, and that she had "paid particular attention to the guys." Jokes about Lewinsky's "big hair," and how she was sent home from the White House because she dressed too provocatively, became instant clichés. When *Vanity Fair* published photos of Lewinsky in glamorous poses, a female acquaintance of mine scrutinized the layout and decreed that the only reason Lewinsky looked so attractive was that the magazine gave her a great makeup job and airbrushed the photos. Clinton himself referred to Lewinsky as "that woman" ("I never had sexual relations with that woman"); with those two words alone he managed to portray her as a classic "slut," a throwaway woman he clearly didn't want to humanize by invoking her name.

A concerted effort to smear Lewinsky as an oversexed, hyperaggressive woman was under way. Speculation abounded that Lewinsky had invented the whole affair in a girlish fantasy; Representative Charles Rangel of New York said, "That poor child has serious emotional problems, she's fantasizing. And I haven't heard that she played with a full deck in her other experiences." In an editorial, the *Wall Street Journal* called her a "little tart." After being portrayed as a stalker who "used emotional blackmail to trap" a married lover by the *New York Post* and a "manipulative, sex-obsessed woman" by the *Daily News,* Fox News released a poll investigating whether the public thought she was an "average girl" or a "young tramp looking for thrills." Fifty-four percent rated her a tramp. Later it was revealed that President Clinton had referred to Lewinsky as a "stalker" with his staff. And all this was months before Independent Whitewater Counsel Kenneth Starr served up his own salacious report depicting Lewinsky as an exhibitionistic, sex-obsessed provocateur.

Personally, I think Lewinsky is a good-looking woman who happens to have a voluptuous figure. Starstruck, she participated in an act that was reckless, foolish, and sad but hardly worthy of such national attention. Originally, she did not want to publicly advertise the affair (as Gennifer Flowers did in 1992 about her own extramarital relationship with the president); indeed, by lying about it initially in an affidavit, she demonstrated respectful discretion. (Her March 1999 interview with Barbara Walters and cooperation with the author of *Monica's Story* were part of a defensive measure to try to counter her image as a tramp.) All in all, I believe, Lewinsky does not deserve to be written off as a *Melrose Place* bimbo.

But even as her name fades from late-night punch lines, there is no doubt that Lewinsky will spend the rest of her life in the shadow of her tarnished reputation. Obviously Clinton's own reputation has also suffered, but most Americans have been disappointed that he lied about the liaison for seven months, not because of the liaison itself. And even those who do find the liaison disturbing tend to describe Clinton as someone who has a "problem" or "disease," suggesting that his sexuality lies beyond his control. Meanwhile many Americans believe that an unmarried woman who capitalizes on her sexuality—to feel good about herself, to capture the attention of powerful men, for recreation—is debased.

But why should sex and femininity necessarily be at odds? Of course, sex is often used in ways that degrade women (rape, sexual harassment, forcible prostitution), and too many women mistakenly perceive that their sexuality is their only source of power. But sex is not always and inherently sexist, nor should it transform women into dirty tramps. When

Clinton and Lewinsky participated in their liaison, the only people who got hurt, as I see it, were Hillary and Chelsea Clinton—and that's for them to decide.

Meanwhile, in the women's locker room at my local Y, semi- and fully naked women walk from their lockers to the showers and then back again every day. But when a repairman recently entered one circumscribed corner of the locker room for less than five minutes (all the while monitored by a female staffer), all hell broke loose. I had to pass that corner to get to the shower, and I didn't feel like waiting. I was wearing one of those gym towels that were clearly not intended for women, since they cover either the breasts or the hips, but not both. But what did I care? In the three years I've belonged to the Y, hundreds of different women had already seen me naked; why was I to be intimidated by the fact that one busy male might catch a quick glimpse of my flesh? Yet two clothed women "tsk-tsked" me as I padded by the repairman in my towel, telling me with a shake of their heads that I had committed some grave lapse in judgment. (He didn't even seem to notice.)

This is the sexual double standard: the idea that women are disgraced by sex outside of marriage, that sex transforms them into "sluts." The 1997 movie *Chasing Amy* illustrates how the sexual double standard effectively sidesteps men's concern about their own sexual abilities. In describing the film, reviewers said it was about the sorrows of a postcollege man who has the misfortune to fall in love with a young, cute lesbian. In fact, the movie says less about lesbianism than it does about the fear of "sluts." Holden is attracted to Alyssa, who is, it is true, a lesbian. When she falls for him too, he assumes he's the first man she's ever slept with. But Alyssa wasn't always a lesbian. It turns out that when she was in high school, Alyssa had considerable sexual experience with boys—including, once, a *ménage á trois* with two male classmates. Holden, who was infatuated with Alyssa when he knew that she had had sex with many women, is now disgusted. Having slept with men transforms Alyssa; it makes her a "slut" rather than a chic lesbian. And so

Holden treats her like a "slut" by asking her to participate in a *ménage* with his best male friend. Deep down, he admits, he is intimidated by and fears her sexual experience with men. He feels inadequate and wants to even the score. Alyssa, who feels cheapened by the proposal, leaves him.

Likewise, in the 1986 Spike Lee movie *She's Gotta Have It*, Mars Blackmon says, "Look, all men want freaks. We just don't want 'em for a wife." Blackmon, played by Lee, is frustrated that his girlfriend, Nola, is sexually involved with two other men as well. All three men want Nola, but do they respect her? No. Boyfriend No. 2 sneers, "A nice lady doesn't go humping from bed to bed." Boyfriend No. 3 snickers, "Once a freak, always a freak." Then he rapes her. But it doesn't matter to Nola whether or not these men respect her: She respects herself. "I am not a one-man woman," she says with defiance.

You, too, might think that Alyssa's and Nola's casual attitude about sex is inappropriate, disgusting, or just wrong. You might be opposed to casual sex in principle, believing instead that sex should be reserved for a meaningful, romantic relationship. That's fine—but beside the point. There should be one sexual standard for both genders—and that applies to older teenagers and to adults over the age of twenty-one. If you think that sixteen-year-olds should not be having intercourse, that includes boys as well as girls. If you think that some sixteen-year-olds are mature enough to express their sexual longings, that includes girls as well as boys. Though sexually active girls alone carry the burden of potential pregnancy, both genders must be treated as equals since they share equally in the heterosexual act.

Holden's low opinion of Alyssa, and Mars's contempt for Nola, is indicative of the continued widespread prominence of the sexual double standard. Three quarters of young men and nearly 90 percent of young women surveyed by the Janus Report agreed that the sexual double standard prevails. Roughly half of American teenagers are sexually active—in 1997, 49 percent of boys aged fifteen to nineteen reported ever having had sexual intercourse, compared with 48 percent of girls—but when it comes to moralizing about the excesses of teenage sexuality, girls alone are ridiculed and made to feel cheap. As Steven, a Rhode Island high school junior, comments, his male friends always hang out with the freshman girls known as "sluts," not because they like those girls but because they can "get some." And like in the 1950s, it's usually girls, not boys, who are on the front lines of making fun of others as "sluts."

"In the eighth grade, I had a boyfriend and we sort of explored things sexually, though we never had intercourse," recalls Hanna Wallace, twenty-five, a magazine editor in New York. "I was quite honest with my best friend, Stacia, and told her about it. Her reaction was that she was disappointed in me. She and another friend got together and wrote me a letter that really upset me. It wasn't that they were worried about me, because everything I did with my boyfriend was consensual. They were chastising me for my behavior, which they thought was disgusting. They were moralizing. I felt: Did I have to hide my sexual relationship from my friends?"

Hanna's friend, Stacia Eyerly, vividly remembers the incident. "We did write her a note," she told me. "We were concerned about whether she was doing the right thing. A little of it was envy, but mostly it was the feeling that she shouldn't have done what she did, that it was inappropriate. But this feeling only applied to girls. It was definitely because she was a girl that I had a problem with it."

Despite humiliating encounters like Hanna's, sexually active "sluts" have an advantage over "good" girls. Once they are singled out for derision, they realize they have little to lose by living up to their reputations. And in defying the "good girl" rules, they develop a necessary critical perspective about love and sex. Unlike most girls, self-aware "sluts" perceive the unfairness of the sexual double standard. They know they are in a double bind: That boys like girls who are a little bit "slutty" but also look down on them as cheap and inferior. They are aware that girls as well as boys experience sexual pleasure;

they know that if they are responsible, they can minimize their risk of disease, pregnancy, and emotional distress. And they recognize that most girls take adolescent romance much more seriously than boys do—too seriously. Sexually active "sluts" think of themselves as independent sexual agents and are less inclined to use sex as a bargaining chip for love and affection. As a result, I would argue, they, and not the "good" girls who call them insulting names, are more likely to have a healthy attitude about themselves and their futures.

"Tell Me More, Tell Me More": Young Women's Locker Room Talk as a Boomer-Feminist Legacy

PAULA KAMEN

Paula Kamen, excerpt from *Her Way: Young Women' Remake the Sexual Revolution*, New York: New York University Press, 2000. Reprinted by permission.

In college, one night there were six or seven girls, our same age, good friends, sitting in a bar and really talking, I mean just how we have orgasms," said Janine, twenty-four. "And this happened to be a masturbation conversation. In the middle of the bar. There were [many] people around us, laughing and learning. It was unbelievable. I guess that's how we figure things out."

Recently, this Florida high school teacher and two of her friends again discussed this topic together in detail. One of them, Tammy, admitted that she never had an orgasm. "They told me how and now I can. I'm healed . . . ," Tammy said. "It's comforting to know that people have experienced similar things or that your friends know and that they understand that it's OK. I guess it's good to know that you're OK."

While all three women are generally open with their parents, their friends fill a distinct need for sexual information and openness—without judgment. "At age sixteen," said Janine, a Catholic from a Cuban-American family, "who was I going to talk to about having sex with my boyfriend? My friends."

While sex education from schools and parents give young women the information they should know, women's locker-room talk gives them what they really want to know. Women's locker-room talk today can be both edifying and trashy, therapeutic and ego-fanning. One's girlfriends are often a constant presence influencing sexual relationships in many roles: as a cheerleader, referee, Internet listserve, crisis hot line, absolving priest, Greek chorus, sister, mom, aunt, RA, RN, MSW, reference book, shameless voyeur, and, sometimes, feminist advocate.

As the rules about sex have changed, so have the rules for talking about it. Feeling less guilty about being sexual beings and taking advantage of strong and sharing friendships, women have cranked open their channels of communication. Instead of remaining silent, and serving only as subjects of conquest for men's "locker-room talk," as was the standard in the past, they have cultivated their own potent and shameless breed. By all accounts, women are even more likely than men to talk about sex, and in more vivid Technicolor detail and more critically.

The pervasiveness of locker-room talk among young women of all backgrounds also reflects the particular feminist legacy of the baby boomers.

They opened the doors to free communication about the most intimate matters of one's life and promoted women's friendships as a nurturing, empowering force. The early personal consciousness-raising of the women's health movement, which was fringe work in the 1960s and 1970s, has now become a part of mainstream life. Like the radical message of the Sexual Revolution—to give women the permission to have sex outside of marriage—the feminists' ideologies of women breaking their silences have slowly been absorbed into the nation's collective psychic bloodstream. Today, although with less political emphasis, "third-wave" feminists (along with women of color of all ages and safer-sex activists) build on their work advocating even more authentic and diverse conversations about the most unspoken aspects of women's lives.

through a hole and they clamp it like a mammo-gram," she says, eyes rolling. "After taking my breast photos in about a thousand different ways they decided they couldn't do it because [the calcifications were] too close to the skin." She snorts. "Have you ever had a mammogram?" she inquires, peering across the table with a half smile on her face. "You wait."

CHAPTER 13

Self-Help Gynecology

BETTY DODSON WAS SHOCKED—a difficult feat to accomplish. The veteran educator and erotic pioneer is usually the one doing the shocking. Her honest, detailed books on sex and orgasm have taught several generations of women about the joys of masturbation and the importance of speaking up for sexual pleasure. She and other health feminists had accomplished so much in terms of educating women about their bodies, and so much progress had been made. And yet here she was, sitting in a room full of affluent, educated young New Yorkers—the sort of women who are supposed to embody the "Sex and the City" sophistication and to even be blasé about sex—and yet Dodson was the only one speaking without giggles and shame. It was a bridal shower, and Dodson was the main event. In spite of herself, she was surprised by the lack of knowledge about bodies and sexuality and the amazing level of discomfort projected by these seemingly modern young women, including the bride, who was too ashamed to make eye contact with Dodson for most of the party.

So when it comes to understanding our genitals and sex organs, have we really come a long way, baby?

One of the most abiding images of the second-wave feminist movement is of young women on college campuses going to meetings or sitting with friends and realizing they had never seen a labia or vagina—let alone their own genitalia—up close. In addition to healthy sexuality, having control and understanding of our bodies promotes better general health, and supports reproductive freedom.

Carol Downer and Lorraine Rothman—two of the pioneers of self-help gynecology—come directly from the Elizabeth Cady Stanton tradition of self-reliance based on practical study and physical dexterity. When Carol considered adding new self-help procedures to her repertoire, she normally weighed their level of difficulty by comparing them to familiar kitchen tasks. In 1977, she considered offering cervical caps—a barrier contraceptive imported from England—

at her health centers: "We can do it," she concluded. "Women can do it . . . it's not harder than stuffing a turkey."

Rothman, who passed away suddenly from bladder cancer in September of 2007, created a device called the "DLM" or "Del Em," a small jar attached to tubing and a syringe that helped women remove their periods and provided an early "at home" alternative to abortions. Cynthia Pearson, the director of the National Women's Health Network, said shortly after Rothman's death that the Del Em "totally turned around the lived experience of women in their reproductive years, giving them control and knowledge of their own bodies."

Self-help gynecology isn't just controversial for opponents of feminism: In 1992, Downer and Rebecca Chalker's *A Woman's Book of Choices* was the object of a massive censorship effort by noted feminist Andrea Dworkin and her companion John Stoltenberg. They asked the authors to delete that prior to *Roe v. Wade*, some states permitted clean abortions if pregnancies resulted from rape, because they feared that rape victims would be charged with making up their experiences in order to secure procedures.

No matter what the political climate, taking control of our sexual organs and of our health is at once the most basic and most radical thing a woman can do. While pioneers like Downer and Dodson are still hard at work, young women must discover the ways in which they still need this vital skill set—which some young activists have started calling guerilla gynecology—and the emerging issues facing new generations of feminists.

Self-Help Gynecology

EDITED BY KOFI TAHA

Carol Downer with Rebecca Chalker, excerpt from "Through the Speculum" in R. Arditti, R. D. Klein, and S. Minden, eds., *Test-Tube Women: What Future for Motherhood?* Boston: Pandora Press, 1984; Lorraine Rothman, "Menstrual Extraction: Procedures," *Quest* 4(3), 1978; Lolly Hirsch, "The Curse: A Cultural History of Menstruation," *The Monthly Extract: An Irregular Periodical* September/October 1976; Rebecca Chalker and Carol Downer, "Menstrual Regulation in the Developing World," in *A Women's Book of Choices,* New York: Seven Stories Press, 1992; Ellen Frankfort, *Vaginal Politics,* New York: Bantam Books, 1973. Reprinted by permission.

At the heart of the women's health movement in the early 1970s was the principle of self-help, which emphasized the importance of reclaiming women's bodies from the medical profession, re-examining conventional knowledge produced by patriarchal institutions about women's bodies, and removing the shroud of mystery, shame, and fear that is socially constructed and instilled in women around menstruation, childbirth, and reproductive health. The Feminist Women's Health Center in Los Angeles was at the forefront of this call for self-help gynecology and was also instrumental in developing a technique called menstrual extraction. Although menstrual extraction was mislabeled "self-abortion" by the mainstream media, was legally challenged in conservative states, and never enjoyed widespread practice, it represents perhaps the most revolutionary aspect of the women's health movement because it was created by women, for women, through research conducted by women, on women, in a nurturing group setting.

The following pieces attempt to recount the history of the self-help movement, explain the procedure and purpose of menstrual extraction, and discuss its applications, both in terms of its practical use and its theoretical challenge to patriarchy.

➤ In "Through the Speculum," Carol Downer, one of the founders of the Feminist Women Health Center in Los Angeles, describes the evolution of the center, the women's health movement, and the importance of information sharing in challenging the social control of women's sexuality and reproduction.

➤ "Menstrual Extraction," by Lorraine Rothman, inventor of the Del Em menstrual extractor, details the procedures, materials, and methods of menstrual extraction.

➤ Lolly Hirsch offers, by way of a poetic description of the experience of menstrual extraction, a critical book review of *The Curse: A Cultural History of Menstruation*, written by Delaney, Lupton, and Toth.

➤ In "Menstrual Regulation in the Developing World," Rebecca Chalker and Carol Downer discuss the related practice of menstrual regulation in developing nations and its potential implications for women's health.

➤ The final piece, from *Vaginal Politics* by Ellen Frankfort, discusses the nature of the resistance mounted against menstrual extraction and the theoretical underpinnings of the women's health movement.

CAROL DOWNER WITH REBECCA CHALKER, EXCERPT FROM "THROUGH THE SPECULUM" IN R. ARDITTI, R. D. KLEIN, AND S. MINDEN, EDS., *TEST-TUBE WOMEN: WHAT FUTURE FOR MOTHERHOOD?* BOSTON: PANDORA PRESS, 1984.

On April 7, 1971, a group of women met in a small women's bookstore in Venice, California. I had acquired a plastic vaginal speculum and wanted to share what I had seen with the group. After I demonstrated its use, several other women also took off their pants, climbed up on the table, and inserted a speculum. In one amazing instant, each of us had liberated a part of our bodies that had formerly been the sole province of our gynecologists. Afterward, in a consciousness-raising discussion, we observed that in this supportive, nonsexist setting, feelings of shame fell away, and we acknowledged the beginnings of feelings of power from being able to look into our own vaginas and see where our menstrual blood, secretions, and babies came from.

This meeting was the genesis of activities that spread and connected countrywide with other women engaged in similar pursuits, which became known as the women's health movement. Collectively we worked to reclaim a huge body of knowledge that had been coopted by the medical establishment; through research and observation, [we] regained the technology for safe abortion, birth, and self-insemination, and redefined our sexual anatomy, which had been distorted, put down, or simply ignored by mainstream sex educators and therapists.

Soon, we began doing referrals to illegal abortion clinics. Then we worked as assistants to physicians who were willing to do safe abortion procedures. By assisting at many abortions, we learned that the uterus is not such a remote, mysterious, inaccessible place and that early termination abortions by the suction method were far less technical and complicated than we had been led to believe. We planned to learn to do abortions ourselves, but the 1973 Supreme Court decision on abortion made the procedure legal to twenty-four weeks of pregnancy. Fifty-three days after that decision, we borrowed $1,200, rented a small house, hired a physician, and opened up the first woman-owned, woman-controlled abortion clinic in the United States.

This clinic became the Los Angeles Feminist Women's Health Center (FWHC). Within three years, similar clinics had started in Santa Ana, San Diego, and Chico, California, and in Atlanta, Georgia. Later, clinics in Portland, Oregon, and Yakima, Washington, joined us on an affiliate basis.

The underlying principle of all of the work of the FWHCs is the strategy of undermining the patriarchal structure of society and male dominance by challenging the social control of women's sexuality and reproduction. The institutions of marriage and the laws which regulate divorce, abortion, prostitution, birth control, and homosexuality isolate women from each other and brutally repress their sexuality and reproductive rights. The FWHCs have worked in national coalitions to support the women's movement's impressive campaigns against these laws.

As we progressed in our understanding of the patriarchy, we saw that in addition to laws that maintain the patriarchal family, all institutions of a sexist society function to reinforce women's inferior status, but the male-dominated medical institutions have the special role of enforcing women's sexual and reproductive compliance. Further, we realized that the external oppressive controls and exploitation of women's sexuality has a subjective expression—intense shame—which deprives us of the strength and vigor to assert our most basic rights. This universal shame, felt by all classes of women, causes us to feel extremely humiliated when we expose our genitals, except in situations which we define as medical or sexually intimate. Even in such situations, women frequently need special surroundings, props, or rituals to allow another person (nearly always a male) to see or touch her genitals. In our clinics, we have directly confronted the medical practice, peculiar to the United States, of draping women for exams, by dispensing with the drape altogether. The drape reinforces our feelings of shame we are supposed to feel and inhibits the free flow of information between a woman and her practitioner.

In the past twelve years, we have held thousands and thousands of self-help clinics and have repeatedly observed the immediate release of energy and the joy we experienced that first night in Venice. At the same moment the self-help clinic breaks down the barriers between women and strips away repression and inhibition, it also provides us with a realistic alternative to total dependence on the medical profession. Women can take direct control of their own bodies from the simplest ability to check an IUD string directly by *looking*, instead of blindly by feeling, to identifying and treating common vaginal conditions with safe, inexpensive home remedies. No one would dream of running to the doctor for every sore throat, yet women are expected to regard each vaginal infection as a problem only a doctor can know anything about.

Through information gained in early self-help clinics in Los Angeles, we were liberated from the oppression of misconceptions and misinformation. We learned that the structure of the cervix is beautifully simple. And by observing ourselves and each other on a regular basis, we learned that the medical definition of "the range of normal" is impossible narrow and restrictive. Such notions as "tipped uteruses," "eroded cervixes," "irregular menstruation," and "vaginal discharge," all considered health problems by our doctors, became obviously absurd. We found that everyone's uterus is "tipped" some way or other and that this term has no medical significance whatsoever. We realized that "eroded cervix" means irritated, although the medical term connotes actual disintegration. We soon discovered that very few women have "ideal" twenty-eight-day menstrual cycles. Unless noticeable signs of ill health are present, a woman's cycle can range normally from less than twenty days to six months, nine months, or even longer.

The first technology self-helpers gained was the ability to perform safe, early abortions in a procedure we called "menstrual extraction." We chose this term deliberately to blur the distinction between removing a menstrual period and terminating a pregnancy. In our society, abortion is used solely as a means to control women's reproduction, but to a woman faced with the possibility of terminating a pregnancy, the important thing is to have her period on time. Lorraine Rothman, a member of our group, invented a simple suction device which we call "Del Em" to extract the contents of the uterus. Through our observations of abortion procedures, we learned that a sterile plastic tube, about the circumference of a pencil, could be inserted into the uterus and the uterine contents, menstrual blood or an early pregnancy, could be suctioned out. Because menstrual extraction has traditionally been practiced in the watchful caring environment of small groups of women, the experiences of women having extractions have been profoundly positive, and few serious problems have been reported.

Medical domination and control of pregnancy

and childbirth has been more subtle than oppressive abortion laws, but is virtually complete in Western countries. The normal human experience of childbirth has been entirely removed from daily life, so that most of us have no direct knowledge of it, and it has been transformed into a dangerous, pathological event, so much so that normal birth is no longer even taught in medical schools.

Self-helpers, other feminists, and home-birth advocates have fought a monumental battle against the medical and legal establishments in the United States to retain the right to choose birth attendants and settings.

Through using the technique of self-examination and information-sharing, we reclaimed important and long-ignored information in the realm of women's sexuality. When we began to write about sex, we discovered a vast disparity between the way medical books and popular sex literature treated the sexual anatomy of men and women. The clitoris has always been considered to be the glands alone, while the penis is described as having many parts which function together to produce orgasm. We studied anatomical illustrations in both European and US medical texts and took off our pants and compared our genitals to these illustrations, some of which date back to the nineteenth century. Our group, comprised of both heterosexual and lesbian women, shared experiences and made photographs and movies of masturbation. Putting all this information together, we *rediscovered* the entire clitoris, which encompasses structures of erectile tissue, blood vessels, glands, nerves, and muscles. We learned that both visible and hidden structures of the clitoris undergo remarkable changes during sexual response including erection. The goal of the redefinition of the clitoris is to give women a concrete understanding of what actually occurs during sexual response and to offer clear explanations for various sexual phenomena.

After running clinics for a few years, we decided we needed to spread our ideas in written form. This decision has resulted in four books, each focused on a different aspect of women's health.

A New View of a Woman's Body (Simon & Schuster, 1981) differs from all other women's health books in that it was researched and written by lay health workers involved in day-to-day health care, and draws on the cumulative experience of more than 100,000 women who have visited our clinics over the past ten years. *A New View* also includes clear and detailed illustrations of women's anatomy, especially the redefinition of the clitoris, and the first color photographs of women's vaginas and cervixes to appear outside of a medical text.

How to Stay Out of the Gynecologist's Office (Peace Press, 1981) discusses in-depth problems that every woman is likely to encounter at some time in her life. We evaluated home remedies, over-the-counter preparations, and medical remedies for effectiveness and possible harmful effects and compiled a glossary of over 1,000 terms used by gynecologists. We also included information women might use when seeking to equalize the very unequal power relationship encountered in a gynecologist's office.

Woman Centered Pregnancy and Birth (Cleis Press, 1984) [is] designed to give women more power and control over their birth experience. We included very detailed information to help women evaluate both the multitude of technological interventions they can be faced with in a medical setting. We also discussed self-defense techniques in the hospital, donor insemination, and resources on how to work for political change in childbirth.

In 1979, in response to a request from Chilean women who were being raped while they were imprisoned, Suzann Gage and other women compiled information on self-abortion techniques. In 1979, we published this manuscript as *When Birth Control Fails . . . (How to Abort Ourselves Safely)* (Speculum Press). This book became the object of a heated public debate, both within the women's community and in the mainstream press. Nevertheless, feminists from around the world, especially in countries where abortion is illegal or difficult to obtain, ordered copies and the entire collection was sold in a very short time.

In researching and writing our books, we have found that our early belief in the power of self-examination has been reinforced and validated. Vaginal self-examination with a plastic speculum, when performed in a group setting, is a direct assault on the shame that has been inculcated in us regarding our genitals and is a powerful, positive act of trust and mutual support between women. After this barrier is broken, the information flows rapidly and voluminously. Myth after myth falls away. Using the format of the self-help clinic, women could rediscover all of the old knowledge which has been ripped away from us. Combining this knowledge with a group study of medical texts, we could question existing medical information and put it in a more sound empirical basis.

LORRAINE ROTHMAN, "MENSTRUAL EXTRACTION: PROCEDURES," *QUEST* 4(3), 1978.

Menstrual extraction is a procedure developed by the Los Angeles Self-Help Clinic women in 1971 which gently removes the contents of the uterus by suction on or about the first day of menstruation.

Materials and Methods

It was evident that women did not have equipment to do menstrual extraction, nor any way to get and safely use what was available. Vacuum aspirators are expensive, large and cumbersome, and produce much more vacuum than is necessary. We had practiced with a portable device used by Harvey Karman, and were impressed with its simplicity (the plastic cannula attached directly to a plastic syringe). We found it difficult to manipulate, however, and it had the potential to accidentally reverse the suction, thus allowing menstrual fluid and possibly air into the uterus. We were concerned about potential complications that might result from reversing the suction. As a member of the Los Angeles Self-Help Clinic, I saw that we needed a simple and inexpensively made device, which

had built-in safety features. I invented the Del Em to suit the group's needs. Vacuum is created in a small bottle which is attached to a small cannula that is inserted into the cervical os, where the cervix opens into the endocervical canal. An automatic valve attachment controls the direction of the air flow and locks in the pressure, eliminating any possibility of pushing menstrual fluid or air back into the uterus.

Menstrual extraction occurs either at the woman's home or at the group's meeting place. A woman will usually choose to have an extraction on or about the first day her period is expected. However, some women have extractions as much as two weeks beyond the expected date of menstruation.

Three women are the key people involved with extractions: the woman who is to have the extraction (she sometimes controls the vacuum pressure), a woman who observes the equipment for proper functioning, and a woman who inserts and moves the cannula. At times, other group members participate in order to learn the procedure.

After the woman who is to have the extraction places herself comfortably on the table or bed, other women in the group perform a pelvic examination to determine the size, location, and characteristics of the woman's pelvic organs. Certain signs are watched for, such as advanced pregnancy, infection, or other problems. Because the group has frequent opportunities at regular meetings to become familiar with one another, a basis for comparison has been established so that any contraindications are more easily recognized.

The woman inserts her own speculum, examines her own cervix, and talks with the group; has others in the group look at her cervix; and then decides whether or not she wants to have the extraction. She talks about her past experiences and purposes for extracting her period, such as relief of menstrual pain. If she suspects she is pregnant, she will discuss her subjective signs and these signs will be evaluated in light of her previous experiences with pregnancies, amount and frequency of exposure to sperm, and her fertility at the time of exposure.

The Del Em consists of a plastic 50-cc syringe that has a valve on the end. The valve prevents air from being injected into the uterus. The syringe is pumped until it becomes difficult to pull the plunger. Air is removed from the bottle in this way creating a vacuum. The cannula is carefully inserted through the undilated cervical os. Often, the inner cervical muscle can be felt against the cannula. If the slender flexible cannula bends, forceps can be attached to the middle of the cannula, giving it more stability. Sometimes a stabilizer is attached to the cervix so that the uterus does not move with the movements of the cannula.

The woman who is having the extraction will tell the other women when she feels the cannula touching the back wall of her uterus. She will continue to relate what she is experiencing as the cannula is moved back and forth making sure, however, that it remains fully inserted. The menstrual material appears within the cannula after a short time.

The cannula is moved within the uterus until either no more menstrual material comes out or the woman having the extraction says she wants to stop. The tubing attached to the cannula is clamped off to avoid any unnecessary discomfort of suction as the cannula is removed through the cervical canal.

Results

Most women who do menstrual extraction do not experience excessive discomfort. Women experience different degrees of cramping during the extraction. Sometimes, women can feel strong cramping when the cannula is inserted through the cervical canal. Most women feel strong cramping at the end of the extraction as the uterus contracts. Menstrual extraction discomfort or pain is seldom as severe or intense as the discomfort or pain from abortions that are done by electrically powered suction machines.

Daily phone contact is the common follow-up method until the group meets again.

LOLLY HIRSCH, "THE CURSE: A CULTURAL HISTORY OF MENSTRUATION," *THE MONTHLY EXTRACT: AN IRREGULAR PERIODICAL* SEPTEMBER/OCTOBER, 1976.

No one can possibly describe a menstrual extraction who has not been there; who hasn't stood shoulder-to-shoulder with her sisters, breathing with the woman on her back, rubbing her forehead, rubbing her legs when they quiver, keeping silent except for interaction concerning the feelings of the woman on her back.

Who could ever describe the shock that happens when the syringe accidentally pulls out with the sound of an explosive rifle crack with everyone laughing in relief at the simplicity of the happening and the lesson of better control over the syringe, unless she's been there?

Who can know the best technique—whether the vacuum is best established before the extraction with a clamped-off tube—or better to assemble the tube, syringe, cannula, and bottle before entering the cervical canal—or after—unless she's tried them all?

Who can describe a group who in unison holds back breathing as the cannula is gently, gently pushed through the cervical canal; the search for a method of keeping the cervix from wobbling or pulling back into the vagina, unless she's been there?

Who could ever describe the sensing of the cannula bumping the back wall of the uterus unless she's felt it—as the manipulator of the cannula and as the woman on her back, unless she's been there?

It's a learning experience unlike all the men's books ever written. It's pure learning; pure, unadulterated, uterine, menstrual knowledge. I can't imagine a group of three women who are an automatic beginning of a self-help clinic writing a book on menstruation who've obviously never been in a self-help clinic or done menstrual extraction.

No woman can know the empathy that flows

through a group of women doing menstrual extraction; the exhilaration of control and power—whether it's just learning the extraction of menses process or whether it's terminating an unwanted pregnancy without suffering financial liability or physical trauma. The transcendental emotion of love, exalted in a group of powerful women demonstrating their power defies description.

The only comparable experience is that moment during a home birth when the baby's head exquisitely turns in the perfectly choreographed rotation at presentation while the mother is conscious and among friends.

These moments are holy.

These moments are moments of being overwhelmed with the powerfulness of being a *woman*.

No one can describe them who has not been there.

REBECCA CHALKER AND CAROL DOWNER, "MENSTRUAL REGULATION IN THE DEVELOPING WORLD," IN *A WOMAN'S BOOK OF CHOICES*, NEW YORK: SEVEN STORIES PRESS, 1992.

At the same time that menstrual extraction was developing in California, international family planning activists began using a nearly identical method of fertility control in developing countries. The technique has had a variety of names: "minisuction," "menstrual induction," and "menstrual aspiration." However, the term most widely used today is menstrual regulation (MR). Like menstrual extraction, the procedure is often done without a laboratory test to confirm pregnancy. MR can also be used for teaching women about their anatomy and fertility, diagnosing uterine cancer, menstrual disorders, and infertility, and for completing self-induced or incomplete abortions.

One distinctive difference between the practices of menstrual regulation and menstrual extraction is in the equipment used. The Del Em used in menstrual extraction is individually assembled, while the kit used in menstrual regulation is commercially produced and marketed. With this kit, the uterine contents are suctioned directly through

the cannula into a syringe while with the Del Em, the contents are suctioned through the cannula and a plastic tube about two feet long into a collection jar.

Early on, it became clear to medical professionals and family planning experts that paramedics and lay people with even minimal education could learn to use hand-generated suction devices safely and effectively. Today, training in most countries typically lasts from one to three weeks, occasionally longer, and is done on both a formal basis, including classroom lectures, demonstrations, and supervised practice; and on an informal basis, often consulting demonstrations only. Trainees may observe from ten to twenty procedures before beginning hands-on training, and then do up to twenty procedures under supervision before doing them on their own. Because of the lack of qualified trainers, and the demand for MR services, trainees sometimes begin doing unsupervised procedures without much hands-on instruction, but this is not recommended.

In developing countries where health education and contraception are not widely available, women who fear they may be pregnant often seek to induce miscarriages with sticks, wires, or other instruments, by drinking toxic substances, or by douching with harmful concoctions. In Nicaragua, for example, women commonly use wire from telephone cables to induce miscarriages. Others resort to poorly trained abortionists who often use stiff, unsterile instruments. As a result, at least 200,000 women die each year, and many more are left infertile or with lifelong health problems. In addition, hundreds of thousands of children are left motherless or with a mother who may be too ill or disabled to provide for them adequately.

Many doctors who do menstrual regulation may use anesthesia, but in some clinics, the only anesthesia that is used is the comforting hand and soothing voice of a counselor. Zarina, a counselor at a woman's clinic in Bangladesh, reports that most of the women who seek MR have already endured childbirth; most say the discomfort from the procedure is quite tolerable, even without anesthesia.

In practice, menstrual regulation is performed up to eight to ten weeks from the last period, but in many countries, the procedure is also done up to twelve weeks from the last menstrual period. There are no reliable statistics on the rate of incomplete procedures in Bangladesh or other countries where MR is in use, but the rate of incompletes appears to be low, according to Zarina because "most women in these countries usually don't come in until they are eight to ten weeks from their last period, when it is easier to determine, by examining the tissue, whether or not an implantation has been missed."

Menstrual regulation is practiced throughout Latin America, Asia, in many African countries, and on a limited basis in the Middle East. In every setting in which this technique has become accessible, the complication rate for self-induced and poorly done abortions has been dramatically reduced. In Indonesia, for example, one study found that the rate of septic abortion was 80 percent higher in areas in which menstrual regulation (in this case, suction curettage) was not available, but that where MR was available, wards formerly reserved for cases of septic abortion were no longer necessary. Clearly, if menstrual regulations were employed more widely, the health of many women—and the lives of many others—would be saved.

In an era that is hostile to reproductive freedom, menstrual extraction and other home health care techniques are profoundly relevant. Women may consciously choose to use menstrual extraction or to take herbs for fertility control for a variety of reasons. When used properly, these techniques are far safer than childbirth, and can put an end to the makeshift methods that desperate women have often used to prevent unwanted pregnancies.

ELLEN FRANKFORT, *VAGINAL POLITICS,* NEW YORK: BANTAM BOOKS, 1973.

There are few genuinely original ideas that come along in a lifetime. Period extraction is one. The fact that no one conceived of removing the menstrual flow all at once and assumed that it was a process that had to take place over a "period" of time, until a group of women started doing it, indicates the revolutionary potential behind the women's health movement.

My own initial reaction to period extraction was concern about the immediate danger or risks of a totally new device being tried out by many women. In fact, I reacted as the medical profession responds to anything new: conservatively. In worrying about the crudeness of the first model, so to speak, I did not see what was truly original—the concept. I still worry about the risks . . . but the kinds of feelings inspired by the demonstration and the talk of the women who are extracting their periods are so impressive that I [have had] some second and third thoughts about period extraction, the whole self-help movement out of which it has come, and the medical profession's response to both. For it is this response which has enabled me to see more clearly my own shortsightedness.

After describing the period extraction in "Vaginal Politics," in the *Village Voice,* I received dozens of letters from doctors about the number of women who would die if this thing caught on and how terribly dangerous and irresponsible it was for me to quote nonprofessional women in something that would be read by many women. (It was the "nonprofessional" that bothered them even more than the "women.") [It appears that] the doctor letter-writers were more upset at the independence that period extraction in particular and self-help in general gave women rather than at the dangers of either. Few argued or even considered that the device could be made safer; none remembered that the first camera or radio or airplane was not perfect and that only in time could a new invention be judged. Had women called in a board of doctors to set up a clinic for period extraction in which the doctors would be the ones to do it, I am sure they would have responded differently. But they saw, quite correctly, that period extraction was developed precisely to give women autonomy over their own bodies and that it was inseparable from the concept of self-help.

Carol Downer's History-Bearing: Brushes with the Law

GENA COREA

Gena Corea, excerpt from *The Hidden Malpractice: How American Medicine Treats Women as Patients and Professionals,* New York: William Morrow, 1970. Reprinted by permission.

Women's efforts to gain control of their bodies have been unsuccessfully challenged in court. In September 1972, ten policemen and a detective in Los Angeles raided the Feminist Women's Health Center. It had been under surveillance for six months. The lawmen issued arrest warrants for Carol Downer, the originator of the self-help concept, and Colleen Wilson, a clinic worker. Wilson pleaded guilty to fitting a diaphragm. She was fined $250 and put on two years' probation. (Fitting a diaphragm, Downer believes, is like fitting a shoe, only one fits it to a different part of the body.)

Downer was charged with practicing medicine without a license. She had practiced medicine, the police alleged, by helping a woman insert a speculum, by observing a vaginal infection, and by helping to apply a home remedy—yogurt—to relieve the discomfort. (During the raid, the police tried to confiscate some yogurt as evidence but released it when a woman protested that it was her lunch.)

Downer went on trial on November 20, 1972, at the New Courthouse in Los Angeles. Money for the defense and telegrams of support poured in from women around the country. Feminist Robin Morgan, referring to the police, telegraphed, "If they think they can burn witches and midwives again, they will be taught a bitter lesson."

As the trial progressed, feminists publicly asked for a definition of medical practice. Was it giving an enema? Was it diagnosing measles? If you de-

cided yogurt might cure a cold or a sore and you put it in your mouth, would that be a crime? Then why did it suddenly become a crime when the yogurt was applied to the vagina? Is it a crime to tell a woman she has a sore on her lip? Then why is it a crime to tell her she has a sore—cervicitis—on her cervix? Is it criminal for a woman to look at her own vagina?

On December 5, after two days' deliberation, the jury found Downer not guilty.

"Women in California now have the right to examine their own and each other's bodies," feminist Deborah Rose commented, ". . . [It is] amazing to me that we have to win that right."

Women also had to win the right to give birth without a physician. In Santa Cruz, doctors had warned midwives at the Birth Center not to "catch" babies because that was practicing medicine without a license. The midwives ignored the warning, asserting that a woman delivers her own baby and has a right to do so wherever she wants.

On March 6, 1974, officials from the State Department of Consumer Affairs, the district attorney's office, the state police, and the sheriff's office raided and closed down the Birth Center. They arrested one midwife there and two others in a private home, charging them with the unlicensed practice of medicine.

At their arraignment, the midwives refused to plead either guilty or not guilty. They demurred, arguing that the charge made against them—attendance at a normal physiologic function—did not constitute a crime. In January 1976, the Federal Appeals Court in San Francisco agreed. It ruled that pregnancy and childbirth were not disease states and that the midwives, therefore, could not have been practicing medicine. The court recommended that the state dismiss the charges. The prosecution is appealing.

Today, the Santa Cruz midwives continue to "catch" babies.

In Florida, roles switched. The Tallahassee Feminist Women's Health Center sued physicians, charging them with harassing its staff.

The Center provides abortions for a thousand women each year at its Woman's Choice Clinic, charging from thirty to fifty dollars less than private physicians. The Center prospered until 1975 when it lost three doctors in four months as a result, it alleges, of intimidation by the medical community. The Center maintained local physicians harassed the clinic doctors by (among other tactics) questioning the "ethics" of any doctor who worked at a clinic that advertised. The feminists suspected that physicians simply disliked competition. On October 1, 1975, the Center filed suit against six local obstetrician-gynecologists and the executive director of the Florida Board of Medical Examiners, accusing them of violating the Sherman Antitrust Act by "conspiring to restrain trade and monopolize women's health care in Tallahassee."

As of this writing, the case has not been settled.

In April 1976, the Center learned that women's health groups around the country were being harassed by physicians. So it joined with seven other health groups to form WATCH (Women Acting To Combat Harassment). WATCH will help women's clinics finance and file antitrust suits.

Empowering the Pelvic Exam

LILA A. WALLIS

Lila A. Wallis, MD, with Marian Betancourt, excerpt from *The Whole Woman: Take Charge of Your Health in Every Phase of Your Life*, New York: Avon, 1999. Copyright © 1999 by Lila A. Wallis and Marian Betancourt.

Historically, pelvic exams were so unpleasant and hurtful that women avoided them at all costs, even if they had symptoms that needed to be checked. There is no reason for a painful pelvic exam—other then the physician's failure to learn how to make it painless.

Few women know that! They have hated the clinical invasion of their bodies, the sight and cold feel of a steel instrument (the speculum) entering that private space. In addition to the dis-

comfort and pain, women resented the frequently unfeeling, brusque, and condescending attitude of the doctor.

The women's health movement of the 1960s, 1970s, and 1980s exposed the patronizing attitudes of many physicians toward their female patients. The pelvic exam became a symbol of female subjugation and abuse. A call was issued for a more meaningful partnership between the physician and patient regarding her care and the examination of her reproductive organs. What follows are suggestions for women who desire more involvement in their gynecological care as well as freedom from the shame and secrecy historically attached to their own bodies.

The doctor should communicate with you as a partner in your care and let you know what will be happening during each step of the examination. The first pelvic examination for a young woman should include an explanation of the anatomy. Ask if there is a plastic model or detailed illustration of the anatomy available to make the instruction clear. This will give you a better idea of what the doctor is going to do during the examination. Hold the speculum in your hands and ask what part of the instrument actually goes into your vagina.

The doctor should ask you about you sexual experience as well, whether or not you are a virgin, if you have had sex, whether any part of it was painful, and if you used contraceptives. The doctor should ask if you have been performing breast self-exams or if you have noticed any changes in your vulva. This lets you know your doctor considers you a partner in your health care.

The physician's hands and instruments must be warm, and he or she should tell you before touching each part of your body. The caring physician should also offer you some choices about how you wish to proceed by asking you some questions.

➤ Do you want to be draped during the exam? The drape is used to avoid exposing your body and to create a sense of privacy. However, if you want to watch the examination or see with the aid of a mirror, then you would not have a drape.

➤ Would you like to watch? If you would, ask if your head can be elevated, the drape displaced. A mirror and lamp can be arranged so that you can see your own vulva, vagina, and cervix. This is the beginning of empowerment. It involves you in the process.

➤ Are you able to relax? It is impossible to be totally relaxed during a pelvic exam, but your physician can teach you some ways to relax your perineal and abdominal muscles. First tighten these muscles, as if you were interrupting urination, and then relax them several times before the instrument or doctor's fingers are inserted. Take deep breaths or a series of panting breaths to relax.

➤ Are you comfortable in the foot brackets? These can be shortened to allow your knees to bend. This helps you bear down when necessary, so the cervix moves closer to the vaginal opening. If you had a condition that made your movements difficult, such as arthritis, you should ask for the foot brackets to be lengthened. If you do not like putting your heel into the cold metal foot bracket, keep your socks and shoes on or ask for foam booties.

Above all, the examination should be gentle. No doctor would consider being brusque or squeezing hard on a man's testicles, so expect the same sensitivity from a physician who is palpating your ovaries and uterus.

WHAT THE PELVIC EXAM INCLUDES

A doctor performing a pelvic examination is following a certain procedure designed to provide information. There is usually a nurse present during the examination because assistance is sometimes needed. You always need to empty your bladder before a pelvic exam because a full bladder makes it difficult for the physician to feel the internal organs. There are five parts to the exam.

EXTERNAL GENITALIA First, the doctor will examine the vulva, clitoris, labia, and glandular ducts to look for anything out of the ordinary. After examining the external genitalia some doctors may wish to do a "mini pelvic," using one finger to identify the position and direction of the cervix for the speculum insertion.

SPECULUM EXAM The speculum is an instrument that is inserted into the vagina and pushes the walls of the vagina apart to allow light and other instruments to be inserted. The speculum should be warmed first by holding it under warm water. As long as they are cleaned and sterilized after each use they don't need to remain sterile; the vagina is not sterile. Some doctors use disposable plastic specula. These are thicker than the ones made of steel, and they make a loud click when they are opened or locked, which might frighten the patient.

A smaller, narrower speculum is used when a girl's hymen is still intact. If insertion is difficult, the doctor might teach the girl how to gently dilate her hymen and have her come back for the completion of the exam.

COLLECTIONS OF SPECIMENS

These specimens are taken for routine laboratory studies. While the speculum is inserted, the doctor can insert instruments such as cotton-tipped applicators, cervical brushes, and wooden scrapers and take scrapings and specimens of secretions from the cervix and vagina or endometrium for various tests, such as a Pap smear and sexually transmitted disease cultures.

BIMANUAL VAGINOABDOMINAL EXAM This means the doctor is using both hands, one inside your vagina and one outside your body, pressing on various locations on your abdomen. The uterus, ovaries, and tubes are located, and any abnormalities are detected. The uterine size might alert the doctor to the possibility of pregnancy, an irregular uterine outline, or to the possibility of fluids. The ovaries and tubes are usually small.

Often they are difficult to palpate either because a patient cannot relax her abdominal muscles, because she is overweight and a layer of fat interferes, or because she has intestinal bloating. In that case, a pelvic sonogram would be needed to visualize the ovaries.

BIMANUAL RECTOVAGINAL EXAM Here the doctor inserts his or her middle finger into the rectum and the index finger into the vagina while pressing with the other hand on the abdomen to recheck the findings of the bimanual vaginoabdominal exam. Ovaries are found in the back of the uterus so they are better palpated on the rectovaginal exam. Standard procedure for this examination is to check any fecal matter on the doctor's glove for blood, which could indicate the presence of ulcerative colitis, a bleeding peptic ulcer, polyps, colorectal cancer, hemorrhoids, or fissures and lacerations from rectal intercourse.

FORMULATION: DIALOGUE WITH THE DOCTOR

Once again, get fully dressed after the examination before you talk with the doctor. One woman told me her doctor discussed his findings with her for ten minutes while she sat naked and vulnerable, having just had a breast exam in the examination room.

Once you are dressed and back in your doctor's office, you will hear what the doctor has to say. I call this step "formulation." This is a summary of what has been found on examination. Your doctor should explain the working—or possible—diagnosis as well as other possibilities, and what additional tests might be needed to confirm the diagnosis. If the working diagnosis is correct, then expect a detailed explanation of recommended treatment.

Now is the time to ask some questions. Don't be embarrassed to ask the doctor to repeat things you missed, to define medical jargon, explain your procedures, draw clear pictures for you, or refer to medical diagrams and illustrations.

Listen carefully and take good notes or have your friend or relative take the notes. If medications are prescribed, write down instructions for their use. Ask about side effects and remind your doctor of other drugs you take, including oral contraceptives or hormone therapy, in case there is potential for additional side effects. Find out if a generic drug can be substituted. Some insurance plans will pay only for generic drugs. Some will pay for certain drugs. Often the newest or most expensive drugs are not included.

If the proposed plan of action interferes with your work schedule or other plans, ask the doctor to work out a more convenient timetable, as long as it does not endanger your health.

Find out when results of your blood and urine tests will be available, and ask that a copy be sent to you, or ask if you may call the doctor the next week and ask about the findings. Ask if you should call the doctor with a report of your condition— for better or worse—in a few days or weeks.

Before you go home, make a follow-up appointment if you need one. As soon as you get home, bring your Woman's Health Record up-to-date.

Once you find a competent, compassionate, considerate, and thorough physician, take good care of her or him. Even if you see this doctor only for yearly physical checkups, you are building a relationship of trust and mutual respect. Now you have the peace of mind of knowing you have someone to call if you are ill.

Self-Helpless Gynecology

CAEDMON MAGBOO CAHILL

In this exploratory paper Caedmon Magboo Cahill spoke to ten college-age women to understand how the women's health movement of the 1970s affected their attitudes growing up in the 1990s, toward the pelvic exam, and the role of the doctor.

The majority of women in this ethnography want to take control over their health and their bodies, yet surprisingly look toward the doctor's validation and expertise to gain this control and to feel normal and healthy. Since the vagina is hidden and therefore can not be compared as easily as hips or breasts—there is no cultural norm of what the vagina should look or feel like—instead young women turn to what the gynecologist has accepted as standard. . . .

Many of my informants feel that once they are at the recommended age for the exam, their reproductive organs are now in the domain of the medical authorities, and have difficulty learning the intricacies and details of their own body on their own. There is an understanding among these women that only through a mastery of women's genitalia, something medical professionals assume, can they then self-diagnose or determine what they feel is normal. The responsibility many of these women feel to "take care of themselves" by their yearly gynecological examination in part stems from this feeling that they are in possession of something far more medically important and medically complicated than to trust themselves. . . .

The women interviewed describe themselves as feeling vulnerable and often embarrassed during the exam; vulnerability they attribute to the doctor's presence, and embarrassment due to the exposure of their vagina. Many women expect this vulnerability and embarrassment and accept it as an inherent part of the exam, yet still feel safer under medical authority, rather than in their own hands.

Many women leave the exploration of their vagina up to the gynecologist entirely. Not only do they not feel comfortable deciding what feels normal or healthy, but they also do not feel comfortable learning about their vagina outside of the doctor's office. It is clear that women depend on the doctor to mediate the relationship between themselves and their pelvis. When asked whether they performed pelvic self-exams all of the women answered no. Most explain that they do not feel capable to perform the exam and some feel uncomfortable even looking into their vaginas. . . .

Visiting the gynecologist allows these women to feel as if they are taking care of themselves and "getting in touch with themselves." Many women, especially those who decided to have a pelvic exam before it is usually recommended, would rather make themselves physically and emotionally uncomfortable so that they may feel satisfied, knowing they are being healthy having a doctor examine them. Some even reserve for the doctor the first touch into their vagina, for the sake of "health" and feeling "normal."

Gynecology, for these young women, is used to sustain the separation between women and their genitalia, and having pelvic exams relieves them of the responsibility of understanding their bodies personally, by their own touch and exploration. What makes gynecology particularly susceptible to this is the fact that women do not yet feel comfortable to understand their genitalia with their own hands, and unlike aches of the stomach, throat, or head, they are reluctant to seek advice outside of the doctor's office either from their mothers or friends. Only when women reclaim themselves and feel a part of their genitalia is complementary gynecological attention most effective. When the separation is diminished between themselves and their reproductive organs during the exam itself and then outside of the exam as well, young women can begin to care for and appreciate their bodies, not as reproductive machines but rather as extensions of themselves.

The Bridal Shower: We Haven't Come a Long Way, Baby

BETTY DODSON, PHD

Betty Dodson, PhD, excerpt from *Orgasms for Two: The Joy of Partnersex*, New York: Harmony Books, 2002.

The email asked if I would be available to give a sex lecture to a group of women at a bridal shower who were all in their twenties. Immediately I thought, "What a great idea." Kitty, the young woman who contacted me, said they considered having a male stripper at first, but that had been done so often. She and her girlfriend Brenda wanted something different. They both decided that having me would be fun as well as informative. Their offer came through my website, so neither one knew anything about me except the opening statement that ended with the sentence: "Join me for an honest, intelligent, and fun-loving exchange of ideas and images about my favorite subject, SEX."

As we talked, I proposed bringing a few sex toys that would enhance women's orgasms alone and with partnersex. I'd also bring some drawings of the female genitals with diagrams of the inner structure, and a dildo to demonstrate how to give a good blowjob. Kitty was thrilled with my proposal. We agreed on an hourly fee and I said the chances were pretty good it would last for three hours.

On Saturday, June 1, 2001, at 8:00 PM, I showed up at an East Side apartment with my bag of goodies. The room was filled with about twenty or so women who were all young, well-dressed, attractive New York professionals. There is nothing I like better than interacting with younger men and women to find out what they are thinking about in the new millennium. My first assumption was that these Generation Xers would be fairly sexually sophisticated, especially living in New York City.

My opening remark—"Your oversexed grand-mother has arrived"—elicited only a few smiles. The rest of them weren't sure how to respond. After all, older women with white hair weren't supposed to be having sex. Kitty, the bright-eyed hostess, bubbled with enthusiasm as she welcomed me and introduced me to the other women. She showed me to a comfortable chair with a small end table in front of it.

As I placed the Magic Wand vibrator, a small battery-operated vibrator, and my Vaginal Barbell on the table, I began by asking if they were all proficient masturbators. There was an outburst of hysterical laughter and no show of hands. Maybe they were laughing at the size of the electric vibrator, so I quickly explained it was meant to vibrate our sweet little clits. More laughter, but I didn't stop. The best way to use a vibrator for masturbation was with a folded washcloth. When they used it with a partner, I recommended putting a washcloth over the top and holding it in place with a rubber band from a bunch of broccoli. They screamed with laughter.

Looking around the room, I realized only a few women were able to make eye contact with me. The future bride kept her gaze intently on the floor. Others were whispering in private conversations with the woman sitting next to them.

Finally Kitty asked why guys always wanted to watch their girlfriends masturbate? Why would she want to do herself when she had a boyfriend? After all, getting her off was his job, not hers. After lightheartedly accusing her of being a "do me, do me" girl, I said maybe men wanted to see how their girlfriends handled their clits so they'd learn something. The same was true for men. A woman could ask her boyfriend to do himself so she would know what he liked. Sharing masturbation was a great way to learn about each other's sexual response. Besides, it's very hot for a couple to watch each other!

Again the room filled with more howls of laughter. At that point I knew it was going to take a while to break through the embarrassment, so I became a bawdy comedian, letting them laugh themselves silly. I dived into the pond of heterosexual romantic love, acutely aware of the absence of sexual knowledge that fills it.

Moving ever upward and onward, I passed out Betty's Barbell, a resistance device that I'd designed and manufactured to work the vaginal muscles. It was made of stainless steel and doubled as a fabulous dildo. After a few women felt the weight of it, someone finally asked why it was so heavy. That's when I explained that the weight kept it from shooting out of the vagina while a woman tightens her pubococcygeus (PC) muscle. After talking about how to locate the muscle, I said that all women would benefit from doing the exercise with the Barbell in place while using some form of stimulation on the clitoris.

Looking at the two pregnant women in the room, I told them their doctors would tell them to do Kegel exercises after giving birth. Actually, a well-toned pelvic floor muscle makes having a baby easier as well as improves a woman's orgasm. One expectant mother said she was already doing her Kegels.

Next I asked if they had all examined their pussies in a mirror with a bright light while using both hands to explore inside and out. Looks of embarrassment combined with more nervous laughter. A few shook their heads. Kitty said several of them had gone to get pussy trims at a salon on 57th Street that she had recommended. They were all perfectly willing to discuss whether they had a bikini wax or they were completely nude, but when I asked if they'd seen their clitorises or knew what type of inner lips they had, no one had any idea. One woman asked, "What are inner lips?"

Out came my book. I opened it up to the pages with the vulva drawings and passed it around. Then I explained how our sex organs are like our faces, with different shapes of noses, eyes, and mouths. Every pussy is as unique as our fingerprints—a significant revelation. When I talked about different genital styles like Classical, Baroque, Renaissance, and Art Deco, several wanted to know which styles guys liked the best. I said the ones that had a hole for penetration. This time I joined in the laughter that was becoming more genuine than nervous.

Brenda, who was sitting to my left, wanted to know why it was so difficult to come during intercourse. Perfect question. I asked the group how many of them could have orgasms from fucking only. A sprinkling of hands rose, including Kitty's. When I asked her what position she used, I halfway expected her to say woman on top. Instead she said missionary position. Then I asked if she was

aware of what was getting her off while they were fucking? Her explanation was clear that it was a grinding motion when she and her boyfriend pressed up against each other's bodies. The next question was whether she thought she was getting indirect clitoral stimulation. She had no idea.

A great segue into my well-loved clitoral rap. How the clitoris is a woman's primary sex organ, with eight thousand nerve endings, and the vagina is the birth canal. Although sisters Jennifer and Laura Berman state in their book *For Women Only* that 80 percent of women do not orgasm from intercourse alone, I suspected the number was closer to ninety percent if we factored in all the women faking orgasm. While a wet pussy provides ideal direct stimulation for a penis, a woman also needs some form of direct stimulation from her boyfriend's fingers or tongue, or her fingers. If she was accustomed to using a vibrator, she could also use it during intercourse.

One of the women asked if maybe that was why she could only have an orgasm with oral sex. Several nodded in agreement. One woman asked when I was going to demonstrate how to do oral sex on a man, and several others nodded in agreement. We had just started discussing female sexual pleasure and already they wanted to know how to please a man. The female role is connected to such ancient programming that it must be encoded in our cellular structure: How can I please him so he'll kill a wooley mammoth and bring it back to the cave to feed the children and me?

Reaching into my bag, I pulled out a Cyberskin realistic dildo with a suction cup on the bottom. Licking the base, I stuck it onto the small end table in front of me. Everyone in the room gasped at the full eight inches of dick except for one woman who said it looked just like her boyfriend's penis. Then I explained that the average-sized penis was around five and a half to six inches erect. The standard is always "bigger is better" when dildos are manufactured or men are cast in X-rated videos. Yet if the truth were known, most women prefer an average-sized penis. It's a shame that so many men are obsessed with penis size, believing their dicks are too small or somehow inadequate. Too bad more men don't realize how few women can orgasm from a penis anyway.

At that point, a woman who had been continuously turning red, gasping, and covering her face finally spoke up. She admitted how embarrassed she'd been in the beginning, but now she wanted to thank me. In the last hour she'd learned more about sex than she had during her entire lifetime. Then she admitted that at twenty-eight she'd never had an orgasm. I assured her she was not alone and advised her to start masturbating so she could learn about her sexuality. Then a woman named Carol joined in, saying she'd never had an orgasm with a partner but she could give herself one. These are magic moments of freeing oneself with the truth. I recommended they both go to my website and get all the necessary information on how to proceed.

My cocksucking demo started with the information that every man is different, just like every woman. A smart lover asks what his or her partner likes. Some men prefer a very light stroke while others want a firm grip. It all depends on how he masturbates. As I spoke, I covered my hands with massage oil and started demonstrating different hand strokes. The laughter and voices talking all at once were causing quite a din in the room. Even I had to admit that watching a grandmother doing a dick with style was pretty outrageous. Yet I also knew I was a well-needed reminder that sex doesn't end for every woman after she turns fifty, sixty, or seventy.

Next Brenda asked what female ejaculation was all about. No longer making assumptions, I asked if anyone had read *The G-Spot*. None of them had even heard of it. Kitty said she'd read in a woman's magazine, *Glamour* or *Cosmo*, that female ejaculation was definitely not urine. It was more like the fluid that came from a man's prostate gland.

Most young women today are getting their sex misinformation from women's magazines, in articles written by young, sexually inexperienced writers who get their information from experts who are basically talking about what they have read in books or tested with a PhD thesis that relied on a questionnaire. As one of those sex experts, I am constantly being misunderstood and misquoted in magazine articles. Is it any wonder that sexual myths and outdated information is so rampant?

Getting out the diagrams from *A New View of a Woman's Body*, I showed them the internal structure of the clitoris and the drawing that showed a model's finger inside her vagina pressing up on the ceiling into the urethral sponge. The sponge protected the urinary tract from getting irritated from the friction of a penis moving in and out of the vagina. Inside the sponge is a small paraurethral gland, which led some to speculate that's where the fluid came from. It had been established that the fluid exits the urethra, not the vagina. One study in which female ejaculators were catheterized concluded the fluid was dilute urine and it came from the bladder.

The whole room went crazy over the thought that female ejaculation might be urine. That was disgusting! However, when they thought it was prostatic fluid similar to male ejaculate, it was desirable because it demonstrated that a woman's level of sexual arousal was so high that it made her "come" like a man. That's why "female ejaculators" repeatedly state, "It doesn't smell or taste like urine." The idea of enjoying urinating during sex was a filthy, dirty, nasty idea, while ejaculation sounded sexy.

We took a break to refill our drinks while Kitty served cake. Ellen, the bride to be, began opening all her presents. It was the usual fare, with sexy lingerie, a few gag gifts, a couple of feather boas, and a book for her wedding photos. I told her she could choose any of the toys I'd brought as a wedding present from me. She chose the Cyberskin dildo. When I asked if she intended to fuck her husband on their wedding night, we all broke up laughing, including Ellen, and we made good eye contact for the first time. Later on, she changed her mind and decided to take the small battery vibrator instead. Of course, I thought that there was a much better choice. I told her clitoral stimulation rather than vaginal penetration takes most of us a lot farther, sexually speaking. Best of all is the combination of both.

Out of curiosity, I asked the women what the favorite kind of birth control was these days. There were only two—the pill and condoms. Several of the women who were living with their boyfriends were still using condoms. They had no idea they were missing the exquisite sensation of a bare penis moving inside a slippery vagina, but what you haven't experienced you can't miss. I told them that as a sex educator, I was dedicated to safe sex, but believe me, if I had a choice, condoms would be at the bottom of my list. The pill fucks around with our hormones, so I'd use a diaphragm and agree to be fluid-bonded. The diaphragm was now a birth control fossil and no one knew the term "fluid-bonded."

My explanation was that any woman on the pill, using a diaphragm, or who was post-menopausal made an agreement with her partner not to exchange any bodily fluids (especially semen) with another person. If either of them ever had sex outside their pairbond, they promised to always use a condom. I emphasized that this arrangement required total trust and honesty. These young women saw monogamy as a fact of life, so the possibility that either they or their boyfriend might want to have sex outside the relationship didn't exist.

Looking back, I remember feeling exactly the same way when I was in my twenties, but neither I nor my partner was ever totally successful at being faithful. Cheating was an excuse to break up to find a new, more exciting lover.

After saying good-bye with hugs and kisses, I walked home thinking about how these women's lives were different from mine at the same age. In the fifties as well as the sixties, a woman had to choose between having a career and raising a family. During the seventies and eighties, women were told they could have it all, which meant holding down two full-time jobs—a career and motherhood. The "have it all" generation waited until they were well into their thirties to have babies.

Another thing different from my generation was that many of us married our high school sweethearts because serial monogamy wasn't an option. When I moved to New York City at twenty, everyone back home assumed I would end up a prostitute if I didn't get married the first year. Back in the fifties, any woman who had more than one or two sex partners was considered a whore, and living with a man before marriage was living in sin. The married women at the party had all lived with their boyfriends before they made it official, and several of the single women were currently living with their boyfriends. That was one of the big differences.

However, many of the old sexual myths prevailed—women having their orgasms from penis/vagina sex, men keeping their promises to be monogamous, and living happily ever after in marital bliss. Although these women were all computer literate and they lived in one of the most sophisticated cities in the world, traditional romance, love, and marriage was still everyone's favorite sexual fantasy.

In other words, we haven't come a long way, baby. Our so-called new information age wasn't getting through on the sexual level. Each new generation still has to rediscover the wheel all over again. We wonder why there is so much violence in America, yet so few have the courage to embrace its opposite—sexual pleasure.

CHAPTER 14

Mind and Body

PSYCHOLOGY AND WOMEN

IN THE PAST CENTURY, science has shown what women have known for a long time: when it comes to health, the mental has a huge impact on the physical. In her landmark 1891 story "The Yellow Wallpaper," Charlotte Perkins Gilman wrote passionately about the way doctors used psychological manipulation to create illness in women. Penning the story shortly after suffering her own severe depression, Gilman told the story of a woman confined to her bedroom by her physician husband for depression and a "hysterical tendency." Slowly, the heroine becomes less able to deal with a world that has literally gotten unbearably small. Breaking down, she unleashes her pent-up anger and frustration on the walls of her confinement, ripping the paper from the room in which she has been a prisoner. The story was a critique of how medicine deals with women's mental health, and it was understood that way. Immediately it garnered censoring criticism from a prominent Boston doctor who claimed that no responsible person would have written such a story. Gilman argued that the piece was literature—the truth embellished to a narrative end. Still, she argued, there was enough truth that she sent a copy to the doctor who had failed her during her own depression, and she considered one of the greatest accomplishments of the tale to be the admittances of physicians that it led them to change their treatment methods.

By the second half of the twentieth century, women were still fighting many of the same battles, being mistreated, over-treated, and dismissed by the psychiatric and medical establishments. Old models of the female psyche and personality were swiftly and irrevocably overthrown during a nine-year period starting in 1968, when Naomi Weisstein first presented her paper "Kinder, Kuche, Kirche as Scientific Law," or "Psychology Constructs the Female."

Naomi Weisstein, an experimental psychologist and founding mother of the women's liberation movement, was teaching in Chicago at Loyola in the 1960s when she got involved politically with Shulamith Firestone and other young radicals. After graduating Phi Beta Kappa from Wellesley and ranking first in her class when she received her PhD from Harvard, Naomi was humiliated—and her consciousness raised through the roof—by her treatment at job interviews. "How can a little girl like you teach a great big class of men?" was one question that she was asked. Sigmund Freud's belief that women are morally inferior to men also infuriated Naomi—especially his claim that because she lacks a penis, a woman possesses an inadequate sense of justice, a predisposition to envy, weaker social interests, and a lesser capacity for sublimation. Weisstein also critiqued the popular theories of Erik Erikson and Bruno Bettelheim. Her audience at the University of California at Davis, where she first presented her findings in 1968, was electrified when she proclaimed, "Psychology has nothing to say about what women are really like, because psychology does not know." This was followed by the publication of Phyllis Chesler's landmark book *Women and Madness* in 1972, which documented the mechanism through which sexism creates mental illness, and forever changed the ways that we understand women's minds. The publication of Jean Baker Miller's *Toward a New Psychology of Women* in 1977 punctuated this revolutionary period.

Today feminist authors struggle with new issues and problems. Several writers, notably Chesler and the young author Leora Tanenbaum, have explored female aggression and the ways that women use psychology to control and intimidate each other. The rising popularity of psychiatric drugs has created new questions about the fine line between individuality and illness and opened up fields of inquiry that can be approached in distinctly feminist terms. Although statistically women suffer from depression at higher rates than men, the marketing of antidepressants in gendered terms—and without sufficient medical reason—has again raised the way we treat depression as a women's issue.

Psychology Constructs the Female

NAOMI WEISSTEIN

Naomi Weisstein, adapted from "Kinde, Kuche, Kirche as Scientific Law," *Women* 1(1): 15–20, 1970. Reprinted by permission.

It is an implicit assumption that the area of psychology that concerns itself with personality has the onerous but necessary task of describing the limits of human possibility. Thus, when we are about to consider the liberation of women, we naturally look to psychology to tell us what "true" liberation would mean: what would give women the freedom to fulfill their own intrinsic natures.

The central argument of my paper is this. Psychology has nothing to say about what women are really like, what they need and what they want, essentially, because psychology does not know. I want to stress that this failure is not limited to women; rather, the kind of psychology which has addressed itself to how people act and who they are has failed to understand, in the first place, why people act the way they do, and certainly failed to understand what might make them act differently.

Psychologists have set about describing the true natures of women with an enthusiasm and absolute certainty that is rather disquieting. Bruno Bettelheim, of the University of Chicago, tells us that

> We must start with the realization that, as much as women want to be good scientists or engineers, they want first and foremost to be womanly companions of men and to be mothers.

Eric Erikson of Harvard University, upon noting that young women often ask whether they can "have an identity before they know whom they will marry, and for whom they will make a home," explains somewhat elegiacally that

> Much of a young woman's identity is already defined in her kind of attractiveness and

in the selectivity of her search for the man (or men) by whom she wishes to be sought. . . .

Some psychiatrists even see the acceptance of woman's role by women as a solution to societal problems. "Woman is nurturance," writes Joseph Rheingold, a psychiatrist at Harvard Medical School." Anatomy decrees the life of a woman. . . . When women grow up without dread of their biological functions and without subversion by feminist doctrine, and therefore enter upon motherhood with a sense of fulfillment and altruistic sentiment, we shall attain the goal of a good life and a secure world in which to live it."

These views from men of high prestige reflect a fairly general consensus: liberation for women will consist first in their attractiveness, so that second, they may obtain the kinds of homes, and the kinds of men, which will allow joyful altruism and nurturance.

What we will show is that there isn't the tiniest shred of evidence that these fantasies of servitude and childish dependence have anything to do with women's true potential; that the idea of the nature of human possibility, which rests on the accidents of individual development of genitalia, on what is possible today because of what happened yesterday, on the fundamentalist myth of sex organ causality, has strangled and deflected psychology so that it is relatively useless in describing, explaining, or predicting humans and their behavior.

It then goes without saying that present psychology is less than worthless in contributing to a vision that could truly liberate—men as well as women.

The kind of psychology which has addressed itself to these questions is in large part clinical psychology and psychiatry, which in America means endless commentary on and refinement of Freudian theory. Here, the causes of failure are obvious and appalling: Freudians and neo-Freudians, and clinicians and psychiatrists in general, have simply refused to look at the evidence against their theory and practice and have used as evidence for their theory and their practice stuff so flimsy and transparently biased as to have absolutely no standing as empirical evidence.

If we inspect the literature of personality, it is immediately obvious that the bulk of it is written by clinicians and psychiatrists, and that the major support for their theories is "years of intensive clinical experience." This is a tradition started by Freud. His insights occurred during the course of his work with his patients.

In *The Sexual Enlightenment of Children* (1963), the classic document which is supposed to demonstrate empirically the existence of a castration complex and its connection to a phobia, Freud based his analysis on the reports of the father of the little boy, himself in therapy, and a devotee of Freudian theory. Now there is nothing wrong with such an approach to theory *formulation*; a person is free to make up theories with any inspiration that works: divine revelation, intensive clinical practice, a random numbers table. But he is not free to claim any validity for his theory until it has been tested and confirmed. Consider Freud. What he thought constituted evidence violated the most minimal conditions of scientific rigor.

It is remarkable that only recently has Freud's classic theory on the sexuality of women—the notion of the double orgasm—been actually tested physiologically and found just plain wrong. Now those who claim that fifty years of psychoanalytic experience constitute evidence enough of the essential truths of Freud's theory should ponder the robust health of the double orgasm. Did women, until Masters and Johnson, believe they were having two different kinds of orgasm? Did their psychiatrists cow them into reporting something that was not true? If so, were there other things they reported that were also not true? Did psychiatrists ever learn anything different than their theories had led them to believe? If clinical experience means anything at all, surely we should have been done with the double orgasm myth long before the Masters and Johnson studies.

Years of intensive clinical experience are not the same thing as empirical evidence.

It has been a central assumption for most psychologists of human personality that human behavior rests primarily on an individual and inner dynamic, perhaps fixed in infancy, perhaps fixed by genitalia, perhaps simply arranged in a rather immovable cognitive network. But this assumption is rapidly losing ground as personality psychologists fail again and again to get consistency in the assumed personalities of their subjects and as evidence collects that what a person does and who he believes himself to be will in general be a function of what people around him expect him to be, and what the overall situation in which he is acting implies that he is. Compared to the influence of the social context within which a person lives, his or her history and "traits," as well as biological makeup, may simply be random variations, "noise" superimposed on the true signal which can predict behavior.

I want to turn now to the second major point in my paper, which is that, even when psychological theory is constructed so that it may be tested, and rigorous standards of evidence are used, it has become increasingly clear that in order to understand why people do what they do, and certainly in order to change what people do, psychologists must turn away from the theory of the causal nature of the inner dynamic and look to the social context within which individuals live.

Before examining the relevance of this approach for the question of women, let me first sketch the groundwork for this assertion.

There is a series of social psychological experiments which points to the inescapable overwhelming effect of social context in an extremely vivid way. These are the obedience experiments of Stanley Milgram, concerned with the extent to which subjects in psychological experiments will obey the orders of unknown experimenters, even when these orders carry with them the distinct possibility that the subject is killing somebody.

Briefly, a subject is made to administer electric shocks in ascending 15-volt increments to another person whom the subject believes to be another subject but who is in fact a stooge. The voltages range from 15 to 450 volts; for each four consecutive

voltages, there are verbal descriptions such as "mild shock," "danger, severe shock," and finally, for the 435- and 450-volt switches, simply a red XXX marked over the switches. The stooge, as the voltage increases, begins to cry out against the pain; he then screams that he has a heart condition, begging the subject to stop, and finally, he goes limp and stops responding altogether at a certain voltage. Since even at this point, the subject is instructed to keep increasing the voltage, it is possible for the subjects to continue all the way up to the end switch—450 volts. The percentage of the subjects who do so is quite high; all in all, about 1,000 subjects were run, and about 65 percent go to the end switch in an average experiment. No tested individual differences between subjects predicted which of the subjects would continue to obey and which would break off the experiment. In addition, forty psychiatrists were asked to predict out of one hundred subjects, how many would go to the end and where subjects would break off the experiment. They were way below actual percentages, with an average prediction of 3 percent of the subjects obeying to the end switch. But even though psychiatrists have no idea how people are going to behave in this situation (despite one of the central facts of the twentieth century, which is that people have been made to kill enormous numbers of other people), and even though individual differences do not predict which subjects are going to obey and which are not, it is very easy to predict when subjects will be obedient and when they will be defiant. All the experimenter has to do is change the social situation. In a variant of the experiment, when two other stooges who were also administering electric shocks refused to continue, only 10 percent of the subjects continued to the end switch. This is critical for personality theory, for it says that the lawful behavior is the behavior that can be predicted from the social situation, not from the individual history.

To summarize: If subjects under quite innocuous and noncoercive social conditions can be made to kill other subjects and under other types of social conditions will positively refuse to do so; if subjects can react to a state of physiological fear by becoming euphoric because there is somebody else around who is euphoric or angry because there is somebody else around who is angry; if students become intelligent because teachers expect them to be intelligent and rats run mazes better because experimenters are told that the rats are bright, then it is obvious that a study of human behavior requires, first and foremost, a study of the social contexts within which people move, the expectations as to how they will behave, and the authority which tells them who they are and what they are supposed to do.

Two theories of the nature of women, which come not from psychiatric and clinical tradition, but from biology, can now be disposed of with little difficulty. The first argument notices social interaction in primate groups, and observes that females are submissive and passive. Putting aside for a moment the serious problem of experimenter bias (for instance, Harlow of the University of Wisconsin, after observing differences between male and female rhesus monkeys, quotes Lawrence Sterne to the effect that women are silly and trivial and concludes that "men and women have differed in the past and they will differ in the future"), the problem with the argument from primate groups is that the crucial experiment has not been performed. The crucial experiment would manipulate or change the social organization of these groups and watch the subsequent behavior. Until then, we must conclude that since primates are at present too stupid to change their social conditions by themselves, the "innateness" and fixedness of their behavior is simply not known. As applied to humans, the argument becomes patently irrelevant, since the most salient feature of human social organization is its variety; and there are a number of cultures where there is at least a rough equality between men and women. Thus, primate arguments tell us very little.

The second theory of sex differences argues that since females and males differ in their sex hormones, and sex hormones enter the brain, there must be innate differences in "nature." But the only thing this argument tells us is that there are differences in physiological state. The problem is whether these differences are at all relevant to behavior. Schacter and Singer have shown that a particular physiological state can itself lead to a multiplicity of felt emotional states and outward behavior, depending on the social situation.

In a review of the intellectual differences between little boys and little girls, Eleanor Maccoby has shown that there are no intellectual differences until about high school, or, if there are, girls are slightly ahead of boys. At high school, girls begin to do worse on a few intellectual tasks, such as arithmetic reasoning, and beyond high school, the achievement of women now measured in terms of productivity and accomplishment drops off even more rapidly. There are a number of other, nonintellectual tests which show sex differences; I choose the intellectual differences since it is seen clearly that women start becoming inferior. It is no use to talk about women being different but equal; all of the tests I can think of have a "good" outcome and a "bad" outcome. Women usually end up at the "bad" outcome. In light of social expectations about women, what is surprising is not that women end up where society expects they will; what is surprising is that little girls don't get the message that they are supposed to be stupid until high school; and what is even more remarkable is that some women resist this message even after high school, college, and graduate school.

In brief, the uselessness of present psychology with regard to women is simply a special case of the general conclusion: one must understand social expectations about women if one is going to characterize the behavior of women.

How are women characterized in our culture and in psychology? They are inconsistent, emotionally unstable, lacking in a strong conscience or superego, weaker, "nurturant" rather than productive, "intuitive" rather than intelligent, and, if they are at all "normal," suited to the home and the family.

In short, the list adds up to a typical minority group stereotype of inferiority: if they know their place, which is in the home, they are really quite lovable, happy, childlike, loving creatures.

My paper began with remarks on the task of discovering the limits of human potential. I don't know what immutable differences exist between men and women apart from differences in their genitals; perhaps there are some other unchangeable differences; probably there are a number of irrelevant differences. But it is clear that until social expectations for men and women are equal, until we provide equal respect for both men and women, our answers to this question will simply reflect our prejudices.

Demeter Revisited

PHYLLIS CHESLER

Phyllis Chesler, excerpt from *Women and Madness,* Garden City, New York: Doubleday, 1972. Reprinted by permission.

ZELDA FITZGERALD (1900-1943)
ELLEN WEST (C. 1890-C. 1923)
SYLVIA PLATH HUGHES (1932-1963)

All of these women were uncommonly stubborn, talented, and aggressive. All were hospitalized for various psychiatric "symptoms" which involved being socially withdrawn. They no longer cared how they "looked"; they refused to eat; they became sexually disinterested in their husbands. Ellen West and Sylvia Plath finally committed suicide when they were in their early thirties. Zelda Fitzgerald was burned to death in an asylum fire.

These women share a rather fatal allegiance to their own uniqueness, which in each case was at odds with "being a woman." For years, they denied themselves—or were denied—the duties and privileges of talent and conscience. Like many women, they buried their own destinies in romantically extravagant marriages, in motherhood, and in approved female pleasure. Their repressed energies eventually struggled free, however, demanding long-overdue, and therefore heavier, prices: marital and maternal "disloyalty," social ostracism, imprisonment, madness, and death. They attempted to escape their enforced half-lives by "going crazy." In asylums, where they were treated as "helpless" and "self-destructive" children, they were superficially freed from their female roles. However, neither madness nor mental asylums offered them asylum or freedom.

Writing of her asylum experience, Plath found few differences between "us in Belsize and the girls playing bridge and gossiping in the college to which I would return. Those girls, too, sat under bell jars of a sort."

Perhaps she was right. She speaks of the bell jar as a glass cage of "femininity" and powerlessness in which many women sit, in and out of asylums, and from which many are trying to escape.

Ellen West was struggling to escape. She was a wealthy, sensitive young married woman. As a girl, she had preferred "trousers" and "lively, boyish games" until she was sixteen. Her childhood motto was "Either Caesar or Nothing," and, in a poem written when she was seventeen, she expressed the desire "to be a soldier, fear no foe, and die joyously, sword in hand." She became an ardent horsewoman, a diarist, and a poet. After feverishly and competently performing a variety of approved female activities (doing volunteer work with children, taking noncredit university courses, engaging in serious love affairs), she developed a fear of eating—psychiatrically interpreted as a fear of becoming pregnant—and finally stopped eating altogether:

> Something in me rebels against becoming fat. Rebels against becoming healthy, getting plump red checks, becoming a simple, robust woman, as corresponds to my true nature. . . . For what purpose did nature give me health and ambition? . . . It is really sad that I must translate all this force and urge to action into unheard words [in her diary], instead of powerful deeds. . . . I am

twenty-one years old and am supposed to be silent and grin like a puppet.

Zelda Fitzgerald's "bell jar" was in many ways reinforced by her husband, writer Scott Fitzgerald, who was extremely jealous of and threatened by her considerable literary talent. He reacted with fury when Zelda completed an autobiographical novel before he had finished his own novel—a "story" of Zelda's life and psychiatric confinement. In a letter to one of her many male psychiatrists, Scott noted that:

> Possibly she [Zelda] would have been a genius if we had never met. In actuality she is now hurting me and through me hurting all of us. . . . [Zelda seems to think] that her work's success will give her some sort of divine irresponsibility backed by unlimited gold. It is still the idea of a high school girl who would like to be an author with an author's beautiful carefree life.

Nancy Milford, in her excellent biography, *Zelda*, reveals that Scott rather hysterically accused Zelda of being a "third-rate writer" and reminded her of his worldwide literary reputation. Milford notes that "Scott had some very fixed ideas of what a woman's place should be in a marriage," and quotes him in a conversation with Zelda:

> I would like you to think of my interests. That is your primary concern, because I am the one to steer the course, the pilot. . . . I want you to stop writing fiction.

Zelda says she does not want to be dependent on Scott, either financially or psychologically. Instead, she wants to be a "creative artist": she wants to work. Only if she does good work can she defend herself against Scott's "bad lies." Her male psychiatrist asks her whether being an outstanding woman writer would "compensate you for a life without Scott"; if that accomplishment "would mean enough to you when you were sixty?"

But Zelda is, in Milford's words, "sick of being beaten down, of being bullied into accepting Scott's ideas of everything. She would not stand it any longer; she would rather be in an institution." (And yet, once she was hospitalized, Zelda's psychiatrists, according to Milford, all try to "re-educate her in terms of her role as wife to Scott.")

Sylvia Plath grew up in Massachusetts and began writing poems and stories when she was very young. Her poems and her autobiographical novel, *The Bell Jar*, describe her battle as an artist with the female condition—a battle she did not necessarily see in feminist terms. Plath attempted suicide, was psychiatrically hospitalized, finished college, published her work, got married, moved to England, and became the mother of two children—all before she was thirty.

She was lonely and isolated. Her genius did not earn for her certain reprieves and comforts tendered the male artist. After separating from her husband, Plath continued to write and keep house for her children. On the night of February 10 or the morning of February 11, 1963, she killed herself.

Were these women really "crazy"? Are the women who continue to outnumber men in American psychiatric facilities at an increasing rate really "crazy"? And why are so many women seeking help, viewing themselves and being viewed as "neurotic" or "psychotic"?

There is a double standard of mental health—one for men, another for women—existing among most clinicians. According to a study by Dr. Inge K. Broverman, clinicians' concepts of healthy mature men do not differ significantly from their concepts of healthy mature adults. However, their concepts of healthy mature women do differ significantly from those for men and for adults. For a woman to be healthy, she must "adjust" to and accept the behavioral norms for her sex—passivity, acquiescence, self-sacrifice, and lack of ambition—even though these kinds of "loser" behaviors are generally regarded as socially undesirable (i.e., nonmasculine).

What we consider "madness," whether it appears in women or in men, is either the acting out of the devalued female role or the total or partial rejection of one's sex-role stereotype. When and if women who fully act out the female role (who are maternal, compassionate, self-sacrificing) are diagnosed or hospitalized, it is for "depression," "anxiety," and "paranoia." When women who reject the female role (who are angry, self-assertive, or sexually aggressive) are diagnosed or hospitalized, it is for "schizophrenia," "promiscuity," or "lesbianism." A woman who curses, or is competitive, violent, or successful, a woman who refuses to do housework is "crazy"—and "unnatural." A woman who cries all day, who talks to herself in low, frightened tones, or a woman who is insecure, timid, filled with self-contempt is a more "natural" woman—but she too is "crazy."

It is important to note that men, in general, are still able to reject more of their sex role without viewing themselves, or being viewed, as sick. Women are so conditioned to need and/or serve a man that they are willing to take care of a man who is "passive," "dependent," or "unemployed" than men are willing to relate to—much less take care of—a "dominant," "independent," or "self-centered" woman.

Researchers Barbara and Bruce Dohrenrend recently stated in "Social Status and Psychological Disorders" that men are really as "psychologically disturbed" as women are: "There is no greater magnitude of social stress impinging on one or the other sex. Rather [each sex] tends to learn a different style with which it reacts to whatever fact has produced the psychological disorder."

I would not so much disagree with this statement as qualify it in several important ways. Certainly, many men are severely "disturbed," but the form taken by their disturbance either is not seen as neurotic or is not treated by psychiatric incarceration. Men—especially white, wealthy, and older men—are permitted to act out many "disturbed" and many nondisturbed drives more easily than women can. American men who are young, poor, and/or black are frequently jailed as "criminals" rather than "psychotics" when they attempt to act out the male role fully.

Women are seeking help because they are really oppressed and unhappy—really confined to a very limited sphere—and because the female social role encourages help-seeking, self-blaming, and distress-reporting behavior. This does not mean that such behavior is either valued or treated with kindness by our culture. On the contrary, both husbands and clinicians experience and judge it as annoying, inconvenient, stubborn, childish, and tyrannical. Beyond a certain point of tolerance, such behavior is "managed." It is treated at first with disbelief and pity, then emotional distance, economic and sexual deprivation, drugs, shock therapy, and, finally, long-term psychiatric confinements.

Recent social trends also account for the fact that today more women are seeking psychiatric help and being hospitalized than at any other time in history. Traditionally, most women performed both the rites of madness and childbirth more invisibly—at home—where, despite their tears, depression, and hostility, they were still needed. This is less true today. While women live longer than ever before, and longer than men, there is less and less use for them in the only place they have been given—within the family. Many newly useless women are emerging more publicly and visibly into insanity and institutions.

The treatment of women in mental asylums—and private therapy—both reflects and perpetuates the sexism in our culture. At their best, mental asylums are special hotels or college-like dormitories for white and wealthy Americans, where temporary descent into "unreality" (or sobriety) is accorded the dignity of optimism, short internments, and a relatively earnest bedside manner.

At worst, mental asylums are bureaucratized families, with the same degradation and disenfranchisement of self that is experienced by the biologically owned female child. In the institution, howere, degradation takes place in the anonymous and therefore guiltless embrace of strange fathers and mothers. In general, therapy, privacy, and self-determination are either minimal or forbidden in psychiatric wards and state hospitals. Experimental or traditional medication, surgery, shock therapy and insulin treatment, isolation, physical and sexual violence, medical neglect, and slave labor are routinely practiced. Mental patients are somehow less human than either medical patients or criminals. They are, after all, "crazy"; they have been abandoned by (or have abandoned) dialogue with their own families. As such, they have no way—and no one—to tell about what is happening to them. They can, of course, tell their father-confessor figures: their doctors.

According to the 1960 and 1970 membership figures of the American Psychiatric Association, 90 percent of all psychiatrists in America are men. These male psychiatrists and clinicians often repeat in treatment the authoritarian role women are taught to respond to in the family situation.

The mental asylum—and private therapy—are mirrors of the female experience in the family. This is probably one of the reasons why Erving Goffman in *Asylums* considered psychiatric hospitalization to be more destructive of self than criminal incarceration. Like most people, he was primarily thinking of the debilitating effect—on a man—of being treated like a woman (as helpless, dependent, sexless, unreasonable—as "crazy"). But what about the effect of being treated like a woman when you *are* a woman? And perhaps a woman who is already ambivalent or angry about just such treatment?

Those women who are more ambivalent about or rejecting of the female role are often eager to be punished for such dangerous boldness in order to be saved from its ultimate consequences—the complete ostracism by society. Many mental asylum procedures do threaten, punish, or misunderstand such women, thereby coercing them into real or wily submission. Some of these women react to such punishment (or to a dependency-producing environment) with increased levels of anger and sex-role alienation. If such anger or aggressiveness persists, the women are isolated, straitjacketed, sedated, or given shock treatment.

One study by four male professionals published in 1969 in the *Journal of Nervous and Mental Diseases* described their attempt to reduce the aggressive behavior of a thirty-one-year-old schizophrenic woman by shocking her with a cattle prod "whenever she made accusations of being persecuted and abused; made verbal threats; or committed aggressive acts." They labeled their treatment a "punishment program" and noted that the "procedure was administered against the expressed will of the patient."

In addition, asylum life resembles traditional family treatment of the female adolescent in its official imposition of celibacy and its institutional responses to sexuality and aggression—fear, scorn, and punishment. Traditionally, all mental hospital wards are sex-segregated. Homosexuality, lesbianism, and masturbation are discouraged or forcibly interrupted. The heterosexual dances initiated in the late 1950s and 1960s were like high school proms, replete with chaperones, curfews, and frustration.

The effect of sexual repression and the shameful return to childhood are probably different for female than for male patients. Women already may have been bitterly, totally repressed sexually. Many, by "going mad," may be reacting to or trying to escape from such repression and the powerlessness it signifies. Male patients, on the other hand, may be "going mad" to escape the opposite pressure, the demands of compulsive and aggressive heterosexuality. Thus, the absence of opportunity for sexual expression is perhaps not as psychologically or physiologically devastating for men confined in institutions as it is for women.

In asylums, female patients, like female children, are closely supervised by other women (nurses, attendants), who, like mothers, are relatively powerless in terms of the hospital hierarchy and who, like mothers, don't really "like" their (wayward) daughters. Such supervision, however, does not protect the female as patient-child from rape, prostitution, pregnancy, and the blame for all three, any more than similar motherly supervision protects the female as female-child in the real world, either within or outside the family. From 1968 to 1970, there were numerous newspaper accounts of the prostitution, rape, and impregnation of female mental patients by male inmates at various psychiatric institutions. And, generally, the women must "bear the consequences"—enforced maternity—even though their "madness" may be due to just such pressures. A study published in 1968 in the *American Journal of Orthopsychiatry* documented a 366 percent increase in the recorded pregnancy and delivery rate among psychiatrically hospitalized women in Michigan state hospitals from 1936 to 1964. Sixty percent of the mental asylums in this study did not and/or would not prescribe contraceptives or perform abortions.

Behind such statistics are the misunderstood women themselves. I interviewed twenty-four of them, ranging in age from nineteen to sixty-five, who had been psychiatrically hospitalized at some time between 1950 and 1970. Twelve clearly reported exhibiting opposite-sex traits such as anger, cursing, aggressiveness, sexual love of women, increased sexuality in general, and a refusal to perform domestic and emotional-compassionate services. Four of these twelve also experienced "visions." The other twelve women reported a predominance of female-like traits such as depressions, suicidal attempts, fearfulness, and helplessness.

Some of these women had committed themselves voluntarily: their lives seemed hopeless, there was no alternative, and their parents or husbands insisted it would be "better" for them if they "cooperated" from the start. But most were committed wholly against their will, through physical force, trickery, or in a state of coma following an unsuccessful suicide attempt:

Carmen: "I was so sad [after my daughter's birth] and so tired. I couldn't take care of the house right anymore. My husband told me a maid would be better than me, that I was crazy . . . he took me to the hospital for what they called observation . . ."

Barbara: "My mother had me put away when I was 13. She couldn't control me. My father had left us; my mother was drinking and crying all the time. I kept running away from bad foster homes, and so she finally committed me to an institution. . . ."

All of the women received massive dosages of such tranquilizers as Thorazine, Stelazine, Mellaril, and Librium, and many received shock therapy and/or insulin coma therapy as a matter of routine, and often before they were psychiatrically interviewed:

Laura: "The first thing they did was give everyone shock treatment. It didn't matter who you were. You walked in and they gave you shock three times a week. . . . I was scared to death. I thought I was going to die. . . ."

Many of the women were physically beaten. Their requests for contact with the outside world were denied. Their letters were censored or not mailed. Legitimate medical complaints generally went untreated or were brushed aside as forms of "attention getting" or "revenge."

Barbara: "I got beat up lots of times. Then I learned the ropes, and they put me in charge of beating up the younger children if they got out of line . . . they were beating up five- and six-year-olds. If I complained about it, they'd do the same to me. . . ."

Those women remanded to state asylums were involved in sex-typed forced labor. They worked as unpaid domestics, laundresses, ward aides, cooks, and commissary saleswomen. If they accepted these jobs, and performed them well, the hospital staff was often reluctant to let them go. If they refused these jobs, they were considered "crazy" and "uncooperative" and punished with drugs, shock treatments, beatings, mockery, and longer hospital stays.

Susan: "I refused to peel potatoes in the kitchen. So they threw me in solitary for a few days."

Priscilla: "When I refused to mop up the ward and put the chronics' shit in the little coffee cans for them, they [the attendants] ganged up on me. They put a sheet over me, threw me down to the floor, and began punching and kicking me."

Only a few of these women received any psychotherapeutic attention. Therapy groups (and therapists) either interpreted their requests for information or release psychodynamically or counseled them to become more feminine and "cooperative."

Only two of the women had any awareness of their legal rights, and of course, both were defeated in court battles and "punished" by further psychiatric incarceration. Only one of the women did not consider herself crazy. Most of the women were humiliated, confused, fatalistic, or naïve about their hospitalization and about the reasons for it. Most dealt with the brutality by (verbally) minimizing it and blaming themselves. They were "sick"—weren't they?

Lucy: "Whenever I'd question something they'd done, criticize them, especially about how they treated some of the other patients, they'd yell at me and lock me in solitude. I'd get emotional and excited, I'm sick like that . . . They're not explicit about what's expected, but you find yourself locked up if you say too many things too loud that they don't like . . . I was sick, no question about it."

Why do these women think they are "sick"? *Are* they "sick"? Or are they just sick and tired of being powerless, of feeling hopelessly trapped in a Cinderella's slipper, a doll's house, or under a "bell jar"?

Dominants

JEAN BAKER MILLER

Jean Baker Miller, excerpt from *Toward a New Psychology of Women*, London: Penguin, 1986. Originally published in 1977 by Beacon Press. Reprinted by permission.

Once a group is defined as inferior, the superiors tend to label it as defective or substandard in various ways. These labels accrete rapidly. Thus, blacks are described as less intelligent than whites, women are supposed to be ruled by emotion, and so on. In addition, the actions and words of the dominant group tend to be destructive of the subordinates. All historical evidence confirms this tendency. And, although they are much less obvious, there are destructive effects on the dominants as well. The latter are of a different order and are much more difficult to recognize.

Dominant groups usually define one or more acceptable roles for the subordinate. Acceptable roles typically involve providing services that no dominant group wants to perform for itself (for example, cleaning up the dominant's waste products). Functions that a dominant group prefers to perform, on the other hand, are carefully guarded and closed to subordinates. Out of the total range of human possibilities, the activities most highly valued in any particular culture will tend to be enclosed within the domain of the dominant group; less valued functions are relegated to the subordinates.

Subordinates are usually said to be unable to perform the preferred roles. Their incapacities are ascribed to innate defects or deficiencies of mind or body, therefore immutable and impossible of change or development. It becomes difficult for dominants even to imagine that subordinates are capable of performing the preferred activities. More importantly, subordinates themselves can come to find it difficult to believe in their own ability. The myth of their inability to fulfill wider or more valued roles is challenged only when a drastic event disrupts the usual arrangements. Such disruptions usually arise from outside the relationship itself. For instance, in the emergency situation of World War II, "incompetent" women suddenly "manned" the factories with great skill.

It follows that subordinates are described in terms of, and encouraged to develop, personal psychological characteristics that are pleasing to the dominant group. These characteristics form a certain familiar cluster: submissiveness, passivity, docility, dependency, lack of initiative, inability to act, to decide, to think, and the like. In general, this cluster includes qualities more characteristic of children than adults—immaturity, weakness, and helplessness. If subordinates adopt these characteristics, they are considered well adjusted.

However, when subordinates show the potential for, or even more dangerously have developed other characteristics—let us say intelligence, initiative, assertiveness—there is usually no room available within the dominant framework for acknowledgment of these characteristics. Such people will be defined as at least unusual, if not definitely abnormal. There will be no opportunities for the direct application of their abilities within the social arrangements. (How many women have pretended to be dumb!)

Dominant groups usually impede the development of subordinates and block their freedom of expression and action. They also tend to militate against stirrings of greater rationality or greater humanity in their own members. It was not too long ago that "nigger lover" was a common appellation, and even now men who "allow their women" more than the usual scope are subject to ridicule in many circles.

A dominant group, inevitably, has the greatest influence in determining a culture's overall outlook—its philosophy, morality, social theory, and even its science. The dominant group, thus, legitimizes the unequal relationship and incorporates it into society's guiding concepts. The social outlook, then, obscures the true nature of this relationship—that is, the very existence of inequality. The culture explains the events that take place in terms of other premises that are inevitably false, such as racial or sexual inferiority. While in recent years we have learned about many such falsities on the larger social level, a full analysis of the psychological implications still remains to be developed. In the case of women, for example, despite overwhelming evidence to the contrary, the notion persists that women are meant to be passive, submissive, docile, secondary. From this premise, the outcome of therapy and encounters with psychology and other "sciences" are often determined.

Inevitably, the dominant group is a model for "normal human relationships." It then becomes "normal" to treat others destructively and to derogate them, to obscure the truth of what you are doing, by creating false explanations, and to oppose actions toward equality. In short, if one's identification is with the dominant group, it is "normal" to continue in this pattern. Even though most of us do not like to think of ourselves as either believing in or engaging in such domination, it is, in fact, difficult for a member of a dominant group to do otherwise. But to keep on doing these things, one need only behave "normally."

It follows from this that dominant groups generally do not like to be told about or even quietly reminded of the existence of inequality. "Normally" they can avoid awareness because their explanation of the relationship becomes so well integrated *in other terms*; they can even believe that both they and the subordinate group share the same interests and, to some extent, a common experience. If pressed a bit, the familiar rationalizations are offered: the home is "women's natural place," and we know "what's best for them anyhow."

Dominants prefer to avoid conflict—open conflict that might call into question the whole situation. This is particularly and tragically so, when many members of the dominant group are not having an easy time of it themselves. Members of a dominant group, or at least some segments of it, such as white working-class men (who are themselves also subordinates), often feel unsure of their own narrow toehold on the material and psychological bounties they believe they desperately need. What dominant groups usually cannot act on, or even see, is that the situation of inequality in fact deprives them, particularly on the psychological level.

Clearly, inequality has created a state of conflict. Yet dominant groups will tend to suppress conflict. They will see any questioning of the "normal" situation as threatening; activities by subordinates in this direction will be perceived with alarm. Dominants are usually convinced that the way things are is right and good, not only for them but especially for the subordinates. All morality confirms this view, and all social structure sustains it.

It is perhaps unnecessary to add that the dominant group usually holds all of the open power and authority and determines the ways in which power may be acceptably used.

Mental Patients' Political Action Committee

ELLEN FRANKFORT

Ellen Frankfort, excerpt from *Vaginal Politics*, New York: Quadrangle Books, 1972. Reprinted by permission.

The boutiquing of America. Somebody ought to write a book. No sooner does a major political event happen than Bloomingdale's sells it on the sixth floor.

In November 1971, the American Psychiatric Association did its boutiquing during its Seventh Biennial Divisional Meeting at the Hotel Biltmore in New York City. Throughout the weekend psychiatrists dropped by at Suite 1738 to "rap" with members of MP-PAC, the Mental Patients' Political Action Committee. Not only was there the thrill of crossing forbidden social barriers, but there also seemed to be a therapeutic component for the psychiatrists as one after another insisted that he, as an individual, was not guilty.

Outside the suite there was talk of a "newly formed coalition with America's *real* silent majority: mental patients." Strange talk for a group that excluded the former mental patients from panels, discussions, and cocktail parties, and even prevented them from obtaining official name cards. In fact, the boutique was there only because MP-PAC had gone to the trouble and expense of renting a suite; it had never been invited by the psychiatrists, who later were busy congratulating themselves on MP-PAC's presence.

MP-PAC is not a self-help group, a recovery group, or Schizophrenics Anonymous. MP-PAC is a group whose members have analyzed the mental patient's role from a political perspective and are dedicated to changing it. As they state in one of their papers, "In modern American society, two institutions of incarceration exist: the prison and the mental hospital. . . . In their essentials, they are quite similar; both are enclosed fortresses in which are incarcerated individuals who have come into conflict with society. In both, the restraints of walls, bars, and locks are used to keep their victims imprisoned. The patient, however, has an additional restraint not imposed on the prisoner, the restraint of *words*. . . . *His* jailors are *doctors* and *nurses*, he is held in a *hospital*, all supposedly in order to *help* him. . . . The prisoner who tells his guards that he hates the institution and longs to leave is seen by them as expressing a normal human desire for freedom; the patient who tells his doctor the same thing only adds on to the length of his indeterminate sentence. The only way out of the mental hospital is to *appear* to cooperate with the semantic fiction while maintaining in the recesses of the mind the knowledge that it is fiction."

Propaganda from yet another activist group? Not quite. In December 1971, thirty-one staff members of the Ohio Hospital for the Criminally Insane were arraigned on charges brought by a grand jury. The charges included the beating of patients after they had been tied to doors or sedated, and sexual attacks on patients by attendants.

However much the psychiatrists wanted personal expiation, most weren't interested in real change. One, a psychiatrist from New York City's Fordham Hospital, wanted something—people with hospital experience willing to work without pay in an underfinanced, understaffed psychiatric ward . . . if they wouldn't upset the applecart, rock the boat, or cause any trouble.

"To the extent that injustice exists, I'm with you 100 percent," the psychiatrist said to MP-PAC.

"Then what are you doing about it?"

"I could ask you what you're doing about the war in Vietnam. When you tell me psychiatrists could be doing more, I'm with you 100 percent, as I said."

"Can we come speak to the patients in your hospital?"

"I told you that if you're a responsible, viable group with a constructive program."

"What does that mean?"

"That's for me to determine. When you live in an

apartment and someone rings the bell, you have to decide whether he can be trusted to be let in."

"Look, the man is scared. He's fucking scared. He won't even let a small group of former mental patients into his hospital."

"Do you let anyone into your apartment?"

"If you're holding people hostage, it's not an apartment."

"You know, if you people were up on trends and directions in psychiatry, you'd know about patient meetings, governing boards . . ."

"We *do* know about them. We've all been part of your meetings and your governing boards. Don't you understand?"

"Are you saying you want to work cooperatively or you want to bash my head in?"

Clearly the man was scared. MP-PAC was not exotica, a boutique, radical chic, or whatever you name it (and the naming is part of the boutiquing). MP-PAC members turned out to know more about what it's like to be a mental patient and what's wrong with mental hospitals than anyone else present. As the psychiatrist began to perceive that, he became concerned. You could almost see the visions of Attica racing through his head.

After three hours of polite dialogue with members of MP-PAC, the psychiatrist said he was not convinced that the group was "viable," that it wouldn't turn into another "fly-by-night affair," or that it wouldn't resort to "rantings and ravings once allowed inside." (All this from a man who decides in fifty minutes whether a stranger is to be committed to an asylum and stripped of all his rights, possibly for life.)

"But I want you to know, in principle I'm 100 percent sympathetic," the psychiatrist said as he got up to leave.

"How can you say that?"

"Why?"

"You don't even trust us to enter your hospital. Let's be honest at least."

"Look," he said, lifting the cuffs of his trousers. "See these? I'm a psychiatrist who wears boots." And then he, his wife, and his colleague's wife all

returned to the convention, officially entitled "Psychiatry: Explosion and Survival."

An Interview with Jules Masserman

KATHRYN WATTERSON

Kathryn Watterson, excerpt from "Afterword: An Interview with Jules Masserman," *You Must Be Dreaming*, Poseidon Press, 1992. Reprinted by permission.

You Must Be Dreaming *sent shock waves through the professional psychiatric community. Kathryn Watterson tells the story of coauthor and singer Barbara Noël, who battles to bring her world-renowned psychiatrist, Dr. Jules Masserman, to justice for his sexual and ethical betrayals. Watterson also includes the stories of several other patients who brought charges and won out-of-court settlements against Masserman.*

Step by painful step, the book details the hidden life of Jules Masserman, past president of the American Psychiatric Association, cochair of psychiatry and neurology at Northwestern University, and author of 411 journal articles and sixteen books. It details how the man who was called "psychiatry's ambassador to the world" systematically and ritualistically injected many of his most attractive and vulnerable female patients with Amytal, a barbiturate, and kept them unconscious for six to eight hours at a time in a little room off his main consultation office. Barbara Noël awoke during one of these sessions as she was being raped, and others recounted breakthrough memories of Masserman kissing and fondling them. In addition, Masserman took many of his female patients to his "home office," where he played the violin for them. He took them out on his sailboat Naiad, Nymph of the Lakes, *gave them gifts, and accepted gifts from them.*

Neither Masserman's abuse of his patients nor the failure of his profession to censure him are unique. The best available data indicate that 6 to 10 percent of psychiatrists and psychologists have had sexual contact with their patients, and that the majority of their colleagues know of such cases but do not intervene. More than half of the psychologists and psychiatrists interviewed in various surveys indicate that they have treated women patients who had been sexually involved with previous therapists.

The American Psychiatric Association responded to You Must Be Dreaming *by issuing a public apology and undertaking a year-long review of its ethical policies and procedures for reporting misconduct. The task force recommended that the job of policing and punishing its members is antithetical to the purpose of promoting the profession, and that the job should be turned over to an independent regulating agency.*

Dr. Masserman looked at me intently and smiled. "Please sit down," he said, indicating the couch. I sat there, behind a coffee table that held a small black tape recorder, a stack of textbooks, and a copy of *Who's Who in the World.* Dr. Masserman sat in an easy chair next to the couch, and Mrs. Masserman sat in a swivel chair facing us.

They set up the conditions of this interview: I could not tape-record it. Mrs. Masserman said, however, that they planned to tape-record, because Dr. Masserman "has suffered so much injustice" and they didn't want his comments "taken out of context." "I'll tell you what," Dr. Masserman said pleasantly, as if he had just lit upon a solution. "If my lawyer approves, after reviewing the tape, of course, then I'll send you a copy." At the time this book went to press, I still had not received a copy of the tape.

Mrs. Masserman turned on the tape recorder and also took notes on a white pad as we spoke. From time to time during the following two and a half hours, she would scribble notes on her pad, signal Dr. Masserman, and hold up the pad to show him what she had written.

Dr. Masserman picked up some papers and began with statements he had prepared. He enunciated his words carefully and formally, without contractions:

"I will be straightforward and honest and give you demonstrable facts. I am a very ethical practitioner, and so I cannot tell you confidential information about my patients. I took a Hippocratic oath, and even though I have retired, I still abide by that oath. . . . For the past forty years, under the aegis and supervision of four different universities, I have treated literally thousands of patients. Until Miss Noël's complaint, not a single previous one of my patients—simply not one—ever made one complaint against me." In 1983, one year prior to Barbara Noël's complaint, a patient, Cheryl Russell, sued Dr. Masserman for needlessly injecting her with Amytal and injuring her in the process. Her lawsuit, civil case No. 83L-10063, was settled against Dr. Masserman, by his insurers, for $50,000 not long after Barbara initially filed her complaint.

I started to ask about his use of Amytal, but Dr. Masserman waved his hand toward the stack of reference books, commenting that his own book "is a classic in the field now."* He pointed out the dozens of plaques on his walls that paid homage to him, and invited me to look at his entry in *Who's Who in the World,* saying, "It's an unusual honor . . . it's a rare honor to be in that book."

Continuing his prepared talk, Dr. Masserman said: "I can say a few things about Barbara Noël's treatment. She profited so greatly from Amytal interviews when necessary. I can't tell you *why* they were necessary, because that would be revealing."

He added, "The only complaint Barbara Noël ever made came on September 24, 1984. Had there been any unethical conduct that morning when she said she was conscious—there were no locked doors in my office. All she had to do was to go into the next office and complain.

"She had been my patient for eighteen years," he said, shaking his head.

---

*In the stack, he had two different editions of *Comprehensive Textbook of Psychiatry* by Freedman, Kaplan, and Saddock; and *The Technique of Psychotherapy* by Louis Wolberg.

"What happened on that day [September 24, 1984] is relevant," Dr. Masserman continued. "She did not call me back and make any complaints. She went to her gynecologist and stated to him that she may have dreamed the whole thing. She went to the police with various allegations. . . . I can assure you, I would have been arrested like *that* had her complaints been true. . . ." Dr. Masserman also mentioned "a prominent Chicago attorney" who "investigated her allegations and then withdrew from the case." Then he sat back in his chair, folded his hands across his chest, and seemed to relax.

"But what about the other lawsuits?" I asked. "Why do you think they surfaced?"

Dr. Masserman, his eyes bright and friendly, smiled sweetly and comfortably. "You put me at a disadvantage because the two other lawsuits—" he said, "I don't know who you talked to—"

I said, "There were five other lawsuits, not two, but of the two I think you're referring to, I talked to both of them."

"Well, the major one—the principal one under my therapy—resumed the practice of law, joined a prominent firm, married a rich client, invited me to her wedding, and publicly proclaimed her gratitude in the presence of her father! Neither woman had made any complaints whatsoever. Both left owing me money, but I had written statements pledging to pay me. . . ."

"Why do you think their accusations surfaced? Do you think they're based on malice, profit, fantasy?" I asked.

"My attorney advised me to say this. . . . Please note that there were no criminal charges filed at any time, let alone rape. The only action filed was to obtain money, to secure money."

Asked if he denied all the allegations, he replied, "Absolutely." Raising his voice in irritation, he added, "I never did anything unethical to any patient."

"Then why did you agree to give up your medical license?" I asked. "Why didn't you fight it?"

"I'm glad you asked that," he said, meeting my eyes. "At the time the suit was settled, I had already given notice to the building where I kept my office that I was retiring at the end of that year." Dr. Masserman said he'd planned to retire because he was "taking a great deal of time dashing home to feed my wife, to take her to the toilet, to get her out of bed," because she needed a hip operation. He said he also was having three operations for prostatic cancer during that time.

"What's your reaction to these lawsuits? How do you feel about all these allegations?" I asked.

"Being a very sensitive person—which I have to be to be a psychiatrist—and now this has come up again—it's been seven years of unjustified tension, which I have withstood. Many another might not have." He looked at me with a wounded gaze, not unlike a child who has been refused a treat.

I asked him why he continued to use Amytal regularly, when most psychiatrists say it fell out of use after the early 1950s because it was never very effective.

"With the Amytal, I followed precisely what I wrote in my textbook and what everybody else writes . . ." he said, pointing again to the textbooks.

I said everybody else seemed to think Amytal should *not* be used regularly . . . that he himself had written that the Amytal interview "was a preferred treatment only in extreme cases . . . and that little could be achieved by drug narcosis that could not also be achieved by therapeutic interviews conducted without its use."

He said, "There are many instances in which I only used talk therapy and I always talked afterwards."

I asked him if he had any colleagues who use Amytal on a regular basis, and he said, "Of course I do . . . many."

I asked, "Who?"

"Among others, Louis Wolberg used it frequently." He gestured to Dr. Wolberg's book.

Referring to my notes, I said, "Well, in fact, Dr. Wolberg writes that Amytal is used only in extreme cases—that it's '*sometimes* employed intravenously as an *emergency* measure in quelling intense excitement. . . .' and you yourself say that it's used for 'morose, evasive, withdrawn patients in early schizophrenic or depressive reactions. . . .'" I said it seemed it was normally used only in a hospital under emergency situations.

"No, no. It was used regularly during World War Two and ever since then. . . ."

I asked him why he used Amytal so regularly.

"I only used it with patients that had serious crises—to prevent suicide when someone was so desperate and needed relief, or to *prevent* a bout of alcoholism. . . ."

I asked, "Didn't you worry about it being addictive?"

"*It's not addictive,*" he said.

I said, "In the *Physician's Desk Reference,* in *Goodman & Gillman's,* in *Martindale's,* and every other drug reference, it says it's habit-forming and carries warnings to that effect. Even Louis Wolberg writes that 'Short-acting barbiturates, Pentothal, Seconal, and Amytal are particularly addictive. They are truly as addictive as heroin or morphine. . . .'"

"Amytal is habit-forming only in the sense that they might try to get drugs on the outside," he said, "and naturally I wouldn't give them any. . . ."

I was reeling from the illogic of that statement, but I asked, "What did the people you prescribed Amytal to have in common?"

"They would be people inclined to very severe anxieties, depressions, melancholy, and temptations toward suicide. . . ."

"In references they say that it's given rarely, and yet you used it repeatedly over the years. One patient recently told me there were many periods she got it every week. Why did you do that? Did they have that many crises?"

"There have been years with no Amytal," he said. "But during the past year with Ms. Noël, before September 1984, there were various crises, more frequent than usual."

"You gave them Amytal to help them through a crisis every time—all that often?" I asked.

"I would have to judge each case. Before I ever gave an Amytal interview, I would call in the family; I would consult the[m]. Sometimes I would give the Amytal instead of hospitalizing the person and sometimes I would hospitalize the person instead. . . ."

"Did you ever recommend that Barbara be hospitalized?"

"I can only say what's positive," he said with an apologetic smile. "I did send her to a friend of mine at Northwestern University who helped her by having her do some music therapy at Northwestern with students. . . . I did refer her to other physicians, which shows that I did consult other medical doctors when it was called for."

I said, "Saddoff and Freedman's textbook says Amytal is used only in extreme cases, in emergency situations. They also say 'narcotherapy is *infrequently* used in clinical practice' and when it's used, it's for '*acute* symptoms.'"

Dr. Masserman waved his hand as if to dismiss all this and said, "There are a great many psychiatrists who are so caught up in analytic thinking that they believe only in talk therapy, without using every known therapy—using drug therapy, diet, behavior therapy—I use them all, whatever is called for."

I asked: "Did you use combined drug therapy and talk therapy with most of your patients, some of them, half of them, or . . . ?

"Less than 1 percent," he said.

"You gave Amytal to *less than 1 percent* of your patients?"

"That's right."

"You mean to say that *all six lawsuits* came from that less than one percent of your patients who had Sodium Amytal?"

"Yes, the six lawsuits were part of that 1 percent. . . ."

I said, "I'm confused about Amytal. . . . From what I understand from talking with others, it's a short-acting barbiturate."

"I never gave barbiturates . . ."

"But Amytal is a barbiturate!"

"Yes, but not in addition to that. I didn't give drugs in therapy. . . ."

"But I'm confused about something . . . The patients I talked to—and in your own descriptions—said they were asleep from like 7:00 AM to 2:00 or 3:00 PM in the afternoon or later, sometimes 4:30 or 5:00, and then afterwards they were often groggy for the entire evening or into the next day—"

"They're not asleep. They're relaxed, at ease. They were conscious, and just in a relaxed state so they could converse. . . ."

"But the people I talked to said they never remembered anything afterwards."

"But they *do*," he said, enunciating the words slowly, and meaningfully nodding his head as he looked at me, as if we two knew the truth. "They *do*. Part of the technique is to talk about it afterward."

"Well, I was wondering, since Amytal is a short-acting drug, did you add a sedative to the Amytal or use a continuous IV drip to help them stay out for that long?"

"No, no, absolutely not! I only gave the standard dose of Amytal."

I said, "One woman I talked with told me that you had recommended she take Amytal when she was pregnant, and another told Barbara Noël that she'd had Amytal and subsequently lost her baby. Did you ever give Amytal to a pregnant patient?"

"She never told me she was pregnant," he said. "None of my patients ever told me she was pregnant."

"Do you think it's ever justified for a therapist to have sex with a patient?"

"Of course not!" he said vehemently. "I have sat in on ethics committees in the past and expressed that view unequivocally!"

"You mention in *Psychiatric Odyssey* that 'perverse sexuality has deprecatory meaning only in Western culture. . . .' Do you think it's only Western culture—that maybe Americans are too repressed and overly concerned about these ethical matters? Do you think in another culture or in Biblical times, these things would be considered normal or harmless?"

Dr. Masserman raised his eyebrows in surprise, but then looked rather pleased and amused. "Well, that is true," he said. "In many cultures homosexuality was preferable, for instance. In Greek classic times, homosexuality was not only acceptable, but was considered preferable. Socrates initiated his apostles and that was considered a normal thing. Even cannibalism was accepted in some cultures. But psychiatrists should not make such broad general statements. I deplore this kind of guerre attitude. . . ."

"In *Adolescent Sexuality*, you mention incest can be harmless and can be a non-neurotic experience if it's treated properly. You say, 'Contrary to many current concepts . . . noninjurious parent-child or intersibling sexual relations, even when verified, usually leave no serious adverse effects, and require only judicious avoidance of social and legal traumata. . . .' Is that still your position?"

"Well, that's true if the child isn't dragged through the humiliation of testifying and all," he said. "Certainly, making the child testify can do a great deal of unnecessary harm. There was one example in that book about a girl whose stepfather molested her. The girl didn't want him to go to jail and break up the family . . ."

I said, "Several of your patients talked about your taking them on boat rides or airplane rides or to your home for home office visits and on trips. . . . Did you do that to broaden their horizons or for what purposes?"

Dr. Masserman said he had never taken any patient out on his boat. "Let me show you something," he said, asking me to stand up. The three of us stood and looked out the window; Dr. Masserman stood close to me. I remembered Barbara, Daniella, and Annie telling me about their trips out on his boat—being rowed from the dock to the boat and back. "See that house?" he said, pointing out the clubhouse. "And the dock beside it? I keep my boat in the harbor, and I have to row from that dock to my boat. . . . If I was stupid enough to take anyone else but my wife out to that boat, she'd know it before I got home!"

"Honey, you didn't mention this," Mrs. Masserman said, picking up a pair of binoculars.

"That's right," he said with a little chuckle. "I'm under surveillance at all times. . . . Not really!" Dr. and Mrs. Masserman both laughed. In depositions, when asked if he had ever taken patients out on his boat, Dr. Masserman had said, under oath, "Yes. Ms. Noël on one occasion." And when he was asked, "Have you taken anyone else on your boat, any of your other patients?" he had answered, "Yes, I have." He had also admitted, under oath, that he had taken female patients flying in his airplane.

"But why would these different people say that they went out on the boat and the airplane with you?" I asked. "Are you saying they were making that up, or having the same delusion or something?"

"See that picture?" Dr. Masserman asked me, pointing out a small oil painting of a gray-blue boat with full white sails listing in rough seas.

"It's nice."

"I have the same picture in my office."

"You do?"

"Yes, and I have a picture of the plane I flew when I was flying, in my office. I have a picture of my playing a violin, in my office. It is one part of one technique called *transference*, which illustrates by personal example that there are many activities in life that can give more satisfactions than drinking or quarreling or competing or seeking revenge. And so people ask me these things:

"Do I sail? What sort of boat? Oh, do you fly? Do you take people up? They can make all sorts of fantasies from their own ends . . ."

"So you say they're fantasizing this?" I interjected.

"That's exactly what I'm saying."

The interview was over and we all stood up. Dr. Masserman invited me to look around his music room—and showed me his beautiful old Albani violin and viola. I thought he was starting to say he would be glad to play something for me, but his wife cleared her throat and interrupted, so he didn't finish his sentence. After I left, I felt an amazing sadness. I gave a lot of thought to Dr. Masserman's defense—and to his magnetism. I thought it was no wonder he charmed Barbara and his other patients into believing him. He was compelling and appeared so genuine that I had actually liked him, even when I was so vividly aware of his wrong-doing.

Later, I called Dr. David Spiegel, MD, professor of psychiatry and behavioral sciences at Stanford University and a leading expert in the field. I asked Dr. Spiegel whether the dose of Amytal Dr. Masserman claimed to have used could possibly have kept anyone out for seven to eight hours. "Not from one dose of Amytal!" he said without pause. "It's a short-acting barbiturate. They might be groggy for an hour or two afterwards, but they wouldn't be that deeply affected by it." When I asked him whether a continuous IV may have been used or a sedative added to the Amytal, he said that would make sense. Dr. Spiegel said he didn't know of anyone who still uses Amytal in the normal practice of psychiatry, and that he had never heard of it being used on a repeated basis, since, of course, it is highly addictive.

Lineal Victims

PHYLLIS L. FINE

Phyllis L. Fine, "Lineal Victims: Family Members of a Perpetrator." Speech adapted for this publication.

With the growing national recognition given to the serious problem regarding abuse by professionals, the therapy community has responded to the needs of the primary victims of the perpetrator, whether they be patient, client, or parishioner. Even the family members of the primary victim are being recognized for the pain they suffer. However, lineal victims—the family members of the perpetrating professional, including the spouse, the children, and the other family members—have until recently been the unrecognized, unacknowledged victims who often suffer for years, if not a lifetime, from the effects of having been connected to the perpetrator.

Just as the patient has been victimized by the perpetrating professional, so have the spouse and the children. Generally, the family has been subjected to years of abuse. Overtly or covertly abused, they have been manipulated and often live in a world filled with deception. The abusive personality one experiences at home and the manipulating personality that was able to seduce the client/patient/parishioner is often not the personality viewed by the outside world. . . . The Jekyll-Hyde personality of the perpetrating professional is brilliantly masked, bringing further pain and confusion to family members. . . . Family members suffer tremendous isolation, desperately needing the connection of others who can understand the overwhelming destruction shattering their lives.

Lineal victims often carry within themselves a sense of shame, that—although it does not belong to them—isolates them from the world. They may fear being judged for having been connected to the perpetrator as well as fear angry repercussions from the primary victims and their families. A triangle of fear is created by the perpetrator, a triangle that separates the victims. . . .

Surviving devastation of this magnitude is exceedingly difficult [because of] the many complicating factors impacting the family. It is often the families who are left struggling financially, especially if the professional should lose the ability to practice. As of recent years, insurance companies have restricted their involvement in malpractice suits to paying only for legal costs. Any resulting damage awards or settlements are the responsibility of the perpetrating professional. Although this may appear to be fair, it is the spouse and children who once again are unjustly left struggling, for it is generally the marital assets which are the source of payment for these damages.

For those who have not been abused, it is difficult to understand why these professionals carry so much power, and even more difficult to understand why spouses stay in abusive situations.

The skillfulness of the narcissistic personality to be able to manipulate and control vulnerable people cannot be sufficiently emphasized.

There are many spouses and families who choose not to remain in denial, but rather choose to face their greatest fears and break the isolation. It is a most difficult and pain-filled journey, and one that needs to be recognized and made less isolating.

Airless Spaces

SHULAMITH FIRESTONE

Shulamith Firestone, *Airless Spaces*, New York: Semiotext(e), 1998. Reprinted by permission.

Refusing a career as a professional feminist, Shulamith Firestone has found herself in an "airless space" since the publication of her first book, The Dialectic of Sex. *Lost women in and out of (mental) hospitals are the lens through which Shulamith Firestone views the cultural shrinking of individuality. Using the small crises in the lives of women who are continually framed inside and outside of institutional walls, Firestone illustrates the limits of experience, consciousness, and space at the end of this century.*

PATCHES

When she came out of the hospital, her Levi's no longer fit her. She dug through her hand-me-downs to find a pair of scruffy light blue jeans with big rips at the knees that she had found thrown out in front of an old brownstone. She wore them through the winter with long johns underneath the rip, until at last when spring came, the rip had widened to way beyond fashionable, and it was time to invest in a new pair. Her figure wasn't going to return eventually. After a confusing and fruitless shopping trip to Canal Jeans, where all three used Levi's were incorrectly sized, and she fled the jammed dressing rooms in despair that she was no longer able to shop, she finally settled on the first pair of jeans about her size she saw on an outdoor rack. They had a hole in exactly the same place as the previous jeans, the right knee, but it was a smaller hole, and since the jeans were a little long she figured unless she wore a belt the tension point of the knee would not fall exactly on the hole and widen it to a rip again. There was a long line waiting for the dressing room, and she didn't have the heart to go through all the jeans in the rack to find the one with a less obtrusive hole, and the very handsome salesboy let her know she couldn't tie up the dressing room any longer even if she wanted to. So she plumped down fifteen bucks, which was the lowest sale price for Levi's anywhere, holes or no holes. Besides, she had already invested $2 in an iron-on patch from Woolworth's for the old pair, but it was the wrong color for the new pair.

Still stiff from the Haldol she was on, she prevailed upon a friend to help her iron the patch on the new jeans before the hole should widen in the wash. Her little ironing board did not hold up, so they had to use a towel on her butcher block kitchen table, unplugging the refrigerator to find a near outlet. But after forty-five minutes the patch began to unpeel around the edges and they had to clumsily sew it on, wrong color, oversized, and scrubby, with no guarantee it wouldn't come out in the wash anyway, since she had neglected to sew together the hole before ironing on the patch.

Thus it was that she went from scruffy fashionable with splits at the knees to pickaninny-in-patches wherever she went.

PASSABLE, NOT PRESENTABLE

She remembered the time before she had gotten sick. When it was a challenge to dress, how good it felt to look just right and be certain of one's appearance. Then came losing her looks in the hospital, and the ghastly difference it made in the way she was received; the way people turned away from her after one glance in the street. And the slow climb back, trying to disguise the stiffness in her gait, and the drooling moronic look on her face that came from the medication. Perhaps this was why the mentally disabled always seemed so bland-looking as a group: they had to strive to look ordinary, to "pass." That little bit of extra aplomb that made one stand out of the crowd was beyond them.

Catfight

LEORA TANENBAUM

Leora Tanenbaum, excerpt from *Catfight: Women and Competition*, New York: Seven Stories Press, 2002. Reprinted by permission.

The more complicated a woman's life becomes, the more likely she is to take stock of her life and compare it with that of other women. And women's lives are complicated indeed. Women born and raised in the wake of modern feminism live in a contradictory cultural climate. We have been taught clashing messages about what it means to be a woman. We are caught in a threshold between two paradigms, the old and the new.

Regarding beauty, we have learned from our parents, magazines, advertising, and other women: It's important to be thin and pretty and wear the latest fashions and always be well groomed. We have also learned (often from the very same sources): such concerns are frivolous. Inner beauty, not superficial appearance, is what counts.

When it comes to romance, we've been told: We need to find a good man and get married. We've also been told: We don't need a man to be complete as a person—and with women's rise in the workplace, we don't need his money, either.

In the workplace: We need to compete like a man to get ahead. And yet: It's important for women to share, to be cooperative, and to be nice—otherwise we are seen as castrating bitches.

What about our source of identity? Becoming a full-time wife and mother is a woman's finest achievement, we have been taught. But at the same time we know: A woman needs a career to pay the bills and to feel fulfilled, regardless of marital and parental status.

With all these mixed messages, women are caught in perpetual vertigo. We face internal battles about the "right" way to live our lives. No matter which path we choose, we are going against something deeply ingrained in us, against a path that many other women we know are following, against a path our mothers may have followed, even against a path we may have followed ourselves in the past. As a result, we feel defensive. To defend ourselves, we go to great lengths to justify our decisions, to validate ourselves, to prove to ourselves and to others that our chosen path is the right one. Along the way, any ambivalence we might have about our life course hardens into certainty that our path is the only correct and appropriate one.

Of course, no one can live her life by checking off a series of boxes. Many women today strive to achieve a balance between the old rules and the new—by wearing lipstick and mascara but unapologetically eating lasagna and ice cream; by getting married but striving for an egalitarian partnership; by mentoring other women but strategically moving up the corporate ladder; by raising children but continuing to put in full-time hours at the office. If juggling all this sounds easy, you probably think that Linda Tripp tattled on Monica Lewinsky to protect her young friend from an unhealthy relationship. Living as a woman today is difficult, fraught with pressures, with many of us desperate for a sense of control and direction. An easy way to delude ourselves into thinking we've achieved mastery over our lives is to compete with other women. By competing, we place ourselves and others into neat little categories—"I'm a doting stay-at-home mom; *she's* a workaholic who neglects her kids" or "I work out four times a week; *she's* let herself get out of shape"—that serve to organize our lives and deliver them from chaos to complacency.

Women also, perversely, compete over who is worst off. We listen to a friend complain about her evil boss, her boyfriend's "commitment problem," and her fat thighs—and then we checkmate her by telling her that we've got all the same problems ourselves, *plus* our mother has broken her hip and our credit cards are maxed out, so of course our situation is truly worse and we deserve more sympathy. Many of us can't help but strive for the Biggest Martyr award. If we can't get the recognition we crave for our achievements, at the very least let us get some recognition for our burdens and sorrows.

Competition, of whatever form, is caused by feelings of inadequacy. When a person feels threatened, her instinct is often to go on the defensive. But the cause is more than psychological. A sense of inadequacy is fostered by a very real societal situation: women's restrictive roles.

Change gender stereotypes and parenting arrangements—by getting men more involved in child care and letting girls grow up seeing a mother who, in addition to being a skillful parent, also has a "valued role and recognized spheres of legitimate control"—and circumstances can be altered. Today, women do have quite a bit of power in the larger world (though still not as much as men). As a result, today's young daughters do not grow up devaluing themselves, as per psychologist Nancy Chodorow's theory. Instead, they grow up brimming with self-confidence—which often deflates when they realize women are not allowed to be as strong as they had supposed.

Psychologist Phyllis Chesler similarly implicates the mother-daughter relationship. To Chesler, all women's relationships with other women are, to some extent, reflective of the mother-daughter bond. "Most women unconsciously expect other women to mother them and feel betrayed when a woman fails to meet their ideal standards," she writes in *Woman's Inhumanity to Woman.* "Most women are no more realistic about women than men are. To a woman other women are (supposed to be) Good Fairy Godmothers, and if they are not they may swiftly become their dreaded Evil Stepmothers."

From Kohn to Nelson, and Gilman to Chodorow and Chesler, many pieces of the puzzle of woman-against-woman competitiveness have been explored. To my mind, however, it is crucial not to overlook the power of gender roles and the effect these roles have on our psyches. No matter how a girl is raised, as she grows up, she finds that the power of gender stereotypes is enormous and incredibly difficult to escape. No matter how egalitarian-minded a woman is, chances are that she still behaves, at least in some aspects, according to the old stereotype of femininity, which dictates that she separate from her mother and define herself in relation to men and to what men want. Thus, we grow up longing for male approval because men are the ones with the power. Many women compete over things they think men value, such as looking sexy. On the other hand, according to the stereotype of masculinity, a man can be self-assured whether or not women value him, so he doesn't need to compete over things he thinks women value, such as remembering an anniversary.

Society still conditions girls and women to believe they are inferior to boys and men—in terms of emotional stability, physical strength, psychological fitness, sexual behavior, mathematical ability. The implications of this message are enormous and far-reaching. The most dangerous outcome of this is self-hatred: girls and women disparage themselves and disassociate from other females. Self-hatred is common among subordinated groups of people. When power is withheld, those with power are resented. Yet their values and norms are internalized. Frantz Fanon, the influential West Indian philosopher, psychiatrist, and revolutionary who analyzed the condition of being black in a white world, wrote in 1952:

> In [children's] magazines the Wolf, the Devil, the Evil Spirit, the Bad Man, the Savage are always symbolized by Negroes or Indians; since there is always identification with the victor, the little Negro, quite as easily as the little white boy, becomes an explorer, an adventurer, a missionary "who faces the danger of being eaten by wicked Negroes.". . . There is identification—that is, the young Negro subjectively adopts a white man's attitude. . . . As a schoolboy, I had many occasions to spend whole hours talking about the supposed customs of the savage Senegalese.[1]

Being black while living in a culture with negative stereotypes of blacks leads to an alienation from and rejection of other blacks. According to Fanon, it leads also to shame, self-contempt, even nausea. "If the signals I get from the dominant culture are that I am a person deserving of disdain," asks writer Jill Nelson, "is it any wonder I begin to hate myself?"[2]

Being a woman of any color in a sexist culture leads to similar responses. The archetypal woman is self-sacrificing, nonintellectual, soft and pretty, and derives utter contentment from taking care of others. I don't identify with these traits, and yet I am not a man. How do I reconcile this paradox? By viewing myself as different from (read: better than) other women who do appear to live the stereotype. A male friend who enjoys wry humor always seems pleasantly surprised when I come up with a well-timed deadpan. "You're the only funny woman I know," he says. It's a compliment to me but an insult to women. Despite myself, I eat it up every time.

When I was growing up, I thought it was cool not to like the other girls but to hang out with the boys: The girls were, well, *girlish* and sort of prissy, while the boys beckoned with their mischief. Many of my girlfriends remember feeling the same way. As women, we come to believe that male approval is more significant than female approval, and that a relationship with a man confers more status than a relationship with a woman. Thus, many women believe that supporting other women is suicidal if they want to achieve success in a male-dominated milieu. It's one small step away from thinking that they should cut down other women who might stand in their way.

WOMEN AND RESENTMENT

It's easy to feel resentful toward someone who appears to have an unfair advantage. It can be difficult to be happy for another woman when she succeeds, because the question nags us: What's stopping me from achieving the same thing? It's not a big leap from resentment to believing she doesn't deserve this success, that she deserves to fail. Nietzsche's notion of resentment is useful in understanding this thought process. Admittedly, it may seem perverse to refer to a philosopher who romanticized competition and survivalism. Nevertheless, his concept of resentment strikes me as helpful in making sense of how one individual can turn on another. According to Nietzsche, resentment occurs when one lacks some value, yearns to be the person who possesses it, and then seeks to undermine that person. It is part of a "slave morality" of the weak, who don't like themselves and attempt to bring down the strong. In *The Genealogy of Morals*, Nietzsche asked:

> Is there anyone who has not encountered the veiled, shuttered gaze of the born misfit, that introverted gaze which saddens us and makes us imagine how such a man must speak to himself? "If only I could be someone else," the look seems to sigh, "but there's no hope of that. I am what I am; how could I get rid of myself? Nevertheless, I'm fed up." In the marshy soil of such self-contempt every poisonous plant will grow, yet all of it so paltry, so stealthy, so dishonest, so sickly sweet![3]

The essence of resentment is a real or imagined powerlessness, which can lead to the denigration of everything you are not. If you are weak and financially struggling, you malign the strong and the prosperous as evil and immoral. After all, you can't *both* be good and moral—and it's not fair if your nemesis is blessed with both a fat bank account and moral virtue. You must be the saint, which explains why the interest due on your credit card exceeds the cost of your purchases.

There is a sense of satisfaction when someone you resent is put in her place. That's how Carolyn Kate's two best friends appear to have regarded their friend. Their example is extreme, yet at the same time completely ordinary. Carolyn likes to wear short skirts, which show off her long legs, with clunky black boots. That's her style, she will defiantly tell you: She likes to look feminine, but with an edge. Several years ago, in her sophomore year of college, Carolyn was raped. And from the way her friends reacted, it was almost as if they were glad that someone had finally taught her a lesson for looking so damn good.

Carolyn woke up in her friend's bed with a strange man on top of her, having sexual intercourse with her. Hours before, she had gone to visit her friend, drank too much, and fallen asleep. Now, at 6:00 AM, Carolyn was in pain and asked the man to stop. He didn't. She was paralyzed with fear and couldn't scream or move. After two more hours, he jumped up, pulled up his pants, and left. Carolyn gathered her clothes and walked home.

When Carolyn mustered the courage to tell her two best friends what had happened, they were far from supportive. The first asked, "What do you expect, getting drunk in those little skirts?" The other queried, "Carolyn, are you sure you're not making this up because you feel bad about a one-night stand?" As Carolyn puts it, "They acted like I did not say the word 'rape' and they would not use that word when mentioning the incident. I felt like I was in the twilight zone." Indeed, it is alarmingly common for rape victims to be disbelieved, even by friends and family.[4] Carolyn didn't want to press charges—part of her believed her friends, that she deserved it—but she did spread the word about the rapist; she wanted to warn other women about him. The only person who was supportive was a gay male friend.

A week later, Carolyn saw the rapist at a club. He was dancing with two women, a smirk on his face, when he spotted Carolyn. He pointed in her direction. The women he was with laughed and called over to her, "Lying bitch." Carolyn was telling me this story over the phone. Her voice lowered to a whisper so that her roommate wouldn't be able to hear; I had to press my ear to the phone. "I overheard one of them say, 'Look at what she's wearing. She was asking for it.' I was horrified because these women were competing with me over a rapist! After that, I became very depressed throughout college and isolated myself for months. I feel very vulnerable about my relationships with other females. I feel that my friends in college betrayed me because they never confronted the rapist."

To Carolyn's friends, and to the rapist's friends, it was easier to believe the man who claimed he was innocent than to believe the woman who said she was the victim of a crime. Even though they could just as easily have been raped themselves, they could not imagine themselves in Carolyn's place. Carolyn, after all, has the audacity to want to look attractive—a quality that, no doubt in the backs of their minds, they wished they could pull off. And so they distanced themselves from her— *she's not one of us.* "Slave ethics," wrote Nietzsche, "begins by saying no to an 'outside,' an 'other,' a non-self, and that no is its creative act. This reversal of direction of the evaluating look, this invariable looking outward instead of inward, is a fundamental feature of resentment."[5] The weak cause the strong to desire weakness, to turn against themselves. And that is precisely what Carolyn's friends did to her: They caused her to doubt herself, to agree that she deserved to be raped.

WOMEN'S ESSENTIAL NATURE

But wait a minute—how can women be so callous? Aren't women supposed to be sensitive and gentle, empathetic and interconnected with people? At least, that's what a large group of feminist scholars says: that there is something special about women's nature, that they are more sharing and caring

than men. Women are commonly believed to operate on a higher moral plane and to be more attuned to others' feelings. After all, only women can be mothers—and mothers, as everyone knows, are more nurturing than fathers. Indeed, in her influential feminist treatise, *Maternal Thinking*, author Sara Ruddick went so far as to maintain that mothers are necessarily pacifist because "maternal attentive love, restrained and clear-eyed, is ill adapted to intrusive, let alone murderous, judgments of others' lives." She contrasts motherhood with the male-controlled military. "Mothers protect children who are at risk; the military risks the children mothers protect."[6]

Psychoanalyst Nancy Chodorow has argued that since mothers are generally the primary parents, their daughters have a role model with whom they can easily identify (albeit a role model who is "devalued" and "passive"), while their sons do not. As a result, this theory goes, girls emerge from childhood with a strong sense of connectedness to others, while boys see themselves as separate from others. Psychologist Carol Gilligan, building on Chodorow's theory, has advanced the idea that females' relational character makes them feel a stronger sense of justice and responsibility to the world than men do. To Chodorow and Gilligan, women's relational character propels them to be, among other considerate things, caring citizens who are active in community affairs and who work to better circumstances for others. These ideas have been so popularized (and watered down) that they seem to be invoked in nearly every lecture, course, and even conversation on the subject of women's and men's supposed essential differences.

Yet it is a well-known fact that women can be appallingly aggressive and violent, toward women and children as well as toward men. In the United States, men are overwhelmingly responsible for violent crime: they commit 90 percent of the murders, 80 percent of the muggings, and nearly all the rapes. But women do their share too: they commit the majority of child homicides, a greater share of physical child abuse, an equal rate of sibling violence and assaults on the elderly, about a quarter of child sexual abuse, an overwhelming number of the killings of newborns, and a fair amount of spousal assaults.[7]

Of course if women alone possess caring characteristics, then men needn't bake the holiday cakes or wake up for the 3:00 AM baby feedings. Carol Tavris, social psychologist and author of *The Mismeasure of Woman*, is concerned about this "growing tendency to turn the tables from us-them thinking (with women as the problem) to them-us thinking (with men as the problem)." She argues that it is "a misguided belief that there is something special and different about women's nature, an attitude that historically has served to keep women in their place. It continues to use the male norm, although this time to define what is supposedly right with women instead of what is wrong with them."[8]

Tavris points out that many people *think* that women are kinder and gentler, so that when they rate themselves on empathy, women score higher than men. While it's true that women, on average, are better able to intuitively interpret male behavior than men are with female behavior, "this is not a female skill," writes Tavris. "It is a *self-protective* skill, and the sex gap fades when the men and women in question are equal in power." Psychologist Sara Snodgrass conducted an experiment that proved this to be the case. She paired men and women in work teams, sometimes assigning the man to be the leader, sometimes the woman. The person in the subordinate position was more sensitive to the leader's nonverbal cues than the leader was to the subordinate's cues—regardless of whether a man or a woman was the leader or follower.[9] Habitually jumping up to serve your husband coffee while he lounges on the sofa is the result of a power imbalance and social conditioning, not hormones. Empathy, in other words, is about power, not gender.

"Much of the stereotype of women's innate advantage in empathy derives from the different jobs that women and men do and their different average levels of power. Women are more likely than men to be the caretakers and monitors of relationships," continues Tavris. "Although there is no question that mothers spend far more time, on the average, than fathers in terms of the daily care of their children . . . it does not follow that mothers are necessarily more empathic about understanding their children's feelings or actions."[10] Feminist commentator and *Nation* columnist Katha Pollitt adds that it's no accident that women may be more "relational" and men more "autonomous": These characteristics are borne from inequitable work arrangements. Most women need to rely on a wage earner so that they can survive, leading them to be more deferential and therefore empathetic, while most men need someone to care for their children and manage their emotional life so that they can do the work, leading them to be more independent and therefore less attached to others.[11]

As a result of the "kinder, gentler" myth, many men come to believe that they don't have to be sensitive and caring to be considered good and decent people. Women, meanwhile, have been encouraged to develop themselves in relation to others, making their rivalries intensely personal.

INDIRECT AGGRESSION

There is another pernicious consequence to the "kinder, gentler" myth: the double standard in competition. Girls and women internalize the idea that being aggressive is acceptable only for men, so we direct our aggression underground. Rather than confront the people whom we feel have wronged or unfairly bested us, we express our aggression indirectly, through social sabotage, gossip, or vague double entendres. Indirect aggression is aggression that appears unintentional, such as when a supervisor pats you on the back and says, "Your report is excellent; I'm so glad you were able to understand the assignment"; a friend exclaims, "Oh, you've lost twenty pounds! How wonderful! Are you going to lose the rest?"; a colleague accidentally-on-purpose misplaces something that you're responsible for, like an important file or phone number. These actions could be interpreted as hostile, but they also could be construed as just clueless—the result of someone who perhaps has good intentions but just doesn't know the proper way to convey them, or of someone who is simply disorganized. Women are masters of this sort of competitiveness.

Indirect aggression is slippery, impossible to nail down; it is disguised beneath a veneer of politeness or gentleness. If confronted, the aggressor has an accessible backdoor: "I didn't mean it the way it sounded" or "Of course I'm not angry with you" or "You're too sensitive" or even "You're paranoid." The recipient is left paralyzed. She has no proof, just her suspicions. If she confronts the aggressor with her doubts, she may very well be blamed for causing conflict herself.

Meg, a manager at an insurance company, relates that Jackie, a woman she supervises, is supposed to show her materials before they are mailed to clients. Jackie often doesn't show Meg the materials beforehand. Meg interprets this as a way for Jackie to undermine her authority. When Meg confronts her, Jackie's reaction is always, "I'm sorry, I forgot to show it to you, but I can't believe you think that I would ever intentionally go behind your back." Meg complains that Jackie never deals with the substance of the accusation. "I end up agreeing with her because it's easier. I end up saying something like, 'I never thought you were against me; I'm just telling you that if you do have a problem, you should come to me to discuss it.'" Jackie puts Meg on the defensive so that she doesn't have to account for her actions. It gives her the upper hand because now she is in a position where she can turn the accusation around and suggest that her supervisor is the one with the problem: She is delusional.

Dana Crowley Jack, author of *Behind the Mask: Destruction and Creativity in Women's Aggression*, observes that:

> Many women feel they cannot overtly express their feelings, oppose others, or exercise their wills. Instead, much like the brightly painted Russian dolls that nest one inside another, they hide their intent inside a different form, and another, and another, placing feelings within charming exteriors that hold surprising contents. The recipient ends up with a doll that appears to be one form, most often that of good femininity, but that contains a complexity of hidden intentions.[12]

Jack identifies the factors that lead women to mask their aggression. First, there is women's unequal amount of power. Many of the women Jack interviewed expressed fear of physical, economic, or emotional retaliation if they openly expressed overt opposition to someone more physically or socially powerful, or they feared negative professional consequences. Second, there is women's socialization. While boys are given permission to punch and kick to express negative feelings, girls are taught to avoid direct conflict. The third cause is cultural expectations. Women told Jack that they masked their aggression in order to give the appearance of being nonaggressive, so that they can conform to the myth of the kinder, gentler female and not come across as bitchy.

Many girls master their hidden machinations of indirect aggression: They know, even at a young age, that they are supposed to appear good and demure and deferential, not overtly aggressive. But of course, says science writer Natalie Angier with exasperation, girls have aggressive impulses that need to be uncorked from time to time. "They're alive, aren't they?" she writes. "They're primates. They're social animals. So yes, girls may like to play with Barbie, but make the wrong move, sister, and ooh, ah, here's your own Dentist Barbie in the trash can, stripped, shorn, and with toothmarks on her boobs."[13] As adults, women are supposed to be sisterly, to "relate" to one another. Feeling angry or hostile toward another can be scary for anyone, but especially for a woman: Since the female role is to prize and nurture relationships, she doesn't want to be regarded as hampering those relationships. She does not feel entitled to express her anger. So what does she do with it? She either suppresses it or she reroutes it.

NOTES

1. Frantz Fanon, *Black Skin, White Masks* (New York: Grove, 1967), 146, 147, 148.

2. Jill Nelson, *Straight, No Chaser: How I Became A Grown-Up Black Woman* (New York: Putnam, 1997), 99.

3. Friedrich Nietzsche, *The Genealogy of Morals III*, section xiv, in *The Birth of Tragedy and the Genealogy of Morals*, translated by Francis Golffing (New York: Doubleday, 1956), 258–59.

4. See Alice Vachss, *Sex Crimes* (New York: Random House, 1993); and Helen Benedict, *Virgin or Vamp: How the Press Covers Sex Crimes* (New York: Oxford, 1993).

5. Nietzsche, *The Genealogy of Morals I*, section x, in *The Birth of Tragedy and the Genealogy of Morals*, translated by Francis Golffing (New York: Doubleday, 1956), 170–71.

6. Sara Ruddick, *Maternal Thinking: Toward a Politics of Peace* (Boston: Beacon, 1989), 150, 148.

7. Patricia Pearson, *When She Was Bad: How and Why Women Get Away with Murder* (New York: Penguin, 1998), 7.

8. Carol Tavris, *The Mismeasure of Woman: Why Women are Not the Better Sex, the Inferior Sex, or the Opposite Sex* (New York: Touchstone, 1992), 60.

9. Sara Snodgrass, "Women's Intuition: The Effect of Subordinate Role on Interpersonal Sensitivity," *Journal of Personality and Social Pscyhology* 49 (1985): 146–55. Cited in *Tavris, Mismeasure of Woman*, 65.

10. Tavris, *Mismeasure of Woman*, 65–66.

11. Katha Pollitt, "Marooned on Gilligan's Island: Are Women Morally Superior to Men?," originally published in *The Nation* in 1992. Reprinted in Katha Pollitt, *Reasonable Creatures: Essays on Women and Feminism* (New York: Knopf, 1994), 42–62.

12. Dana Crowley Jack, *Behind the Mask: Destruction and Creativity in Women's Aggression* (Cambridge, Mass.: Harvard University Press, 1999), 196.

13. Natalie Angier, *Woman: An Intimate Geography* (New York: Houghton Mifflin, 1999), 239.

Women and Madness: A Feminist Diagnosis

PHYLLIS CHESLER

Phyllis Chesler, "Women and Madness: A Feminist Diagnosis," *Ms.*, November/December 1997. Reprinted by permission.

Twenty-five years ago Phyllis Chesler's book Women and Madness *challenged the psychotherapeutic community's routine pathologizing of women. She documented the patriarchal straitjacketing of women's mental health and urged sweeping reforms in both the theories and the practices. In this excerpt from the introduction to the special anniversary edition of this landmark work, Chesler reflects on what has and has not changed.*

When I started writing *Women and Madness* I immersed myself in the psycho-analytic literature, and located biographies and autobiographies of women who'd been psychiatrically treated or hospitalized—women who were unable to leave home, or to lead lives outside the family. I read novels and poems about sad, mad, bad women; and devoured mythology and anthropology, especially about goddesses, matriarchies, and Amazon warrior women. I interviewed the real experts: women who had been psychiatric and psychotherapy patients. I interviewed white women and women of color, heterosexual women and lesbians, middle-class women and women on welfare, women who ranged in age from seventeen to seventy women whose experiences in mental asylums and therapy spanned a quarter century.

And so I began to document how patriarchal culture and consciousness had shaped human psychology for thousands of years. I was charting the psychology of human beings who, as a caste, did not control the means of production or reproduction and who were in addition routinely shamed—sexually and in other ways. I was trying to understand what a struggle for freedom might entail, psychologically, when the colonized group was female.

Women and Madness received hundreds of positive reviews, and over the years more than two and a half million copies were sold. However, those in positions of institutional power either ignored the challenge this book posed, or said that, by definition, *any* feminist work was biased, "neurotic," and "hysterical." (Yes, our critics psychiatrically pathologized an entire movement and the work it inspired—much as individual women were pathologized.) Some said my feminist views were "strident" (how they loved that word), "man-hating," and "too angry."

Piffle.

What has really changed since I wrote this book? The answer is too little—and quite a lot. Although there has been enormous progress—a sea change even—the clinical biases I first wrote about in 1972 still exist today. Many clinical judgments remain clouded by classism, racism, anti-Semitism, homophobia, ageism, and sexism. I have reviewed hundreds, possibly thousands, of psychiatric and psychological assessments in matrimonial, criminal, and civil lawsuits. The clinical distrust of mothers, simply because they are women, the eagerness to bend over backward to like fathers, simply because they are men, is mind-numbing. Mother-blaming and woman-hatred fairly sizzle on clinical pages.

Even many of those clinicians who are less likely to gender-stereotype still exhibit (often unconscious) preference for men over women. Their sexism may be sophisticated, subtle. Often, female clinicians are much harder on women than are male clinicians. They may feel they have to be—as a way of distancing themselves from a despised group. One 1990 study confirmed that there was less gender-stereotyping among psychiatrists in 1990 than in 1970. However, more of the female psychiatrists rated "masculine" traits as optimal for female patients while more male psychiatrists chose "undifferentiated, androgynous" traits as optimal for both male and female patients.

Continuing clinical bias affects women in at least five important areas: women (and to a lesser extent, men) with medical illnesses are often, and wrongfully, psychiatrically diagnosed and medicated. Women who allege sex discrimination, harassment, rape, incest, or battery are being ordered into therapy and/or diagnostically pathologized at trial. Women (and men) who have no money and no insurance cannot afford therapy nor are they always respected or understood by therapists who are middle-class in orientation. Women of color, Jewish and other Semitic women (and to a lesser extent, men) still face an extra level of clinical fear and hostility. Psychotherapist-patient sexual abuse still exists.

While society has changed, it also remains the same. For some, family life has changed radically in the last twenty-five years. Nearly half of all marriages end in divorce; many mothers are daring to leave men who abuse them and their children. Lesbians and gay men are creating alternative families and raising children.

Nevertheless, most girls and boys continue to experience childhood in father-dominated, father-absent, and/or mother-blaming families. Sex-role stereotyping still exists in many homes, as does, though to a lesser extent, maternal and paternal child abuse. Incest and family violence remain epidemic but have, increasingly, been depoliticized. First, by women who believe that "going public" might help them. Second, by the media, which are all too happy to capitalize on the entertainment value of their public confessions. And third, by the understandable but misguided belief in the power of individual "therapeutic" solutions as opposed to collective legal or social justice solutions.

The cumulative effect of being forced to lead circumscribed lives is toxic. The psychic toll is measured in anxiety, depression, phobias, suicide attempts, eating disorders, addictions, alcoholism, and such stress-related illnesses as high blood pressure and heart disease. It is therefore not surprising that many women still behave as if they've been colonized.

The image of women as colonized is a useful one. It explains why some women cling to their colonizers the way a child or a hostage clings to an abusive parent or a captor; why many women blame themselves, or other women, when they are captured (she really "wanted" it, she freely "chose" it); and why most women defend their colonizers' right to possess them (God or nature has "ordained" it).

In *Women and Madness,* I described asylums as dangerous patriarchal institutions. Tragically, such snake pits still exist in the United States today, in which patients are wrongfully medicated, utterly neglected, and psychologically and sexually abused.

Women who have been repeatedly raped in childhood—often by authority figures in their own families—are traumatized human beings; as such, they are often diagnosed as borderline personalities. If they are institutionalized, they are rarely treated as the torture victims they really are. On the contrary, in state custody, women are more, not less, likely to be raped again (and each time is more, not less, traumatic). Instead of being trained to understand this, most institutional staff—psychiatrists, psychologists, nurses, and attendants alike—do not believe the rape victims, nor do they think of a rape as a lifelong trauma.

There is no excuse for subjecting institutional inmates to the same awful conditions that existed in the nineteenth century. By this, I am referring to solitary confinement, restraints, unending physical and psychological cruelty, and criminality unrestrained among the inmates by overworked or punitive staff.

Institutional psychiatry may fail us, but madness still exists. I said so in 1972, but I also said that most women were not mad, merely seen as such. My own and other historical accounts of asylums strongly suggest that most women in asylums were not insane; that help was not to be found in doctor-headed, attendant-staffed, and state-run institutions; that what we call "madness" can also be caused or exacerbated by injustice and cruelty, within the family and society; and that freedom, radical legal reform, political struggle, and kindness are crucial to psychological and moral health.

On the other hand, the family members and friends of people who suffer from schizophrenia or manic depression know that something is seriously "wrong" with a relative who can no longer eat or sleep, hears voices, can't work, is afraid to leave the house, has become suicidal, or verbally and physically aggressive. They see they are suffering, learn that they cannot help them or even continue to live with them. Families of the mentally ill often see major improvements with psychiatric medication and psychotherapy and are concerned about the right to treatment.

Obviously, consumer education and legal action remain crucial in the struggle to humanize both institutional and noninstitutional life.

Often those who condemn institutional psychiatric medication, shock therapy—any kind of therapy-for-hire—do not feel responsible for the female casualties of patriarchy. Such critics, even if well-intentioned, may be confusing the fact that quality mental health care is not available to all who want it with the question of whether quality mental health care exists at all.

So what did I mean when I said that quite a lot has changed in the last twenty-five years? For one thing, we've learned more about the genetic and chemical bases of mental illness. We've learned that those suffering from manic depression, depression, or schizophrenia often respond to the right drug at the right dosage level; that all drugs have negative side effects; that we shouldn't prescribe the same drug for everyone, especially without continually monitoring the side effects; and that supportive therapies are often impossible with such medication.

Despite the progress in biological psychiatry, both women and men are still wrongfully or overly medicated—or denied proper medication—by harried psychiatrists and psychopharmacologists. Psychiatric inpatients are often overly medicated for the convenience of staff, who do not always treat the to-be-expected side effects with compassion or expertise.

As bad as many institutions are, turning the mentally ill loose, into the streets, is not the solution; it is merely another unacceptable alternative. People do have a right to treatment, if that treatment exists. I realize this statement is almost laughable today, given how insurance and drug companies, managed care, and government spending cuts have made quality psychotherapy totally out of reach for most people. This means that just when we know what to do for the victims of trauma, there are very few teaching hospitals and clinics that treat poor women in feminist ways.

Medication by itself is never enough. Women who are clinically depressed or anxious also need access to feminist information and support.

What does a feminist therapist do that's different? A feminist therapist tries to *believe* what women say. Given the history of psychiatry and psychoanalysis, this alone is a radical act. When a woman begins to remember being sexually molested as a child, a feminist does not conclude that the woman's flashbacks or "hysteria" prove that she's lying or "crazy."

A feminist therapist *believes* that a woman needs to be told that she's not "crazy"; that it's normal to feel sad or angry about being overworked, underpaid, underloved; that it's healthy to harbor fantasies of running away when the needs of others (aging parents, needy husbands, demanding children) threaten to overwhelm her.

A feminist therapist believes that women need to hear that men "don't love enough" before they're told that women "love too much"; that fathers are equally responsible for their children's problems; that absolutely no one—not even feminist, self-appointed saviors—can rescue a woman but herself. A feminist therapist *believes* that self-love is the basis for love of others; that it's hard to break free of patriarchy and that the struggle to do so is both miraculous and lifelong; that very few of us know how to support women in flight from, or at war with, internalized self-hatred and violence against women and children.

A feminist therapist tries to listen to women respectfully, and does not minimize the extent to which a woman has been wounded. A feminist therapist remains resolutely optimistic because no woman, no matter now wounded she may be, is beyond the reach of human community and compassion.

A feminist therapist does not label a woman mentally ill because she expresses strong emotions or is at odds with her "feminine" role. Feminists do not view women as mentally ill when they engage in sexual, reproductive, economic, or intellectual activities outside of marriage. We do not pathologize women who have full-time careers, are lesbians, refuse to marry, commit adultery, want divorces, choose to be celibate, have abortions, use birth control, have a child out of wedlock, breast-feed against expert advice, or expect men to be responsible for a full 50 percent of the child care and housework.

Some feminist theorists and therapists have been moved by the radical liberation psychology in *Women and Madness*. They agree that women's control of our bodies is as important as sexual pleasure, and that we must be able to defend "our bodies, ourselves" against violent or unwanted invasions like rape, battery, unwanted pregnancy, or unwanted sterilization.

As feminist clinician Janet Surrey says, "The work of feminist healers is to integrate our minds and our bodies, ourselves and others, human community and the life of our planet. I question our profession's fear of feminism. I practice psychology within a feminist liberation theology."

In *Trauma and Recovery*, psychiatrist Judith Lewis Herman models a new vision of therapy and of human relationships, one in which we are called upon to "bear witness to a crime" and to "affirm a position of solidarity with the victim." Herman's ideal therapist cannot be morally neutral but must make a collaborative commitment, and enter into an "existential engagement" with the traumatized. Such a therapist must listen, solemnly and without haste, to the factual and emotional details of atrocities, without flight or denial, without blaming the victim, identifying with the aggressor, or becoming a detective who "diagnoses" ritual or satanic abuse after a single session, and without "using her power over the patient to gratify her personal needs."

While the love and understanding of relatives, friends, and political movements are necessary, they are not substitutes for the hard psychological work that victims must also undertake with the assistance of trained grassroots professionals; in fact, even enlightened professionals like Herman cannot themselves undertake this work without a strong support system of their own.

Make no mistake: feminists have learned what works, what must be done. Nevertheless, the most important feminist work has been "disappeared" or never made its way into the graduate and medical school canon. This is truly astounding given that contemporary mental health professionals did not learn about incest, rape, sexual harassment, wife-beating, or child abuse from graduate or medical school textbooks but from feminist consciousness-raising and research, and from grassroots activism. We all learned from the victims themselves, who had been empowered to speak not by psychoanalytic but by feminist liberation.

When I began writing *Women and Madness,* there were few feminist theories of psychology and virtually no feminist therapists. Now we are everywhere. Feminists have established journals, referral networks, conferences, and workshops—programs that are both psychoanalytic and anti-psychoanalytic in orientation. We have served incest and rape survivors, battered women, batterers, mentally ill and homeless women, refugees, alcoholics, drug addicts, the disabled, the elderly—and each other. Feminists have also published many extraordinary books and articles.

Today, there are feminist psychopharmacologists; forensic experts; lesbian therapists; sex therapists; family therapists; experts on recovered memories, race, and ethnicities; and, perhaps the truest sign of having arrived: feminist critics of feminist therapy!

Despite such progress, most feminists in mental health understand how much remains to be done. But we have come a long way.

We now understand that women and men are not "crazy" or "defective" when, in response to trauma, they develop post-traumatic symptoms. We recognize that trauma victims may attempt to mask these symptoms with alcohol, drugs, overeating, or extreme forms of dieting.

We now understand more about what trauma is, and what it does. We understand that chronic, hidden family/domestic violence is actually more traumatic than sudden violence at the hands of a stranger, or of an enemy during war. We understand that after even a single act of abuse, physical violence is only infrequently needed to keep one's victim in a constant state of terror, dependent on her captor and tormentor.

We understand that rape is not about love or even lust, but about humiliating another human being through forced or coerced sex and sexual shame. The intended effect of rape is always the same: to utterly break the spirit of the rape victim, to drive the victim out of her (or his) body and to make her incapable of resistance and quite often out of her mind. The effects of terror on men at war and in enemy captivity are equivalent to the trauma suffered by women at home in "domestic captivity."

What do victims of violence need to ensure their survival and to maintain their dignity? Bearing witness is important; being supported instead of punished for doing so, especially by other women, is also important. Putting one's suffering to use, through educating and supporting other victims, is important; drafting, passing, and enforcing laws is important. However, as Judith Herman has written, "The systematic study of psychological trauma . . . depends on the support of a political movement. . . . In the absence of strong political movements for human rights, the active process of bearing witness inevitably gives way to the active process of forgetting."

In my view, in addition to therapy and political

movement, we also need rape prevention education, i.e., compulsory self-defense training for girls. And more: military training for girls; swift, effective prosecution of rapists; a nonstop series of successful civil suits for monetary remuneration, in addition to criminal prosecution. Perhaps most important, we need to support women who have fought back against their rapists and batterers and who are wasting away in jail for daring to save their own lives.

Despite my own early critique of private patriarchal therapy geared primarily to high-income clients, I have come to believe that women can and do benefit from feminist therapy. Some feminists have questioned whether any therapy, including feminist therapy, is desirable. They have noted, correctly, that "therapism" may indeed siphon activist energies. They are right, but severely traumatized women cannot always rise to the occasion of political action. For example, an incest survivor with insomnia or panic attacks often cannot sit in a room long enough to have her consciousness raised; an anorexic or obese woman who is obsessed with losing weight may not be able to notice others long enough to engage in fund-raising; a woman on a window ledge or in an alcoholic daze may not have the peace of mind to analyze her fate in feminist terms.

Being traumatized does not necessarily make one a noble or productive person. Some women rise above it; others don't. Some women want to be "saved"; others are too damaged to participate in their own "redemption."

As feminist author bell hooks writes: "It had become more than evident that individual black females suffering psychologically were not prepared to go out and lead the feminist revolution. . . . Working with women, especially black women, I have found that many of us are willing to acknowledge the evils of sexism, the way it wounds and hurts everyone, but are reluctant to make that conversion to feminist thinking that would require substantive changes in habits of being."

This applies to women of all colors. As feminist psychotherapist E. Kitch Childs said: "We need a whole new level of consciousness-raising groups and networks. We must learn how to speak our bitterness about each other to each other. It will liberate our energies to keep on working together."

We need a Feminist Institute of Mental Health that is both local and global, a learning community that lasts beyond our lifetimes, a clinical training program that is not patriarchal, a spiritual retreat with an intellectual agenda, a health club with a political agenda, a place where feminists can come together to both learn and teach in ways that are inspired, rigorous, humane, and healing.

I wanted to create such an institute from the moment *Women and Madness* was on the way. It was too soon. Now, at last, I and many others have begun to do so. For example, the Cambridge Hospital Victims of Violence (VOV) Program was co-founded in Massachusetts in 1984 by psychologist Mary Harvey and Judith Herman. It offers crisis intervention, supportive therapy, and group support to "survivors of rape, incest and childhood sexual abuse, domestic violence, and physical abuse/assault." A multidiciplinary staff develops programs, presents workshops, and conducts in-service trainings. VOV offers support groups in Trauma Information, Parenting for Mothers with Trauma Histories, Time-Limited Rape Survivors Groups, Male Survivors of Childhood Trauma, etc.

We need such programs in every city, every community, worldwide.

I am currently associated with the Choices Mental Health Center, which, as the Women's Medical Center, Inc., started a rape crisis center in 1991, and became a fully licensed mental health clinic in 1995. Since 1971, women had been coming to the Choices Women's Medical Center for abortions and other reproductive health services; they talked about being raped, battered, drug-addicted, and victims of incest. Choices has now begun to offer short-term, crisis-oriented feminist therapy for the adult victims of violence on an HMO, Medicaid, or fee-for-service basis. The center is also beginning to work with children and with batterers who are court-ordered into treatment. We envision creating and consulting on similar programs both nationally and internationally.

Freedom and justice do wonders for one's mental health. So, in response to my brother Sigmund Freud's infamous query, what do women want? For starters, and in no particular order: freedom, food, nature, shelter, leisure, freedom from violence, justice, music, poetry, nonpatriarchal family, community, compassionate support during chronic or life-threatening illness and at the time of death, independence, books, physical/sexual pleasure, education, solitude, the ability to defend ourselves, love, ethical friendships, the arts, health, dignified employment, and political comrades.

Maud

NELL CASEY

Nell Casey, "Maud," 2008. Original for this publication.

The challenge of dealing with a mentally ill family member impacts not only the way we experience our family life, but the way we see ourselves. Journalist and author Nell Casey writes about her sister Maud's struggle with manic depression and her own efforts to keep herself and her family together during hospitalizations and her sister's darker moments.

My sister, Maud, was eighteen years old when she was hospitalized for the first time. Diagnosis: manic depression. I was sixteen. When I visited her, we sat at a round table in a cafeteria-like room filled with cigarette smoke and she asked me if she had a tampon in her spleen. I reassured her, *No, no Maud, there is no tampon in your spleen. You do not have cancer. Dad is not dead.* I used to remember this experience as having a fairy-tale end—the doctors gave her medication, the strange behavior got a little less strange, and soon after, Maud got well again. I used to think of this as a neat little chapter in our exotic, dysfunctional family life.

At twenty-nine, though, Maud was institutionalized again. This time—eerily aware that she was about to stop understanding reality—she decided to check herself in and asked a friend to accompany her to a hospital in Queens. She'd secretly quit taking the lithium that she'd been on for eleven years. She wanted to feel something from before, an unencumbered emotion, and didn't want to believe that she was a personality made up of medication. Slowly, unfairly, her mind unraveled.

"I'm happiest here," Maud told my mother and me in the hospital. "This is the only place where I can really be myself." We were sitting on orange plastic chairs, inches away from the other patients and their families, all of us in our tight huddles of concern.

My own sanity, I realized later, must've seemed like magic to Maud in those moments. "You're so strong," she said then, eyeing me with suspicion and awe. The truth is, though, I am like Maud. We are both an erratic mix of fragility and strength. We are both worried. But I am a different breed—all wiry energy and dizzying panic attacks. Once, at the height of my distress over Maud's second hospitalization, I couldn't read the menu at a restaurant. The words just stopped being reasonable. I wasn't convinced I'd officially learned the English language in the first place. *How do you live with a mind that can't hold on?*

In the beginning of Maud's second breakdown, however, I felt pure, heroic strength. I pictured those women you hear about who suddenly take on otherworldly powers in an emergency and lift trucks off their children. In mobilizing around Maud's roiling emotion, I was able to give my own a purpose. I dealt with doctors and medical paperwork, waited patiently on the phone while Blue Cross had me on hold, made the seventy-minute subway ride to the hospital in Queens almost every day after work and arranged for others to go when I couldn't make it. I informed friends and relatives about the situation, saying too much with a kind of dire rapture. (*Maud burned her arm with a cigarette! They put her in restraints last night!)* Sometimes, I found myself consoling the person I'd just made cry with the grisly details. I admit a small part of me was spellbound, but mainly I hoped that telling friends everything would make it all more manageable, maybe even nudge the story along, encourage it to end.

And, through therapy, medication, and a month and a half in a hideous psychiatric hospital, Maud did become grounded again. That is, grounded in the sense that she no longer believed there was a bomb in the bed, but not in the sense that she was, once again, Maud. After she reined it in and focused on life as we're asked to experience it on a daily level, she hurtled in another direction.

I want so much to explain the absence of my sister during her depression. The hidden, shadowy terror of devouring misery. The hollow lifelessness of her pupils, exaggerated into large, black pools from medication. The listless physicality. I have watched Maud shuffle down hospital corridors— dirty sweatsocks, toes knocking into the backs of her ankles as she saunters up and down to nowhere. *Oh, for chrissakes, pick up your feet!*

Maud came to see me—with those hungry, medicated pupils—right away after she was released from the hospital in September. I cried in my bed all night afterward. It was impossible to decipher a real person in her. She seemed so tiny. She's not tall to begin with—maybe five-three—and she'd lost a lot of weight, but, most alarmingly, her spirit had vanished. She came over that night with all the trappings of a new lease on life, armed with a Gap bag full of clothes. She tried on a pair of army-green pants she'd bought and slowly twirled in front of the mirror. The too-tight pants pulled awkwardly against her body as if everything now was conspiring to show how difficult it would be for her to reenter this world.

She was walking, talking, making sense, and somehow this was worse. There was enough of her there to imitate a functioning, viable person in the world (able to shop at the Gap), but the sum of these parts only added up to a ghostly version of the person she used to be. She crawled into my bed. She was like a strange infant of sadness in my arms. Her tenderness—able to reign over such intense misery—struck me hard. That, and my own first flash of bottomless doubt. *Maybe this is it. Maybe this is as well as she gets.*

When it did find a voice, Maud's depression opened up new worlds of insecurity: *Should I live in New York? Do I know enough about history? Have I said the right thing? In the right language?* We had these conversations on the phone at night, sitting on the sidewalk (when she was too seized with anxiety to continue walking down the street), in our cramped New York apartments. I mostly gave practical, soothing answers, but I was frighteningly close to asking myself the same questions Maud kept firing away. One moment, I had total compassion—*this, this* is what it's like to be Maud. The next, the feelings were eating me alive, threatening to hurl me downward as well. I had the taste of this thing on the tip of my tongue.

I wanted to be there for Maud, I knew that was what she needed (the one thing people always say about depression is that stubborn, consistent support helps even when it seems like it doesn't), but I didn't have the sturdiness of my own character to rely on. We were both young—with the amplified longings and alarms of people in their twenties. I had spent so much of my own life too heartily entertaining turbulent emotion, it seemed dangerous to peer into Maud's black hole of doubt. Sometimes it felt like a trade-off: I had to throw my life over in order to save hers.

No one is a stranger to despair. It takes a resourceful mind to see, again and again, the purposeful good in broken-down ideals and renegotiated expectations. And, still, there are always private suspicions in the presence of the depressed: Is this person just spiritually weaker? Am I stronger? Couldn't it be worse? You have life! You have your health! I wondered if Maud was clinging to her sadness, stubbornly digging her heels in on a life that had become unwieldy and disappointing. In tearful conversations with friends, I thrashed about (*I think*

I might . . . be . . . having . . . some kind of . . . emotional collapse) and, then, in the presence of Maud, I wondered if she just wasn't trying hard enough.

At some indiscernible point, though, things did start to get better. Maud's life started to take shape again. She made efforts that had once seemed impossible in her feeble state. She cooked dinner for friends. She went on a few dates with a young psychiatrist she met at a party. (Even Maud has to raise an eyebrow at this.) She got an agent for her novel. She stopped telling me about the medications once they were settled.

As she pulled back—to regain composure, privacy—I lurched forward. I worried at the same fever pitch I had during the worst of her depression. I finished her sentences, laughed too hard at my own jokes when we talked, leaped forward at parties to help with conversations when she was doing just fine on her own.

For a while, there was not enough of us all to go around, but, as I said, at some inscrutable moment things did right themselves. In December, at her thirtieth birthday party, Maud wryly commented to a group of friends that she hoped the coming year would be better than the last. It marked a new, hopeful phase.

In February, at the doorway of the East Village bar I was headed toward, I saw an impressive woman in a belted leather jacket. A spark of jealousy went off in me. *I need a leather jacket.* She was the kind of beautiful woman that throws me into a superficial tizzy, makes me reevaluate my life. *I shouldn't work such long hours at the office. I should really dress up more for these parties. I need to go shopping.* As I got closer, I saw it was Maud.

She was talking to our friend Hank about her novel. Editors were interested. There was going to be a conference call with her agent to discuss it the next day. Hank was praising. Maud was gesticulating. Her eyes were lived-in again, wise. Yes, I remember now, this is Maud.

I had a teetering, uncharitable moment: *That's it? You're better now?*

I wanted nothing more than to have Maud back, than to have Maud have Maud back, but now I didn't want to *forget*. Happiness was no longer an expectation, something big and looming to strive for, but actually right there in front of me, plain and simple, ready to be taken for granted again. Here was happiness: Maud standing before me in muscular exuberance. But Maud had also conjured the trembling subconscious of life (*I'm not real, I'm not here*). And watching it slink back to its hiding places, I needed to know that if we let it go, it wouldn't be roused again. It took me time not to want to needlessly slip the story into my conversations, yell it out all day long, to sternly remind Maud and myself how hard it had all been. I wanted to resuscitate the sadness if only to ward it off. Until slowly it dawned on me that Maud's sadness wasn't ever going away—it was right there in every swell and turn of my consciousness, smuggled always into our everyday lives. There it was in the curve of Maud's outstretched hand, rising up with her voice in conversation with Hank, settling down now in her hard-earned, knowing demeanor.

Yes, I remember now. *This* is Maud.

Addiction by Prescription: Women and the Problem of Tranquilizers

ANDREA TONE

Andrea Tone, excerpt from *The Age of Anxiety: A History of America's Turbulent Affair with Tranquilizers*, New York: Basic Books, 2008. Reprinted by permission.

On May 22, 1978, some seventeen million viewers of NBC's national evening news broadcast learned the medical misfortune of Cyndie Maginnis, a prescription drug addict. Like millions of other American women, the thirty-two-year-old wife and mother of three had struggled with the challenges of a busy life. When she discussed her difficulties with her gynecologist, he prescribed tranquilizers. When her problems got worse, he prescribed more. Maginnis soon discovered that she had become a prisoner of prescription pills, taking increasingly higher doses to keep calm. Breaking her tranquilizer habit proved difficult. "My body was completely out of whack," Maginnis told the NBC reporter. "Why did you wait so long before you got hooked?" the reporter asked. "I thought I was taking medicine," Maginnis replied.[1]

Maginnis's story represents one of hundreds of tranquilizer narratives recounted in newspapers, magazines, courtrooms, government investigations, and television studios across the United States in the 1970s and 1980s. Although the circumstances that turned anxious patients into drug addicts varied, "all" these narratives offered a chilling account of medicines and patients veering out of control.

The pessimistic and cautionary climate that propelled women such as Cyndie Maginnis onto the evening news was at odds with the heady optimism that had informed attitudes to tranquilizers only a few decades earlier. In the 1950s, researchers, journalists, and physicians had hailed meprobamate, the first of the minor tranquilizers, launched in 1955, as a triumph of American pharmaceutical science. The decade as a whole was characterized by widespread faith in the possibilities of pharmaceutical research; the reception and popularity of meprobamate must be understood in this historical context. Companies had recently made available a host of new prescription drugs, including antibiotics and synthetic hormones. Children who survived what a few years earlier might have been a deadly bout with bacterial pneumonia, adults with rheumatoid arthritis who were liberated from wheelchairs because of cortisone; these well-publicized triumphs seemed to provide tangible evidence of the wonders wrought by pharmaceutical medicine. Nor was there, as yet, public debate on the safety and efficacy of prescription medications. The thalidomide tragedy and DES disaster had yet to occur. In a society where "ethical" drugs enjoyed cultural currency and reports of drug-induced injuries were infrequent, the debut of an antianxiety pill induced much excitement.

Sold under the brand names Miltown and Equanil, meprobamate was flaunted as a safe and easy way to handle unproductive stress and anxiety. An article in the family magazine *Town Journal* typified the enthusiasm of the era. "Science has discovered an amazing new drug that effectively controls anxiety,"[2] it proclaimed. It "brings sleep to the sleepless, relaxation to the tense, tranquility to the nervous." The Hollywood tabloid *Uncensored!* reassured patients that they could take Miltown and Equanil with confidence because "they are not habit-forming and even a severe overdose can't kill you."[3] Word from prominent doctors was equally sanguine. Psychiatrist and researcher Dr. Nathan Kline, director of New York's Rockland State Hospital, told readers of *Business Week* that in its potential benefit to Americans, the advent of minor tranquilizers was "equal in importance to the introduction of atomic energy, if not more so." Meprobamate restored "full efficiency to business executives" and put artists and writers "suffering from long periods of nonproductivity because of 'mental blocks'" back on track.[4]

This kind of hyperbole had commercial and medical repercussions. Only fourteen months after it was made available, meprobamate had already become the country's largest-selling prescription drug.[5] By 1957, meprobamate was selling at a rate of one prescription per second.[6] With sales topping the $200 million mark, meprobamate became the first psychotropic wonder drug in medical history.[7]

In the 1950s housewives, but also male athletes, celebrities, and executives, were quick to praise their "tranks." While minor tranquilizers would later be discredited as mother's little helpers, their initial success stemmed from their use by a wide portion of the population. Indeed, the drug's fanatical following among businessmen in this decade earned it the nickname "Executive Excedrin." Pharmaceutical companies encouraged doctors to prescribe meprobamate to men, for firms had no financial incentive to confine tranquilizers to half the population. The surest path to profits was to position tranquilizers as a drug suitable for all anxious Americans. In advertisements for tranquilizers published in medical journals in the 1950s, the gender of the "anxious" patient was just as likely to be male as female.[8] From the male patient's perspective, moreover, there was as yet no reason for men to feel awkward or embarrassed about taking tranquilizers. As the "Executive Excedrin" label suggests, tranquilizers were very much a man's drug. The stigma of mother's little helper, which linked the feminization of prescription drug-taking to a rhetoric of dependence, emasculation, and societal decay, had not yet taken hold. In such a gender-neutral milieu, men remained avid users and outspoken proponents, effectively stoking patient demand.

By the 1970s, however, minor tranquilizers, which now included the best-selling benzodiazepine tranquilizers Librium, launched in 1960, and Valium, first marketed in 1963, had been recast as dangerous "women's" drugs. They were recklessly prescribed, aggressively promoted, and carelessly consumed, less a sign of the triumph of pharmaceutical science than a commercial bonanza achieved at women's expense. In Washington DC, Senator Edward Kennedy opened a 1979 hearing on the "Use and Misuse of Benzodiazepines" by warning that tranquilizers had "produced a nightmare of dependence and addiction, both very difficult to treat and recover from."[9]

What had caused this change? By the 1970s the pharmacological management of everyday nerves was a well-established tradition. In addition, studies documenting the addictive potential of meprobamate and benzodiazepines had been in print for almost a decade. What had changed, in short, was not the fact that Americans took tranquilizers—a whopping 800 tons in 1977—or that, like Cyndie Maginnis, many had a tough time when they stopped.[10] What was new in the 1970s was that Americans were, for the first time, anxious about their prescription drug behavior.

In the late 1960s, the United States was engulfed by worries that the cultural and therapeutic popularity of anxiolytics such as Valium made things

worse. The thalidomide tragedy and nagging doubts about the safety of oral contraceptives had burst the bubble of confidence in pharmaceutical panaceas. Patients across the country contemplated the extent to which drugs could hurt as well as heal. Thousands got caught up in the burgeoning women's health and consumer movements, which shared common ground in their suspicion of pharmaceutical and medical interests and their demands that patients be better apprised of the risks of all medical technologies, including drugs.

Tranquilizers previously lionized for their ability to patch social fissures were disparaged as disruptive and politically dangerous. Like Timothy Leary's LSD disciples, tranquilizer takers were "tuning out" the realities of the world. The fact that users got their drugs from doctors rather than on the streets made them no less dangerous. Indeed, it made the "drug problem" that much more far-reaching and ominous, for it meant that mind-altering agents had penetrated the "safe" inner sanctum of middle-class suburbia.

By the early 1970s, the media had seized on this image of chemical contamination to promote the idea of widespread but secret middle-class addiction. "Condemnation of drug abuse has been primarily directed against hippies and narcotics addicts," Leonard S. Brahen, the director of medical research and education in the Nassau County department of drug and alcohol addiction, told participants in the 1972 meeting of the New York Sate Medical Society. "We now recognize the abuse of mood changing drugs is more extensive, involving people in all socioeconomic classes. Most middle-class housewives use such agents legally and consciously. . . . There is [even] evidence that a smaller number of suburban housewives have experimented with marijuana.[11]

In this cacophony of concern, nothing was more disturbing than the realization that stay-at-home moms, sentimentalized symbols of wholesome family values, were drug users. "The typical woman who uses drugs to cope with life is not a fast-living rock star, nor a Times Square prostitute, nor a devotee of the drop-out-and-turn philosophy," reported the *Ladies Home Journal* in a 1971 exposé, "Women and Drugs: A Startling Journal Study."[12] "She is an adolescent, confused by the stresses of impending adulthood. She is a newlywed, by turns anxious and depressed by strains of adjustment to a new relationship and new responsibilities. She is a once-busy housewife, her youngsters grown, who finds her days increasingly empty and her thoughts obsessed with the inexorable passing of the years." She was, in short, "an average, middle-class American—one of the folks next door. She could even be you."

Women as a group consumed twice as many minor tranquilizers as men, but studies showed that it was non-wage-earning women aged thirty-five and over who consumed the most. A divorcée from Topeka took them for insomnia. "It does the trick," she told a reporter. A Des Moines housewife who got nervous at parties popped a Valium before heading out to put herself at ease. A mother of five found tending to her kids imposed "a lot of pressure." She took four pills a day, and was grateful for the relief. "I never feel jittery."[13]

Some researchers made these findings part of a broader feminist critique of society's mistreatment of women. The real problems, they averred, were the circumstances that led women to seek escape. Why, indeed, should a woman feel calm minding five children alone? How fulfilled could a woman be cleaning dirty floors and toddler spit-up? Why did society expect women to look and act a certain way? Tranquilizer use was a logical corollary to an unhealthy ordering of gender roles. Canadian sociologist Ruth Cooperstock found in her research for the Addiction Research Foundation that wage-earning women were significantly less likely to take tranquilizers than were women who stayed at home.[14] Cooperstock suggested that employment had a positive effect on women's well-being. It made them less anxious and "less apt to commit suicide." Sociologist Pauline Bart of Chicago's Abraham Lincoln School of Medicine reported that women often got locked into roles that made them unhappy. Isolated at home, they felt powerless to change their situations. "Instead of getting rid of the real constraints in their lives," Bart said, women take drugs "so they'll be better able to bear the pain."[15]

In a different time and place, these analyses might have fomented a political discussion of the mistreatment of women and a blueprint to help housewives experience their full potential as humans. But America's anti-drug fervor favored simple rationalizations over complicated explanations that shared the blame. Visionary thinking on this issue was left to the feminist movement and the women's health movement. The mainstream media instead projected a straightforward and ultimately more reassuring message that discounted women's grievances. They blamed pharmaceutical firms for excessive drug promotion and for cultivating an "unnecessary" market for tranquilizers for everyday problems. At the 1979 hearings on the use and abuse of benzodiazepines, Senator Edward Kennedy told the audience that "the whole pitch appears to be to sell and market, to sell and market."[16] Companies had medicalized something that could not be fixed with a pill.

These explanations resonated with Americans because, in part, they were true. Doctors had prescribed tranquilizers carelessly; companies had promoted them excessively. At the same time, media reports erased the nuances of a complicated history of drug development, diffusion, and everyday use. They did not, for instance, detail the commercial restraint that had characterized Miltown's release. Nor did they discuss the cultural and institutional enthusiasm for minor tranquilizers in the 1950s and early 1960s. Rarely did they mention that evidence of the drug's dependence liability had been well documented since 1961. Nor did they try to sort out the difficult question of what seemed to make Americans, particularly women, anxious in the first place, or what had prompted millions to endeavor to placate their troubles with something as seemingly simple as a pill.

NOTES

1. NBC evening news broadcast, May 22, 1978, located at Television News Archives, Vanderbilt University, Nashville, Tennessee.

2. Howard La Fay, "All Wound Up? Here's a New Drug to Calm You Down," *Town Journal* (May 1956), 72; Susan Speaker, "From 'Happiness Pills' to 'National Nightmare': Changing Cultural Assessments of Minor Tranquilizers in America, 1955-1980," Journal of the History of Medicine and Allied Sciences 52 (1997): 338-76.

3. Victor Schmidt, "What You Should Know about Those New 'Happiness Pills!,'" *Uncensored*, Oct. 25, 1957, 37.

4. Kline quoted in "Soothing—But Not for Drug Men" *Business Week*, March 10, 1956, 32.

5. "Tranquilizers—Successors to Aspirin?" *Chemical Week*, August 25, 1956, 18; La Fay, "All Wound Up?" 72.

6. Francis Bello, "The Tranquilizer Question," *Fortune* (May 1957), 162.

7. Thomas Whiteside, "Onward and Upward with the Arts: Getting There First with Tranquility," *The New Yorker*, May 3, 1958, 99; Elizabeth McFadden, "Tension Busters," *Newark Sunday News*, May 19, 1957, 17.

8. Jonathan Metzl, *Prozac on the Couch: Prescribing Gender in the Era of Wonder Drugs* (Durham and London: Duke University Press, 2003).

9. *The Use and Misuse of Benzodiazepines: Hearing Before the Subcommittee on Health and Scientific Research of the Committee on Labor and Human Resources*, United States Senate, Ninety-Sixth Congress, First Session on the Examination of the Use and Misuse of Valium, Librium, and other Minor Tranquilizers (GPO: Washington, D.C., 1979), 1.

10. Edward Shorter, *A Historical Dictionary of Psychiatry* (New York: Oxford University Press, 2005), 42.

11. Leonard S. Brahen, "Housewife Drug Abuse," *Journal of Drug Education* 3 (Spring 1973), 13.

12. Carl D. Chambers and Dodi Schultz, "Women and Drugs: A Startling Journal Survey," *Ladies Home Journal* (November 1971): 191.

13. "The Prisoner of Pills," *Newsweek*, April 24, 1978, 77; Penelope McMillan, "Women and Tranquilizers," *Ladies Home Journal* (November 1976): 164–67.

14. Ruth Cooperstock, "Sex Differences in Psychotropic Drug Use," *Social Science Medicine* 12 (July 1978): 179–86; Ruth Cooperstock and Henry L Lennard, "Some Social Meanings of Tranquilizer Use," *Sociology of Health and Illness* 14 (December 1979): 331–47; "Non-Working Wives Over 34 Are Biggest Users of Tranquilizers, Research Shows," nd., Hoffman-La Roche Manufacturers Files, FDA History Office.

15. Bart quoted in McMillan, "Women and Tranquilizers," 165.

16. Kennedy quoted in *Use and Misuse of Benzodiazepines*.

Women and Drug Addiction

STEPHEN R. KANDALL

Stephen R. Kandall, MD, excerpt from *Substance and Shadow: Women and Addiction in the United States*, Cambridge, Massachusetts: Harvard University Press, 1996. Reprinted by permission.

By 1782, it was common practice for the women of Nantucket Island to "take a dose of opium every morning." A century or so later, "although drug use was known to exist among women of all social classes, the stereotypical picture was that of a genteel white, middle- or upper-middle-class Southern lady much like the ennobled morphine-addicted Mrs. Henry Lafayette Dubose portrayed in Harper Lee's novel To Kill a Mockingbird.*" In every generation, physicians prescribe mind-numbing drugs to affluent female patients, but the roster of "respectable" products changes over time, depending, it seems, on who has the economic and political influence to determine what will be designated as "licit" or "illicit." In the nineteenth century, women relied on opiates, cocaine, chloral hydrate, and cannabis to numb their mental and physical pain; in the twentieth century, Dexedrine, Nembutal, Valium, Prozac. In the twenty-first, self-medication with legal but "alternative" treatments such as herb-based pills, tinctures, and teas—including ginseng, St. John's wort, valerian, chamomile, ginkgo biloba, and kava—may overtake the prescription market.*

The inability of contemporary society to deal with addiction in women in effective and comprehensive ways recapitulates the failures of the past. Historical information on women and drug use in the United States is far less accessible than comparable information on men. Precise statistical data on female addicts for the last half of the nineteenth century is lacking, and much of the available information is buried in physicians' anecdotes and pharmacy records. A few early surveys provide limited, if sometimes contradictory, information on this population. Given the primitive epidemiology of the time, the easy accessibility of unregulated "patent" medicines, and the fact that women's opiate addiction was often unknown to their families, or if known, quietly tolerated, this scarcity is not surprising.

A number of major themes recur throughout the following chapters. The central one is that in a society where drugs have been available from early times, women have always made up a significant portion, and at times a majority, of America's drug users and addicts. Popular stereotypes notwithstanding, addicted women have come from a variety of racial, geographic, and socioecominic backgrounds, and these factors have affected individual patterns of drug use. If these women share any common bond, it is that their addiction has not yielded to treatment. Despite their intentions, guilt and shame, both self-imposed and societal, have pushed them to the margins of society.

A second theme is the inappropriate and often excessive medication of women by physicians and pharmacists, which, along with women's own self-medication, has been a significant component of the female addiction problem. Voltaire once said that "doctors pour drugs, of which they know little, for diseases, of which they know less, into patients—of whom they know nothing." Throughout recent history, women have been thought to need "special protection" and were regarded as less able to bear pain and psychic discomfort, whether because of "women's diseases" and "neurasthenia," as in the Victorian era, or the modern-day stresses of running a busy household, competing in a male-dominated workforce, or attempting to conform to society's slender, youthful ideal. The fact that physicians, physicians' wives, and nurses have been disproportionately afflicted by addiction, and are thus less likely to view it as a "problem, has resulted in the under-estimation of its gravity. In addition, the number of female physicians, who might be expected to be more sensitive to women's needs and life stresses, has increased only in recent years.

A third theme is the unique role of women as childbearers, child rearers, and child medicators. Throughout the nineteenth century, concerned voices called attention to the dangers of the opiate-laden homeopathic and allopathic (or "conventional") medications mothers and nurses gave to children at home. Until such drugs were regulated in the early years of this century, women were held increasingly responsible for their inappropriate administration. (This theme resurfaces with new virulence in the prosecution of women for drug use during pregnancy in the 1980s.)

A fourth theme is the link between female sexuality and drug use. The association is an ancient one. Within the context of the past century and a half, it has pervaded the issues of prostitution, the perceived or proclaimed sexual threats to women from minorities, the glamorization of drug-associated sex, the connection between psychedelic drug use and "free love," and the contemporary drug-using mother's "triple curse": minority status, HIV-positive diagnosis, and children who are "drug babies."

A fifth theme is that, although concern about women's drug use has been raised, and to some degree acknowledged, for over a century, the specific issue of helping drug-addicted women was not directly confronted until the early 1970s. Before the Second World War, much of the attention focused on women and drugs came from the less-than-objective press and from the movie industry, which, by sensationalizing the threat posed to women by socially marginalized groups such as Chinese immigrants, Southern black males, and Mexican migrant workers, both mirrored and shaped society's attempts to control these "socially deviant" groups. While it is true that some women were passive beneficiaries of such drug treatment efforts as sanitariums, drug clinics, and methadone maintenance programs, not until the 1970s, following the emergence of the Women's Movement and various self-help initiatives, did addicted women finally begin to receive attention in their own right. Even then, drug-using women, especially those belonging to racial and ethnic minorities, faced hostility, prejudicial reporting to legal and child protection authorities, and criminal prosecution for drug-related conduct during pregnancy. The story of women and drugs in the United States is an ongoing one and there is, unfortunately, no end in sight.

Silver Hills

ERICA WARREN

Erica Warren, "Silver Hills," 2008. Original for this publication.

As we come as a society to understand addiction as a phenomenon with both physiological and genetic components, Erica Warren examines the effect of her aunt's years of alcoholism and subsequent rehabilitation in the context of the changing lives of four generations of women in her family. As her grandmother struggles to understand her daughter's problems, her mother to heal her ailing sister, and Erica's sister to begin raising her infant daughter, the author tries to find her role and legacy amidst these other brave women.

The talking heads buzz: ". . . with little relief in sight. The heat will continue as we get into next week, with a slight break around Thursday, when highs will only reach the lower nineties . . ."

"Turn off that TV, we're ready to go!" my mother's voice announced through the wall from the kitchen, an order given over a loudspeaker. I heard her bound through her room to grab the final batch of last-minute items: sunglasses, road map, cough drops.

I returned to the living room with my own necessary items, and was confronted by my mother, sister, and niece waiting for me. Child, mother, and grandmother stood silhouetted against the bay windows, waves of heat visible on the far side of the glass. I handed the binky over to Crystal, who popped it into her daughter's mouth in one swift, unthinking motion.

". . . and now we turn from the Weather Center to more local cover—"

Crystal cut the newscaster off by the press of a button.

"I'll probably lose it before we get very far," she admitted as we moved outside.

The car had been running long enough to cut the harshest of the heat, but the short walk from the front door of the house to this chilled haven proved to me that the air is a real, tangible, living thing. Crystal strapped her daughter in the back seat, my mom took the steering wheel, and I folded myself in next to her.

Annabelle's necessary traveling supplies—bags of diapers, multiple changes of clothes, blankets, toys, and so forth—filled the unused spaces in the back, flanked by the baby's car seat and her mother. My necessary traveling supplies—a book and, according to my mother, my license—nestled between my feet. I figured I could use the license as a bookmark, since it wouldn't be of much use otherwise. I doubted I would be getting carded anywhere.

A close friend once told me not to put the organ-donor sticker on my driver's license.

"Seriously, it's true," he insisted. "This situation rarely happens I'm sure, but all things being equal between two patients, the paramedics will take the non-organ donor to the hospital first if you're ever in a car wreck."

I put the organ donor sticker on my driver's license.

Although I don't know what use my organs would be after my mangled body flew through the windshield on impact, ricocheting off the offending tree, guardrail, embankment, before slapping the asphalt with a crack and a thud. Whatever force—intentional or otherwise—that led to the accident would leave my bones in shards, my flesh smeared across the ground in a manner more resembling some unfortunate woodland creature than a nineteen-year-old on a pointless errand with her family.

Maybe they could salvage something from the

wreckage of my body; I would be sacrificed to save the irresponsible. Those who thought they could separate their lives from those around them would learn that their bodies belong to us as much as to them. No one would have to worry about what my aunt Liz's drinking was doing to her liver; she could have mine. There would be no more concern over Ellen's refusal to go on dialysis after her kidneys failed. I would end the self-destructive tendencies of my kin; stop them from tearing my family apart. And I wouldn't have to watch my mother cry anymore, I wouldn't have to hear her sob "I just don't want another sister to die."

A blinding ray of sunlight reflecting off the car ahead of us jolted me out of my reverie: my flesh was intact, Ellen was dead, and everything else was falling apart.

I pulled the visor down, trying to shield some of the blinding rays from my face. I hadn't planned on sun. I figured that the weather should empathize with my mood and my mission, cast heavy clouds and gusty winds, interspersed with eerie stillness. The clouds should be of the kind that compel mothers to send their children inside to play, to take the laundry in (even if it's still a bit damp at the end)—but nothing would fall from the heavens to quench the parched earth, to feed the stunted corn that flew past our car. "'Knee-high by the Fourth of July,' my mother always used to say," Mom announced into the stream of cool air blowing into her face. Her immediate response to my puzzled stare was to jerk her head toward the fields, like she was trying to get water out of her ear. "The corn, it should be taller by now."

"Yeah, well it should have gotten a lot more rain." Against my deeper feelings, I continued the trivial chatter we kept circling through. The more she talked, the less she'd have to think.

"Well, we're lucky it's such a sunny day." My mother trailed off, less interested in what was happening around her. I mumbled in agreement, although I secretly believed that luck had little to do with the weather. A more likely culprit was the confluence of certain meteorological phenomena

that led to not only a severe drought but the longest heat wave New England had seen in some time.

"How much longer until we get there?" Crystal whispered from behind me, having finally convinced Annabelle that it would be better to sleep through most of the ride.

"I don't . . ." my mother trailed off. She was equally mesmerized by the two figures swimming through the atmosphere in front of us. "I'm sorry, what did you say?"

The heat waves shimmered on the road, revealing reflections in distant, imaginary lakes.

"How much longer until we get there?" my sister repeated from behind me.

"Well, we have reservations at Mulino's at six-thirty tonight, so we should be at your grandmother's house no later than five."

The mirage I had been staring at evaporated before we had traveled much further.

"Mom, we . . . aren't we stopping to see Liz first?" Crystal looked puzzled.

"Oh, right." My mother sighed, knowing that she could not get away with feigning amnesia. "Well, Gramma said that we should meet her there at one. We'll have lunch with Liz, and then we're going back with Gramma to meet Jack before dinner."

False reality tried to reassert itself in front of me in the form of a liquid highway. But now it only reinforced the memory of the heat hovering just outside the pane of glass next to my face. I leaned back in my seat and closed my eyes.

My toes played with the air conditioning vent. The cover of the one to my right was missing. Well, it was not so much missing as shattered into pieces too small to be of any use. I tried to imagine my aunt Liz's hand as it slammed into the rigid plastic of the vent on the passenger side. She was probably screaming and fighting with my mother as her flailing leg found its way through the windshield, at which point the air conditioning was more or less a moot issue. My mom had to drive the rest of the way to the hospital with the car in that condition, with my aunt in that condition.

Mom wouldn't talk about it, though. She just

returned home that night last week with her puffy eyes and went to bed. Only later did I divine the story from brief explanations and whispered details around the house.

A blood alcohol level of .08 will get you arrested for drunk driving. A blood alcohol level of .15 shows highly noticeable lack of coordination; one is clearly drunk at this point. A blood alcohol level of .40 will most likely kill you. My aunt Liz had a blood alcohol level of .30 when my mother took her to the hospital that night. She doesn't remember what she did to our car, but this was certainly not the first time Liz had blacked out and damaged something after a binge. Usually it was just herself she endangered.

Even though my mother is one of six children, the task of taking care of Liz has fallen to her. Her brothers—Chris and Dave—have moved too far away to be of much help. Her youngest sister, Pattie, tries, but she tends to fall apart when faced with conflict. Yet, while my youngest aunt's tears will fall at the shortest notice, the only time I can remember seeing my mother cry is when she got hit in the thigh with a softball when I was twelve. It left a bruise the size of a dinner plate. That was until this summer, though.

Her sixth and oldest sibling, Ellen, died less than a month ago.

My grandparents live about twenty minutes away from their daughter Liz, but after the relatively unexpected death of their first-born child, one can hardly expect them to be strong enough to deal with her alcoholic mishaps. So my mother has been making the hour and a half drive down from our house in western Massachusetts about two or three times a week since Ellen passed away in early June to try to prevent Liz from following their sister into the ground.

When my mother returned from the last trip, she was driving a rental car. She had gotten a hysterical call from my grandmother the night before, eventually finding her sister in the highly intoxicated state I've already mentioned. Liz's demolition of my mother's car from the inside occurred on the way to the emergency room. Upon arrival the doctors stabilized her enough to ensure that she'd make it through the night without dying, but my mom and grandmother insisted on checking her out when they learned that she would go to a locked ward for detox. Instead they took Liz home and did the detox themselves, holding her down when her shaking body threatened to fling itself out of the bed.

At least seeing the horror of her life infect the lives of those around her was enough to inflict a modicum of sense into Liz's psyche. Once her mother and sister explained to her what she had done, Liz even admitted (for the moment) that she had a serious problem. At least seriously endangering someone besides herself got her to admit herself to a rehab program. She had been at Silver Hills Hospital for almost a week by the time we were allowed to trek down for a highly supervised luncheon. Or (as my mother explained when she told me what today's agenda would be), since we were "going to be in the neighborhood anyway for Gramma's birthday, we might as well drop in and say hello."

Silver Hills is another two hours south of Gramma's house. Also, I didn't ever recall going to celebrate her birthday as a family too often in the past.

"Keep your eyes peeled for a drugstore or a supermarket or something," Mom urged us. "When I talked to Liz last night she said that she had such a craving for chocolate."

"Good time for a stop anyway," my sister chimed in from the back seat, "Annabelle is getting fussy and could use a diaper change."

Annabelle was born about four months ago. Crystal's difficult pregnancy—preparing for the single mom thing in the rare moments when she was not racked with bouts of nausea—necessitated a scheduled, induced birth in early March. This was vicariously thrilling for me, as it occurred during my spring break from college, and I had never seen a person that brand-new before.

Those two weeks were surreal for me; I actually

saw my sister transform into a mother before my eyes. There is nothing more inspiring than watching someone rise to a difficult situation with grace.

While Annabelle's actual birth was well planned, her conception was much less so. A little over a year ago my sister gathered my family to announce that she, at twenty, was pregnant and going to be having a baby. My grandmother cried for a week when she found out that Crystal had no plans to get married to Annabelle's father. My mother was upset about this as well, but accepted Crystal's decisions more quickly than my grandmother did. At least Mom kept quiet about her discontent a little more successfully. Outwardly my mother would only complain that my sister was just "a bit young," and that she herself would be a grand-mother at the unthinkable age of forty-four.

With my sister only being a year older than me, I struggled at times with the gulf that had formed between our daily lives. I had to worry about things like writing papers, declaring a major, and getting through another boring day of filing at an office that summer. My sister had to worry about diapers and health insurance, finding a safe place to raise her daughter, and getting a decent job while still being able to afford day care.

Thankfully, it only took a moment to cut our way through the heavy atmosphere of the parking lot and reach the front of "Big K," as the store is now titled. The cool air wafting in through the au-tomatic doors calmed Annabelle, her attention immediately diverted from her discomfort to the bright lights, moving people, and layered sounds of commerce. Crystal and Annabelle followed the arrow under a sign marked "Restroom," and got swallowed by the crowd.

As we approached the register I grabbed some-thing dropping from Mom's arms. She was loaded with an assortment of goodies: hard peppermint candies, chocolate caramel chews, Starbursts, and wintergreen chewing gum in one arm, a dozen almond Hershey's bars and a bottle of hair-spray in the other. It must have looked like we were going to some crazy midsummer Halloween party, not visiting my aunt in rehab. I hoped everyone would be wearing a costume.

"Liz said they took away her hairspray," she ex-plained as if I had asked. "I don't know if they will let me give her some, but I want her to see that I tried."

We made our way through the sea of humidity to the car, where Crystal had already started the air conditioning and was strapping her daughter in for the second leg of our journey. Clean and cool, Annabelle was back to her usual spunky self, waving around an old set of metal measuring spoons—her favorite toy. The spoons clanked and rattled in the air as we approached the car, and Annabelle greeted her grandmother and aunt with a series of "ooooahhhhheeee" and "thhhhh-hbbbbbbbtsssss."

Back on the road. The parched landscape flew by, and my eyelids began to droop. I'd never been a fan of waking up at seven in the morning only to spend four hours cramped into a bucket seat flying down a road through violently green expanses of midsummer tobacco farms.

Mom, her eyes still focused on the road, asked, "Can you open the glove compartment and get out the directions to the hospital and tell me which exit we have to take?"

I complied with her orders and fished through the maps and papers until I found the pamphlet. "Silver Hills Hospital, founded in 1931, is a na-tionally recognized, not-for-profit psychiatric hos-pital with an outstanding record and tradition." It reassured me.

"Exit ten," I informed my mother. I read on in the pamphlet. Apparently we couldn't bring Liz hairspray. Or much else for that matter. I looked under the heading "Barrett House: Transitional Living—Chemical Dependency for Women." The photograph looked quaint, "a beautiful campus-like setting" nestled in "sixty idyllic acres in the New England countryside." At first glance you would think it was my fancy liberal arts college, with some great history of academic excellence behind it. To my knowledge, however, they don't have to lock you in at college. Guests generally don't have to be searched. Escorts aren't required whenever students leave their dormitories, and they are generally allowed to have such commodities as hairspray, cologne, cough syrup, and candy.

Liz was not in some ivy-league academic institution. As my father's brother Jack, a recovering alcoholic himself, would explain to us later, Liz was in denial. If she can have hairspray and makeup then she looks good, and she's not in rehab, and she doesn't have a problem. If she looks like shit then she's a lush and her sister is dead and she's running trains over her parents and siblings. It's an important step for the forty-two year old to accept the reality of her life.

"Mental development basically stops when someone becomes an alcoholic," he explained, sitting on the peach and sea green couch in my grandmother's living room. "I don't know if it's a proven fact, but at the very least it's a good metaphor for her state right now."

Jack will meet up with us later in the day, after our little visit with Liz. My mother invited him to dinner, ostensibly to spend time with the family.

"While she may be forty-two in reality, I highly doubt that she believes that's how old she is. Mentally she's thirty-four, twenty-six—whatever age she started her addiction."

I soon realized that the real purpose of the visit was to let him talk to my grandparents. No one else would be able to understand what Liz was going through right now; maybe not even Liz herself.

"Right now she's on a 'pink cloud,' as many people call it. Her time spent in rehab will help her get out of denial about her addiction, but it will also give her a sense that she is in control and can take care of anything."

"That's good, though . . . right?" my mom asked from her position on the other side of the room. She was flanked by my grandmother, sister, and niece on one side; my grandfather and aunt Pattie

on the other. My father and brother were around somewhere in the house.

"Well, it's not really good or bad. Yes, taking control of her life is important, but things aren't as easy in the real world as they are for her at the hospital. Control is part of the problem, because this is something she can't control."

My grandmother made a face.

"Do you believe this is a disease?" Jack looked toward my grandmother, but he was asking us all.

"Well . . . I suppose she could have certain genetic predispositions . . ." Gramma trailed off, unwilling to follow through with the argument welling inside.

"You have to understand that this is not something she chooses to do if you want to be of any help to her. It's as much a disease as Ellen's diabetes was."

"I know, I know, that is what the people at Silver Hills keep telling me. But . . . I don't know. I just don't understand why she doesn't just make up her mind and stop drinking!"

Jack paused, letting us all absorb that statement. "So you think it's just a matter of will power?"

"That has to be a part of it."

"Well, it's like I was saying before. Alcoholics are some of the most willful people in the world. I bet Liz is the type of person who'll go to work no matter how sick she is. If there is something she wants to do, she'll do it."

"Yeah, that's definitely her," my mother chimed in.

"Well, that's part of her problem with alcoholism. It's something she can't control, but that lack of control just makes her feel worse about herself, so she'll continue to want to 'self-medicate' with alcohol."

While Jack's case—sober longer than I've been aware—would offer some hope when we would need it, the statistics do not.

"With modern psychiatry and medications," he explained, "maybe a third of alcoholics in the United States reach what would be considered some kind of remission or recovery. Most go back to drinking at some point. No one ever really gets over it."

My grandmother was skeptical, but Jack continued.

"Even though I haven't had a drink in years, it's still something I have to deal with every day. It was a while before I admitted to myself that I can never have another drink."

He took a sip of his root beer.

"I even ran into a psychologist at an event a few months back," Jack continued. "He said that he was studying alcoholism, so I told him I am a recovering alcoholic. After I told him my story, he had the nerve to say to me, 'Well, you should have a drink. I'm sure after all of this time you could just have one.' I didn't know what to say. That's the problem, I *can't* just have one. And neither can Liz."

Annabelle began to wake up as we pulled into Silver Hills's Visitor Parking Lot. She stretched and yawned, blinking her dark blue baby eyes in the sun. We held our breath collectively, waiting for the wail that generally follows awakening from a nap. Who could blame her, leaving a dreaming state for our real world can be traumatic.

There were no tears this time though. She reached for a stuffed piggy, and as my mother turned off the engine Crystal took her daughter, piggy and all, out of the car seat. Annabelle waggled the stuffed animal in the air, laughing as she dropped it in the dust. It was a laugh that can come solely from one who knows only the moment, someone who understands the importance of the little things: a full stomach, a restful nap, a warm hug from a loved one. I smiled, despite myself.

As we walked up the hill to the front gate, I could spy my grandmother waving to us. She had a lot of energy for such a small woman. I always thought that she seemed to get smaller every time I saw her because I was growing. Lately I've realized that she's been shrinking all the while. At this point she couldn't have been taller than five feet.

"Happy birthday, Gram," I wished her as we approached.

"Oh, thanks so much sweetie," she bubbled. Her small, round frame was clothed in her trademark outfit: a brightly colored sweatshirt with matching stirrup pants, finished off with a white pair of Keds. Today the ensemble was of a lighter shade and material than usual.

"And there's Annabelle!" she cheered as her face lit up. Crystal handed the baby over to her great-grandmother.

"Annabelle says happy birthday too," Crystal assured her.

"Well, thank you very much," my grandmother crooned to Annabelle.

Annabelle played with her great-grandmother's necklace.

"Have visiting hours started yet?" my mother asked as she approached us.

"They're just about to. I was just waiting for you all to get here. They are serving lunch up in the main building, where Liz is waiting for us."

It was a bit of a hike up from the front gate. The main building was placed on the highest part of the land, and when we reached the top I stopped to look around. The view would have been grand if it weren't for the haze from the heat.

My grandmother was looking west.

As we entered the foyer of the building a uniformed man stopped us.

"I need to look through your bags for contraband," he said with a stern glare.

"Well, I brought these for my sister." My mom handed over the bag from K-Mart. The guard rumbled through the contents, removing everything except for the hard candies.

"They are not allowed," he said, gesturing to the hairspray and candy bars on the table next to him. "You can leave them here and pick them up before you leave."

With that he pressed a blue button on the wall next to his table. A long buzz sounded, accompanied by the click of the lock as the main door opened.

"Hi everybody!" the excited voice of my aunt Liz sounded as the door swung open. We shuffled forward into the main room. The building was basically a very large house, and we were standing in the living room area. It was well furnished and full of little groups of people hugging and talking in hushed voices. It could almost have been a conference center, if it weren't for the security guard studying us in his booth by the door.

Liz ran forward to hug us all. She looked better than I expected her to, but then again I don't know what I was really expecting. Was she supposed to look on the outside the way I imagined she looked on the side?

No, she was just Liz, as much like I remembered her as possible. She was definitely my mother's sister—same nose, same smile, same hair. My mother—having given birth to three children—had a rounder figure than her younger sister, but the resemblance was still striking.

Liz came up and hooked me in a strong embrace. "It's so good to see you," she said.

"It's great to see you too," I eked out over her tight hold. "How . . . How are you?" It was out before I thought about the ramifications of this question. It's usually such a harmless thing to ask.

"I'm . . . I'm working on it."

The group of us moved into the dining room, where a buffet lunch was set out for the patients and their guests. I was blown away by the spread. There were sandwiches and fruit and cheesecake. They had any sort of soft drink or juice you could imagine, squished between Caesar salad and bagels. All of this was served on real dinnerware with full place settings at each table. Cloth napkins too.

Unfortunately I wasn't really in the mood to chow down, so I just got a drink and half a plate of salad to play with while my family ate their midday meal. The meeting was rather uneventful. Liz went for Annabelle as soon as she could, and held the baby for as long as she would stay away from her mother.

"What a darling," Liz repeated over and over again, while Annabelle played with the bread on her plate.

"Yeah, she's the cutest baby ever," my mom chimed in. "It's really wonderful to have her around all of the time."

"Even at three in the morning?" Liz chuckled.

"Well, Crystal takes care of that."

Liz told us a little of what she had been doing at Silver Hills—the meetings, the psychiatrists, the other patients. The conversation generally moved away from these details as quickly as they were mentioned.

"So how are you, Erica?"

"I'm not too bad, just working this summer."

"Oh really? That's good, keeps you busy."

"I suppose."

"What are you doing?"

"Nothing interesting, just working at an office filing and filling in for the receptionist."

"I was a receptionist when I was your age," my grandmother said wistfully. "I was very good at it too. I always liked typing, answering phones, things like that. I couldn't work very long though. They tried to get me to sign a contract that said I wouldn't get married for five years, or at least say that I wouldn't have any children for that long. But I was seeing your grandfather then." She trailed off a bit. "And once . . . once the children came along, I had to stay home with them."

"I wish I could stay home with Annabelle all of the time," Crystal said. "That would be ideal. But money doesn't grow on trees, right?"

"That's why I'm glad I only had three kids," my mom said. "Once you kids were all in school it was no problem for me to go back to work."

I got a piece of chocolate cake before we left, but barely had time to finish it. Visiting hours were quickly coming to a close, we realized, as people in the same uniforms as the guard by the door guided guests out. They were not pushy, but certainly had authority with the patients. We said our good-byes.

A step out of the door reminded me how much I had come to depend on air conditioning. *At the very least,* I thought to myself, *Liz doesn't have to worry about this heat much, being locked inside most of the day.*

We worked our way down to the car, sitting under a nearby tree while my mother opened the doors for it to cool down. In a few minutes we were back on the road for the trip northward, to my grandmother's house.

My mother turned the radio on with a click.

" . . . after this break for a news update from our local . . ."

"That wasn't so bad," my mother sighed.

"No, it wasn't. She looked good," Crystal proclaimed from the back.

" . . . heat continues to be a problem throughout New England . . ."

"Eeeahhhhh!!" Annabelle added self-assuredly.

"Lunch was pretty good," I shrugged.

"Yeah, just a stop at Gramma's before dinner, then we should be back home by ten tonight," my mom updated us.

"And then back to work tomorrow," I sighed.

"Back to normal."

" . . . relief from a storm system developing just west of us . . ."

CHAPTER 15

Rape and Violence Against Women

FOR MANY YOUNG WOMEN, it is an introduction to feminist activism: a large college march called "Take Back the Night." Laura Eldridge well remembers her first one at Barnard College in the spring of her freshman year in the late 1990s. It had been raining that day, and the air was still misty. Hundreds of women gathered together, many holding homemade signs, to walk around their New York City neighborhood and declare their rights to be on the street. It was an amazing environment to find herself in—the sense of women coming together to make a change was palpable. It is, I think, the closest that many young women come to having a taste of what it must have been like to be a part of the energy and passion of second-wave activism.

After the march, Laura sat on the lawn of the college, still damp from the day's drenching, and listened for hours as women got up to tell their stories—of sexual abuse as children, of rape, of unthinkable sexual violence experienced in their lives. For those who had been lucky enough to avoid such tragedy, it was eye-opening. All women spoke not just to the brutality of the crimes committed against them, but to the power of sharing their stories in helping them to heal. Laura and her friends sat closely together on a beach towel and hoped not to recognize the voice of a friend.

Susan Brownmiller changed the face of activism on the issue of violence against women with her landmark book *Against Our Will*, originally published in 1975. A former civil rights activist, Brownmiller got involved with the women's movement after the Miss America protests in Atlantic City in 1968. The book, still unequalled on the subject, created a psychological and historical profile of rape and led to great anti-violence work on the part of women's movement activists.

The college campus still remains, unfortunately, an environment where rape is not only possible, but one where rapists are often protected by school administrations wary of having their statistics rise and scare potential students and their parents. Ask any young woman about the incidence of rape on her campus and you're likely to get the same answer—officially there are none. But every woman I know can name a friend or a peer who has gone through this horrible ordeal. Some campuses even lack rape crisis facilities. Young women have responded to this need with enthusiasm and energy. Helen Lowery and Nicole Levitz attended Boston University, an immense urban school with over thirty thousand students but no rape crisis center. While still seniors, the two girls changed this by organizing a "Take Back the Night" march and starting a family justice center.

Violence against women inside their families and communities continues to be a major challenge facing women.

Margaret Lazarus's Academy Award–winning 1994 documentary *Defending Our Lives* presents the stories of several women who share a terrible secret. It's not, as you might imagine, that they are victims of domestic abuse, although they are, and their harrowing stories make the movie one of the most compelling treatments of the subject. The secret the women share is that they are in prison for killing their abusers. Legal definitions of murder involve thinking about "premeditation" that ignores the psychology of the battered woman. Because many women kill or maim abusers while they sleep or are similarly indisposed—a clear sign that they planned the attack—they are often held accountable for the greater crime of murder without regard to the terrible violence done to these women, many of whom were held prisoner by partners who would most likely have eventually killed them.

The issue of domestic violence is a personal one for me. For many years, I was abused by my second husband, a man who seemed to friends and relatives to be the picture of a charming, loving man. After being hospitalized—again—after one of his attacks, a thoughtful nurse figured out what was going on and asked me if I was in danger. Her questions got me on the road to leaving my batterer and also made me start thinking about how we could change the ways that hospitals deal with women when abuse is suspected. Rather than relying on vague questions, women should be asked directly if they are being beaten and if they would like help.

Unfortunately, not all women were as lucky as I was. Hedda Nussbaum's tragic story made headlines in the late 1980s when her partner of over a decade, Joel Steinberg, beat their adopted daughter Lisa to death. Nussbaum herself had endured years of unthinkable abuse at Steinberg's hands, followed by years of scrutiny from the press and even feminist activists who felt she was little better than a drug addict who had let her daughter die. From this catastrophe, Nussbaum has recovered herself and her life, and has written a riveting book about her experiences, *Surviving Domestic Terrorism*. Her writing and her activism have helped many other women identify potentially deadly partnerships.

Judith Herman's *Trauma and Recovery* has been described as the most important new psychiatric book since Freud. A compassionate thinker and a lovely writer, Judy has greatly influenced the thinking of her colleagues, as well as the general public. Several selections in this chapter, including some from Herman's groundbreaking book, have been consciousness-raising.

Against Our Will: Men, Women, and Rape

SUSAN BROWNMILLER

Susan Brownmiller, excerpt from *Against Our Will: Men, Women and Rape*, New York: Simon & Schuster, 1975. Copyright ©1975. Reprinted with the permission of Simon and Schuster.

VICTIMS: THE SETTING

The rape fantasy exists in women as a man-made iceberg. It can be destroyed—by feminism. But first we must seek to learn the extent of its measurements.

Male sexual fantasies are blatantly obvious in the popular culture. Female sexual fantasies are quite another matter. Rarely have we been allowed to explore, discover, and present what might be some workable sexual daydreams, if only we could give them free rein. Rather, our female sexual fantasies have been handed to us on a brass platter by those very same men who have labored so lovingly to promote their own fantasies. Because of this deliberate cultural imbalance, most women, I think, have an unsatisfactory fantasy life when it comes to sex. Having no real choice, women have either succumbed to the male notion of appropriate female sexual fantasy or we have found ourselves largely unable to fantasize at all. Women who have accepted male-defined fantasies are often quite uncomfortable with them, and for very good reason. Their contents, as Helene Deutsch would be the first to say, are indubitably masochistic.

What percentage of women fantasize about sex? Frankly, I do not know the answer, nor would I care to hazard a guess. I know of no objective studies that deal with the nature and prevalence of women's sexual fantasies. Kinsey did not delve into this area; nor, as yet, have Masters and Johnson. I am vehemently hostile to suggestions that some known, popular sex fantasies attributed to women are indeed the product of a woman's mind. I am thinking here of the scurrilous, anonymous pornographic classic *The Story of O* and its dreary catalogue of whips, thongs, bonds, and iron chastity belts that represents the pinnacle, or should I say the nadir, of painful masochism. I first became acquainted with *O* when it made the rounds of my college dormitory. It was during finals week, as I recall, and I was looking for some diversion. I nearly retched before I closed the book and handed it back to the giver. A few years ago, when I was working for one of the TV news networks, a fellow writer earnestly presented this same book to me as "the truest, deepest account of female sexuality" he had ever encountered. I am sorry I behaved with such civility at my second refusal of *O* and "her" story.

Because men control the definitions of sex, women are allotted a poor assortment of options. Either we attempt to find enjoyment and sexual stimulation in the kind of passive, masochistic fantasies that men have prepared us for, or we reject these packaged fantasies as unhealthy and either remain fantasy-less or cast about for a private, more original, less harmful daydream. Fantasies are important to the enjoyment of sex, I think, but it is a rare woman who can successfully fight the culture and come up with her own non-exploitative, nonsadomasochistic, non-power-driven imaginative thrust. For this reason, I believe, most women who reject the masochistic fantasy role reject the temptation of all sexual fantasies, to our sexual loss.

Given the pervasive male ideology of rape (the mass psychology of the conqueror), a mirror-image female victim psychology (the mass psychology of the conquered) could not help but arise. Near its extreme, this female psychosexuality indulges in the fantasy of rape. Stated another way, when women do fantasize about sex, the fantasies are usually the product of male conditioning and cannot be otherwise.

Two extreme examples of male fantasy that were commercially palmed off as female fantasy in recent years have been the pornographic movies *Deep Throat* and *The Devil in Miss Jones,* and I cannot deny I know a few women who claim they enjoyed seeing them. However I am not talking about such obvious junk; I am talking about the normal run of the mill books and movies with the theme of man as the conquering sexual hero, works that influence the daydreams of women as well as men.

I do not mean to suggest that a woman's basic erotic fantasy, through cultural conditioning, is a fantasy of being raped. Rape is simply a noticeable marker near the end of a masochistic scale that ranges from passivity to death. And I do not intend to limit this discussion to specific erotic fantasies. At issue here is Everywoman's attitude toward her sexuality, her being, her attractiveness to men.

I owe it to Helene Deutsch to quote from her writings, since she was the first to define the female rape fantasy. Deutsch writes

> The conscious masochistic rape fantasies are indubitably erotic, since they are connected with masturbation. They are less genital in character than the symbolic dreams, and involve blows and humiliations; in fact, in rare cases the genitals themselves are the target of the act of violence. In other cases, they are less cruel, and the attack as well as the overpowering of the girl's will constitute the erotic element. Often the fantasy is divided into two acts: the first, the masochistic act, produces the sexual tension, and the second, the amorous act, supplies all the delights of being loved and desired. These fantasies vanish with the giving up of masturbation and yield to erotic infatuations detached from direct sexuality. The masochistic tendency now betrays itself only in the painful longing and wish to suffer for the lover (often unknown). . . . Many women retain these masochistic fantasies until an advanced age.[1]

The combination of perception and dogma contained in the above paragraph continues to amaze me no matter how many times I read it through. The conscious rape fantasy is offered as proof of inherent female masochism; masturbation is seen as an adolescent stage to be "given up." Yet despite these rigidities in her thought, Deutsch perceives that the female rape fantasy is no simple matter: For some, the rape of the will constitutes the erotic element; yet for others, the sufferance of a physical attack, or mental abuse, is a necessary prelude to the acceptance of love and affection. These two quite different sets of responses might have given Deutsch a clue that the most significant factor of all lies precisely in the lack of a uniform response. I would conclude that both sets of responses, or utilizations of the rape daydream, indicate a pitiful effort on the part of young girls, as well as older women, to find their sexuality within the context of the male power drive. This effort is the crux of woman's sexual dilemma.

NOTE

1. Helene Deutsch, "The Conscious Masochistic Rape Fantasies," *The Psychology of Women*, New York: Grune Stratton, 1944–1945, p. 225.

Rape Doesn't End with a Kiss

PAULINE BART

Pauline Bart, "Rape Doesn't End with a Kiss," *Viva*, June 1975. Reprinted by permission.

In November 1974, Viva *magazine published a questionnaire asking readers who had been victims of rape to help gather information about this widespread yet highly misunderstood crime. Dr. Pauline Bart analyzed the enormous response from over a thousand women—the most wide-ranging survey ever taken in this country.*

Psychiatrists say a gun is a substitute phallus. After reading and analyzing the stories of 1,070 rape victims I find the reverse to be true. When it comes to rape, a phallus is a substitute gun. Rape is a power trip, not a passion trip. The rapist is more likely to rape in cold blood, with contempt and righteousness, than with passion. And women don't relax. They don't enjoy it. They don't much trust or like men afterward—a long time afterward. And they don't forget it. It haunts their lives.

As one woman wrote, "The rape and attempted rape . . . have combined to foul up my relationships with men to the point where I react irrationally when angered. All men, my present husband and son included, lose their identity in my eyes and become walking penises."

Who gets raped? Every female is a potential victim, as are some men (the 1,070 cases include several men who recounted homosexual assaults). The ages ranged from four to forty-seven years, but the percentage increased dramatically between twelve and sixteen, with most rapes perpetrated on women between sixteen and twenty. Unmarried status was much more common in the group than in the US female population at large. Twenty-two percent of the victims were under fifteen, with 7 percent under twelve.

Ninety-seven women, or 9 percent, suffered gang rape. Although gang rapes were no more likely to result in physical injury than being raped by one man, the victims were more likely to feel hostility towards men afterward.

Eighty-four women (8 percent) were raped on more than one occasion, sometimes both as a child and as an adult. In some cases, two or even three rapes took place in adulthood. For seventy women, the rape was attempted but not completed. These women who were able to fend off the attempts were less seriously affected than those who were raped.

Who is the rapist? In the most frequent scenario, the rapist is a total stranger. When the attacker was known, he was most likely to be an acquaintance (23 percent) or a date (12 percent). But rapists could also be friends, men known by sight, relatives, ex-lovers, lovers, or husbands. State laws are usually written in such a way that even the most brutal sexual attack by a husband is not considered rape. Nevertheless, four women named their husbands as their rapists.

Rapists averaged older than their victims. About 70 percent were white. Contrary to racist stereotypes, most rapes in the society at large are not perpetrated on white women by nonwhite men. Even in this selective sampling, 700 of the rapes were intrarace—71 percent of the white women being raped by white men and 68 percent of the nonwhite women being raped by nonwhite men.

Almost half the attackers were calm or matter-of-fact; about a quarter were contemptuous, angry, and righteous; on the other hand, 11 percent seemed frightened. While some victims mentioned that the attacker was drunk, very few noted that the attacker was sexually hungry or passionate.

Given the fact that the rapists averaged considerably taller and heavier than their victims, it is a tribute to women's courage that 88 percent of them resisted, 70 percent of them physically. Those who did not resist often gave reasons. "I allowed the man who raped me to do it without trying to fight him," explained one woman, "because he could have done me great physical damage." In many states, a woman must prove she resisted in order for the rapist to be prosecuted and convicted. Fortunately, feminist groups have succeeded in changing some such laws and are working to change others.

Where and when do most rapes occur? No time is safe. Rape takes place at all hours of the day and night. The fewest took place in the morning between 6:00 and 12:00 AM; fully half were in the six hours between 9:00 PM and 3:00 AM. Over half of the women were attacked inside—one-fifth in their own homes and one-fifth in the man's home. Only 161 of the women (15 percent) were actually raped outside—in the streets, alleys, and parks.

What happened to the victims as a result of the rape? Plenty. Almost half suffered a loss of trust in male-female relationships. About a third were affected sexually, had nightmares, and felt hostility toward men. About a quarter said they felt a loss of self-respect, and a similar number received psychiatric care. Sixteen percent had suicidal feelings, 16 percent felt a loss of independence, and 14 percent had physical injuries.

Not all the effects were bad. Over half of the women felt more strongly about standing up for themselves, 16 percent learned self-defense, and 6 percent joined women's groups.

More often, there is an aftermath of guilt and misery. "I was too ashamed to tell anyone in my family about it because of my puritanical upbringing," wrote one woman. "When I decided to tell my minister about my having been raped, I was told never to show my face in the house of God again."

Even when the woman is treated sympathetically after the rape, she still frequently suffers sexually.

An eighteen-year-old was raped by her cousin when she was fifteen. As is frequently the case when the assailant is a family member, she didn't report the rape because it would cause a family scandal.

> The pain! For six months I didn't go out with guys at all. Later I could go out but sex was completely out of the question. After almost a year of that, I decided to block it completely out and make love with someone. It didn't work. Every time a guy and I would start to get it on, he would touch me in a certain way and flash! I froze. All I could see was my cousin on top of me, hitting me, hurting me—and it was all over for me and my guy. My boyfriends became frustrated, and eventually left me in search of girls not as "cold" as me.
>
> Now I can enjoy sex most of the time, but once in a while my partner touches me the wrong way and, baby, it's all over.

The more intimately the victim has known the attacker, the more likely she is to suffer sexual problems after the attack.

To be raped by a stranger is a violation of your body; to be raped by someone you know adds an even crueler violation of trust.

Young victims, those under fifteen, were much more likely to have their sexuality affected. This may be because they were more likely to be raped by someone they knew and thus more likely to have their trust violated.

Another factor affecting the woman sexually is whether or not the rapist is legally convicted. Forty-one percent of those women whose rapists were *not* convicted were affected sexually. One policy implication of this study is that in order to diminish the effect of rape on women's sexuality, more vigorous efforts should be made to apprehend and convict the rapists.

Women who reported the rape to the police were substantially less likely to lose trust in male-female relationships than women who did not.

This result is probably dependent in part on whether or not the police were sympathetic.

Women who were raped by men who were righteous and contemptuous were substantially more likely to be hostile to men afterward than were women raped by men not holding those attitudes. The reason is probably that righteous and contemptuous rapists think they are *entitled* to sexual access regardless of the women's feelings.

The last factor significantly associated with hostility to men was the attitude of the police. A woman who was raped twice by the same man said: "I can only commend the Seattle police. I talked to nine (at least ten different people). . . . [They were] very sympathetic and willing to offer whatever aid or counseling I might find necessary." She reports that her feelings about the two incidents are "anger and rage against the man who raped me; *not against all men* [my italics]."

It is important not only that the police were sympathetic but that she was treated in a special rape relief center in the Seattle hospital. Such specialized centers at hospitals, most notably at Philadelphia General Hospital and Jackson Memorial in Miami, are performing a vital function, and the anti-rape movement is working hard to make such centers available in all cities.

About a quarter of the women lost self-respect as a result of the rape—a classic example of the way women are taught to blame themselves for whatever happens and to turn their anger inward rather than against the aggressor.

It is not surprising that almost a quarter of the women had psychiatric care of some type as a result of the rape. This does not necessarily mean that they were *helped* by the care; 35 percent of those who had such care said they were helped. The remaining 65 percent were not. Almost one-half were helped by other sources. For example, 132 women who reported they had had psychiatric care but were not helped by it received help from women's groups.

Quite possibly because of the greater number of anti-rape groups, hotlines for rape victims, and other women's support groups, more recent victims have alternatives to psychiatric care which were previously not available.

Women who resisted physically or by screaming were *more* likely to be physically injured than those who didn't—although it is unclear which caused which—and those who resisted by talking were *less* likely to be physically injured.

The following letter from a woman who was raped at knifepoint is an example not only of why women do not resist but also of the possible physical effects of rape—in this case, gonorrhea and severe pelvic infection. The letter also explains why she, like two-thirds of the women who answered the questionnaire, did not report the rape to the police:

I tried to talk my way out of the situation, but he put his knife in his sleeve, put his arm around me, and ordered me to walk with him without a sound—I never once imagined that I was allowing this man to walk me right into my own rape!

I refused to go to the police out of fear. When I went to a gynecologist, I found I had become infected with gonorrhea. I was treated immediately with antibiotics.

The shame stayed. I talked to some friends—that seemed to help. Then one day I felt a terrible pain in my stomach. I realized I had a high fever and I rushed to the hospital, where I was found to have a severe pelvic infection resulting from the original gonorrhea. I was hospitalized for ten days. It took me two years to get back on my feet physically—and I am afraid that I may never be able to have children.

Some women reacted constructively: they felt more strongly about standing up for themselves, they joined anti-rape groups. Women belonging to anti-rape groups (which provide victims with the kinds of legal advice and emotional support necessary for them to endure the court ordeal and testify effectively) are more likely to report the rape

to the police and the attackers are more likely to be arrested *and* convicted.

In order for the victim to be treated she has to see a physician, and in order for the rapist to be arrested she has to go to the police, and in order for him to be convicted she has to appear in court. Yet most victims don't do any of these things. Why? Perhaps this account, by a woman who was raped by her sister's ex-boyfriend, helps explain why so many women prefer silence to dealing with these institutions.

From the moment the police came it was just one question after another. After they got all the important information, I was taken to my family doctor. When he found out I had my period, he skipped most of the examination.

After five minutes at the doctor's office (most of it spent dressing and undressing), I was taken to the police station. I made a full statement, which took two and a half hours. I had to undress in front of four policemen to look for semen and bruises. They took pictures of me naked.

Now, the district attorney tells me that the man who raped me, thanks to a fancy lawyer who changed his plea three times, will more than likely get parole. I did my duty and reported the crime—and for my trouble they are going to set him free.

Everything I went through was for nothing. So help me God, if I ever get raped again I'll never lift a finger to help the police. It's just not worth what you go through. All this has taught me is that a lot of money and a good lawyer will get you out of any trouble.

Stories of official indifference are becoming less frequent. Our findings indicate not only that women *should* go to the police but that the police have become more sympathetic. Police are more sympathetic if the attacker is unknown and if the victim resisted by screaming. Perhaps surprisingly, we could not find any differences in police attitude associated with the race of either the attacker or the victim. Police, at least in this sampling, were just as likely to be sympathetic to nonwhite women, whatever the race of their attackers. The presence of policewomen is noted as helpful.

Hospitals, however, have lagged behind the police in sensitive treatment of rape victims.

> The hospital personnel made it quite clear they were examining me only for presence of semen. The nurse rudely yanked my legs into the stirrups. The doctor who examined me stated, "You're lucky you take the pill." I was never told whether they found semen. I was never offered any tranquilizers, and the surface wounds were never examined or X-rayed. I was told to see my personal physician for a VD test. . . . The final coup came about two months later when I received a bill from the emergency room.

Why do I believe that rapes should be reported in spite of these horror stories? Because it makes a difference. Of those rapes reported to the police, 38 percent of the rapists were arrested. Of those arrested, 44 percent were convicted of rape. As word gets out that the police and courts are more sympathetic, more victims will choose to report their rapes, and as a consequence more rapists will be taken off the streets.

What can we learn from this study? It is amazing how insensitive our society has been to rape victims. The women's movement has been able to bring about changes in the victims and in the institutions with which they have to deal; but clearly, many men, often including the husbands of victims, are unaware of rape's impact. One respondent's husband crossed out his wife's responses to the question, "In what ways would you say your life has been affected?" and wrote: "I helped my wife fill out this form, and I don't believe she was honest about this." Women's feelings about their rapes must be seen as valid, and their reality supported. Men have to realize this for their own welfare as well as the welfare of the women they relate to. This kind of support is what the rape crisis lines, rape counselors, and feminist therapists provide.

Rape need not be always with us. It may simply be something that we are set up for because of the way our society is put together and the way boys and girls are brought up. The solution lies not in changing our biology but in changing our society so that, as one woman wrote, "God willing, maybe someday a woman can walk down a dark alley or sit in her home . . . without fear of rape."

Rape in Great Art

AUDREY FLACK

Art editor, Judith Kletter. Based on a slide lecture prepared and given by the author. Reprinted by permission.

Many men—as well as women—attest that Audrey Flack's slide lecture on misogyny and violence against women in great art has deeply shaken, disturbed, and ultimately enlightened them. A world-renowned photo-realist painter and sculptor of contemporary, neoclassical goddesses, for years Flack was a persistent feminist voice at the American College Art Association.

Looking at art in a great museum such as the Metropolitan Museum of Art can be a wonderful and uplifting experience, but the average woman doesn't realize that she is seeing rape all around her. She takes it for granted, looks at the paintings, and walks right on. Our vision has been so coerced that we accept scenes of brutality and abduction as part of out historical memory. What I am hoping for is an enlightened vision.

THE *VENUS OF WILLENDORF*

When I lecture or write on the Goddess, I go way back to ancient times and reference statues like the *Venus of Willendorf* (Fig. 1). The Venus has become a favorite of many women, including myself, but she must be examined more thoroughly and viewed through a new lens in order to be under-

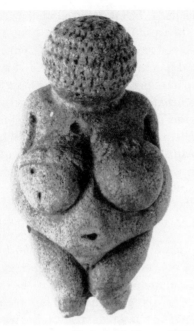

Figure 1: *The Venus of Willendorf*
[© Naturhistorisches Museum Wien.
Photo by Alice Schumacher]

or protect herself. She is completely defenseless.

And so is the lovable *Venus of Willendorf.* People like her because she is not a threat, she is not a sexual object. Her body has been used a great deal. She is probably a very strong woman who survived childbirth without the help of a male obstetrician. And not just one birth: you can imagine how many women died in childbirth in those days. Thin women, women with not enough fat or poor immune systems, probably perished immediately.

The *Venus of Willendorf* is a survivor, a giver of life. Her breasts nurtured many children, and she became an object of worship. I believe that the *Venus of Willendorf* was sculpted by a woman for other women, to be held and carried as a magic charm, transmitting much-needed healing energy during childbirth or other life-threatening situations. We love her because she is a survival object, delivering life forces to us even to this day.

But large, pendulous breasts ache and can cause back problems, and we all know the dangers of being overweight. Like tiny bound feet, big breasts burden us, tie us down; nevertheless, women put their own health at risk to enlarge their breasts with implants. I wonder if men would think about putting implants in their testicles. How would it feel having those testes hanging down to their knees? Would women find it attractive? I doubt it. Images of beauty must be reevaluated and reimaged. Double standards must be exposed and questioned.

THE EXPULSION OF ADAM AND EVE FROM THE GARDEN BY MASACCIO

In this wonderful painting by the fifteenth-century Italian master Masaccio, an angry angel is pointing a finger at the two sinners (Fig. 2). Adam is covering his eyes. Eve's face has a pained expression. She is covering her breasts and genitals in shame, but Adam remains exposed. What exactly is the terrible act she has committed? Let's think about it.

She took the apple from the tree of knowledge. She wanted information. She wanted to know what to do when she gave birth to her children.

stood. She is one of the oldest goddesses to be uncovered, a small figurine with breasts so voluminous it would be hard for her to walk. Her belly is enormous and protrudes in front of her. She has something on her head, I have never been quite sure what, either a cap of curled hair or a tight-fitting hat, but in either case, she has no face. You cannot see her eyes or her expression—she just is.

Her feet are very small, not unlike the big-breasted women with tiny feet that the famed sculptor Gaston Lachaise creates. There is one always on display in the garden of the Museum of Modern Art. It would be difficult, if not impossible, to support such a body with such malformed feet.

I am reminded of Chinese girls who for centuries had to endure their feet being bound in order to keep them from growing to a normal size. Tiny feet were considered a symbol of beauty. These women became cripples who could barely walk, all for the sake of male adulation. But it is more like male *domination,* for such a woman could not run away

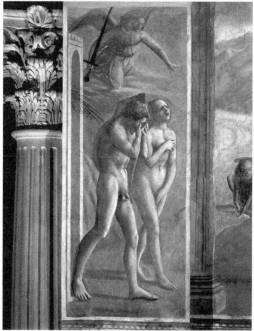

Figure 2: *The Expulsion of Adam and Eve from the Garden* by Masaccio [Scala/Art Resource, NY]

She needed to be informed about the process and what she was in for. It's the most basic question any woman can ask. A baby would grow inside of her and had to come out. She didn't even know what part of her body it would emerge from. Her desire for knowledge was considered a sin. Her only other alternative was to remain childlike and dependent, not in control of her body, her life, or her death. It is important to reassess early biblical and mythological stories and analyze how women are portrayed.

LEDA AND THE SWAN BY MICHELANGELO

Myths about ancient goddesses are filled with tales of rape and violence. The male god is never held accountable. Why does Zeus, the most powerful of all the gods, have to deceive and rape women? Can't he get them any other way?

In this painting he transforms himself into an excessively long-necked swan and somehow man-

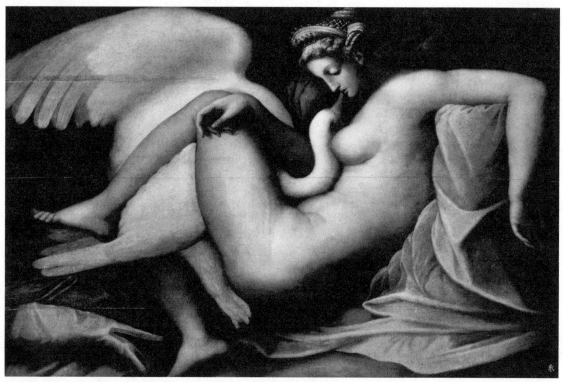

Figure 3: *Leda and the Swan* by Michelangelo [Alinari/Art Resource, NY]

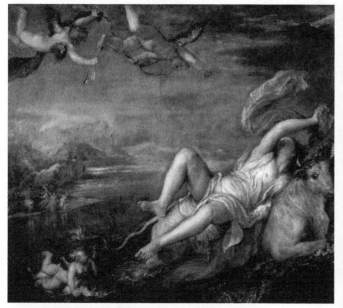

Figure 4: *The Rape of Europa* by Titian [Isabella Stewart Gardner Museum, Boston]

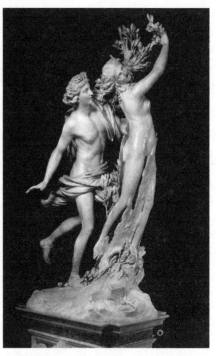

Figure 5: *Apollo and Daphne* by Bernini [Alinari/Art Resource, NY]

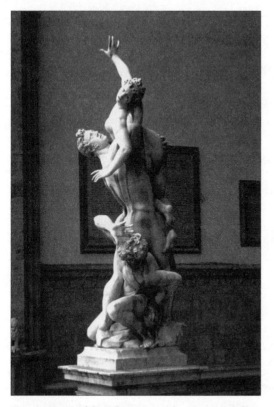

Figure 6: *Rape of the Sabine Woman* by Giovanni Bologna [photo by Manrico Romano]

ages to impregnate Leda (Fig. 3). While the image of a white-feathered giant swan twisting its body and elongated neck around a nude Leda may appear to be glamorous, imagine what a woman would *really* feel if she were penetrated against her will by an overgrown waterfowl.

THE RAPE OF EUROPA BY TITIAN

Here we see Europa lying flat on her back on top of a bull (Fig. 4). Her legs are spread wide apart facing the viewer in anticipation of receiving her abductor rapist. Europa's rapist is, once again, Zeus, who has transformed himself into a ridiculous, drooling white bull, decorated with garlands of flowers around his neck and horns, as if that would make him more appealing. The reality of being raped by a bull is grotesque, and yet this painting is considered delightful.

Museums all over the world are filled with images that glamorize and romanticize rape, and we have come to accept these images as part of the nature of things. Most often the woman looks like a helpless but willing victim. At other times she appears to be enjoying her situation.

In reality a woman confronted by a rapist will close her legs rather than open them, shield her body rather than expose it; she will fight her attacker using any means—scratching, clawing, kicking, gouging. She will not submit willingly. All rapists are ineffectual men who force sex in a misguided attempt to secure love. But even a rapist knows that no weapons or threat of power can force love from a woman against her will.

RAPE OF THE SABINE WOMAN BY GIOVANNI BOLOGNA

Rape is the subject of many great works of art—for example, Reubens' *Rape of the Daughters of Leucippus* or Bernini's *Apollo and Daphne* (Fig. 5)—though it may not be part of our conscious perception. The women's nude bodies are painted in pale tones, in sharp contrast to the ruddy, healthy-looking men who are either draped or fully clothed and armed with breastplates, shields, and swords.

I have looked at Giovanni da Bologna's *Rape of the Sabine Woman* (Fig. 6) for decades—I even saw the original in Florence—but only recently did I realize that this beautiful statue is a brutal rape scene. Throughout my entire art education I was taught to admire the lavish curves of the women's nude bodies, the graceful swing of their arms, and the expressiveness of the woman's hand in the air, but I was never once led to ask, "Why is her hand up in the air?" I will tell you why: she is imploring God, a patriarchal deity with a white beard, to descend from the heavens and come to her aid. He never does.

IRIS, MESSENGER OF THE GODS BY RODIN

This is another image that disturbs me (Fig. 7). Rodin exposes the model's genitals by spreading her legs apart as if she were on an examining table in a doctor's office. Rodin was a voyeur

and a womanizer. This image is not surprising in our culture—we are used to women being displayed. Men would be embarrassed and upset to have their bodies portrayed in a similar manner. I'm not talking about nude statues. I'm talking about voyeurism and the double standard.

LUNCHEON ON THE GRASS BY MANET

This is one painting that has always made me uncomfortable (Fig. 8). The men are sitting around fully clothed, having a picnic on the grass, and the woman with them is completely nude. The men are fully dressed, in suits and ties no less. Whenever I look at this painting, I think, isn't she cold? Her bare bottom is on the grass with all the bugs and dirt. Isn't the breeze affecting her? She is so vulnerable. Manet's purpose was to shock but also to titillate his male viewers.

PERSEUS WITH THE HEAD OF MEDUSA BY CELLINI

According to mythology, Medusa was a hideous gorgon with fangs, scales, and claws. Live snakes writhed in her hair. She was so ugly that any man who looked at her turned to stone. Freud even claimed that men were frozen with terror because Medusa's head looks like a huge bloody vagina, symbolizing castration.

In Cellini's sculpture, Perseus is stepping on Medusa's body as she writhes in pain, twisted and deformed (Fig. 9). He has just cut off her head by sneaking up behind her, not looking directly at her face, but instead looking at her reflection in his shield, which acts as a mirror. He holds her head up triumphantly as blood spurts from her neck. He is a hero. But look again—there is more to this story. . . .

THE ANCIENT GORGON AND COLOSSAL HEAD OF MEDUSA

When I first began to research the story of Medusa and went back to Ovid, I found that a lot had been left out (Fig. 10). Medusa was one of triplets. Her sisters were hideous gorgons, but she was a

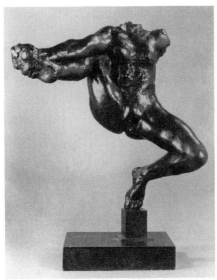

Figure 7: *Iris, Messenger of the Gods* by Rodin [Los Angeles County Museum of Art, gift of B. Gerald Cantor Art Foundation]

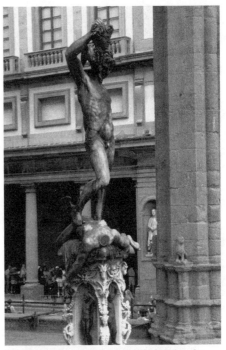

Figure 9: *Perseus with the Head of Medusa* by Cellini [Photo by Manrico Romano]

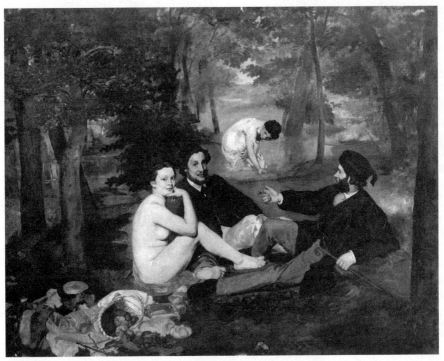

Figure 8: *Luncheon on the Grass* by Manet [Giraudon/Art Resource, NY]

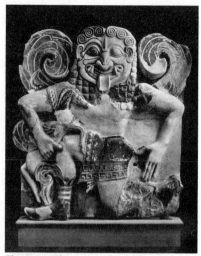

Figure 10: *The Ancient Gorgon*
[Alinari/Art Resource, NY]

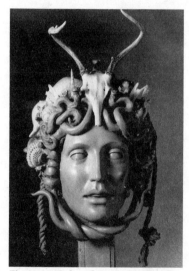

Figure 11: *Colossal Head of Medusa* by
Audrey Flack [Photo by Steve Lopez]

that her temple had been defiled that she turned Medusa's hair into snakes. The innocent Medusa is thus twice victimized, once by rape and once by Athena's punishment.

I think that Athena was really trying to *empower* Medusa by guaranteeing that she would never be raped again: if any man harassed her, he turned to stone. But this empowerment is double-edged. Medusa never wanted to *kill* anyone, yet because men die at the sight of her, she can never again have sex. The same is true of victims of rape, who often cannot enjoy sex anymore, or at least not for a long while.

It took me twenty years to understand the story of Medusa from a woman's perspective, to see her as she truly was: a frightened young woman who had been brutally abused, so ashamed of the way she looked that she hid in her lair at the end of the world. But she isn't ugly; on the contrary, she is ravishingly beautiful. And this is how I portray her, waking up from her sleep just before the cowardly Perseus beheads her (Fig. 11).

There are wonderful men out there—considerate, kind, gentle men who know that the only way to save the planet is to share the power with women. But they need to base their masculinity on new role models, not on so-called heroes like Poseidon, Zeus, or Perseus. They need to be able to hear the women speak.

Very often I portray goddesses with their lips slightly parted, as if they are about to speak. I want to give them a voice. It's time for them to speak out and show their true beauty. It's time to set these ancient myths straight.

Working to End Sexual Violence on College Campuses

HELEN LOWERY AND NICOLE LEVITZ

Helen Lowery and Nicole Levitz, "Starting the Boston University Coalition for Consensual Sex," 2008. Original for this publication.

beautiful sea creature with long, flowing hair. She looked like a goddess and sang like a siren.

When Medusa was a young woman—I imagine her as a girl really, about fourteen years old—Poseidon, god of the sea, fell in love with her. And he did what all gods do when they fall in love: he raped her. The violation took place in Athena's temple. According to myth, Athena was so angry

The Coalition for Consensual Sex is a student group we created to address issues of rape and sexual assault. The idea of the Coalition grew out of a conversation we had with our roommates about the lack of sexual assault resources on our campus. We decided to do something about it.

We spent the summer researching. We found out about programs at other schools and local resources. We also spoke with a number of professionals who worked on this issue who gave us feedback on our ideas and suggestions for how best to proceed. By the end of the summer, we were armed with plenty of information and were ready to start making changes on the campus. Our original plan was a full-service rape crisis center on campus, a campus public education program, a student-run crisis hotline, and an official university sexual assault policy designed to support victims. We had to alter our wonderful plan with practicality, because the responses involved money and politics. Universities, like people, are slow to change. You have to be flexible and work with them, not against them, to make things happen, though sometimes you have to push them before they are ready to move.

We didn't wait for the school to start the program; we found speakers ourselves and brought them to campus. The school said it was not in the budget to hire a counselor to run a support group, so we worked with the local rape crisis center to get their counselors to campus to run a group. We compiled a list of area sexual assault resources and went door-to-door handing it out so students would have the information. We really shocked people with our "I Heart Consensual Sex" T-shirts. People started talking about the issue. Starting dialogue is a great catalyst for change.

In April, sexual assault awareness month, we took on the duty of informing the campus. In addition to launching an informational campaign, putting on an "I Rock for Consensual Sex" concert, and forming a walk team to raise money for the local rape crisis center, our group hosted a "Take Back the Night" on the Boston Common. It was the first event of its kind in the area, a citywide in-tercollegiate event. Normally college campuses hold their own annual "Take Back the Night" events, which makes sense for isolated schools, but we were lucky enough to be in a city full of college campuses with active students. For years, there had been talk of doing an event bringing the campuses together, but no one would step forward to organize it—that year we did. We applied for a permit for the Boston Common and started calling everyone we knew at local universities. We had representatives from fifteen area schools at the event. The event had a unique power, because it wasn't the same people—there were new faces with new energy. We had our sisters (and brothers) in arms from around the city who cared about our issue.

Then, as luck would have it, the federal government gave the city money to build the Family Justice Center. The Boston Police Department Sexual Assault Unit and the assistant district attorney were moving their offices into the center. In addition, there was space for the local rape crisis center to provide services on the premises. The site for the center was at the western edge of our campus, right by a large cluster of freshman dorms. It was perfect. We immediately got involved doing what we could to help facilitate conversation between the center, the local rape crisis center, and our school. When we were asked to participate in some of the planning and negotiating for the partnership between the school and the organizations within the center, we were confident that we could make a meaningful contribution because we had learned so much over the year.

It was an amazing year. We were seniors saying goodbye to college, working, and enjoying our friends. The Coalition grew out of those experiences and became a piece of our lives. The key point being that it was a part, but not all of, our lives. Though it did not turn out exactly how we wanted it, we achieved in a year almost exactly what we set out to do.

Trauma and Recovery

JUDITH HERMAN

Judith Herman, excerpt from *Trauma and Recovery,* New York: Basic Books, 1992. Reprinted by permission.

A single traumatic event can occur almost anywhere. Prolonged, repeated trauma, by contrast, occurs only in circumstances of captivity. When the victim is free to escape, she will not be abused a second time; repeated trauma occurs only when the victim is a prisoner, unable to flee, and under the control of the perpetrator. Such conditions obviously exist in prisons, concentration camps, and slave labor camps. These conditions may also exist in religious cults, in brothels and other institutions of organized sexual exploitation, and in families.

Political captivity is generally recognized, whereas the domestic captivity of women and children is often unseen. A man's home is his castle; rarely is it understood that the same home may be a prison for women and children. In domestic captivity, physical barriers to escape are rare. In most homes, even the most oppressive, there are no bars on the windows, no barbed wire fences. Women and children are not ordinarily chained, though even this occurs more often than one might think. The barriers to escape are generally invisible. They are nonetheless extremely powerful. Children are rendered captive by their condition of dependency. Women are rendered captive by economic, social, psychological, and legal subordination, as well as by physical force.

Captivity, which brings the victim into prolonged contact with the perpetrator, creates a special type of relationship, one of coercive control. This is equally true whether the victim is taken captive entirely by force, as in the case of prisoners and hostages, or by a combination of force, intimidation, and enticement, as in the case of religious cult members, battered women, and abused children. The psychological impact of subordination to coercive control may have many common features, whether that subordination occurs within the public sphere of politics or within the private sphere of sexual and domestic relations.

Former prisoners carry their captors' hatred with them even after release, and sometimes they continue to carry out their captors' destructive purposes with their own hands. Long after their liberation, people who have been subjected to coercive control bear the psychological scars of captivity. They suffer not only from a classic post-traumatic syndrome but also from profound alterations in their relations with God, with other people, and with themselves.

A NEW DIAGNOSIS

Most people have no knowledge or understanding of the psychological changes of captivity. Social judgment of chronically traumatized people therefore tends to be extremely harsh. The chronically abused person's apparent helplessness and passivity, her entrapment in the past, her intractable depression and somatic complaints, and her smoldering anger often frustrate the people closest to her. Moreover, if she had been coerced into betrayal of relationships, community loyalties, or moral values, she is frequently subjected to furious condemnation.

Observers who have never experienced prolonged terror and who have no understanding of coercive methods of control presume that they would show greater courage and resistance than the victim in similar circumstances. Hence the common tendency to account for the victim's behavior by seeking flaws in her personality or moral character. Prisoners of war who succumb to "brainwashing" are often publicly excoriated. Sometimes survivors are treated more harshly than those who abused them. In the notorious case of Patricia Hearst, for instance, the hostage was tried for crimes committed under duress and received a longer prison sentence than her captors. Similarly, women who fail to escape from abusive relationships and those who prostitute themselves or betray their children under duress are subjected to extraordinary censure.

The propensity to fault the character of the victim can be seen even in the case of politically organized mass murder. The aftermath of the Holocaust witnessed a protracted debate regarding the "passivity" of the Jews and their "complicity" in their fate. But the historian Lucy Dawidowicz points out that "complicity" and "cooperation" are terms that apply to situations of free choice. They do not have the same meaning in situations of captivity.

DIAGNOSTIC MISLABELING

This tendency to blame the victim has strongly influenced the direction of psychological inquiry. It has led researchers and clinicians to seek an explanation for the perpetrator's crimes in the character of the victim. In the case of hostages and prisoners of war, numerous attempts to find supposed personality defects that predisposed captives to "brainwashing" have yielded few consistent results. The conclusion is inescapable that ordinary, psychologically healthy men can indeed be coerced in unmanly ways. In domestic battering situations, where victims are entrapped by persuasion rather than by capture, research has also focused on the personality traits that might predispose a woman to get involved in an abusive relationship. Here again no consistent profile of the susceptible woman has emerged. While some battered women clearly have major psychological difficulties that render them vulnerable, the majority show no evidence of serious psychopathology before entering into the exploitative relationship. Most become involved with their abusers at a time of temporary life crises or recent loss, when they are feeling unhappy, alienated, or lonely. A survey of the studies of wife-beating concludes: "The search for characteristics of women that contribute to their own victimization is futile. It is sometimes forgotten that men's violence is men's behavior. As such, it is not surprising that the more fruitful efforts to explain this behavior have focused on male characteristics. What is surprising is the enormous effort to explain male behavior by examining characteristics of women."

While it is clear that ordinary, healthy people may become entrapped in prolonged abusive situations, it is equally clear that after their escape they are no longer ordinary or healthy. Chronic abuse causes serious psychological harm. The tendency to blame the victim, however, has interfered with the psychological understanding and diagnosis of a post-traumatic syndrome. Instead of conceptualizing the psychopathology of the victim as a response to an abusive situation, mental health professionals have frequently attributed the abusive situation to the victim's presumed underlying psychopathology.

An egregious example of this sort of thinking is the 1964 study of battered women entitled "The Wife-Beater's Wife." The researchers, who had originally sought to study batterers, found that the men would not talk to them. They thereupon redirected their attention to the more cooperative battered women, whom they found to be "castrating," "frigid," "aggressive," "indecisive," and "passive." They concluded that marital violence fulfilled these women's "masochistic needs." Having identified the women's personality disorders as the source of the problem, these clinicians set out to "treat" them. In one case they managed to persuade the wife that she was provoking the violence, and they showed her how to mend her ways. When she no longer sought help from her teenage son to protect herself from beatings and no longer refused to submit to sex on demand, even when her husband was drunk and aggressive, her treatment was judged a success.

While this unabashed, open sexism is rarely found in psychiatric literature today, the same conceptual errors, with their implicit bias and contempt, still predominate. The clinical picture of a person who has been reduced to elemental concerns of survival is still frequently mistaken for a portrait of the victim's underlying character.

Concepts of personality organization developed under ordinary circumstances are applied to victims, without any understanding of the corrosion of personality that occurs under conditions of prolonged terror. Thus, patients who suffer from the complex aftereffects of chronic trauma still commonly risk being misdiagnosed as having personality disorders. They may be described as inherently "dependent," "masochistic," or "self-defeating." In a recent study of emergency room practice in a large urban hospital, clinicians routinely described battered women as "hysterics," "masochistic females," "hypochondriacs," or, more simply, "crocks."

This tendency to misdiagnose victims was at the heart of a controversy that arose in the mid-1980s when the diagnostic manual of the American Psychiatric Association came up for revision. A group of male psychoanalysts proposed that "masochistic personality disorder" be added to the canon. This hypothetical diagnosis applied to any person who "remains in relationships in which others exploit, abuse, or take advantage of him or her, despite opportunities to alter the situation." A number of women's groups were outraged, and a heated public debate ensued. Women insisted on opening up the process of writing the diagnostic canon, which had been the preserve of a small group of men, and for the first time took part in the naming of psychological reality.

I was one of the participants in this process. What struck me most at the time was how little rational argument seemed to matter. The women's representatives came to the discussion prepared with carefully reasoned, extensively documented position papers, which argued that the proposed diagnostic concept had little scientific foundation, ignored recent advances in understanding the psychology of victimization, and was socially regressive and discriminatory in impact, since it would be used to stigmatize disempowered people. The men of the psychiatric establishment persisted in their bland denial. They admitted freely that they were ignorant of the extensive literature of the past decade on psychological trauma, but they did not see why it should concern them. One member of the Board of Trustees of the American Psychiatric Association felt the discussion of battered women was "irrelevant." Another stated simply, "I never see victims."

In the end, because of the outcry from organized women's groups and the widespread publicity engendered by the controversy, some sort of compromise became expedient. The name of the proposed entity was changed to "self-defeating personality disorder." The criteria for diagnosis were changed, so that the label could not be applied to people who were known to be physically, sexually, or psychologically abused. Most important, the disorder was included not in the main body of the test but in an appendix. It was relegated to apocryphal status within the canon, where it languishes to this day.

NEED FOR A NEW CONCEPT

Misapplication of the concept of masochistic personality disorder may be one of the most stigmatizing diagnostic mistakes, but it is by no means the only one. In general, the diagnostic categories of the existing psychiatric canon are simply not designed for survivors of extreme situations and do not fit them well. The persistent anxiety, phobias, and panic of survivors are not the same as ordinary anxiety disorders. The somatic symptoms of survivors are not the same as ordinary psychosomatic disorders. Their depression is not the same as ordinary depression. And the degradation of their identity and relational life is not the same as ordinary personality disorder.

The lack of an accurate and comprehensive diagnostic concept has serious consequences for treatment, because the connection between the patient's present symptoms and the traumatic experience is frequently lost. Attempts to fit the patient into the mold of existing diagnostic constructs generally result, at best, in a partial understanding of the problem and a fragmented approach to treatment. All too commonly, chronically traumatized people suffer in silence; but if they complain at all, their complaints are not well understood. They may collect a virtual pharmacopoeia of remedies: one for headaches, another for insomnia, another for anxiety, another for depression. None of these tends to work very well, since the underlying issues of trauma are not addressed. As caregivers tire of these chronically unhappy people who do not seem to improve, the temptation to apply pejorative diagnostic labels becomes overwhelming.

Even the diagnosis of "posttraumatic stress disorder," as it is presently defined, does not fit accurately enough. The existing diagnostic criteria for this disorder are derived mainly from survivors of circumscribed traumatic events. They are based on the prototypes of combat, disaster, and rape. In survivors of prolonged, repeated trauma, the symptom picture is often far more complex. Survivors of prolonged abuse develop characteristic personality changes, including deformations of relatedness and identity. Survivors of abuse in childhood develop similar problems with relationships and identity; in addition, they are particularly vulnerable to repeated harm, both self-inflicted and at the hands of others. The current formulation of post-traumatic stress disorder fails to capture either the protean symptomatic manifestations of prolonged, repeated trauma or the profound deformations of personality that occur in captivity.

The syndrome that follows upon prolonged, repeated trauma needs its own name. I propose to call it "complex posttraumatic stress disorder." The responses to trauma are best understood as a spectrum of conditions rather than as a single disorder. They range from a brief stress reaction that gets better by itself and never qualifies for a diagnosis, to classic or simple post-traumatic stress disorder, to the complex syndrome of prolonged, repeated trauma.

Although the complex traumatic syndrome has never before been outlined systematically, the concept of a spectrum of post-traumatic disorders has been noted, almost in passing, by many experts. Lawrence Kolb remarks on the "heterogeneity" of posttraumatic stress disorder, which "is to psychiatry as syphilis was to medicine. At one time or another [this disorder] may appear to mimic every personality disorder. . . . It is those threatened over long periods of time who suffer the long-standing severe personality disorganization." Others have also called attention to the personality changes that follow prolonged, repeated trauma. The psychiatrist Emmanuel Tanay, who works with survivors of the Nazi Holocaust, observes: "The psychopathology may be hidden in characterological changes that are manifest only in disturbed object relationships and attitudes towards work, the world, man and God."

Many experienced clinicians have invoked the need for a diagnostic formulation that goes beyond simple posttraumatic stress disorder. William Niederland finds that "the concept of traumatic neurosis does not appear sufficient to cover the multitude and severity of clinical manifestations" of the syndrome observed in survivors of the Nazi Holocaust. Psychiatrists who have treated Southeast Asian refugees also recognize the need for an "expanded concept" of posttraumatic stress disorder that takes into account severe, prolonged, and massive psychological trauma. One authority suggests the concept of a "posttraumatic character disorder." Others speak of "complicated" posttraumatic stress disorder.

Clinicians who work with survivors of childhood abuse have also seen the need for an expanded diagnostic concept. Lenore Terr distinguishes the effects of a single traumatic blow, which she calls "type 1" trauma, from the effects of prolonged, repeated trauma, which she calls "type 2." Her description of the type 2 syndrome includes denial and psychic numbing, self-hypnosis and dissociation, and alternations between extreme passivity and outbursts of rage. The psychiatrist Jean Goodwin has invented the acronyms FEARS for simple posttraumatic stress disorder and BAD FEARS for the severe posttraumatic disorder observed in survivors of childhood abuse.

Thus, observers have often glimpsed the underlying unity of the complex traumatic syndrome and have given it many different names. It is time for the disorder to have an official, recognized name. Currently, the complex posttraumatic stress disorder is under consideration for inclusion in the fourth edition of the diagnostic manual of the American Psychiatric Association, based on seven diagnostic criteria (see box). Empirical field trials are under way to determine whether such a syndrome can be diagnosed reliably in chronically traumatized people. The degree of scientific and intellectual rigor in this process is considerably higher than that which occurred in the pitiable debates over "masochistic personality disorder."

As the concept of a complex traumatic syndrome has gained wider recognition, it has been given several additional names. The working group for the diagnostic manual of the American Psychiatric Association has chosen the designation "disorder of extreme stress not otherwise specified." The International Classification of Diseases is considering a similar entity under the name "personality change from catastrophic experience." These names may be awkward and unwieldy, but practically any name that gives recognition to the syndrome is better than no name at all.

Naming the syndrome of complex posttraumatic stress disorder represents an essential step toward granting those who have endured prolonged exploitation a measure of the recognition they deserve. It is an attempt to find a language that is at once faithful to the traditions of accurate psychological observation and to the moral demands of traumatized people. It is an attempt to learn from survivors, who understand, more profoundly than any investigator, the effects of captivity.

SURVIVORS AS PSYCHIATRIC PATIENTS

The mental health system is filled with survivors of prolonged, repeated childhood trauma. This is true even though most people who have been abused in childhood never come to psychiatric attention. To the extent that these people recover, they do so on their own. While only a small minority of survivors, usually those with the most severe abuse histories, eventually become psychiatric patients, many or even most psychiatric patients are survivors of childhood abuse. The data on this point are beyond contention. On careful questioning, 50 to 60 percent of psychiatric inpatients and 40 to 60 percent of outpatients report childhood histories of physical or sexual abuse or both. In one study of psychiatric emergency room patients, 70 percent had abuse histories. Thus abuse in childhood appears to be one of the main factors that lead a person to seek psychiatric treatment as an adult.

Survivors of child abuse who become patients appear with a bewildering array of symptoms. Their general levels of distress are higher than those of other patients. Perhaps the most impressive finding is the sheer length of the list of symptoms correlated with a history of childhood abuse. The psychologist Jeffrey Bryer and his colleagues report that women with histories of physical or sexual abuse have significantly higher scores than other patients on standardized measures of somatization, depression, general anxiety, phobic anxiety, interpersonal sensitivity, paranoia, and "psychoticism" (probably dissociative symptoms). The psychologist John Briere reports that survivors of childhood abuse display significantly more insomnia, sexual dysfunction, dissociation, anger, suicidality, self-mutilation, drug addiction, and alcoholism than other patients. The symptoms list can be prolonged almost indefinitely.

When survivors of childhood abuse seek treatment, they have what the psychologist Denise Gelinas calls a "disguised presentation." They come for help because of their many symptoms or because of difficulty with relationships: problems in intimacy, excessive responsiveness to the needs of others, and repeated victimization. All too commonly, neither patient nor therapist recognizes the link between the presenting problem and the history of chronic trauma.

Survivors of childhood abuse, like other traumatized people, are frequently misdiagnosed and mistreated in the mental health system. Because of the number and complexity of their symptoms, their treatment is often fragmented and incomplete. Because of their characteristic difficulties in close relationships, they are particularly vulnerable to revictimization by caregivers. They may become engaged in ongoing, destructive interactions, in which the medical or mental health system relicates the behavior of the abusive family.

Survivors of childhood abuse often accumulate many different diagnoses before the underlying problem of a complex posttraumatic syndrome is recognized. They are likely to receive a diagnosis that carries strong negative connotations. Three particularly troublesome diagnoses have often been applied to survivors of childhood abuse: somatization disorder, borderline personality disorder, and multiple personality disorder. All three of these diagnoses were once subsumed under the now obsolete name *hysteria*. Patients, usually women, who received these diagnoses evoke unusually intense reactions in caregivers. Their credibility is often suspect. They are frequently accused of manipulating or malingering. They are often the subject of furious and partisan controversy. Sometimes they are frankly hated.

These three diagnoses are charged with pejorative meaning. The most notorious is the diagnosis of borderline personality disorder. This term is frequently used within the mental health professions as little more than a sophisticated insult. As one psychiatrist candidly confesses, "As a resident, I recalled asking my supervisor how to treat patients with borderline personality disorder, and he answered, sardonically, 'You refer them.'" The psychiatrist Irvin Yalom describes the term "borderline" as "the word that strikes terror into the heart of the middle-aged, comfort-seeking psychiatrist." Some clinicians have argued that the term "borderline" had become so prejudicial that

it should be abandoned altogether, just as its predecessor term, *hysteria*, had to be abandoned.

These three diagnoses have many features in common, and often they cluster and overlap with one another. Patients who receive any one of these three diagnoses usually qualify for several other diagnoses as well. For example, the majority of patients with somatization disorder also have major depression, agoraphobia, and panic, in addition to their numerous physical complaints. Over half are given additional diagnoses of "histrionic," "antisocial," or "borderline" personality disorders. Similarly, people with borderline personality disorder often suffer as well from major depression, substance abuse, agoraphobia or panic, and somatization disorder. The majority of patients with multiple personality disorder experience severe depression. Most also meet diagnostic criteria for borderline personality disorder. And they generally have numerous psychosomatic complaints, including headache, unexplained pains, gastrointestinal disturbances, and hysterical conversion symptoms. These patients receive an average of three other psychiatric or neurological diagnoses before the underlying problem of multiple personality disorder is finally recognized.

All three disorders are associated with high levels of hypnotizability or dissociation, but in this respect, multiple personality disorder is in a class by itself. People with multiple personality disorder possess staggering dissociative capabilities. Some of their more bizarre symptoms may be mistaken for symptoms of schizophrenia. For example, they may have "passive influence" experiences of being controlled by another personality, or hallucinations of the voices of quarreling alter personalities. Patients with borderline personality disorder, though they are rarely capable of the same virtuosic feats of dissociation, also have abnormally high levels of dissociative symptoms. And patients with somatization disorder are reported to have high levels of hypnotizability and psychogenic amnesia.

Patients with all three disorders also share characteristic difficulties in close relationships. Interpersonal difficulties have been described most extensively in patients with borderline personality disorder. Indeed, a pattern of intense, unstable relationships is one of the major criteria for making this diagnosis. Borderline patients find it very hard to tolerate being alone but are also exceedingly wary of others. Terrified of abandonment on the one hand and of domination on the other, they oscillate between extremes of clinging and withdrawal, between abject submissiveness and furious rebellion. They tend to form "special" relations with idealized caretakers in which ordinary boundaries are not observed. Psychoanalytic authors attribute this instability to a failure of psychological development in the formative years of early childhood. One authority describes the primary defect in borderline personality disorder as a "failure to achieve object constancy," that is, a failure to form reliable and well-integrated inner representations of trusted people. Another speaks of the "relative developmental failure in formation of introjects that provide to the self a function of holding-soothing security"; that is, people with borderline personality disorder cannot calm or comfort themselves by calling up a mental image of a secure relationship with a caretaker.

Similar patterns of stormy, unstable relationships are found in patients with multiple personality disorder. In this disorder, with its extreme compartmentalization of functions, the highly contradictory patterns of relating may be carried out by dissociated "alter" personalities. Patients with multiple personality disorder also have a tendency to develop intense, highly "special" relationships, ridden with boundary violations, conflict, and the potential for exploitation. Patients with somatization disorder also have difficulties in intimate relationships, including sexual, marital, and parenting problems.

Disturbances in identity formation are also characteristic of patients with borderline and multiple personality disorder (they have not been systematically studied in somatization disorder). Fragmentation of the self into dissociated alters is the central feature of multiple personality disorder. The array of personality fragments usually includes at least one "hateful" or "evil" alter, as well as one socially conforming, submissive, or "good" alter. Patients with borderline personality disorder lack the dissociative capacity to form fragmented alters, but they have similar difficulty developing an integrated identity. Inner images of the self are split into extremes of good and bad. An unstable sense of self is one of the major diagnostic criteria for borderline personality disorder, and the "splitting" of inner representations of self and others is considered by some theorists to be the central underlying pathology of the disorder.

The common denominator of these three disorders is their origin in a history of childhood trauma. The evidence for this link ranges from definitive to suggestive. In the case of multiple personality disorder the etiological role of severe childhood trauma is at this point firmly established. In a study by the psychiatrist Frank Putnam of one hundred patients with the disorder, ninety-seven had histories of major childhood trauma, most commonly sexual abuse, physical abuse, or both. Extreme sadism and murderous violence were the rule rather than the exception in these dreadful histories. Almost half the patients had actually witnessed the violent death of someone close to them.

In borderline personality disorder, my investigations have also documented histories of severe childhood trauma in the great majority (81 percent) of cases. The abuse generally began early in life and was severe and prolonged, though it rarely reached the lethal extremes described by patients with multiple personality disorder. The earlier the onset of abuse and the greater its severity, the greater the likelihood that the survivor would develop symptoms of borderline personality disorder. The specific relationship between symptoms of borderline personality disorder and a history of childhood trauma has now been confirmed in numerous other studies.

Evidence for the link between somatization disorder and childhood trauma is not yet complete. Somatization disorder is sometimes also called Briquet's syndrome, after the nineteenth-century French physician Paul Briquet, a predecessor of Charcot. Briquet's observations of patients with the disorder are filled with anecdotal references to domestic violence, childhood trauma, and abuse. In a study of eighty-seven children under twelve, Briquet noted that one-third had been "habitually mistreated or held constantly in fear or had been directed harshly by their parents." In another 10 percent, he attributed the children's symptoms to traumatic experiences other than parental abuse. After the lapse of a century, investigation of the link between somatization disorder and childhood abuse has only lately been resumed. A recent study of women with somatization disorder found that 55 percent had been sexually molested in childhood, usually by relatives. This study, however, focused only on early sexual experiences; patients were not asked about physical abuse or a more general climate of violence in their families. Systematic investigation of the childhood histories of patients with somatization disorder has yet to be undertaken.

These three disorders might perhaps be best understood as variants of complex posttraumatic stress disorder, each deriving its characteristic features from one form of adaptation to the traumatic environment. The physioneurosis of posttraumatic stress disorder is the most prominent feature in somatization disorder, the deformation of consciousness is most prominent in multiple personality disorder, and the disturbance in identity and relationship is most prominent in borderline personality disorder. The overarching concept of a complex posttraumatic syndrome accounts for both the particularity of the three disorders and their interconnection. The formulation also reunites the descriptive fragments of the condition that was once called hysteria and reaffirms their common source in a history of psychological trauma.

Many of the most troubling features of these three disorders become more comprehensible in the light of a history of childhood trauma. More important, survivors become comprehensible to themselves. When survivors recognize the origins of their psychological difficulties in an abusive childhood environment, they no longer need attribute them to an inherent defect in the self. Thus the way is opened to the creation of new meaning in experience and a new, unstigmatized identity.

Understanding the role of childhood trauma in the development of these severe disorders also informs every aspect of treatment. This understanding provides the basis for a cooperative therapeutic alliance that normalizes and validates the survivor's emotional reactions to past events, while recognizing that these reactions may be maladaptive in the present. Moreover, a shared understanding of the survivor's characteristic disturbances of relationship and the consequent risk of repeated victimization offers the best insurance against unwitting reenactments of the original trauma in the therapeutic relationship.

The testimony of patients is eloquent on the point that recognition of the trauma is central to the recovery process. Three survivors who have had long careers in psychiatric treatment can speak here for all patients. Each accumulated numerous mistaken diagnoses and suffered through numerous unsuccessful treatments before finally discovering the source of her psychological problems in her history of severe childhood abuse. And each challenges us to decipher her language and to recognize, behind the multiplicity of disguises, the complex posttraumatic syndrome.

The first survivor, Barbara, manifests the predominant symptoms of somatization disorder:

> I lived in hell on earth without benefit of a doctor or medication. . . . I could not breathe, I had spasms when I attempted to swallow food, my heart pounded in my chest, I had numbness in my face and St. Vitus dance when I went to bed. I had migraine headaches, and the blood vessels

above my right eye were so taut I could not close that eye.

[My therapist] and I have decided that I have dissociated states. Though they are very similar to personalities, I know that they are part of me. When the horrors first surfaced, I went through a psychological death. I remember floating up on a white cloud with many people inside, but I could not make out the faces. Then two hands came out and pressed on my chest, and a voice said, "Don't go in there."

Had I gone for help when I had my breakdown, I feel I would have been classified as mentally ill. The diagnosis probably would have been manic depressive with a flavor of schizophrenia, panic disorder, and agoraphobia. At that time no one would have had the diagnostic tools to come up with a diagnosis of [complex] post-traumatic stress disorder.

The second survivor, Tani, was diagnosed with borderline personality disorder:

I know that things are getting better about borderlines and stuff. Having that diagnosis resulted in my getting treated exactly the way I was treated at home. The minute I got that diagnosis people stopped treating me as though what I was doing had a reason. All that psychiatric treatment was just as destructive as what happened before.

Denying the reality of my experience—that was the most harmful. Not being able to trust anyone was the most serious effect. . . . I knew I acted in ways that were despicable. But I wasn't crazy. Some people go around acting like that because they feel hopeless. Finally I found a few people along the way who have been able to feel OK about me even though I had severe problems. Good therapists were those who really validated my experience.

The third survivor is Hope, who manifests the predominant symptoms of multiple personality disorder:

Long ago, a lovely young child was branded with the term *paranoid schizophrenic*. . . . The label became a heavy yoke. A Procrustean bed I always fit into so nicely, for I never grew. . . . I became wrapped, shrouded. No alert, spectacled psychologist had trained a professional mind upon my dull drudgery. No. The diagnosis of paranoid schizophrenic was not offered me where I could look kindly back onto the earnest practitioner and say, "You're wrong. It's really just a lifetime of grief, but it's all right."

Somehow the dreaded words got sprinkled on my cereal, rinsed into my clothes. I felt them in hard looks, and hands that inadvertently pressed down. I saw the words in the averted head, the questions that weren't asked, the careful, repetitious confines of a concept made smaller, simpler for my benefit. The years pass. They go on. The haunting refrain has become a way of life. Expectation is slowed. Progress looks nostalgically backward. And all the time a lurking snake lies hidden in the heart.

Finally, dreams begin to be unlocking. Spurred on by the fresh, crisp increase of the Still, Small Voice. I begin to see some of what those silent, unspoken words never said. I saw a mask. It looked like me. I took it off and beheld a group of huddled, terrified people who shrank together to hide terrible secrets. . . .

The words "paranoid schizophrenic" started to fall into place, letter by letter, but it looked like feelings and thoughts and actions that hurt children, and lied, and covered disgrace, and much terror. I began to realize that the label, the diagnosis, had been a handmaid, much like the letter "A" Hester Prynne embroidered upon her breast. . . .

And down all the days and all the embroidered hours, other words kept pushing aside the badge, the label, the diagnosis. "Hurting children." "That which is unseemly." "Women with women, and men with men, doing that which is unseemly. . . ."

I forsook my paranoid schizophrenia, and packed it up with my troubles, and sent it to Philadelphia.

CHARACTERISTICS OF COMPLEX POST-TRAUMATIC STRESS DISORDER

A history of subjection to totalitarian control over a prolonged period (months to years). Examples include hostages, prisoners of war, concentration camp survivors, and survivors of some religious cults. Examples also include those subjected to totalitarian systems in sexual and domestic life, including survivors of domestic battering, childhood physical or sexual abuse, and organized sexual exploitation.

1. ALTERATIONS IN AFFECT REGULATION

➤ Persistent dysphoria
➤ Chronic suicidal preoccupation
➤ Self-injury
➤ Explosive or extremely inhibited anger (may alternate)
➤ Compulsive or extremely inhibited sexuality (may alternate)

2. ALTERATIONS IN CONSCIOUSNESS

➤ Amnesia or hyperamnesia for traumatic events
➤ Transient dissociative episodes
➤ Depersonalization/derealization
➤ Reliving experiences, either in the form of intrusive post-traumatic stress disorder symptoms or in the form of ruminative preoccupation

3. ALTERATIONS IN SELF-PERCEPTION

➤ Sense of helplessness or paralysis of initiative

➤ Shame, guilt, and self-blame
➤ Sense of defilement or stigma
➤ Sense of complete difference from others (may include sense of specialness, utter aloneness, belief no other person can understand, or non-human identity)

4. ALTERATIONS IN PERCEPTION OF PERPETRATOR

➤ Preoccupation with relationship with perpetrator (includes preoccupation with revenge)
➤ Unrealistic attribution of total power to perpetrator (caution: victim's assessment of power realities may be more realistic than clinician's)
➤ Idealization or paradoxical gratitude
➤ Sense of special or supernatural relationship
➤ Acceptance of belief system or rationalizations of perpetrator

5. ALTERATIONS IN RELATIONS WITH OTHERS

➤ Isolation and withdrawal
➤ Disruption in intimate relationships
➤ Repeated search for rescuer (may alternate with isolation and withdrawal)
➤ Persistent distrust
➤ Repeated failures of self-protection

6. ALTERATIONS IN SYSTEMS OF MEANING

➤ Loss of sustaining faith
➤ Sense of hopelessness and despair

How to Befriend a Battered Woman

BARBARA SEAMAN AND LESLYE E. ORLOFF

Barbara Seaman, excerpt from "Domestic Violence: What the Doctor Should Do," Anne D. Lopatto and James Neely, eds., *The Lawyer's Manual on Domestic Violence*, Supreme Court of the State of New York, Appellate Division, First Department, ©1995; Leslye E. Orloff, "Effective Advocacy for Domestic Violence Victims: Role of the Nurse-Midwife," *Journal of Nurse-Midwifery*, 41(6): 473–494, 1996. Reprinted by permission.

BARBARA SEAMAN ON DOMESTIC VIOLENCE: WHAT THE DOCTOR SHOULD DO

Public health, as well as law enforcement, authorities have come to recognize that "wife beating" is not only a crime, but also a major cause of death and injury to women. Many battered women who fear accessing the police and courts do, of necessity, access health facilities, especially hospital emergency departments. One physician compares sending a domestic violence victim home to "tossing a burn victim back into a fiery house." According to the American Medical Association, "Seventy-five percent of battered women first identified in a medical setting will go on to suffer repeated abuse."

A woman may be safer on the streets at night than at home with her own husband. The AMA accepts the estimate that more than half of female murder victims are killed by current or former partners, and that 8 to 12 million women in the United States are at risk of abuse:

> Domestic violence also known as partner-abuse, spouse-abuse, or battering, is one facet of the larger problem of family violence. Family violence occurs among persons within a family or other intimate relationships, and includes child abuse and elder abuse as well as domestic violence. Family violence usually results from the abuse of power or the domination and victimization of a physically less powerful person by a physically more powerful person. Changes in traditional services, including medical care, are needed to meet the needs of abused women.

As these changes, for which the regulatory underpinnings are now in place, come into full expression, the health care system will likely be recognized as a logical first point of intervention in battery, not as a mere adjunct. Ultimately, health care can do better than legal services at rescuing battered women, because the health provider's duty is solely to the patient, and is unambiguous. Unlike the police and the courts, protective efforts of the doctor or other health provider are not constrained, delayed, or inhibited by "he says/she says" conflicting explanations of the victim and the perpetrator. The AMA's Council on Ethical and Judicial Affairs has concluded that the principal of "beneficence" requires physicians to intervene in cases of domestic violence, and warns that if an injured woman is treated by a physician who does not inquire about abuse or who accepts an unlikely explanation of the injuries and she then returns to the abusive situation and sustains further injuries, the physician could be held liable.

MEASURING THE MEDICAL RESPONSE During the 1980s, a handful of women physicians began to collect evidence that emergency departments and other medical facilities were failing to give appropriate care to most of the battered women who apply for treatment, and that only a fraction of domestic violence victims are correctly identified when they enter the system. At the typical emergency department, no more than 2 to 5 percent of women presenting with injuries are recorded as having had them deliberately inflicted, while the true figure ranges from one-fifth to one-third. A corner was turned in 1985, when then-US Surgeon General Everett Koop, persuaded by the new research, announced his conclusion that more women are injured by battery than by rape, muggings, and accidents combined.

THE TIME FRAME It took a dozen years or more, from the first stirrings of the "battered women's movement" in the early 1970s, until Koop's acknowledgment in 1985, to the identification of "wife beating" as a major source of both morbidity and mortality—the leading single cause of injury to women.

From 1985 to 1992, the government, public health, and organized medical authorities, under the national leadership of Koop and his successor, Antonia Novello, developed a blueprint for sweeping changes in the medical response to domestic violence. Although regulations are insufficiently publicized to lay persons, by 1993 most health care facilities throughout the United States were subject to national, state, and local regulations requiring that suspected victims of both domestic violence and elder abuse receive attention and processing which is quite similar to that afforded to victims of rape and to abused children.

The president of the AMA gives domestic violence education the highest priority, while the American College of Obstetrics and Gynecology is also deeply committed. It is now recognized that: many males first commence battering when their wives or girlfriends are pregnant; one in six pregnant women is battered; pregnant adolescents are apt to experience multiple beatings, at the hands of parents as well as sex partners.

Our society is now allocating resources to carry out the new requirements. A national objective of the US Public Health Service is that by the year 2000, at least 90 percent of hospital emergency departments have procedures for routinely identifying, treating, and referring victims of spouse abuse. If this goal is met, it will have taken domestic violence from a private sin and sorrow, outside the concern and purview of medical practitioners, into as unquestioned a public health responsibility as the requirement that surgeons scrub their hands before performing surgery. And, like the adoption of sterilized operating procedures, the enforcement of laws against drunk driving, and other successful programs in public health, the relative cost of enhanced domestic violence identification will be modest. However, knowing what to do with that information is another matter. Health providers need training in a new set of skills, procedures, and resources, as Dr. Nancy Kathleen Sugg's study of primary care physicians in Seattle clearly demonstrates. Faced with a possible domestic violence situation, the doctors readily acknowledged that discomfort, fear of offending, powerlessness, time constraints, feelings of inadequacy, and above all fear of opening either "Pandora's box" or a "can of worms" (both phrases

were used repeatedly), inhibited them from making appropriate interventions. Many pointed to the complexity of the problems and complained that they had "no tools" to help. Sixty-one percent complained that they had had no domestic violence training whatsoever in medical school or residency, or in continuing medical education courses. Thirty-nine percent conceded that identification with patients might blind them from considering the possibility of domestic violence in their own social class.

REGULATIONS In recent years, regulations—state, local, and national—have required emergency departments to identify, treat, and refer battered women, while compiling an evidentiary record and taking steps to secure their safety. In 1990, the American Medical Women's Association became the first major medical group to pass resolutions concerning physician responsibility toward victims of domestic violence. In the same year, the New York State Health Department became one of the first to issue domestic violence protocols for hospital emergency services.

Effective January 1992, the Joint Commission on Accreditation of Healthcare Organizations (JCAHO) revised its *Accreditation Manual for Hospitals* to require that "standards previously addressed only to the management of child abuse and rape victims be expanded to include victims of spousal and elderly abuse." JCAHO, which has the power to close down a hospital for noncompliance, acknowledges that more than 1 million women every year use emergency departments for treatment of immediate injuries from battery.

The following four-step intervention strategy is suggested for use by all health care providers who treat female patients. It includes specific steps to take if a patient discloses the abuse.

1. IDENTIFY battered women by interviewing all female patients alone and out of earshot of any accompanying partner. Ask directly, for example, "Are you in a relationship where you have been physically hurt or threatened by your partner?"

2. VALIDATE her experience. Believe what the battered woman tells you. Offer positive messages such as "You are not alone" and "You don't deserve this." Document her injuries and symptoms in the medical record.

3. ADVOCATE for her safety and help her expand her options. Assess for safety by asking: "Is it safe for you to go home?" and "Is there somewhere else you can go—a friend or family member?" Be prepared to refer her to domestic violence service providers who can assist her in finding emergency shelter. In all identified cases, offer written and verbal information about local domestic violence services.

4. SUPPORT the battered woman in her choices. Recognize that she is the best judge of what is safe for her. Your intervention is a success if she is talking about the violence and beginning to explore her options. Remember that for most battered women, leaving is a long and difficult process. Most battered women leave and return six to eight times before leaving for good.

RECOGNIZING AND TREATING VICTIMS OF DOMESTIC VIOLENCE

It is important to recognize that the primary goal of all interventions for battered women and their children must be their safety. The following is based on the American Medical Association's Diagnostic and Treatment Guidelines on Domestic Violence.

If you treat women, whether in private practice or in a hospital, you are almost certainly treating some patients who are victims of domestic violence. The following decision tree is designed to help you assess a patient's risk of domestic violence and offer appropriate help to those in need of it.

IDENTIFYING VICTIMS OF DOMESTIC VIOLENCE

Although many women who are victims of abuse will not volunteer any information, they will discuss it if asked simple, direct questions in a nonjudg-

mental way and in a confidential setting. *The patient should be interviewed alone, without her partner present.* You may want to offer a statement such as: "Because violence is so common in many women's lives, I've begun to ask about it routinely." Then you can ask a direct question, such as "At any time, has your partner hit, kicked, or otherwise hurt or frightened you?"

If the patient answers yes, the following steps are suggested:

ENCOURAGE HER TO TALK ABOUT IT: "Would you like to talk about what has happened to you?" "How do you feel about it?" "What would you like to do about this?"

LISTEN NONJUDGMENTALLY. This serves to begin the healing process for the woman and to give you an idea of what kind of referrals she needs.

VALIDATE: Victims of domestic violence are frequently not believed, and the fear they report is minimized. The physician can express support through simple statements such as: "You are not alone." "You don't deserve to be treated this way." "You are not to blame." "What happened to you is a crime." "Help is available to you."

DOCUMENT: The patient's complaints and symptoms as well as the results of the observation and assessment (complaints should be described in the patient's own words whenever possible); the patient's complete medical and trauma history and relevant social history; a detailed description of the injuries, including type, number, size, location, resolution, possible causes, and explanations given; an opinion on whether the injuries were consistent with the patient's explanation; results of all pertinent laboratory and other diagnostic procedures; color photographs and imaging studies, if applicable; if the police are called, the name of the investigating officer and any action taken (the police should be called if patient exhibits a reportable injury).

ASSESS THE DANGER TO YOUR PATIENT: Assess your patient's safety *before she leaves the medical setting.*

The most important determinants of risk are the woman's level of fear and her appraisal of her immediate and future safety. Discussing the following indicators with the patient can help you determine if she is in escalating danger: an increase in the frequency or severity of the assaults; increasing or new threats of homicide or suicide by the partner; threats to her children; the presence or availability of a firearm.

PROVIDE APPROPRIATE TREATMENT, REFERRAL, AND SUPPORT: Treat the patient's injuries as indicated. In prescribing medication, keep in mind that medications which hinder the patient's ability to protect herself or to flee from a violent partner may endanger her life. If your patient is in imminent danger, determine if she has friends or family with whom she can stay. If this is not an option, ask if she wants immediate access to a shelter for battered women. If none is available, can she be admitted to the hospital? If she doesn't need immediate access to a shelter, offer written information about shelters and other community resources. Remember that it may be dangerous for the woman to have these in her possession. Don't insist that she take them if she is reluctant to do so. It may be safest for your patient if you write the number on a prescription blank or an appointment card. You may wish to give her the opportunity to call from a private phone in your office.

If the patient answers no, or will not discuss the topic:

BE AWARE OF CLINICAL FINDINGS THAT MAY INDICATE ABUSE: injury to the head, neck, torso, breasts, abdomen, or genitals; bilateral or multiple injuries; delay between onset of injury and seeking treatment; explanation by the patient which is inconsistent with the type of injury; any injury during pregnancy, especially to the abdomen or breasts; prior history of trauma; chronic pain symptoms for which no etiology is apparent; psychological distress, such as depression, suicidal ideation, anxiety, and/or sleep disorders; a partner who seems overly protective or who will not leave the woman's side.

IF ANY OF THE ABOVE CLINICAL SIGNS ARE PRESENT, IT IS APPROPRIATE TO ASK MORE SPECIFIC QUESTIONS. BE SURE THAT THE PATIENT'S PARTNER IS NOT PRESENT. Some examples of questions that may elicit more information about the patient's situation are: "It looks as though someone may have hurt you. Could you tell me how it happened?" "Sometimes when people come for health care with physical symptoms like yours, we find that there may be trouble at home. We are concerned that someone is hurting or abusing you. Is this happening?"

IF THE PATIENT ANSWERS NO: If the patient denies abuse, but you strongly suspect that it is taking place, you can let her know that your office can provide referrals to local programs, should she choose to pursue such options in the future.

DON'T JUDGE THE SUCCESS OF THE INTERVENTION BY THE PATIENT'S ACTION. A woman is most at risk of serious injury or even homicide when she attempts to leave an abusive partner, and it may take her a long time before she can finally do so. It is frustrating for the physician when a patient stays in an abusive situation. Be reassured that if you have acknowledged and validated her situation and offered appropriate referrals, you have done what you can do to help her.

LESLYE E. ORLOFF ON EFFECTIVE ADVOCACY FOR DOMESTIC VIOLENCE VICTIMS

Many battered women become trapped in abusive relationships because abusers lower their victims' self-esteem and convince their victims that they deserve the abuse, that it is normal, or that no one will believe them if they seek help.

Nurse-midwives and other health care professionals are uniquely situated to help abuse victims bring an end to the domestic abuse they experience. Health professionals are often the only professionals with whom abuse victims have continuing contact from the time before they learn that they may obtain help leaving their abusers, through failed attempts to leave, and after they survive the abusive relationship.

Health care professionals, particularly midwives, generally establish long-term trusting relationships with their patients. These trusting relationships make battered women more likely to disclose abuse and seek help and support from a midwife long before she might be ready to seek social services or legal relief. The midwife may be the first, and only, source of ongoing support for many abused women and their children. Nurse-midwives, whether they realize it or not, often see women before and after they are abused. Workers in the health care system are perhaps the only professionals who have regular contact with abuse victims at *all* stages of the abuse continuum. Frequently, the midwife or the physician is the only professional with whom the abuser will allow the battered woman to have contact.

It can therefore be seen that health care professionals have a special responsibility to abuse victims to identify abuse early, provide what may be the first message that abuse is not normal or tolerated in our society, treat victims' injuries, offer referrals to legal and social services, and support the victim as she goes through what may be a lengthy struggle to leave an abuser. For these abuse victims, the health care provider's office may be the only safe place they can go when they seek a break from ongoing violence. Midwives must be aware of this and make patients aware that their office will always be a place where they can find safety.

The most important roles for the nurse-midwife are identifying the domestic violence, documenting the abuse for subsequent legal proceedings, referring the victim to social and legal services, and supporting the victim through the frustrations she may encounter as she turns to police, prosecutors, and the courts for help.

BARBARA SEAMAN ON WHAT THE NEIGHBOR SHOULD DO

More American women are injured by battery than by rape, muggings, and accidents combined. Think of that! A woman is safer roaming the streets at night than snuggled up on the couch at home reading a book with her husband stewing in the den.

An American crisis? Yes, because so many of us who are tuned in to the media have heard it all (think of Nicole Brown Simpson and Hedda Nussbaum) but just don't know what to do. Haven't you seen some signs around you? Sunglasses and heavy makeup in the elevator? A cheerful co-worker who becomes inexplicably depressed and suffers a limp due to recurring "accidents"? Or it may be thuds on your ceiling. And of course you have doubts ("Frank? He always has those annual barbecues . . ."). But remember, 82 percent of batterers are Jekyll-and-Hyde types. When acquaintances doubted that a person as likable as my batterer (whose main method of assault was to run at me and knock me down, as in a football tackle) could have broken my ankle and smashed out my teeth, the downstairs neighbors set them straight.

Not wanting to probe in people's "personal" lives, we often gape at the puffy eye and remain silent. But, as Keith Haring put it, "Silence equals death"; we must reach out to these battered women (or men or children) in order to save their lives (and save America). It can feel so hard to do, so awkward, right? Well, here are a few tips on how to befriend a battered woman: Take her aside and quietly ask, "Are you safe at home? or "Did someone hurt you?" If she doesn't acknowledge it, ask again next time. Keep telling her, "No one has the right to hurt you." Many battered women are brainwashed into blaming themselves. Comments such as "He must be crazy" have the power to break through the haze. Don't ask her what she did to provoke him. When a batterer reaches the boiling point in his compulsive cycle, the excuse can be anything . . . or nothing. My batterer once beat me up after we returned home from the opera because I'd toted a purse that he considered too large and "day-timey." Don't ask why she doesn't leave. She may be well aware that escaping is apt to escalate the danger. Instead, help her devise a safety plan.

So the next time you see a locker mate at the gym with a suspicious black-and-blue handprint on her thigh, start talking. It just may work.

Fifty Ways Not to Leave an Abusive Spouse

ELAINE WEISS

Elaine Weiss, "Fifty Ways Not to Leave an Abusive Spouse," *Hadassah*, December 1998. Reprinted by permission.

Domestic abuse conjures up the image of a bruised, depressed, timid woman tiptoeing through her house while her unemployed husband swigs beer and throws furniture. The full horror of domestic abuse is this: Women in abusive marriages look like everyone else. They look like me.

I am the daughter of a physician father and a college-educated mother. My Judaism was as integral to my identity as my tendency to be picked first for spelling bees and last for volleyball. I had best girlfriends. I also had boyfriends; mostly bespectacled Jewish boys who played chess or clarinet. I fell in love with one during my sophomore year in college. We married in the summer of 1967. Eight years, seven months, and twenty-one days later I left.

I have spent twenty years trying to unravel the tightly woven threads of physical and verbal abuse that made the fabric of that marriage. Why bother? Why not just be grateful that I found the strength to leave? Because I still have nightmares. Because, beautiful though *Carousel* is, I can't watch Billy Bigelow hit Julie Jordan—and watch her forgive him. Because I cry when I see Charles Boyer methodically driving Ingrid Bergman slowly mad in *Gaslight*. And because after O. J. Simpson's arrest, I overheard a woman in the beauty parlor proclaim,

"you know, the women who let themselves be abused are just as sick as the men who abuse them. She should have walked out the very first time he raised a hand to her. That's what I would have done."

She should have—our glib answer to abused women. Miep Gies, who helped hide Anne Frank and her family, heard this in Amsterdam. "If these terrible things are happening to the Jews, they must be doing something very bad." These days we know enough not to blame the woman directly; instead, we say she should have gotten therapy. She should have called the police. She should have been more assertive. She should have been more accommodating. So as if the pain of the relationship weren't enough, we tell women it is their fault. They hear she should—never he should. It's "She should have stood up to him"—which, ideally, she should—but never "He should have stopped being abusive."

I know it's not that simple. I know that men who batter are themselves in pain. I know their behavior is a desperate attempt to feel in control. I know they can't just stop, that they need professional help. And I sympathize, just as I sympathize with alcoholics and drug addicts. I'm no longer angry with my former husband (this took years to accomplish). But I am hotly, fiercely angry when I hear, "Why don't these women just leave." To me, this is as meaningless as asking the victim of a train wreck, "Why didn't you just drive to work that morning?" Here is my answer.

I didn't leave because abuse wasn't supposed to happen to women like me. In 1967 the term spouse abuse didn't exist. No one thought to join those two words, since no one accepted that it happened. Or if it did, it happened only to uneducated women who were married to unemployed alcoholics. It certainly didn't happen to nice Jewish girls from Westchester County, New York; they went to college, married nice Jewish boys, then started a family. They didn't have to worry about abuse because Jewish men don't beat their wives. So when the abuse started—within a week of the wedding—I had no way to frame what was happening.

I didn't leave because I thought it was my fault. My only experience of marriage was the seventeen years in my parents' home, where I saw kindness and love. If my marriage looked nothing like theirs, I assumed I was doing something wrong. My husband would throw me against a wall—then berate me for "egging him on." Lying in bed at night, I would try to pinpoint the moment I had gone wrong. I always found it. I should have laughed when he told me the dinner was disgusting. I should have ignored it when he called me a fat dummy. I shouldn't have cried when he announced he wanted to sleep with other women—and if I didn't like it, I was insecure and possessive.

I didn't leave because I believed I could fix it. During our courtship he was tender and affectionate. He told me I was the most wonderful "girl" in the world. So I held on to the image of the man who was once my loving boyfriend. He told me I had changed, that I was no longer the pure, bright girl he had married—and I imagined he must be right. Since rational people don't suddenly turn violent without provocation, I must be provoking him. I thought that if I could just get it right, he would be nice to me again.

I didn't leave because I told myself I was overreacting. Yes, he would occasionally punch me in the stomach or choke me—but at least he never gave me a black eye or a broken arm. Yes, he would delight in pointing out an obese woman on the street and saying, "your ass is even bigger than hers"—but perhaps I did need to lose weight (I was then, as I am now, a size 6). Yes, he would indicate another woman, tall, blond, buxom, and leggy, and scold "Why can't you look like that?" But this was the 1960s, when the Beach Boys wished we all could be California girls, and maybe a petite brunette couldn't hope to be seen as attractive. Yes, he would occasionally put a pillow over my face while I slept, then watch with detached interest as I woke up half smothered—but I had to be imagining that, didn't I?

I didn't leave because there was no place I could tell my story and be told "It's not you—it's him. There's no way you can get it right because he desperately needs you to get it wrong." I never confided in a rabbi, since everyone knows Jewish men don't beat their wives. Instead, we saw a psychiatrist. I tried to find the words to pin down my husband's actions: He goes through a door ahead of me and gives it an extra push to make it swing back and hit me. He tells me I'm so ugly that his new nickname for me is uggles. I feel like I'm constantly walking on eggshells. The psychiatrist insisted my husband couldn't function without me, that I must learn to become that sort of wife he would want to treat well. We spent two years in weekly visits to this man. Nothing changed.

I didn't leave because I grew accustomed to living a lie. Maintaining our loving appearance became a conspiracy between us. He called it "not airing our dirty linen" and I agreed. After all, I was to blame for his behavior and he would treat me well if I could make him happy. A wife who doesn't know how to make her husband happy—why would I want that to become public knowledge? I agreed to the charade and played my part well. Which probably explains why, when I left, no one believed I had any reason to escape such a wonderful marriage.

And then one day I left. A total stranger was the catalyst. My husband was working at a prestigious New York law firm and I had started graduate school at Columbia University. One afternoon as we stood at a downtown crosswalk, I spotted a lovely old building with a magnificent garden on its terraced roof. "Isn't that building beautiful?" I said. "Which one," he sneered, "you mean the one that looks exactly like every other building on the street?" A woman standing beside us turned abruptly. "She's right, you know. The building is beautiful—and you are a horse's ass." As the light changed and she stalked off, I suddenly realized this man was never going to change. Within a year I announced I was leaving.

Yes, it took more than this one encounter. Fellow students became close friends. With professional and personal successes, it became easier to shrug off my husband's abuse. The day I told him the marriage was over (my twenty-eighth birthday), he cried and begged me to stay. He swore he would change. He painted an idyllic picture of the new life we would build. I barely heard him.

I am one of the lucky ones. He didn't threaten me. He didn't stalk me. He didn't murder me. Some men do. I am one of the lucky ones. I didn't commit suicide. I didn't become homeless. I didn't turn to drugs or alcohol. I didn't enter into a series of abusive relationships. Some women do.

Instead, I earned a doctorate and developed a successful consulting practice. I remarried. My husband and I have a strong marriage and *shalom bayit*—domestic tranquility. Life is good. But I still have nightmares. I still can't watch movies that show violence against women. And I still, and probably always will, feel anguish when I hear someone ask, "Why don't these women just leave?"

Out of Control

NORMA FOX MAZER

Norma Fox Mazer, excerpt from *Out of Control,* New York: Morrow Junior Books, 1993. Reprinted by permission.

Saturday morning, Rollo, Candy, and Brig play cutthroat, two-on-one, switching partners after each game. They play hard for a couple of hours.

Afterward, standing in the showers, Brig analyzes their games and instructs Rollo about his mistakes. "There's such a thing as hitting too hard. You can't hit the ball and not think about the next shot."

Rollo turns off the shower. Okay, he powers the ball, but that's what he has going for him—power and muscle. He loves to let go and smash the ball. He loves the sound of the ball smacking against the racket. He isn't swift and showy like Brig, who likes to run up the walls and kill every ball, and he isn't a precision player like Candy.

"This is a game of strategy, not strength."

"I got strategy," Rollo says.

"Where, in your ass? You see the ball and your muscles start popping and pow, you send it to kingdom come. That's why we lost that third game to Candy." Brig punctuates his words with snaps of the towel. "All you did was set Candy up. You kept sending the ball right back to him."

"Hey, that was my superior playing that won that game," Candy says. He's in front of the mirror, towel knotted at his waist, blow-drying his hair.

Brig zips up his pants. "Why didn't you call me back last night, Rollo? I was waiting."

"Last night?" Rollo dives into his locker for his shirt. "I didn't talk to her," he mumbles. "I'll do it, I'll call her today, you can count on it. Just remind me—"

"I'm not reminding you of anything!" Brig's face twitches, and he walks away toward the washroom.

Rollo looks at Candy. "He wanted me to call Arica for him."

"He's really cut up over her. He got too involved."

A group of men walk in and noisily get their gym bags out of their lockers and walk out again.

"You know how I started going with Arica?" Brig says, coming back from the washroom. "She was hanging around my locker. She was giving me the eye. She was saying cute things." He drops down on a bench. "What am I talking about her for? I don't want to talk about her. It's all over." He punches his leg, and he's crying.

Rollo has never seen Brig cry. It's terrible. Brig is making these hoarse, choking sounds, and Rollo can hardly stand it. He pats his friend's shoulder over and over. "I'm sorry, Brig. I'm really sorry. I should have called her. Brig, I'll do it."

"Forget it, I said. I don't care."

"That's the way," Candy says, hovering over Brig, too. "Just forget her. What do you care about her?"

"I don't. I don't care about her."

"Good. You can get another girl."

"Right," Rollo says. "There's a lot of other girls."

"They're like fish in the ocean," Candy says. "Brig just has to drop his line."

Brig slaps at Candy halfheartedly. "What do you know about it, Candrella? You ever have a girlfriend?"

"Plenty."

"You did?" Rollo says. "When was that?"

"When was that?" Candy mocks, sitting down next to Brig. "You think you know everything about me?"

Rollo lets his mouth drop open and shakes his head like a rube. He's playing dumb, doing it for Brig, to cheer him up. And it seems to be working. Brig is almost smiling.

They sit on the benches facing each other, their knees banged in together, and talk about how many years they've been friends and all the things they've done together. They talk about the other night, how crazy it was the way Brig and Rollo drove down into Union, and the way they faced off with Mark Saddler.

Candy brings up the time he and Rollo broke into the guardhouse near the quarry. And after that they go over the famous night when they all sneaked out of their houses at midnight. "We stayed out until two in the morning," Rollo says.

"No, it was three o'clock," Brig says.

"Don't laugh, you guys," Candy says "I know what I'm going to say is corny, but you know what I'm thinking sitting here listening to all this?" He looks from one to the other of them. "I'm thinking how our friendship is more important than any girl."

Rollo's eyes get damp. He gets his arms around Brig and Candy and sort of hugs them. Then they're all hugging, and their faces are close. Close enough to kiss, Rollo thinks. A weird thought, but maybe Candy has the same weird thought, because suddenly he pounds Rollo on the leg, really pounds him hard, and says, "Hey, cream puff! Hey, you big cream puff!" And they all laugh and break apart.

The hall is empty. The three of them stand still for a moment, then Brig walks quickly to the stairs. Rollo and Candy follow. When they turn the corner, they hear footsteps on the stairs.

"Let's get her," Brig says, and they run up the stairs. They run up the stairs quickly and quietly.

Maybe Brig doesn't say anything. Maybe Rollo only thinks he hears Brig say that. Maybe it goes like this: They hear footsteps on the stairs, and no one says anything, but they run up the stairs anyway. They run up the stairs after her. They are fast, they are quiet. They are taking the stairs two at a time. They are running up the stairs quickly and quietly.

On the second-floor landing, they listen, and they hear the footsteps still going up. Going up to the third floor. They follow. They go up after the footsteps. After Valerie Michon's footsteps. They don't talk about it, they just do it.

It's a game. Fun. They glance at each other, and they take the stairs swiftly, grinning. It's a game, and then, too, it's like a dream. Rollo feels something dreamlike in the way he is running up the stairs, running after Brig so smoothly, so swiftly, and the way Candy is running after him, and the way they are all running up the stairs after the footsteps.

Maybe there is nobody there, Rollo thinks. Just for a moment he thinks that—nobody there, no body, no person, no Valerie Michon. Nobody, just the footsteps leading them on.

Then they are on the third floor and they see her.

Her back is turned to them. She is at the end of the corridor in front of the window that looks out over the woods behind the school.

She doesn't seem aware of them. She's leaning forward, her hands on the windowsill, looking out.

She's like a shadow against the window, like cardboard, a dark cutout against the wintry white light flooding in from outside.

They trot toward her. They are not so quiet now.

She turns and looks at them. She says "What do you want?" Her eyes flicker one way, then the other.

She starts to move around them and Brig grabs her. And then they all grab her. They just do it, all together. It happens fast, so fast. It's like reading each other's minds. Let's get her. Did Brig say it? They don't say anything now, they just grab her, and you can't tell who does what, whose hands are where.

"Stop! Quit! Oh, damn, no—oh—oh—stop—"

Rollo hears panting. Maybe it's himself. He hears grunts, and he's aware of his hot breath. His face and hands are burning, and his hands are on Valerie: he has some part of her in his hand, some soft flesh, some thrilling part of her.

She's twisting around, trying to get away, trying to get free, but they have her.

Rollo's sweating and grinning. He can feel the grin stretched across his face, and he remembers slipping and sliding down the winding road into Union, the car skidding through the snow—dangerous, thrilling—You know you should stop but you keep going, you don't want to stop, you just want that thrill—that thrill—

Valerie is flailing and yelling. She wrenches free, her arms swing wildly, and she stumbles and crashes to her knees. Then Brig is trying to straddle her, trying to get on her back, and she's jerking around frantically.

A bell rings and it shrills into Rollo's brain.

He blinks and stumbles back, breathing hard.

Candy pulls at Brig. Valerie is up on one knee. Her hair is down around her face.

They leave. They walk down the hall, tucking in their shirts.

The auditorium is still dark. The play is still going on. The same characters that were onstage when they left are still onstage, sitting around the laden table: Tiny Tim, Scrooge, the "baby" in the high chair—

Rollo moves quietly toward his seat. He tiptoes, lifting one foot at a time, the way you do when you're entering a room full of people, and you're trying not to disturb anyone. You pick up each foot carefully, put down each foot carefully, and carefully lower yourself into your seat, hoping the floor won't squeak, the seat won't creak.

He sits and looks up at the stage. Denise Dixon is there, her head tilted to one side. Any moment now Tiny Tim will say, God bless us all. Rollo stares at Denise Dixon, and for a moment everything

blurs. Nothing is distinct. The stage and everyone on it, the auditorium and everyone in it, collapse into a smear of sound and light. He looks at his friends. Brig is leaning back, legs out, arms crossed over his chest. He catches Rollo's eye and nods soberly. Candy seems absorbed in the play, bent forward, chin in hand.

Rollo's heart slows down, his breath is quiet. He watches the stage.

From the corner of his eye, he sees a door open on the other side of the room. A bar of light appears. Someone leans into the auditorium, someone else rises. All the way across the dark room, Rollo senses whispers, ripples of movement. The door closes again.

"God bless us all!" Tiny Tim cries.

A moment later, a hand taps Rollo on the shoulder, Mr. Maddox's tall and slightly bent form is standing over him. "Come with me," he whispers. He taps Brig on the shoulder, then Candy. The auditorium is clapping. The three of them follow Mr. Maddox into the hall and down the corridor.

"Where are we going?" Rollo says.

Mr. Maddox glances at him. "Principal's office."

It's not much of a walk, just over the bridge into the addition, down three steps, and around the corner, but it seems long, because no one says anything after that. Brig whistles quietly. The only other sound is the muted thump of their feet on the wooden floor.

In the outer office, the secretaries look up when they enter. A printer is spitting out paper. A phone rings. One of the secretaries answers, and another phone rings. Each time, Rollo's stomach lurches a little.

Mrs. Andresson, the one with gold hair and two chins, nods to Mr. Maddox and says, "I'll say you're here." She raps on the door beyond the counter that says *S. Ferranto, Principal,* opens it, and goes in. When she comes out a moment later, she tells the boys to sit down. "Thank you, Mr. Maddox," she adds.

Mr. Maddox bends over Rollo and looks into his face. Like Coach at the end of the season, he goes to each of them and bends close, but, unlike Coach, he makes no speeches. He only stares, as if he's trying to understand something incomprehensible.

He leaves. The door shuts quietly behind him.

Candy, who's sitting between Rollo and Brig, says, "What do you think?"

"Michon must have told," Rollo says.

"Right." Candy glances at the women working behind the counter. "What do you think she said?" he asks quietly.

"A bunch of lies," Brig says.

Rollo can't get comfortable on the wooden bench. He crosses and uncrosses his legs. He's hungry again. He watches the women working behind the counter. He wishes Mrs. Andresson would smile at him. He likes her. She never raises a fuss when he needs a pass or forgets his locker key.

They sit there for a long time. People look at them, but nobody talks to them.

Our Guys

BERNARD LEFKOWITZ

Bernard Lefkowitz, excerpt from *Our Guys: The Glen Ridge Rape and the Secret Life of the Perfect Suburb,* Berkeley and Los Angeles: University of California Press, 1997. Reprinted by permission.

Bernard Lefkowitz's book Our Guys *evokes the lives of some high school athletes in an affluent New Jersey suburb and that of a developmentally disabled young woman whom they raped with a baseball bat and a broom stick. In this excerpt he recounts his first visit to the town and compares it to what he found when he wrote an earlier book,* Tough Change, *about poor youngsters in Newark, New Jersey.*

The sense of social nihilism expressed by many youngsters in Newark was attributable, at least partially, to their economic condition and the social devastation it created. The immutable condition they all shared was poverty. Being poor was the ongoing trauma of their childhoods. You could draw a line from the rubble of the streets to the rubble of their lives.

Of course, Glen Ridge was different. It was a town where almost everybody was pretty well off. If I decided to write about this place, I would have to readjust my perspective. The prosperity of Glen Ridge didn't negate the impact of economics on the values of young people in this suburb. But instead of writing about the sense of impotency arising from generations of poverty I might be writing about how affluence and privilege could inflate the self-importance of otherwise unremarkable young men, not always with good results.

This was all surmise from a distance. Before I decided to write about Glen Ridge, I wanted to take a closer look at the boys involved in the alleged rape, at the residents, and at the town. In the late afternoon of June 23, 1989, I boarded a number 33 DeCamp line bus from the Port Authority bus terminal in New York City. Forty minutes later, I got off at the intersection of Bloomfield and Ridgewood Avenues in Glen Ridge. I followed the crowd that was walking toward the field behind the high school, where the graduation ceremonies for the Class of '89 were about to begin.

My first mental snapshot: Glen Ridge was a squeaky-clean, manicured town that liked to display its affluence by dressing its high school graduates in dinner jackets and gowns. What impressed me most was the orderliness of the place. The streets, the lawns, the houses—everything seemed in proportion. There were no excesses of bad taste, no evidence of neglect or disrepair.

Although graduation was an emotional ritual, made more intense by the recent arrest of four seniors on rape charges, there were no outbursts of feeling, no overt expressions of anger, grief, or remorse. The adults and their progeny exercised near-perfect restraint.

It was if these graduates had fulfilled the first requirements of a master plan for their lives. Their parents' success had secured them a place in this charming town. Now they would follow their parents down the same road, passing all the trailmarks that led to achievement, security, and fulfillment. The constrast with Newark was overwhelming. The youngsters I met there had no idea what they would be doing tomorrow, let alone five years from now. The teenagers in Glen Ridge seemed to exude confidence in the future. It was a future that included more years of higher education, then entrance into an occupation or career. After that, marriage, children, and, perhaps, residence in Glen Ridge or a place very much like it.

They were secure in the knowledge that they would be protected as they made their passage into adulthood. Most of them would have their college board and tuition paid by their parents. If they needed to buy new clothes or a car or to pay a doctor's bill, they could depend on a check from home. Most of them had the luxury of easing into independence.

That's what I thought on the first night I visited Glen Ridge. But I also recognize that, even with all these advantages, kids don't always fulfill their parents' expectations. Some people have the benefit of wealth and nurturing parents and a good education, and still wind up morally and financially bankrupt. There are no foolproof master plans for success. I knew that because of what had happened three months before in this town, only a few blocks away from where I was sitting on this warm, humid night in June. What I didn't know was why it happened. If I found that out, I might have an interesting theme for a book.

Later that night I got my first glimpse of some of the boys who had been in the basement. They showed up for one of several parties that the town was holding for the graduates. As these thick-necked, broad-shouldered young men circulated in the crowd of students and chaperones, I felt a surge of recognition. I knew these kids! I had seen them all my life. They were the kids on my block who had developed faster than all the other boys of their age. They were out driving cars and dating

and having sex while I was still fussing with my stamp collection. They were the guys in the jock clique of my high school, louder and tanner than the students who never saw sunlight because they were always home studying so they could win the Nobel Prize in chemistry before they turned fifty.

The kids in Newark, black and brown, speaking Spanish, hoods over their heads, wheeling their stolen cars over to the local chop shop—they were aliens in America. Strange, forever separate and separated from the American ideal. But these Glen Ridge kids, they were pure gold, every mother's dream, every father's pride. They were not only Glen Ridge's finest, but in their perfection they belonged to all of us. They were Our Guys.

And that was the way they were being treated that night at the graduation party. Parents and kids collected around them, slapping them on the back and giving them big, wet, smacky kisses. Who would have guessed from this reception that some of them had been charged with rape and more of their pals would soon be arrested? In the bosom of their hometown, they were greeted like returning warriors who had prevailed in a noble crusade. Or, if you prefer, martyred heroes.

It may have all been a bravura show of solidarity by a bunch of scared people who saw their world crashing down on them. But it looked real to me. The accused looked like a bunch of carefree kids who had just wrapped up high school and were heading off to the shore for some sun and fun before they started college. Then I heard a voice next to me saying, "It's such a tragedy. They're such beautiful boys and this will scar them forever." The man who said that drifted away before I could ask him a question, but others I spoke to repeated this sentiment, "It's such a tragedy." Often they identified the victims of the tragedy. It was a short list: the young men who had been arrested, their families, and the good name of Glen Ridge. The list, more often than not, omitted the young woman in the basement and her family.

The Campaign to Free Charline

JENNIFER GONNERMAN

Jennifer Gonnerman, "The Campaign to Free Charline," *The Village Voice,* December 10, 1996. Reprinted by permission.

Marvin Brundidge told his wife repeatedly that he would kill her. Instead, she killed him.

Marvin, forty-six, and Charline, thirty-seven, had been together for seven years. From almost the beginning, he abused her physically, verbally, and sexually. On the night of April 21, 1985, they went out drinking together at a few bars near their Rochester home. Following a familiar pattern, Marvin became paranoid and possessive, accusing his wife of cheating on him. He said he wanted her to "get the fuck out" of their house.

Back in their bedroom, Marvin grabbed Charline by the throat, shoved her down on their bed, and started slapping her face. He called her a "whore" and a "bitch." Charline kicked him off and staggered away. "His eyes and his nostrils were flared," she later said. "It was like he was foaming at the mouth."

Marvin, who weighed 250 pounds and stood 6 feet, 2 inches tall, picked up his wife by the hair and smashed her head against the wall so hard it left a visible dent. Seven inches shorter and only 130 pounds, Charline was at a marked disadvantage. She grabbed on to the dresser to keep from falling.

While Charline slumped bleeding against the dresser, Marvin undressed, wrapped a maroon bathrobe around his naked body, and lay on their bed. Then he called the police. Dialing 911 and pretending to need protection was one of his favorite ploys, according to Charline's attorney. This way, Marvin could beat up his wife until the police arrived and then avoid arrest by blaming her.

"My wife is leaving," Marvin told the dispatcher, according to a police tape of the incident. "I just want them to be here if she come[s] back, 'cause I don't want her."

While Marvin was on the phone, Charline reached into the top drawer of the dresser and pulled his .38 caliber revolver out of its leather holster. From a few feet away, she unloaded five bullets into Marvin's head and chest. His body crumpled. She picked up the phone and found the dispatcher still on the line.

"Send the police here," she said. "I just shot my husband."

Today, Charline Brundidge is one of thousands of battered women across the country who killed their abusers during the 1970s or 1980s and are still incarcerated. She has served ten years already and, with a fifteen-years-to-life sentence, will not be eligible for parole until 2001. But much has changed in the ten years since "domestic violence" became an everyday term.

Many prosecutors now consider a defendant's history of abuse before charging her, thereby increasing the chance she will be charged with a lesser crime—manslaughter, say, instead of murder—that carries a shorter sentence. When cases go to trial, judges are far more likely to allow testimony about past abuse. And the defense now often includes an expert witness on domestic violence.

As a result, jurors are better informed, and more sympathetic, than ever before. For example, a Rockland County grand jury declined last year to indict a woman who had stabbed her husband to death with a fishing knife. And this summer, a Bronx woman who shot her husband in the throat—but didn't kill him—got only probation. If Charline Brundidge—or the many like her—had committed her crime this year, her sentence might have been far less stiff.

There is now a statewide movement to free Charline. More than fifty lawyers, legislators, and antidomestic violence activists, as well as the judge who sentenced her, have written to Governor George Pataki urging him to commute her sentence. Charline even has the support of Libby Pataki, the governor's wife, who met last month with Charline's lawyer. Were the governor to grant clemency, he would probably do so around Christmas.

If Charline is freed, she will be the first victim of domestic violence in New York to benefit from a nationwide movement to release women imprisoned for killing their batterers. Since 1978, governors in twenty-three states have granted clemency to more that one hundred women. In 1990, Ohio's governor commuted the sentences of twenty-five battered women. Maryland's governor released eight domestic violence victims in 1991.

Charline's current lawyer, Mary Lynch, has spent more than two years building Charline's case. While Charline refuses to talk to the media, she did let the *Voice* view a fifteen-minute videotaped interview that she has submitted along with her written petition. The picture that emerges from this videotape—plus interviews with Charline's friends and family, hospital records, police reports, and trial transcripts—is of a woman who is neither bitter nor angry, only eager to be reunited with her family.

When Charline was growing up in Gulfport, Mississippi, in the 1950s, she says, she often saw her father hit her mother. The lesson she learned from the older women around her was that "the man loved you if he beat you," Charline says in her interview. "My mother told me I should be able to take a lick."

Throughout her marriage to Marvin, this is exactly what Charline did.

Charline met Marvin through her sister when she was thirty years old. She'd already been married twice and had a fourteen-year-old daughter, Tyra. The two moved to Rochester in the fall of 1978 to live with Marvin, who ran a local bar. Charline eventually worked as a typist and then a clerk at the state Department of Agriculture, where she collected glowing performance evaluations.

"Everything that first year was beautiful," Charline says in her videotape. But it did not stay that way for long. "I really realized something was changing when Marvin started becoming really physical with me, beating me up," Charline says. "It was like his normal behavior. He wasn't talking to me anymore; he was always hitting me. All that we had in the beginning—all of that openness and him talking—that was gone. His size, [his]

legal permit to carry a gun, his temper, and his ability to use it all was very intimidating."

Charline wore sunglasses to hide her bruises, but she could not keep the battering secret. Five former co-workers attested to her abuse in letters they wrote supporting her clemency request.

Like many abusers, Marvin monitored his wife constantly. When Charline attended seminars for work, Marvin came along to watch her from the back of the room. He demanded she return home or to his bar immediately after work each day. And he timed her to make certain she did not make any stops. The drive home from work was about twenty minutes. If Charline took longer, Marvin would accuse her of having an affair.

As the beatings worsened, Charline's confidence crumbled. With violent, controlling behavior, Marvin crushed her sense of self. "I wasn't even me anymore," she says. "He had literally destroyed me. I didn't know who I was."

Charline tried to leave Marvin many times. Sometimes she hid in the attic. Other times she escaped to motels. Once she fled to her family in New Jersey, but Marvin tracked her down and enticed her to return with promises that he would change.

"The times that I did leave him, it was like he could find me anyway," she says in her videotape. "It seemed like I couldn't get away from him no matter where I went."

Marvin's blows sent Charline to the hospital several times. He burned her with cigarettes, held a butcher knife to her face, and raped her. In the two years before Charline shot Marvin, the police were called to their house at least four times. Often, the officers did no more than advise the couple to "stay away from each other." One time, when Charline showed up at the emergency room with a busted lip, a police officer asked who had hit her. "Nobody," Charline said, as Marvin glared at her from nearby.

Today, this scenario is likely to play out differently. Police and hospital workers across the state are trained to interview battered women in private.

Moreover, under a policy that went into effect in January, officers are required to make an arrest when they break up a domestic dispute if there is evidence of a crime.

When a case involving a batterer now reaches the district attorney's office in the county where the Brundidges resided, it goes to a prosecutor who specializes in domestic violence. This lawyer contacts victims, urges them to press charges, and offers information about a hot line and shelter. If this program had existed a decade ago, it might have saved Charline, and Marvin.

Charline was first convicted of murder in September 19, 1985. Her defense was that she suffered from an "extreme emotional disturbance." At the time, few attorneys had developed expertise in defending battered women. Charline's lawyer, John Speranza, did not call many witnesses who had seen Marvin abuse his wife. A jury found Charline, who had no prior criminal record, guilty of second-degree murder.

In a rare move, the judge set aside Charline's conviction a few days later because the wife of a juror stepped forward to say her husband could not have been impartial because he too was a batterer.

While waiting to be retried, Charline stumbled across a newspaper story about Charles Ewing, a lawyer and forensic psychologist from Buffalo, who had just written *Battered Women Who Kill*. From Monroe County Jail, Charline wrote to Ewing about her predicament. He agreed to testify for free as an expert witness in her second trial.

Speranza developed a new strategy. He argued the murder was an act of self-defense and emphasized Charline's suffering as a domestic violence victim. A slew of new witnesses testified that they had seen Marvin hit her. Ewing told jurors that Charline had reason to believe her life was in danger. He also explained that she suffered from battered woman's syndrome, which left her feeling so helpless that she no longer viewed leaving as a viable option.

But the jurors, who may have been hearing about domestic violence for the first time, might not have realized how much pain Marvin had in-

flicted. Moreover, Judge Eugene Bergin refused to let the jurors see portions of hospital records reporting that Charline had said her trips to the emergency room were caused by Marvin's abuse. The prosecutor, Charles Siragusa, claimed that Charline was not a "real" battered woman. "If slaps, pushes, and shoves amount to a basis for a syndrome, then I know sisters at the grammar school I went to . . . that are in deep trouble," said Siragusa, who is now a judge. Charline's current attorney, Mary Lynch, says, "It's a characterization that I don't think today would be appealing to a jury."

Despite the new defense, Charline was again convicted of second-degree murder. The judge gave her the minimum sentence of fifteen years to life. "Charline didn't fit some of the stereotypes that people had about battered women," Ewing told the *Voice*. "There was a belief that battered women were small physically. That they were unattractive, stay-at-home women—not assertive in any aspect of their life. And that they didn't have careers or interests of their own."

Starting in October 1988, Charline's home was a 6-by-10-foot cell at Bedford Hills Correctional Facility, a maximum security prison in Westchester County. She lived behind a steel door with a Plexiglas window. Wakeup time was 5:00 AM. At Bedford Hills, she spent her days working as a typist, clerk, tailor, and kitchen helper.

A model prisoner, Charline eventually landed a coveted job conducting orientation classes for new inmates. "She kept her nose clean, minded her own business, read her Bible," says David McCoach, who ran the prison's skills assessment program and supervised Charline for more than three years. "She received respect from not only her fellow inmates, but state employees as well."

Behind bars, Charline has earned both an associate's degree and a bachelor's degree. "I'm really proud of her," says her daughter Tyra. "She's accomplished a lot of things that she wanted to accomplish when she was married to [Marvin], but wasn't able to."

For many battered women like Charline, prison

is the haven they never had. They don't have freedom, but at least they no longer have to worry about being awakened in the night by the punches of an angry boyfriend or husband. "This has been like a shelter for me—a healing period in my life," Charline says in her videotape. "While I have been incarcerated, I have found myself."

Mary Lynch, an Albany Law School professor, first heard about Charline more that two years ago. As director of the school's domestic violence clinic, Lynch had been looking for an ideal battered woman on whose behalf to file a clemency petition. Charline fit the bill.

There are no rules about how to write a clemency plea. Even a note scrawled to the governor on a piece of toilet paper will do. As prepared by Lynch and her interns, Charline's clemency petition runs 337 pages and includes everything from her high school report card to a photo of the dent in the wall made by her head.

Lynch's team tracked down dozens of Charline's friends, relatives, and former coworkers, who wrote letters testifying to her character and her abuse. Perhaps the most persuasive letter is from Judge Bergin, who presided over Charline's second trial. Writes Bergin: "This, in my view, is the only case I have ever experienced that merits commutation in thirty-two years as a prosecutor and judge."

Nonetheless, there are people who firmly believe the governor should not free Charline. "I think she should stay in for the rest of her life because she took a life she could have avoided taking," says Archie Brundidge, Marvin's sixty-year-old brother. Richard Keenan, first assistant district attorney for Monroe County, says, "We would hope that she would serve out her minimum sentence."

No one knows exactly how many women are incarcerated in New York State for killing their abusers. Estimates range from 30 to 200. One of the goals of Charline's petition is to draw attention to these women. Says Lynch, "We convicted them, sentenced them, and forgot about them."

There is no trace of resentment in Charline's voice as she talks on the videotape, made earlier this year. "I feel the loss of Marvin," she says. "I take full responsibility for my actions. He played a huge part in our marriage that didn't work. And I played a huge part in our marriage." About the night she shot Marvin, Charline says, "It's a day I don't want to remember."

Charline, now forty-nine, grows most excited when she talks about daughter Tyra, now thirty-one, and her grandchildren. Charline has not seen Tyra for ten years. "I don't like prisons," explains Tyra. And until recently, Tyra and her husband, an Air Force sergeant, lived on the West Coast.

"It would mean a lot to me to be there with my daughter's family," Charline says. "I talk to my [grandchildren] when I call Tyra and they call me 'Grandma Charline.' Have you ever heard a little voice on the telephone say, 'Hi, Grandma'? I just want to be there to hold that little person where that little voice came from."

Charline has never met two of her three grandchildren, who were born after she was jailed. But if Pataki commutes Charline's sentence, she will join them in Delaware, where she plans to work as a counselor for domestic violence victims. If her clemency request is denied, Charline will not be eligible for parole until 2001.

"She was in prison when she was married to Marvin," says Tyra. "I feel now she's being doubly punished. She's done her time."

Governor George Pataki awarded clemency to Charline Brundidge on December 23, 1996. She was released from prison a month later and moved to Delaware to live with her daughter's family.

Surviving Intimate Terrorism

HEDDA NUSSBAUM

Hedda Nussbaum, excerpt from *Surviving Intimate Terrorism*, PublishAmerica, 2005. Reprinted by permission.

When six-year-old Lisa Steinberg was found brutally beaten and nearly brain-dead in her Greenwich

Village home, the story garnered national attention. After Lisa died in a New York City Hospital, the media frenzy grew surrounding the parents, successful lawyer Joel Steinberg and former book editor Hedda Nussbaum, who illegally adopted her shortly after her birth. It was soon clear that not only had Steinberg beaten little Lisa to death, but that he had subjected Nussbaum to over a decade of unthinkable abuse. The havoc wreaked on both Nussbaum's body and mind were so severe that New York County District Attorney Robert Morganthau decided not to prosecute her despite the fact that she had failed to call 911 after Lisa was knocked unconscious. Now a writer and domestic violence advocate, Nussbaum bravely tells her almost unfathomable story with elegance and honesty. Her hope is that other women in her situation will understand her experiences and seek help before it is too late.

THE FIRST TIME

How it first happened, I can't recall. It was a major change in the relationship, but I hadn't a clue. In fact, I decided pretty quickly that it had brought us closer together. In case you haven't guessed, I'm talking about the first time Joel hit me.

We were in the bedroom—I recall that much. That's where most of our interactions took place: sex, "therapy" sessions, crossword puzzle sharing, and finally, assaults. I have no idea what led up to it, what sort of exchange we'd had. All I can recall is the impact, the blow with the heel of his right hand, karate style, to my left eye. Blammy! That's all.

And then he embraced me, held me close. To me, that meant he was sorry, although he never uttered those words. It was just a fluke, I thought, something that'll never happen again. After all, no one who claimed to love me had ever hit me before, not even one of my parents when I was a child.

The next day I got ready for work, just like I did every weekday morning, but with one difference: I had a black eye and a cut under it.

After I'd exclaimed that I couldn't go to work looking like *that*—what would I tell everyone in the office?—Joel had insisted, with what I now consider incredible hubris, "You don't have to tell them anything. You don't owe anybody an explanation. It's your own business and none of theirs."

So I went. But I did feel a need to explain.

"Would you believe I was mugged *on East 57th Street?*" I told everyone.

In fact, I had been to that posh street the day before, and that's why it was so easy to come up with that particular story.

"Did you call the police?" I was asked.

I don't recall what I said in response to that question. However, whether I said yes or no, I'd already lied. And that was something I rarely, if ever, did. It just wasn't my way to tell an untruth to anyone. Oh, maybe at first I'd avoided telling my parents that I'd been living with Joel or, when I was fourteen, that the piano teacher had taken a quick feel, stuff like that, which I'd thought they couldn't handle. Although Joel considered those "lies," I never had before. He kept telling me, "The sin of omission is just as great as the sin of commission." So I now considered those kinds of things "lies" too. But to deliberately make up a story, no, not Hedda.

Anyway, about three or four days later, I started to see lights flashing from that eye, which scared me but good. Was I about to lose my vision? When my co-workers suggested I ask the company nurse to have a look at the eye, I did. And she advised me to get on over to an emergency room. I did that too.

I chose an ER not far from Random House, where I worked, in a hospital that specialized in eyes and ears. Being truthful by nature, as I just said, I told the female doctor that "my boyfriend hit me." But as I saw her writing that down, I immediately regretted my words. *They could get Joel in trouble, especially since he's a lawyer*, I thought.

So I quickly recanted, "No, no, cross that out!" And she did.

I'm sitting here now, as I write this, looking at a copy of that ER report. The doctor had written:

Thurs nite hit ~~by boyfriend~~ fist . . .
"black eye & laceration." . . . sutured . . .

Actually, "by boyfriend" had scribbles through it, not just one line like that. But those words were still visible, and yet, no one ever followed up on the report. This, you must remember, was March, 1978, when the battered women's movement was just beginning. And as I now say in my talks about domestic abuse, oddly using an expression I picked up during my years with Joel, "In 1978 it was 'domestic WHAT?'"

So, neither the hospital staff nor I, the patient, was acting in my best interest. Since I valued Joel so highly, I thought of him first. But had you told me a few years earlier that I'd behave in this way, I'd never have believed you.

One summer evening while I was living with Risa a few years before I met Joel, I heard a terrible ruckus emanating from an apartment in my building. I knew that the man who lived there was an alcoholic, but I didn't know that he sometimes became violent towards his wife. That night, the wife ran into the street in her robe, and Risa and I, like many others in the building, peered out the window at the scene. The wife stayed in front of the building and didn't return inside until the police had arrived, even though her husband kept up a steady stream of abusive hollering at her. Two policemen escorted her back in, she packed a bag, and left him that night. You can imagine how completely shocked I was when I saw her return the next day. I absolutely couldn't understand her. I remember saying to myself, *If my husband ever hit me, even once, I'd be out in a minute, never again to return.*

When the reality of the situation faces us, we don't act in such idealistic ways. Love often interferes with reason, and because of my intense feelings for Joel, I dealt with the circumstances in a way that may seem mystifying. I now think about what I did like this: I put the incident in a drawer in the back of my mind and shut the drawer. And there the incident stayed for a long, long time.

THE CYCLE OF ABUSE

I've learned that there are definite phases in the cycle of abuse, and they've been observed and studied. Although it's a mystery to me how any man "follows" the pattern, Joel surely did. He had a Tension Building Phase followed by a Serious Battering Incident, and then came a Honeymoon Phase where he treated me just like he might on a honeymoon—it was all sweetness and love. But soon the tension began again, and the cycle continued indefinitely.

Early in our relationship, it often took Joel months or even years to complete a cycle. But as time went on, the cycles got shorter and shorter.

The so-called Honeymoon Phase, when he was attentive and loving, could sometimes last for months, and sometimes only weeks or days. But it always roused in me the abiding hope that our early, idyllic era would return. Need I add that it never did?

And I really couldn't see the approach of a battering incident. Some women can see a man's aggression escalating, know that an assault is coming, and get away—anywhere—before they get hurt. But not me. The periods when Joel's offensive behavior was intensifying were short and so very subtle that I never realized that an attack was close at hand.

One day, for example, Joel had been doing some mild complaining—nothing to write home about. Hours later, while I was in the living room with Lisa in her playpen and Joel and Al Gross were in the bedroom installing a new telephone system that Joel had acquired from a doctor friend of his (the ob-gyn who eventually got us our little boy), the phone rang. I answered it in the living room and called Joel in to talk to a client. I was standing directly behind him when he picked up the phone. With no warning or provocation at all, and without even looking, he lifted his leg karate style and kicked behind him. It was a perfect hit. He got me right in the eye, that same left eye his right hand always smashed.

The force of the blow knocked me to the floor, and blood spurted from under my eye. I just sat there completely stunned, but Joel cut his conversation short and called to Al for aid.

I'd tripped on the shell of an old phone on the floor and fallen on one of the cradle prongs, Joel told him. As always, I backed the story. The old, large black phone minus its insides, now a toy for Lisa, lay right where I'd fallen.

With Joel directing his friend, the physician, they treated my wound and washed the eye all night long—literally. Al kept urging Joel to take me to an emergency room, but Joel always had an excuse. Time has erased from my mind his justifications for keeping my injury away from educated eyes, but you can be sure they were excellent. The cut below my left eye eventually healed, leaving no apparent scar; I credited this miracle to Joel's magical healing powers.

Only recently, some eighteen years later, a small scar has appeared in that very spot. Mornings when I'm putting on my makeup and looking closely at my face in the mirror, I recall the incident and feel the fury I didn't experience back when it happened. It's a fury that's meant not for just this one tiny scar, but for all the scars—on my body and within my heart—that I wear because of Joel Steinberg.

CHAPTER 16

Women in Sports

MOST WOMEN PROBABLY don't realize how Title IX changed their lives. When congressperson Patsy T. Mink helped pass this act into law in 1972, most people thought its implications would mostly have to do with school activities, more specifically sports. While it certainly did, the implications of the act were far-reaching, ensuring that "no person in the United States shall, on the basis of sex, be excluded from participation in, be denied the benefits of, or be subjected to discrimination under any education program or activity receiving federal financial assistance." That meant not just sports, but housing, health care and even quota systems that kept women out of academic programs they should otherwise have been admitted to.

It seems fitting that an act that is known to be about athletics should end up affecting all aspects of women's education. One of the things the women's health movement believes is that the health of the body affects the rest of a person's life. The fact that athletics have been historically associated with men, seems to be another way to entrench the notion that healthy bodies are male, while female bodies are always already abnormal.

When women embrace physical activity in any form, they reject this notion. They provide an example of health and strength that is distinctively female. When we understand ourselves as athletes, we can also learn the potential fitness issues that are distinctively female. For example, Dr. Rose Frisch writes that when women have too little body fat, they can find they are unable to conceive—a problem that can be better remedied by gaining five pounds than by resorting to dangerous fertility drugs.

Women in Motion

LUCINDA FRANKS

Lucinda Franks, excerpt from "Women in Motion," in Maggie Tripp, ed., *Woman in the Year 2000*, New York: Arbor, 1974. Reprinted by permission.

Turn your thoughts back about twenty-five years. When the Total Human had not yet been born and the average body was just a neglected dormitory for the mind. Try to remember those sedentary days when the finely tuned work of art called the human anatomy was pounding and screaming to get out from under dimpled scalloped layers of fat, sagging muscles, and aching bones entering the final and fatal stages of benign neglect. Who would have thought then that society would rediscover a secret as old as civilization, a secret that would intensify a human's joy in life, that would cleanse the brain and turn agitation and unrest into peace of mind.

Now that we are in the year 2000, with modern technology and a rebirth of the age of reason having joined forces to put a world hurtling toward catastrophe back on course, it is hard to move back in time—to recall a period when there were no integrated golf and baseball teams, when women athletes were not vying for football scholarships, when indeed it was not known that women are capable of being as strong pound for pound as men and, with equally strenuous training, can match or surpass them in many sports.

Lest we forget, however, there *was* a time when Little League and high school ball teams were all-male, with coaches swearing they'd dynamite the field before letting girls in and actively defying court orders for integration. There *was* a time when women were regarded, in the words of one sports philosopher of the seventies, as "truncated males, which should be permitted to engage in such sports as men do—but in foreshortened versions."

Somewhere around the mideighties, sports finally became an "in" thing. Suddenly the concept of sports had changed, and the very word shifted in its connotations. Just as in the seventies good nutrition suddenly became faddish with "natural and health foods," so did exercise and games skyrocket in status. They no longer evoked images of smelly locker rooms, tile floors, exhaustion, and former ninety-nine-pound weaklings with muscles the size of watermelons. And female athletes all at once were transformed from "Amazon Lesbos" to "goddesses," thanks to the appearance of Billy Jean King and other coolly feminine tennis pros, who started Americans down the road to female sports-star worship.

At the heart of this change was a realization of what coordinated bodily movements, as expressed in a sport, could do for a sense of well-being. The idea was as old as man. The Greeks had known that a sound mind is inside a sound body. People began to examine the generally well-balanced state of mind that many athletes seem to have. Statistics were taken, polls and studies were made, and the reasons were sought. Athletes came forth with personal descriptions of the almost religious feeling that came upon them after they had stretched their bodies to the limit.

It could not be denied that exercise improve clarity of thinking, alertness, ability to absorb complex ideas; it increased blood flow to the brain, strengthened the cells, and without a doubt acted on the regions of the brain to decrease anxiety and induce confidence and inner harmony.

And then "gamesmanship" was redefined. In the seventies, the need to win, and the need to have one's favorite team win, was crucial—so crucial, in fact, that the means used, the art of the game itself, was secondary. Now the conquering of one's opponent is not the prime mover in games; it is conquering *one's self.*

Both spectators and participants have now come to place less emphasis on winning or losing than on the way the game is played. Older children's games are structured in a way that lets everybody win. The Harris Games, named after Dr. Dorothy V. Harris of Pennsylvania State University (Penn State), are designed to reverse two traditional but still disquieting facts about sports: there are many more losers than winners, and the ones who need to win most generally lose. The Harris Games are intricately structured so they do not discriminate against the weak, the fat, the clumsy, or the slow. Instead, the complicated series of games favors each player and brings out the one particular thing each can do better than anyone else: the fat child wins the game where weight is important; the small boy, where smallness is crucial.

In the old days, people used to pass the time having parties, drinking liquor, and watching television. If they did venture outdoors, it was to rest on park benches and on beaches. Only the kids, sometimes with their fathers, played games. Now, of course, people celebrate their bodies. School gymnasiums, neighborhood baseball diamonds, and playing fields have replaced the corner cafés and "singles bars" as adult hangouts.

Much of the credit for all these changes belongs to women. Their full and equal entry into the sports arena, after years of chipping away at this narrow and selective male-dominated field, expanded it into a healthful and consciousness-raising pastime for everyone. It is ironic that women should be at the forefront of the "body movement," having launched their modern liberation campaign in the sixties and seventies with a demand for men to stop ogling the female body and start paying attention to the female mind. Once it was generally accepted that the female mind was as sound as the male mind, the battle turned back to the body—to prove that it was more than just a pleasure trove for man.

The array of myths about women and sports fell like dominoes. It was proven that, up until menopause, a woman's bones, though smaller, were no more fragile than a man's, that a woman was *not* more likely to be injured while playing than a man, and that in fact the injury rate per participant was generally lower for girls than boys—in both contact and noncontact sports—because of the girls' extra padding of fat. Breast pads were soon devised for women athletes, similar to men's jock straps. Coaches were convinced by medical testimony that the well-guarded uterus was one of the most shock-resistant internal organs in the body and that strenuous activity actually increased muscular support around the pelvis. Similarly, it was accepted that vigorous exercise helped both menstruation and pregnancy (the US Olympic Committee stopped advising its swimmers and other athletes to use the pill to prevent menstruation from coming during their contests). The scientific discovery that men also enjoy monthly cycles, with attending emotional highs and lows, also helped to dash the legend of the "female curse." The widely held belief that women athletes developed bulging muscles turned out to be scientifically unprovable—a woman's physique is genetically determined at birth, and no amount of exercise and training can radically change it. When women began to train strenuously for serious athletics in the eighties, it turned out that with the same amount of training they developed less musculature than men and instead used a higher percentage of already-existing fiber. Those shot-putters with bowling-ball shoulders turned out to have had the basic bulges in the first place.

Centuries of ignorance about and lack of research on the female physiology were overcome. Women, exhilarated with this new sense of physical power, began the slow process through the seventies and eighties of throwing over the "femininity game"—luring, baiting, and netting a husband—for the far simpler and honest games that men had enjoyed for years.

After long research into the female physiology, there now appear to be only a few sex-linked differences between the male and female performance in the sports arena. The average female is still born smaller than the average male and thus is at a disadvantage when a random sample women are pitted against a random sample of men. Moreover, she is at a disadvantage when performing in a climate where heat and humidity are high, since the body temperature of a woman must rise two to three degrees higher than that of a man before she begins to perspire and cool off. It was this discovery that led to the successful movement to have lacrosse and field hockey meets postponed form the traditional spring and summer season to late fall and winter.

Women athletes who have undergone steady and rigorous training also have overcome the historical heat dissipation handicap of the average female—that is, that the female has fewer functional sweat glands than the male. It was definitively established that women in fact had, in earlier times, not exercised as much as men had and had thus lost the use of a high percentage of their sweat glands; these needed to be reactivated, and were, by rigorous exercise. The change in conditioning has not altered a basic difference in the female frame, however, and her wider hips and lower center of gravity still place her at a disadvantage in some sports. Nevertheless, women keep closing the gap between men's and women's world records.

Back in 1974, when the bulk of research on female physiology could barely have filled one small library shelf, it was recognized that the trained woman athlete could always beat the untrained man. But given a man and a woman of the exact same build and training, it was believed that the man would always win because of his greater muscle mass, larger maximal oxygen uptake—or aerobic power—and proportionately bigger heart and lungs. Women were believed to have less stamina and less potential for reaching the heights of male athletes. It took a long time, but eventually it was recognized and accepted by coaches—who had long been as movable as the Pyramids on the issue—that women's physical inferiority was the result less of physiology than of a lifetime of deprivation. It had been so socially unacceptable for a woman to engage in strenuous activities, and she had been encouraged so often to depend on others to defend her—to act as her arms and legs—that she did not know she was capable, for instance, of even lifting a television set.

At first it was thought that even if this conditioning were removed and woman given opportunities to develop in the same way as man, her innate biological inferiority would prevent her from ever being able to compete with the male athlete. It took research by physical education scientists at Penn State, the University of California, and others to finally break the last ball and chain of opinion that was holding sportswomen down.

Until the late seventies, an athlete's maximum aerobic power (the capacity to extract oxygen from the air and deliver it to the working muscles) had been measured relative to his total body weight and was considered the best indication of his endurance capabilities. According to tests, the aerobic power of the female was only 70 to 75 percent of that of the male.

A number of scientists decided that it would be fairer to measure aerobic power in relation to fat-free body weight—in other words, the working muscle. It was found that square inch for square inch of muscle, women are as efficient as men in the use of oxygen. The discovery that at least in the laboratory women had as great an aerobic work capacity as men led to other tests to see if women's muscle power pound for pound was also as great. Not only were women found to be as strong as men in relation to lean body weight (total weight minus the weight of fat), in many tests their muscles proved to be stronger.

The fact that men have about twice the muscle mass of women was finally discovered to be meaningless. Just as men and women utilize only a small percentage of brain cells, so they use only about a quarter of their muscle fiber. This discovery put an end to the practice in the sixties and seventies of feeding female athletes, especially in the eastern European countries, steroids. Women athletes who trained as strenuously as men were found to slowly increase use of muscle fiber and reduce fat. Today, there is virtually no difference in strength between the average-trained male athlete and the average-trained female of the same body weight. It appears that the sedentary lifestyle of women has been largely responsible for the long-standing belief that nature meant her to be weaker.

Little League teams now generally have a preponderance of girls. At the high school level, all sports are integrated and there are no longer "boys" and "girls" squads.

On the college and university scene, the passage of the Education Amendments of 1972 forced educational institutions receiving federal assistance—virtually every college in the nation—to give early equal treatment to men and women. . . . The universities, after much rancor and protest, were forced to cut back their men's athletic budgets and skimp on the revenue-producing sports such as football and basketball to give the women a greater share. Women, freed from having to throw bake sales to raise funds for their travel, spent more time in rigorous training and eventually reached levels in which they could compete with men.

On the professional circuit, there used to be a vicious circle in the seventies whereby tournaments of women's golf, tennis, and bowling would not get television coverage unless there was a big purse offered, but sponsors wouldn't provide the big purse unless the tournament was televised. That catch-22 of women's sports was soon ended, and by the eighties men and women were earning equal prize money.

Women have come a long way in twenty-five years. Perhaps that is why all this uproar is happening now. Men are frightened by the sight of all these lean compact women—most young girls today do look like they stepped out of an Egyptian fresco. It is not that women no longer look like women—their muscles, though more outlined, are no bigger, and the sloping feminine lines are sill there. It is the uniform absence of a *traditional* thickness in the female form that seems to be disquieting to the people making the most noise. "You can't pinch women anymore, you can't even get hold of them," grumbled one of the leaders of the new male chauvinism [NMC] movement recently. And it is true that flesh seems to be the sole province of the over-forty these days. The NMC complains that women have usurped every last asset unique to males: "First, women have a stronger constitution and a longer life—their survivability

is superior to ours. Then they equal us mentally, and moreover claim they have the secret of the universe stashed somewhere in their consciousness. They give birth to life, and now they're saying they're just as strong as, if not stronger than we are." One of the more legitimate concerns of the NMC movement is the fear that with the decreasing fatty tissue in active, exercising young women today, a danger is being posed to the species. If the female fat layer is not there to protect sex tissue and the stomach during pregnancy, they ask, are we not raising a generation of female bodies that will be unable to protect their unborn babies? Are we gradually making female fat obsolete, and will the reproductive organs be the next to go? NMC sportswriters are calling sportswomen puppets, charging that they are mimicking males instead of being what they are best at. They are demanding that women quit competing with men. The hue and cry is great. You would sometimes think we were back in the seventies.

The Athletic Triad: A Dangerous Triangle

LILA A. WALLIS

Lila A. Wallis, MD, with Marian Betancourt, excerpt from *The Whole Woman: Take Charge of Your Health in Every Phase of Your Life*, New York: Avon, 1999. ©1999 by Lila A. Wallis and Marian Betancourt. Reprinted by permission.

The "athletic triad" is the combination of excessive athletic activity, weight loss, and menstrual abnormalities. With continued excessive exercise and excessive weight loss, the estrogen level drops, causing menstruation to stop and leading to bone loss. Young ballet dancers and other athletes often get what we call march fractures in the feet and ignore them until pain becomes insufferable. These are hairline fractures that usually cannot be detected without an X-ray. The healthy physiologic limit that should be imposed on the vigorous exercising of young women should be absence of side effects. Young women who exercise excessively might experience several side effects.

Intense physical activity leads to injuries of the musculoskeletal system. Thirty-five to 65 percent of runners are injured per year; the risk of injury increases with the total distance run per week. The critical level varies from one individual to another. Exercise that leads to injury is too much exercise.

The pleasant mood associated with physical activity is a great benefit, but a dangerous point is reached when an athlete's "high" makes her disregard physical discomfort and drives her to increasing amounts of exercise. Watch out for these feelings and behavior.

All in all, the dangerous athletic triad occurs in only a small fraction of young girls, while the malignant "pentad" of physical inactivity, overeating, obesity, accelerated chronic illness, and premature death affects millions of people in our country—between a third and a half of the female population. Physical inactivity and obesity constitute a far more serious public health problem than the athletic triad.

Patsy Mink on Title IX

INTERVIEW BY TANIA KETENJIAN

Congresswoman Patsy Mink (D-HI) served in the House of Representatives from 1990 until her death in 2002. This interview was conducted in June 1999.

TK: In *The Conversation Begins,* you discuss other issues you were working on when you were first elected. As a politician, what are the things that you've tackled that you're the most proud of?

PM: I was one of the principal advocates for Title IX, the provision in our education laws that says that all educational institutions—from universities all the way down to kindergarten—cannot discriminate against females in their selection of participants for programs, scholarships, fellowships, postdoctorates, and so on. Title IX has probably transformed all educational opportunities for women in the United States. It has opened up law schools, medical schools, all of the professions; certainly it has had a major impact in sports, as young women now typically star in all of our Olympics programs. That's probably been the most phenomenal piece of legislation that I helped to get through. We're still making sure it isn't watered down or changed in any way.

TK: Do you feel Congress now has a greater female presence?

PM: Oh no, we certainly can use many more women. At the moment, we're somewhere around 58 or 59 of the total number and, while that's a lot more than when I started many years ago, this still falls short of our representational entitlement in the country; many, many more women need to consider politics as a tremendous opportunity for participating in our society.

TK: Has there been a failure to address women's issues as a result of that lack of presence?

PM: Definitely, for example, five years ago, we passed the Brady law, which said that a licensed gun dealer had to do a background check on customers with a waiting period of five days. The gun shows were never included in the Brady law, so we were trying to include them because, as the Brady law went into effect, the criminals who didn't go to the gun dealers were going to the gun shows to purchase their illegal weapons. So we felt it was really critical to close that loophole in the sales traffic. But unfortunately, we lost this very simple amendment. Although all of the women of the House literally stood up together—we were all there on the floor at precisely the same moment to make our statement—the amendment was lost. So, yes, the presence of more women would be critical, I think, in a close fight like the one we had last night.

Why Feminists Are in Such Good Shape

AMELIA RICHARDS

Amelia Richards, "Ask Amy," an online advice column at www.feminist.com. Reprinted by permission.

Amy fields approximately twenty questions per day on topics ranging from women's health, to research papers on feminism 101, to young women in need of a friend.

Q: Hello. I know that you do not know me but I would like to take only a moment of your time. I am 5 feet, 4 inches and weigh approximately 107 pounds. I don't like to weigh over 103 pounds, but lately I have gotten lazy. I would like to know what my ideal weight is. I don't want to be extremely thin but I have this constant fear of becoming fat. I would like to also know what exercises will help me with my problem areas, which are my lower stomach and my thighs. If you will please reply and help me. Thank you for your time.

—Sincerely, Dawn

A: I am by no means a fitness expert or a physician, so I can't answer your questions from that level of expertise, but I can add personal insight.

First, I would hardly call 107 pounds "lazy"—if that's lazy then I am absolutely totally pathetic, and I know I'm not that. The thing about weight and body image is that there is no set formula. Every body—and everybody—is unique. By trying to fit yourself into a set pattern, you are ignoring the fact that life isn't that predictable—nor is your metabolism. As for weight, I am shorter than you (5 feet, 1 inch) and I weigh a little more than you (110–15 pounds—I don't keep track). I run two times a week and walk whenever possible—for sanity of mind more than sanctity of body. Of course I have days where I think I am bordering on obese, but in general I am comfortable with my body and my health. Body image isn't as much about "poundage" as it is about a mental state—

and false comparisons. It took me many years—with a little bulimia mixed in, although I didn't know that what me and my friends did after eating a pint of ice cream had a name—to realize that my body wasn't meant to be like Kate Moss's and my thighs would never look like those women in the Nike ads. What those years also taught me was that, thank goodness, I don't look like everyone else that's five feet one inch.

As for specific exercises—you need to figure out what you like to do, because the minute you start to do something purely to lose weight or stay in shape, it becomes a "must" and not a "want to," and therefore more drudgery than pleasure. So find out what you like—walking, swimming, running.

I've often thought of a comic: "Why feminists are in such good shape. . . . " We work in a profession that doesn't pay that well, so we are forced to walk everywhere—good for the legs and the cardiovascular; we always have to defend ourselves and our beliefs, so we always have to have lots of literature on hand too—heavy bags help build up our arm muscles; we can't drink beer, because these ads are offensive to women, or eat Domino's pizza, because they support Operation Rescue; we can't eat dairy products, because we are educated enough to know that animal fat can cause cancer. I still need to work this out, but I hope you see my point.

If you think you might possibly have an eating disorder, it is best to speak to an expert. If you think this is the case, you can try using our database of women's services to find an eating disorder treatment center near you. Be well.

CHAPTER 17

Body Image

WHEN LAURA ELDRIDGE BEGAN her freshman year of college, she quickly discovered that around 75 percent of the girls on her dorm floor had something in common: they had or had suffered from an eating disorder. These were bold, educated young women who were—unlike many of their counterparts around the country—almost unanimously identified with feminism, savvy to the history of women's rights struggles and sympathetic to the rejection of rigid social codes for female beauty. If you had asked them, they would have given an articulate, angry speech about expectations for attractiveness and the importance of cultivating the mind over the abs. And yet their bodies told a different story. All the knowledge in the world couldn't stop many of these young women from starving themselves or secretly purging after the dining hall.

Few issues affect so many women on a daily basis as body image, and have proved so impervious to education and consciousness-raising. On a basic level how we feel about how we look affects the way we move through the world.

In 1980 author Marcia Millman wrote a book that would become one of the few serious looks at what it means to be fat in a country that has a deeply unresolved relationship with overweight people. Housing a population that is more obese than almost anywhere else in the world and yet absolutely fetishizes thin bodies, America struggles to understand how and why it feels the way it does about weight. Millman interviewed children at "fat camp" and adult members of Overeaters Anonymous and the National Association to Aid Fat Americans. She asked important questions about sexuality and obesity, the psychological effects of living as a fat woman in America, and negative cultural messages and mythologies ranging from assumptions of self-hatred to a lack of self-control.

Today, little has changed. If anything, the notion that overweight people pose a societal health burden has only gained momentum, and being fat is seen as a character flaw rather than a factor of genetics, economics, and cultural patterns. We are swimming in a sea of diet books and weight loss products, but rarely stop to dig into or question the deep, convoluted cultural meanings inscribed in body size. Meanwhile, we struggle with rising obesity rates and resulting health problems, including rampant type II diabetes.

It is increasingly necessary to talk about these issues in a world that not only continues to overvalue thinness but has begun to recode the language when talking about bodies and beauty. Aesthetic values, once a cornerstone of sentiments about obesity, have been replaced with notions about health. Rather than implying that someone should lose weight to look good, we are told you should focus on "being healthy." While there is certainly a lot of scientific truth to back the value of exercise and the maintenance of a somewhat lower body weight, all too often conversations about beauty are recoded into conversations about health and well-being.

Fat Is a Feminist Issue

SUSIE ORBACH

Susie Orbach, excerpt from *Fat Is a Feminist Issue,* New York: Berkeley, 1978. Reprinted by permission.

PREFACE

In March 1970, I went to the Alternate U on Sixth Avenue and 14th Street in New York City to register for a course on compulsive eating and self-image—women only. I walked into a room jammed with forty women of various sizes talking about their bodies and their eating habits. It was the first time since the beginning of the women's liberation movement that women had dared to come forward for discussion groups specifically dealing with body image. The call for the course had seemed to me almost like a travesty—feminists concerned about how they looked! At the time we were used to rejecting male ideals of how we should look as

projected in advertisements and movies. We were ostensibly happy in our blue jeans and work shirts. We were not used to discussing clothes or body size with our female friends; there was, in fact, a widespread feeling of relief that we could relax in our bodies and not worry about what was especially fashionable, provocative, or appealing. We wore the clothes of rebellion and did not care what others thought. Or did we? . . .

I was hesitant to explore the topic of compulsive eating outside the context of a political vocabulary—a vocabulary that looked at the relationship between patriarchy and Western society with the family as the linchpin. I was uneasy but held on to the slogan that the personal is political.

I would not have gone back but for one thing. Despite my discomfort, I also experienced a relief to be in a group with women, fat and thin, who were all compulsive eaters. The problem had been named, and perhaps I did not have to feel quite so ashamed. In the last year or so I had become quite used to talking about very personal topics in consciousness-raising groups, and I was quite excited that we [were going to] discuss in the same way a subject that had been so hidden and so private.

We had taken the formula of a women's group, and one by one we shared how we felt about our bodies, being attractive, food, eating, thinness, fatness, and clothes. We detailed our previous diet histories and traded horror stories of doctors, psychiatrists, diet organizations, health farms, and fasting. We knew enough to know that all our previous attempts at getting our bodies the right weight and shape had not worked. We wondered *why* we had wanted them so right, *what* was so powerful about looking a particular way that we had all tried and succeeded in losing weight dozens of times. We did not understand why we could not keep "it" off, why every time we neared the goal "it" would creep up, or why we always broke our diets. Why were we so plagued by our body size and shape?

We began asking new questions and coming

up with new answers. We were a self-help group at the time when energy from the women's liberation movement sparked us all into rethinking many previously held assumptions. The creativity of the movement prepared a fertile soil in which feminist ideas, nurtured and developed in countless consciousness-raising groups, in mass marches and demonstrations, in organized political campaigns, found new applications and usefulness. Compulsive eating was one such area.

Compulsive eating is a very painful and, on the surface, self-destructive activity. But feminism has taught us to be wary of this label. Feminism has taught us that activities that appear to be self-destructive are invariably adaptations, attempts to cope with the world. In our group, we turned our strongly held ideas about dieting and thinness upside down. Slowly and unsurely we stopped dieting. Nothing terrible happened. My world did not collapse. Maybe we did not want to be thin. I developed a new political reason for not being thin—I was not going to be like the fashion magazines wanted me to be; I was a Jewish beatnik, and I would be *zaftig*. I relaxed, ate what I wanted, and wore clothes that were expressive of me. But why was I afraid of being thin? The things I was frightened of came into vision. I confronted them, always asking myself—how would it help to be fat in this situation? *What* would be more troublesome if I were thin? As the image of my fat and thin personality conflated, I began to lose weight. I felt a deep satisfaction that I could be a size that felt good for me and no longer obsessed with food. I promised myself I would not be responsible for depriving myself of the food I liked. I had learned a crucial lesson—that I could be the same person thin as I was fat. Satisfied, I left the group six months later. I no longer defined myself as a compulsive eater, and I had stabilized at a weight I found acceptable. It turned out to be rather higher than my previous Twiggy-like fantasies. Food no longer terrified me, and I could live in my body.

Obesity and overeating have joined sex as central issues in the lives of many women today.

In the United States, 50 percent of women are estimated to be overweight. Every women's magazine has a diet column. Diet doctors and clinics flourish. The names of diet foods are now part of our general vocabulary. Physical fitness and beauty are every woman's goals. While this preoccupation with fat and food has become so common that we tend to take it for granted, being fat, feeling fat, and the compulsion to overeat are, in fact, serious and painful experiences for the women involved. Being fat isolates and invalidates a woman. Almost inevitably, the explanations offered for fatness point a finger at the failure of women themselves to control their weight, control their appetites, and control their impulses. Women suffering from the problem of compulsive eating endure a double anguish: feeling out of step with the rest of society and believing that it is all their own fault.

The number of women who have problems with weight and compulsive eating is large and growing. Owing to the emotional distress involved and the fact that the many varied solutions offered to women in the past have not worked, a new psychotherapy to deal with compulsive eating has had to evolve within the context of the movement for women's liberation. This new psychotherapy represents a feminist rethinking of traditional psychoanalysis. A feminist perspective to the problem of women's compulsive eating is essential if we are to move on from the ineffective blame-the-victim approach and the unsatisfactory adjustment model of treatment. While psychoanalysis gives us useful tools to discover the deepest sources of emotional distress, feminism insists that those painful personal experiences derive from the social context into which female babies are born and within which they develop to become adult women. The fact that compulsive eating is overwhelmingly a women's problem suggests that it has something to do with the experience of being female in our society. Feminism argues that being fat represents an attempt to break free of society's sex stereotypes. Getting fat can thus be understood as a definite and purposeful act; it is a directed, conscious or unconscious challenge to sex-role stereotyping and the culturally defined experience of womanhood.

Fat is a social disease, and fat is a feminist issue. Fat is not about lack of self-control or lack of willpower. Fat is about protection, sex, nurturance, strength, boundaries, mothering, substance, assertion, and rage. It is a response to the inequality of the sexes. Fat expresses experiences of women today in ways that are seldom examined and even more seldom treated. While becoming fat does not alter the roots of sexual oppression, an examination of the underlying causes of unconscious motivation that lead women to compulsive eating suggests new treatment possibilities. A new therapeutic approach does not reinforce the oppressive social roles that lead women into compulsive eating in the first place. What is it about the social position of women that leads them to respond to it by getting fat?

The relegation of women to the social roles of wife and mother has several significant consequences that contribute to the problem of fat. An emphasis on presentation as the central aspect of a woman's existence makes her extremely self-conscious. It demands that she occupy herself with a self-image that others will find pleasing and attractive—an image that will immediately convey what kind of woman she is. She must observe and evaluate herself, scrutinizing every detail as though she were an outside judge. She attempts to make herself in the image of womanhood presented by billboards, newspapers, magazines, and television. The media present women either in a sexual context or within the family, reflecting a woman's two prescribed roles, first as a sex object and then as a mother. She is brought up to catch a man with her good looks and pleasing manner. To do this she much look appealing, earthy, sensual, sexual, virginal, innocent, reliable, daring, mysterious, coquettish, and thin. In other words, she offers her self-image on the marriage marketplace. As a married woman, her sexuality will be sanctioned and her economic needs will be looked after. She will have achieved the first step of womanhood.

Since women are taught to see themselves from the outside, they become prey to the huge fashion and diet industries that first set up the ideal images and then exhort women to meet them. The message is loud and clear: the woman's body is not her own. The woman's body is not satisfactory as it is. It must be thin, free of "unwanted hair," deodorized, perfumed, and clothed. It must conform to an ideal physical type. Family and school socialization teaches girls to groom themselves properly.

Furthermore, the job is never-ending, for the image changes from year to year. In the early 1960s, the only way to feel acceptable was to be skinny and flat chested with long straight hair. The first of these was achieved by near starvation, the second, by binding one's breasts with an Ace bandage, and the third, by ironing one's hair. Then, in the early 1970s, the look was curly hair and full breasts. Just as styles in clothes change seasonally, so women's bodies are expected to change to fit these fashions. Long and skinny one year, petite and demure the next, women are continually manipulated by images of proper womanhood, which are extremely powerful because they are presented as the only reality. To ignore them means to risk being an outcast. Women are urged to conform, to help out the economy by continuous consumption of goods and clothing that are quickly made unwearable by the next season's fashion styles in clothes and body shapes. In the background, a ten-billion-dollar industry waits to remold bodies to the latest fashion. In this way, women are caught in an attempt to conform to a standard that is externally defined and constantly changing.

But these models of femininity are experienced by women as unreal, frightening, and unattainable. They produce a picture that is far removed from the reality of women's day-to-day lives. The one constant in these images is that a woman must be thin. For many women, compulsive eating and being fat have become one way to avoid being marketed or seen as the ideal women: "My fat says 'screw you' to all who want me to the be perfect mom, sweetheart, maid, and whore. Take me for who I am, not for who I'm supposed to be. If you are really interested in me, you can wade through the layers and find out who I am." In this way, fat expresses a rebellion against the power-lessness of the woman, against the pressure to look and act in a certain way and against being evaluated on her ability to create an image of herself. Becoming fat is, thus, a woman's response to the first step in the process of fulfilling a pre-scribed social role which requires her to shape herself to an externally imposed image in order to catch a man. A second stage in this process takes place after she achieves that goal, after she has become a wife and mother.

For the compulsive eater, fat has much symbolic meaning which makes sense within a feminist context. Fat is a response to the many oppressive manifestations of a sexist culture. Fat is a way of saying no to powerlessness and self-denial, to a limiting sexual expression which demands that females look and act a certain way, and to an image of womanhood that defines a specific social role. Fat offends Western ideals of female beauty, and, as such, every "overweight" woman creates a crack in the popular culture's ability to make us mere products. Fat also expresses the tension in the mother-daughter relationship, the relationship which has been allocated the feminization of the female. This relationship is bound to be difficult in a patriarchal society because it demands that the already oppressed mothers become the teach-ers, preparers, and enforcers of the oppression that society will visit on their daughters. A woman's psychological development is structured in such a way as to prepare her for a life of inequality, but this straitjacket is not accepted lightly and invariably causes a "reaction." Psychological disturbance often distorts a person's physiological capacity: ability to eat, sleep, talk, or enjoy sexual activity.

I suggest that one of the reasons we find so many women suffering from eating disorders is because the social relationship between feeder and fed, between mother and daughter, fraught as it is with ambivalence and hostility, becomes a suitable mechanism for distortion and rebellion. An examination of the symbolic meanings of fat provides insight into individual woman's experience in patriarchal culture. Fat is an adaptation to the oppression of women, and as such, it may be an unsatisfying personal solution and an ineffectual political attack. It is to this problem that our com-pulsive-eating therapy speaks within a feminist context.

Such a Pretty Face: Being Fat in America

MARCIA MILLMAN

Marcia Millman, excerpt from *Such a Pretty Face: Being Fat in America*, New York and London: W. W. Norton and Co., 1980. Reprinted by permission.

SET APART: THE FAT PERSON AS AN ANTISOCIAL FIGURE

A common and important point is made by The National Association to Aid Fat Americans (NAAFA), Overeaters Anonymous (OA) and children's diet camps: despite their differences, the very existence of each organization is evidence of how fat people are isolated and set apart from "normal" society. But why does this happen? What sentiments and reactions do fat people arouse in others that would make them respond so negatively? A few clues to this puzzle can be found in some stories told to me by a friend (a woman of average size) who de-scribed her reactions to some very fat women she saw in public settings.

Walking through a store, my friend Barbara re-cently found herself staring at the massive arms (bared by a sleeveless dress) of a woman who weighed over 300 pounds. To Barbara's eyes this flesh was so white, so spongy that she thought, surely this woman must spend most of her waking hours eating, as if she were cultivating herself, like a giant mushroom. In this case, my friend associated the size and texture of the woman's flesh with a kind of self-absorption. She also recalled a different reaction to another fat woman: As she sat one day on a San Francisco municipal bus, Barbara became fascinated and repelled by the sight of a hugely fat passenger. Asked how old the woman was, my friend shrugged her shoulders, as if to say the woman's massive size had somehow made her age either irrelevant or indeterminable, but finally she guessed the woman was somewhere in her thirties. What had impressed her was that the woman wore a dress she had obviously made for herself out of a bedspread. The pattern of the material was very large, and Barbara noted with some interest that the bold pattern seemed appropriate given the size of the dress and the woman. The woman was carrying two vinyl suitcases, one in each hand (she appeared to be returning from a trip) and my friend thought the luggage looked like little wings on a giant beetle.

The woman maneuvered herself and the suitcase with obvious difficulty. Rather than move very far into the bus she sat in a front seat reserved for the elderly and the physically handicapped. Both my friend and the fat passenger rode all the way to the same suburban station, where each placed a telephone call for someone to pick them up. Barbara, still curious about the fat woman, was surprised that she dialed a number from memory, as if to a husband or another very close person, for she had imagined during the bus ride that this woman must lead an isolated life.

Barbara explained that at first she had felt great pity for how hard the woman's life must have been. Thinking about what it must be like to have to make one's own dresses out of bedspreads, or to have such trouble moving about and carrying packages, my friend imagined that being fat must have cost this woman tremendous effort and energy. But her pity had soon turned into anger at what she believed the woman was doing to herself by being so fat. She wanted to shake the woman and tell her to pull herself together, do something about it.

Other friends have admitted a similar anger at fat people because they take up more than a fair share of space. In their eyes, fat people seem to aggressively intrude beyond proper boundaries. This reaction corresponds with criticisms appearing with increasing frequency in newspapers that fat people use up too many resources. Claims are made by Blue Cross and government officials that obese people drive up the cost of health care and nutritionists admonish that fat people eat enough excess food to fuel several American cities. Another friend recalled that when she was recently at the airport she saw a man who must have weighed 400 pounds. He was chain-smoking and sweating profusely and my friend thought to herself, this man is killing himself and we're all going to pay for it.

Such depth of feeling is puzzling. It is somewhat understandable that fat people might be resented for driving up health costs (although the costs due to obesity are actually miniscule compared with the costs of cancer caused by environmental and occupational hazards or the enormous profits of the health industry). But the health cost argument is not a sufficient explanation for the sentiments aroused. A person with heart disease who smokes or works too hard may be criticized by friends for his habits, but he does not inspire the horror, loathing, speculation, repugnance, and avoidance that very fat people do.

Perhaps mere visibility plays a part. Some would argue that smoking doesn't make a person physically unattractive, but fat does. Even so, there is more to the process of perceiving fat people as characters who are disturbingly unresponsive to social control.

Being slim is highly valued in our society. A fat person violates that value and therefore offends society's expectations. This is especially true for women whose worth and achievement are judged largely on the basis of how they look. And when expectations are violated, explanations and interpretations inevitably follow. Because of these further interpretations, the fat person's differentness comes to be perceived as more than physical.

Responses vary according to the perspective of the viewer. People who used to be fat or fear gaining weight often confess to a sense of horror when they see an obese person. The dreaded "lack of self-control" lurks perhaps in themselves. Those who were never fat and can't imagine becoming so often project onto fat people a willful laziness and self-indulgence. How could a person let herself "go" like that? But in both cases it is the interpretation that the fat person violates norms (whether from weakness or defiance) that lurks behind the reactions of loathing and horror.

Furthermore, by its very nature deviance has a tendency to become generalized: once a person is perceived as deviant at all, nothing about her is trusted or taken for granted and the trait that distinguishes her seems to color her entire being in the eyes of others. As the stories of fat people vividly demonstrate, being overweight and the interpretations surrounding it wind up affecting all of a person's life, pushing the fat person into a special, marginal relationship to the world. Frequently she is clearly excluded, but even when included with others there is always tension, qualification, uncertainty, self-consciousness, and uneasiness between herself and "normals." Are others thinking about her weight? Indeed, she wonders, too, how far she can go in claiming the rights and privileges of "normal" human beings, and where she must not presume to cross the line.

Our earliest experience of social conventions and control is in the family. For many fat people, the family was the first social setting where their weight defined them as deviant, abnormal, and problematic. Fat children often struggle with their parents over food and eating. Conflict over eating habits is of course common among all American parents and children, but in the case of fat children the arguments take on added significance and eating becomes closely associated with autonomy, control, and love.

To parents a fat child is an embarrassment, being viewed in our society as a poor reflection on the parents themselves. If obesity is an expression of something gone wrong with the child, there must be something wrong with the parents as well, and the way they treated the child. Until adolescence, children are not regarded as responsible, so fat children are more pitied and their parents blamed. Many parents therefore not only fight bitterly with their overweight children about their eating habits but also (like the parents of NAAFA member Laura Campbell) let their children know that they are embarrassed and repelled by them. However much some children may experience triumph in defying their parents with eating, they are also devastated by their parents' repugnance. Knowing that even one's parents are ashamed to be seen with oneself is an early and most powerful experience for a fat person. These feelings were nicely captured on an episode of CBS's *Magazine Show* in an interview with the family of a fat teenaged girl. The girl explained that her mother had stopped taking her places. When asked by the interviewer if she was embarrassed by her overweight daughter, the mother refused to answer the question whereupon the father cut in: "The answer is: of course we're embarrassed. And we try to communicate in this family. I've said to her, 'We're not proud of the way you look; don't expect us to pretend we are.'"

It is not just in the home that a fat child comes to think of herself as deviant and set apart from normal society. Not even sympathetic parents, sincerely proud of their child, can assuage the differentness and inferiority a fat child sees in the eyes of their peers. For girls this problem of course grows as the child reaches puberty and adolescence and is increasingly evaluated as to acceptability for mixed-sex activities.

It is not simply the dating question that excludes fat children. Being victimized by other children and always the last to be chosen for any team, they often turn to solitary activities such as reading or they befriend adults. Indeed, many fat children experience a premature or precocious adulthood. Many women who were fat as children recall that their mothers treated them as peers or confidantes rather than children. The loss of childhood and the failure to fit in is further dramatized by clothes—the fat child can't even fit into children's sizes and must often wear clothes made for adults.

When the marginality of the fat child becomes even more pronounced at puberty, when dating and male and female gender roles become more salient, some adaptations characteristically arise in the lives of fat girls. One is to become precociously "sexy." Many overweight women developed secondary sexual characteristics earlier than their friends, and always looked older than their real age because of their size. This led to older boys or men treating them in a sexual manner earlier than other girls their age. Others befriended boys rather than girls, becoming "one of the boys," since they were not regarded by either boys or girls as being like "regular" girls. And probably the most common adaptation of all was for the fat adolescent girl to take on the role of the de-sexualized but sympathetic "listener" or chaperone for other girls.

But even when a child assumes a special role, such as confidante, and so creates a place for herself in the social world, her position is still defined by her weight. Even if she is not completely isolated, her participation is marginal and partial and her experience vicarious. As the confidante she only knows life from the distance of an observer. And her marginality and separation are increased because she is always self-conscious about her weight, always wondering what others are thinking about it while not really wanting to know.

In trying to decide what they may and may not risk, many fat people experience life as double jeopardy. In every situation they must guess whether or not others view them as deviant. There is risk either way they decide: If they presume that others see them as normal and act like a normal person (for example, getting up to dance at a party or eating a nondietetic meal or acting flirtatiously), they run the risk of being called ridiculous. On the other hand, if they never take the risk of presenting themselves as normal, they relinquish any chance of ratification, of participating in the world and its pleasures.

If the fat person is uncertain about how much she can get away with in trying to "pass" for normal, then so are the people around her uneasy, thinking always about her weight but feeling guilty, defensive or conflicted about letting her know it. In many ways, weight becomes a taboo topic, a river that can't be crossed between the fat person and others.

Sometimes the fat person feels an obligation to break the ice by being the first to mention her weight. She may make a point of saying that she is dieting, that she would like to lose weight. These are ways of bridging the gap, of showing others that she sees things the way they do, that she is trying to observe the rules. Conversely, some fat people are so sensitive and humiliated about being fat that they treat the subject of weight as unmentionable and lose all composure when it is brought up by someone else. If they lose weight, they are ambivalent about having people notice, for they are both glad of the compliments and humiliated that their former obesity had really been silently noticed all along.

Because of all the exclusion and the tension of social life, the fat individual often finds it easier to give up, to abandon a world that doesn't want her anyway. She retreats instead to the pleasures of eating in solitude. But being frozen out of the "normal" world and labeled as deviant, everything in her privatized life takes on an illicit or furtive quality. As several women explained, because it is pursued in secret, eating often feels to them either like calculated, premeditated stealing, or like engaging in a shameful perversion. And indeed, one of the stereotypes of fat people is that they surreptitiously and perversely substitute eating for normal human contact and even sexuality.

We started by looking at the feelings and associations that are aroused in thin people by the sights of a very fat person, and we have come full circle to the fat person's response to the world. If the society has a horror of fat people and sees them as basically antisocial characters who are greedy, secretive, isolated, or self-absorbed, and if fat people are excluded as early as childhood from the ranks of normal society, so does the fat person naturally come to feel more comfortable being alone, set apart from others, privately gratifying herself by eating. If the world treats the fat person with hostility, so does she come to feel embattled with her environment. A correspondence is finally constructed between the image and the reality.

The Beauty Myth

NAOMI WOLF

Naomi Wolf, excerpt from *The Beauty Myth: How Images of Beauty Are Used against Women,* New York: William Morrow, 1991. Reprinted by permission.

During the past decade, women breached the power structure; meanwhile, eating disorders rose exponentially and cosmetic surgery became the fastest-growing medical specialty. During the past five years, consumer spending doubled, pornography became the main media category, ahead of legitimate films and records combined, and 33,000 American women told researchers that they would rather lose ten to fifteen pounds than achieve any other goal. More women have more money and power and scope and legal recognition than we have ever had before; but in terms of how we feel about ourselves physically, we may actually be worse off than our unliberated grandmothers. Recent research consistently shows that inside the majority of the West's controlled, attractive, successful working women, there is a secret "underlife" poisoning our freedom; infused with notions of beauty, it is a dark vein of self-hatred, physical obsessions, terror of aging, and the dread of lost control.

It is no accident that so many potentially powerful women feel this way. We are in the midst of a violent backlash against feminism that uses images of female beauty as a political weapon against women's advancement: the beauty myth. It is the modern version of a social reflex that has been in force since the Industrial Revolution. As women released themselves from the feminine mystique of domesticity, the beauty myth took over its lost ground, expanding as it waned to carry on its work of social control.

The contemporary backlash is so violent because the ideology of beauty is the last one remaining of the old feminine ideologies that still has the power to control those women whom second wave feminism would have otherwise made relatively uncontrollable: It has grown stronger to take over the work of social coercion that myths about motherhood, domesticity, chastity, and passivity no longer can manage. It is seeking right now to undo psychologically and covertly all the good things that feminism did for women materially and overtly.

The beauty myth tells a story: The quality called "beauty" objectively and universally exists. Women must want to embody it and men must want to possess women who embody it. This embodiment is an imperative for women and not for men, which situation is necessary and natural because it is biological, sexual, and evolutionary: Strong men battle for beautiful women, and beautiful women are more reproductively successful. Women's beauty must correlate to their fertility, and since this system is based on sexual selection, it is inevitable and changeless.

None of this is true. "Beauty" is a currency system like the gold standard. Like any economy, it is determined by politics, and in the modern age in the West it is the last, best belief that keeps male dominance intact. In assigning value to women in a vertical hierarchy according to a culturally imposed physical standard, it is an expression of power relations in which women must unnaturally compete for resources that men have appropriated for themselves.

Sacrificing Ourselves for Love

JANE WEGSCHEIDER HYMAN
AND ESTHER R. ROME

Jane Wegscheider Hyman and Esther R. Rome, excerpt from *Sacrificing Ourselves for Love: Why Women Compromise Health and Self-Esteem . . . and How to Stop,* Freedom, California: The Crossing Press, 1996. Reprinted by permission.

THE CULTURAL IDEAL

Changes in the beauty ideal for women often mirror social changes; ironically, when social rights are expanded, the ideal image tends to become unhealthfully slim. The shift in ideal from plump to slender began around 1920, at about the same time that the woman's suffrage movement triumphed and the First International Birth Control Congress was held. Elizabeth Taylor's figure was considered the ideal in the 1960s, but by 1976 the ninety-one-pound Twiggy had taken her place. The angular fashions of the 1970s suggested that only males—or male impersonators—could enter the world of professional workers and pursue the traditional male goals of independence, personal achievement, and self-control. In the 1980s, muscles became stylish. The "new woman" was not only thin but had firm, shapely muscles, like those of professional dancers or athletes. Thus, the fashion in body shape and clothes became increasingly at odds with the general biological shape of female bodies. In the 1990s, the basic message remains the same: We could all become as straight and lean as athletic boys with breasts if we only tried hard enough.

As the ideal has shrunk, the actual average weight of women under thirty in the general US population has increased. The average US woman is 5 feet, 3.7 inches tall and weighs 144 pounds, a far cry from the average 5 feet, 8 inches and 123 pounds of fashion models.

LEARNING ABOUT LOOKS AND FOOD

Girls tend to become increasingly sensitive to social expectations and to the opinions of others. At puberty, many are proud of their developing breasts and other signs of womanhood, but are dismayed at a normal increase in fat, especially the fuller hips and thighs so characteristic of women's bodies. Some adolescent girls develop eating disorders when they lose weight through dance, gymnastics, or sports and try to maintain the lower weight; some are told to lose weight for these activities The majority of adolescent girls and high school and college women want to lose weight regardless of what they actually weigh.

Boarding schools and colleges often breed dysfunctional eating. A school environment can be competitive academically and socially, and living in close quarters may encourage a woman to compare her body with those of her housemates. In the close quarters of a college campus or boarding school, we often teach each other how to starve, binge, and purge.

THE EXPERIENCE OF STARVATION

Undernutrition can change body chemistry and affect physical and psychological functioning. Low-calorie diets can alter the functioning of the hypothalamus, which helps control sensations of hunger and fullness. As a result, the brain may lose some of its normal control of hunger and satiety: some women who have starved never feel hungry; some feel constantly hungry even if they have resumed eating meals that would have been filling in the past; some begin eating in uncontrollable binges.

When the cells do not receive enough fuel to burn from food, they feed on both body fat and other sources of calories, such as muscles. Even in moderate undernutrition there is a loss of muscle tissue—including heartmuscle—and a loss of tissue in all organs except the brain.

THE ROLE OF BODY FAT

Body fat is not a useless mass that we can add or

carve off without consequences. Fat stores energy, protects organs, and may be crucial to our ability to bear children. Body fat also helps produce and store the sex hormones that control our fertility. In addition to its effects on our reproductive organs, estrogen produced by fat tissue regulates bone metabolism, the synthesis of vital proteins in the liver, and to some extent, even behavior. How the hypothalamus receives its signal is unclear; it may be through estrogen. Estrogen levels gradually rise along with body fat during puberty. And the estrogen in body fat accelerates the secretion of other hormones necessary for a fertile menstrual cycle.

ANOREXIA NERVOSA

Women who tend toward highly obsessive thoughts and compulsive actions are particularly at risk when they diet. Women who are starving during a food shortage become increasingly fatigued, weak, and listless; in contrast, women with anorexia nervosa are extremely active because of their fear of fat. They often have intense exercise regimens, such as running five to ten miles a day or doing lengthy aerobic activities. Some women with anorexia nervosa become reluctant to sit down, fearing that the inactivity of sitting will cause weight gain. In extreme cases, the intensity of her fear can cause a starving woman to pace ceaselessly.

BULIMIA NERVOSA

Some women with a tendency to obsessive behavior develop an extreme form of bulimia—eating in compulsive and uncontrollable binges, then vomiting and purging. They fear that they will be unable to stop eating and actually feel unable to stop. Often they are anxious or depressed and consider suicide. Virtually all who suffer from this type of binge eating are obsessively preoccupied with food and with body shape and weight, and all were once stringent dieters.

Those of us with bulimia nervosa like the sensations associated with dehydration. These sensations include feeling washed out, drained, or empty; having loose clothes; having a flat abdomen; having protruding bones (especially cheek or hip bones); and feeling light or lightheaded. . . . Many of us who have bulimia nervosa abhor any sensation of food in the stomach—for us starvation is the ideal state.

THE HAZARDS OF ANOREXIA AND BULIMIA

Women who suffer from anorexia or bulimia face the same health risks as women on self-starvation diets, but some of the risks are intensified. They are more likely to have trouble with dehydration, diabetes insipidus, vulnerability to heat and cold, bone loss, and fertility. Cycles of binge eating and purging can cause tooth erosion and tooth loss, disruption of the body's metabolism, spasmodic seizures of the jaw muscles, inflammation of the salivary glands, kidney damage, and, in rare cases, rupture of the stomach and esophagus. Large doses of laxatives and diuretics can deplete the body of potassium and sodium.

FIGHTING BACK

As more women and researchers realize that dieting is not a trivial problem and that unhealthful food restriction can cause a lifetime of problems, more of us are actively opposing thinness and body "control" as requirements for social acceptance.

Ideally, prevention should begin in elementary school, with educational programs that reveal the social influences behind our unrealistic and unhealthy weight and body image goals. Unfortunately, many professionals still have misconceptions about what factors actually determine a woman's fatness and leanness. Therefore, it is important for those of us concerned and informed to organize programs on our own or create individual projects for the sake of our health and the health of our daughters.

CHAPTER 18

Body Parts

WHEN BARBARA CREATED the first incarnation of this anthology—her half of the massive *For Women Only!* (2000)—she imagined a book filed with the voices of health activists spanning decades, much like the one you hold in your hands today. Her original vision was different, however, in that she wanted the writings to be structured around various parts of the body. Instead of using topic as an organizing principle, the book would be assembled corporally, with each piece—the eyes, skin, hair, mouth, arms, etc.—receiving its own section. As the book evolved and grew larger, this framework fell away. The "Body Parts" section remained, but was no longer the central piece of the book. When we returned to reedit the anthology, starting in 2007, we pulled more pieces out to put in sections where they now seemed more properly to belong. It is only right, however, that "Body Parts" remains. It illustrates Barbara's original design and makes the point that all of our parts play dramatic, unexpected and important roles in our health and well-being. Barbara wanted sections for the exclusively female parts—the breasts and vagina for example—but she wanted them for the other parts as well. This section has changed and been reorganized and looks totally different than it did at the start, much like the women's health movement. (L.E.)

FACE

Aging (balm for a 27th birthday)

ERICA JONG

Erica Jong, "Aging (balm for a 27th birthday)," in *Fruits & Vegetables: Poems by Erica Jong*, Hopewell, NJ: Ecco Press, 1997. Originally published in 1968 by Holt, Rinehart & Winston. Reprinted by permission from Erica Jong.

insights which clear-eyed 22 has no inkling of
promising   certain sure-thighed things in bed
certain fingers on your spine & lids

                                              but

it's only the beginning   as ruin proceeds downward
lingering for a while around the mouth   hardening the smile
into prearranged patterns (irreversible!)   writing furrows
from the wings of the nose   (oh nothing much at first
          but "showing promise"   like your early poems

                                        of deepening)

Hooked for two years now on wrinkle creams   creams for
crowsfeet   ugly lines (if only there were one!)
any perfumed grease   which promises   youth   beauty
not truth   but all I need on earth
          I've been studying   how women age

                                        how

it starts around the eyes   so you can tell
a woman of 22 from one of 28 merely by
a faint scribbling near the lids   a subtle crinkle
          a fine line
extending from the fields of vision

                                        this

in itself is not unbeautiful   promising
          as it often does

The No-Nonsense Approach to Cleaning Your Face

DEBORAH CHASE

Deborah Chase, "The No-Nonsense Approach to Cleaning Your Face," *Ms.*, November 1974, with a new introduction by the author, 1999. Reprinted by permission.

When the medically based *No-Nonsense Beauty Book* was first published in 1976, the formulas for beauty products had changed little in over 100 years. Although researchers were beginning to learn more about the causes of a wide range of skin and hair problems, cosmetic companies seemed reluctant to use this new knowledge to develop truly helpful products.

This lack of progress did not inhibit manufacturers from making grandiose claims of performance. These would range from the literary ("turn back the hands of time") to the mystical ("channels the spirit of a legendary Hungarian beauty"). In a regulatory climate diplomatically described as lax, such claims went unchallenged. When I brought insupportable claims for turtle oil, royal bee jelly, and sea salts to consumer agencies I found that they were considered "harmless puffery." The prevailing attitude was that if a woman was dumb enough to believe such promises, then she deserved to buy useless products.

Claims substantiation was made difficult by lack of ingredient labeling. An advertisement promised to cure acne or eliminate lines and wrinkles but would not provide a list of ingredients by which a woman could judge its effectiveness. Up to 1976, one could only guess at ingredients in skin and hair products. I had to help a reader figure out the formulation by its name, feel, and directions on the package.

In 1976, several months after the book's publication, Senator Thomas Eagleton of Missouri successfully introduced a bill requiring all beauty care products to print their entire list of ingredients on the back of each label. Women were now able to search for ingredients to deliver promises or, equally important, to avoid substances to which they were allergic. For the first time, women could make an informed choice about ingredients and price in skin and hair care products.

THE SMALL CHANGE THAT HAS MADE A BIG DIFFERENCE

Looking back over twenty years of writing about beauty, I am especially delighted at the sea change in a woman's relationship to the sun. In 1976 a deep dark suntan was the ultimate beauty treatment. The fact that getting such a tan was arguably the worst thing that one could do to the skin seemed too unfair to accept. While women who read my book accepted most of the advice, they drew the line at tanning. In fact, a large cosmetic company approached me to design a line of No-Nonsense skin care products. In addition to developing formulations that contained the most effective active ingredients, I insisted that they be enhanced with sunscreens. We took the concept out on the road in focus groups through the Midwest. It totally bombed. Women completely rejected anything that would interfere with their relationship to the sun.

Today women of all ages now routinely use pow-erful sunscreens with SPF of 30 to 60. Sunblocks are now a common ingredient in day creams and moisturizers and viewed as a value-added benefit in foundations, eye make-up, and lipstick. It is exactly the kind of lifestyle change that the women's health movement believes can result from a bit of basic beauty science and a list of useful ingredients so that women can make informed choices that were once unimaginable.

Despite the enormous advances made in the fields of biology and medicine in the past 50 years, cosmetics manufacturers, on the whole, have been unwilling to invest the time and money in the research required to come up with a truly revolutionary soap or facial skin care product. Still, there are many safe commercial products that can really help the skin. The trick is knowing which to buy and how to interpret the labels.

CLEANSING

Of the huge array of products offered for cleansing, each has different properties and should be applied to different types of skin.

SOAP

Basic toilet soap consists of a mixture of fat, alkali salt, and water.

Superfatted soap, containing extra amounts of oil and fat, is good for people with normal or slightly dry skin.

Castile soap contains olive oil as its main fat. It is no less drying or richer than basic toilet soap.

Transparent soap, made with glycerin and alcohol—both of which draw water from the skin—is best for people with normal skin.

Deodorant soap contains antibacterial chemicals that kill the bacteria present on the skin's surface. Since there are no apocrine glands on the face, these soaps serve no special purpose for that part of the body.

French milled soap has been specially processed to reduce alkalinity. A low alkalinity makes the soap less drying.

Floating soap floats because it contains extra water and has air trapped in it. It has no special properties for the skin.

Detergent soap is synthetic or "soapless" soap. The cosmetic chemist can adjust the properties of a detergent soap to make it less alkaline, less dehydrating, and less irritating than plain soap to sensitive skin.

Soap with fruit, vegetable, or herb extracts: whatever vitamins or enzymes these ingredients may possess in the raw state are usually destroyed in the manufacturing process.

Cocoa butter soap: cocoa, while not giving any special property to the soap, has sometimes been associated with skin allergies.

CREAM AND LOTION CLEANSERS

Cold cream is made up of mineral oil, wax, and borax. When the cream is taken off with tissues, an oil film that contains some dirt may remain.

Cleansing cream is made of wax, mineral oil, alcohol, water, and some kind of soap or detergent. The soap remains in a film that coats the skin, damaging it and drying it out.

Cleansing lotion is made of the same ingredients, but contains more water. It has the same drawbacks.

Washable cream and lotion are made of ingredients similar to those described above. They do a thorough but gentle job of cleansing and are best for normal and dry skins. They do not have enough degreasing power for oily skin.

Milky cleanser is made of soap, water, alcohol, and mineral oil and contains more soap and less oil than washable creams or lotions. Since they are primarily soaps, they are good for normal and slightly oily skin, but are too harsh for dry skin.

Scrubbing cleanser is soap with tiny, hard grains that rub off the surface of the skin. It should be used daily on oily skin, weekly on normal skin, and monthly on dry skin.

OIL-BALANCE CONTROL

Day cream is made of wax, water, oil, and soap, or soaplike chemicals—to make the cream less greasy so that it does not dissolve makeup. The soap in these products makes them bad for dry skin.

Daytime lotion, frequently called moisturizer, is healthier for the skin. It contains more water and much less soap. Excellent products for dry skin, they should be used judiciously on normal skin and avoided for oily skin.

All-purpose hand, body, and face lotion is made with four basic ingredients: water, wax, oil, and glycerin. Although somewhat oilier, they usually do not contain chemicals that encourage the skin to hold water. An important question to ask is what oil it contains.

There are three categories of oils, all of which are meant to coat the skin and delay the evaporation of water. None have any special power to delay aging or prevent lines and wrinkles:

Of all the oils, *animal fat*—particularly lanolin—most closely resembles the natural human oil. The most expensive animal fats, mink and turtle oil, do the same job as cheaper ones. *Vegetable oil* protects the skin well enough, but it is not as good as animal oil. *Mineral oil* has a tendency to dissolve the skin's own natural oil, and can thereby increase dehydration.

Night cream: More nonsense has been written about night cream than any other beauty product. A night cream merely helps the skin to retain a better supply of water. It does not rejuvenate the skin, prevent lines or wrinkles, reach deep down into the pores, or wake up sleepy complexions. Some night creams, containing estrogens and other water-holding substances, do a better job of retaining water in the skin. Night creams are good for dry skin, not necessarily helpful for normal skin, and not needed for oily skin.

TONING

A *toning lotion* can temporarily shrink facial pores, make the skin look firmer, and reinforce a healthy coloring.

A *skin freshener* is an alcohol compound with various additives, such as herb extracts and camphor or menthol. It can be irritating to normal and dry skin.

An *astringent* contains water, less alcohol than skin fresheners, and, most importantly, aluminum or zinc salts. The salts, by causing a slight puffiness or swelling of the skin around the pores, makes them seem smaller. Beware of astringents that cause sharp, stinging sensations. These products probably contain only camphor or menthol.

A *clarifying lotion,* also known as an exfoliating lotion, contains water, alcohol, glycerin, and a chemical that dissolves the keratin that makes up most of the skin's top layer of dry, dead cells. The skin looks brighter and cleaner after using a clarifying lotion. These lotions include salicylic acid, resorcinol, and benzoyl peroxide, which presently must by law be listed on the label. Papain, an enzyme extracted from papayas, and bromelin, an enzyme extracted from pineapples, can also dissolve keratin, but neither has to be listed on the label. Both are very powerful agents and have been associated with allergies and chemical burns.

Masks come in two basic forms—clay and gel. A *clay mask* picks up the cellular debris and gives the skin a smooth, even texture. The tightening action stimulates circulation and makes the skin glow. The clay contains mild bleaching agents that cause a gentle lightening of the skin. Clay also soothes the skin, reducing any inflammation and soreness. A *gel mask* is especially good for restoring water or rehydrating normal, normal to dry, and dry skin. Most of the value of a mask is based on the clay or gel base that forms the mask itself. Although certain ingredients are useful, like mint or vitamin A, many commercial masks have other exotic ingredients that do not perform any function.

Saunas: These are marvelous for every type of skin.

Susan Brownmiller on Appearance and Makeup

INTERVIEW BY CARRIE CARMICHAEL

Susan Brownmiller is and adjunct professor of women's and gender studies at Pace University. Her most recent book is *In Our Time: Memoirs of a Revolution.* This interview was conducted in May 1999.

CC: You have chosen a makeup-less life. How did you decide that? When did you decide that?

SB: I never looked good in makeup, and I never was handy at it. I'm less artistic and more verbal, so I was never good at painting my face. In the mid- to late 1960s, when feminism was starting, I used to wear lipstick. Then lipstick color lightened. First they did the white thing, and then the pink thing, and then it was just gloss, so it was very easy for me to get rid of the one thing that I did do, which was put on lipstick. When I had my book jacket photo taken the other day, I decided to err on the side of caution—I had a makeup person do the whole number. Her pictures are very nice, but it's me made up. It's me facing the public under a mask. So I was nervous. I was nervous to go before the camera without makeup. That's dangerous. It's not as though you want to hide and be something else for the photo, but you know what the camera sees, what the camera picks up. I was terrified.

CC: Is that about age?

SB: Certainly it's about age.

CC: Did that experience with the makeup for your photo ease your mind about it?

SB: No. But I'll tell you a funny experience. I went from the photo shoot to visit a sick friend, and when I got there, she had no food, so I had to go out to the local grocery store. We decided we'd make a meal of spaghetti and meatballs. So I was ordering from the guy behind the deli counter, and I asked for some meatballs, and the guy said to me, "Is that all I can do for you?" I said, "Yeah, I just need the meatballs." And he said, "Are you sure? You are so appealing." And I said, "Sir, it's the makeup." I mean this was a full-dress makeup. I guess women don't walk into the grocery store like that—I certainly never walk into the grocery store like that. It reminded me of the time I was on the road for *Against Our Will*. I'd go from city to city, and in the course of the day, every television station would slap on more of the stuff and I was bright orange it seemed to me, totally exaggerated, by the time I got on the plane at night to go to the next city. I'd get on that plane, and guys from other rows would be fighting each other to sit next to me. Their feeling must have been, "She knocks herself out so much for us. She is sending out all of these signals. Wow! I want to be near her." And I had forgotten that totally until I had this experience of walking into the grocery store in full makeup a couple of weeks ago.

CC: Do you choose not to wear makeup because you really don't want that kind of invasion?

SB: No, that's not the reason. I just felt that it didn't add anything to my face when I was young. And there was a time when you didn't have to do any of it, thanks to feminism. I didn't care for any of the procedures. In fact, when this professional makeup person did put on the makeup, she came at me with the eyelash curler, and I practically screamed. I hated to go through that torture, which I remembered full well. I let her tweeze my eyebrows though. So it just depends on what you are willing to endure or not endure. And I was always willing to endure a minimum amount. I just didn't have the capacity to endure a lot. Same thing with shoes. I just don't have the capacity to hobble on high-heeled shoes and risk corns and damaging my toes.

CC: As a city person I call them cab shoes. I can't walk very far in them, and they're too expensive, and it's crippling.

SB: But you know how many people do struggle with it all of their lives, and then they have foot pains.

CC: Do you think that one of the benefits of the women's movement in its current incarnation is that we are able to combine the image of femininity, femaleness, and power? Where are we when it comes to those qualities all in the same woman?

SB: I don't think that you can speak for a "we." I urge you to look at *Bust* magazine. They are kind of neofeminists at *Bust* magazine, and they have an article that a young woman wrote, a little chart about all of the things that she must buy, she must do, in order to present herself to the world. And they're still grappling with it, and they don't get it. They don't know why it costs them more to be a woman in society than it costs men to be men.

CC: There was a time when we felt that the only way that you could present yourself as a strong, serious, thinking woman was to not have any of the trappings of the former Barbie doll image. It's different now.

SB: Yes, that's right. There was a lot of excess. Everything was thrown out. And then they came back.

CC: Do you think concern with appearance has come back and taken over? Where do you think we are in terms of things being in some kind of balance?

SB: Well it's not that it's taken over. It's that our movement raised many, many issues. The ones I concentrated on were violence against women and the right to reproductive freedom, and there has been no retreat on those fronts, although the problems are still with us. But around appearance, saying, "God damn it, I won't do the thousand things I'm supposed to do to feminize my body," there's been a total retreat.

CC: But there are those who would quarrel with your statement.

SB: Oh, sure they would. They'd say it's done now for fun. You can do it or not do it. And that's true. There's a lot more freedom out there: to wear pants, to wear jeans, to go makeup-less. There's a lot more freedom than there was in the 1950s and the early 1960s.

CC: To be seen as female, as feminine, is not just defined as manipulation and being false.

SB: Well, it still is. But there are options. You don't have to be that way all the time, but it should be in your wardrobe.

HAIR

Body Hair: The Last Frontier

HARRIET LYONS AND REBECCA ROSENBLATT

Harriet Lyons and Rebecca Rosenblatt, "Body Hair: The Last Frontier," *Ms.*, July 1972. Reprinted by permission.

Actress Faye Dunaway boldly reveals her unshaven armpits for a photograph in a national magazine, and says that that's the way she will appear in all future film roles.

Eunice Lipton, an art historian in her thirties, strokes the growth on her legs and says, "It may seem ugly, but it's me."

Graduate student Grace Boynton, twenty-three, explains that she has thrown away her razor because "I got insulted that my natural body processes were considered disgusting by society. . . ."

While cosmetics imply the real woman is not enough, shaving says that the real woman is too much. There is probably nothing more tedious, messy, or hazardous in the feminine beauty regimen than the removal of hair from underarms, legs, eyebrows, lips, chin, and breasts. . . .

An emerging feminist consciousness tells us that all this punishing depilation reflects the depth of our socialized distaste for our bodies. We slavishly remove body hair and substitute artificial scents for natural body odors because we dare not expect approval if we look or smell as we really are.

Despite the all too familiar bother and pain—as well as the new feminist mandate to let it all hang out—the custom of depilating is still alive and well. Those who do vastly outnumber those who don't, but discussions of female body hair reveal disquieting associations.

In psychoanalytic parlance, hair is the accepted symbol of the genitals, so sexual behavior and hair-removal rituals are closely associated. Hairiness, in this lexicon, is translated as unrestrained animal sexuality. Conversely, extremes of haircutting and shaving are symbolic of castration or the repudiation of the very existence of sex. Anthropological evidence linking shaving customs to celibacy and ceremonial mutilation rites (such as the cutting off of finger joints) supports this symbology.

With hairiness equated to animal sexuality, the unchecked or uncovered appearance of hair in the armpits and on the legs of women collides with the culture's premise of female sexuality as passive. The implication that a woman's underarm and leg hair are superfluous, and therefore unwanted, is but one embodiment of our culture's preoccupation with keeping women in a kind of state of innocence, and denying their visceral selves. Some women will even shave pubic hair, thereby emulating the infantile sexlessness of a little girl. And only within the last year has the men's magazine *Playboy* conceded that adult women have pubic hair at all.

The acceptance of hairiness in men, like its suppression in women, is connected to animality, but, ironically the association is misguided, Man/woman is the only animal sexually active beyond the need to reproduce; the only animal that can experience orgasm at times when conception is impossible. We are both the most sex-driven and the least hairy of the animal kingdom, yet we persist in equating sexuality with furriness. The bald or non-hairy-chested man suffers a minor discrimination all his own.

While our puritanical attitude makes the hairless female body the quintessence of femininity, our obsession with cleanliness works to modify the acceptance of hairiness even in men. Long hair and beards are for dirty hippies. The clean-shaven and the crew cuts satisfy the American ideal.

Hair shares with feces, urine, semen, menstrual blood, spittle, and sweat a centuries-old association with impurity. As a result, fastidious women throughout history have felt obliged to remove hair that appeared anywhere but on the head or pubis. In the 1850s, women were so devoted to their hygienic images that they inflicted skin ulcers upon themselves by reckless use of depilatories made from lime, arsenic, and potash. . . .

Race and class, with their attendant prejudices, determine special cultural attitudes toward body hair. The connotation of dirty foreigner vs. clean American has always been evident in our national thoughts on hair. A young woman involved in a bicycle accident was asked by a New York policeman examining her injured, unshaven leg, "You're not Puerto Rican, are you?"

It's true that, in Puerto Rico, women do not remove body hair unless they are upwardly mobile or mainland-oriented. In France, only lower-class or provincial women remain hairy. Even the sup-posedly earthy Italian women have begun shaving underarms to conform with standards of chicness. In Spain, a mustache on a woman is considered sexy, but not necessarily well bred.

Hair underscores the various myths and mys-teries which have arisen from our different skin colors. Intimidated racial groups try to lose their identity by adopting the hair texture and styles of the majority or ruling class. The kinky hair of American-born blacks has been obscured for gen-erations by straighteners, pomades, and pageboy wigs. In Sweden, where most women are fair enough to make shaving a nonissue, dark-com-plexioned women shave to be less conspicuous in the homogeneous population.

The afro-coifed black woman, and the unshaven woman, regardless of her color, nationality, and class, make of their personal grooming a political statement. They reject an image of beauty and acceptability imposed by the society and risk the censure reserved for the rebel.

In America in the seventies, the hirsute woman is not yet an idea whose time has come. The shaving of body hair by women stubbornly defies extinction. Given the convoluted symbolism of the ritual and the repellent stares directed at the unshaven woman, we are not surprised to discover that even the most liberated women backslide when beach weather arrives.

But more and more individual women are risking those stares to affirm their natural female-ness. Eventually, this small but intimate tyranny will be resisted, so that one more oppressive hang-up can be retired forever and the hirsute will live happily with the hairless.

All Hair the Conquering Heroine

LOIS GOULD

Lois Gould, excerpt from *Not Responsible for Personal Articles*, New York: Warner Books, 1973. Reprinted by permission.

Kimberley Ann, nine, has just decided what she wants to be when she grows up: a part-time cocktail waitress with frosted blond streaks. It is probably just a coincidence that Kimberley Ann's mother recently graduated from law school and lopped off her two-tone gold ringlets right at the dark roots.

Kim's classmate Janice, who is still eight, has her heart set on becoming a file clerk who ties up her hair in a severe bun that can be shaken free, with a single lightning stroke, into a quivering mass of raven tendrils. (Janice's mother is a secu-rities analyst, with a naturally frizzled pepper-and-salt pageboy.)

Nina, ten-and-a-half, plans to be a schoolteacher with a firm grip and frosted blond highlights. And twelve-year-old Stephanie, the cynic, intends to become a frosted blond highlight, period.

Clearly, a fair number of feminists' daughters are having "role model" trouble. The cause seems to be a sudden and widespread cultural confusion about the difference—if any—between a role model and a hair model. As I understand it, a role model is an adult person of your own gender whom you admire and want to be like: a president, an astronaut, a nuclear physicist, a private eye. Whereas a hair model is a stunning, raven-haired president; a luscious red-headed astronaut; a blond bombshell of a nuclear physicist; a frost-streaked poster pinup of a private eye.

It would be easy to blame the confusion on television's newest rage—the female "action-adventure" star who can either ride a motorcycle, toe-tap on a skateboard, shoot straight, do heavy lifting, or figure out how to trap a criminal while wearing a dripping wet bunny costume. After all, no matter what else these new wonder women do besides wonders—and part-time file clerking, school teaching, cocktail waitressing—the thing they all do *best* is their hair.

So it would be easy to blame TV, but, as one of our stunning, raven-haired ex-presidents used to say, "It would be wrong." The truth is, we have always had a little trouble spotting the subtle line between a heroine and a hairdo. In a highly unscientific recent survey, mothers of nine- to twelve-year-olds, selected solely on the basis of shampoo, color tint, and permanent wave length, were asked the following question: When you were between nine and twelve, who was your "role model," and why?

➤ 17 percent answered "Esther Williams, the swimming star, because she could do fifteen minutes of flawless underwater sidestroke with gorgeous flowers twined in her braided coronet."

➤ 5 percent named Brenda Starr, the comic-strip girl reporter, on the basis of her sensational headline set in bold-type curls the color of "a five-alarm fire," an "Irish setter," or a "*saumon fumé*."

➤ 12 percent had idolized Sonja Henie, the Goldilocks of the ice, because she skated like a wind-up Christmas angel; her hair and feet set off "matching sparks of white light"; she was an "animated gold sequin."

➤ The remainder chose a wide assortment of heroines ranging from the Dragon Lady (dangerous mastermind set in a black curtain of silk hair) to Amelia Earhart and Dale, Flash Gordon's dauntless copilot, both of whom had their heads in clouds of wispy gold tendrils escaping from under their flying helmets.

Nobody had a role model with nonterrific hair.

Film historian Molly Haskell has noted that the long, sexy tresses of movie queens in the hard-boiled dramas of the 1940s was the female equivalent of a gun—an ultimate woman's weapon in a tough man's world of crime and carnality. The new "action" heroines of the seventies, operating in the same man's world, actually get to wield both weapons—the hair and the gun. But it's the same old game: Everything, including the girls, is still owned and operated by the fellow who runs the beauty parlor. Body, soul, gun and frost job, they are strictly *Charlie's Angels*.

Armed with this valuable knowledge, I recently watched my first episode of the TV series *Charlie's Angels*, accompanied by two hard-core nine-year-old fans, Nicole and Sandy. Here's how it went:

Me: Tell me about the "angels."

Nicole: Well, first off you have to know which is which. Sabrina is the smart one, Kelly is strong, and Jill is beautiful. Mostly her hair.

Me: But they're *all* beautiful.

Sandy (patiently): Of *course*. But Sabrina is beautiful *and* smart. Kelly is beautiful *and* strong. Jill is *just* beautiful. Mostly her hair.

Me: Oh. (Pause. On the screen, three women are flashing guns, hair, sexy clothes, and dazzling smiles, like armed stewardesses serving plastic filet mignon.) Which would you rather be—the smart one, the strong one, or the beautiful one, with the hair?

Nicole: Definitely not the beautiful one.

Sandy: Obviously.

Me: Why obviously?

Nicole: Because even if she has the most hair, she has the smallest part. (Sandy nods solemnly.)

Me: What if you had a choice, I mean in real life? You could be smart and strong—or you could be beautiful. Which would you choose?

Sandy: Why couldn't we be all three?

Me: Well, first off, because hardly anybody gets to be all three. And hardly anybody even gets to have a choice. So I'm giving you a choice. Beautiful, but dumb and weak. Or smart and strong, but ugly. Ugly *hair*, especially.

Sandy (frowning): Hmmm.

Nicole (cocking her head so that her long mane of naturally frosty curls tumbles gently around her shoulders): *How* ugly?

Femininity

SUSAN BROWNMILLER AND CARRIE CARMICHAEL

Susan Brownmiller, excerpt from *Femininity*, New York: Simon and Schuster, 1984. Reprinted by permission. Subsequent interview with Susan Brownmiller by Carrie Carmichael, May 1999. Reprinted from *For Women Only!*, ed. Gary Null and Barbara Seaman, New York: Seven Stories Press, 1999.

From time immemorial, hair has been used to make a visual statement, for the body's most versatile raw material can be cut, plucked, shaved, curled, straightened, braided, greased, bleached, tinted, dyed, and decorated with precious ornaments and totemic fancies. A change in the way one wears one's hair can affect the look of the face and alter a mood. A uniform hairstyle can set a group of people apart from others and signify a conformity or rebellion, devotion to God or indulgence in sensual pleasures. Hair worn in a polarized manner has served to indicate the masculine and the feminine, the slave and the ruler, the young, the old, the virgin, the married, the widowed, the mourning.

There was a time that stretched over many years when I placed myself in permanent bondage to Elizabeth Arden. There, two lunch hours a week, I was shampooed and curled with setting lotion, winding papers, plastic rollers, and metal clips, gently cushioned around the ears and forehead with absorbent cotton, tied in a pink hairnet and placed under a hot dryer for 35 minutes. Mercifully released, I was unpinned, unwound, brushed out, teased, and fluffed into fair approximation of the season's latest fashion. After a blast of noxious spray I was sent out the door in a forged state of feminine chic that lasted for the rest of the day— that is, if it didn't rain. I always felt like a poseur at Arden's. Not once did I let them shape and polish my nails, not once did I submit to the ritual of the pedicure, the waxing of the legs, or the mysterious rites of the Full-Day Treatment. They must have sensed my lack of commitment. But they had a powerful hold on my hair. They tugged at the roots of my deepest insecurity.

SB: I would say one of the biggest problems women have is the obsession with the hair on their heads. Of course, I fall for it too.

CC: We've been obsessed as a nation with Hillary Clinton's hair.

SB: I've never seen such a demonstration of feminine insecurity, due to trying to break the mold in so many ways, as Hillary Clinton. Because she cannot be comfortable with one image. She's been in such agony over "the look" of her hair, and indeed also "the look" of her clothes. And she seems to have no idea how she might look good. Because otherwise she would say, "Hey, this looks good on me. That doesn't. No, I won't do that." But she seems constantly at the mercy of other people's idea of her image in hair and clothes.

CC: I think your point about her insecurity is key. In her politics, no one tells her how to think or what to do.

SB: Unbelievable the get-ups that have been foisted on her, or that she chose, thinking that, "This looks like power. This looks like efficiency. This looks like femininity." She's got all of these advisers. When I was reading the George Stephanopoulos book that shows the role of all these advisers and how the President triangulates, I was trying to think of Hillary Clinton in the White House with the access that she must have to very good fashion advisers, and how it still comes out wrong all of the time. Now I know basically underneath it's not just simply that she is a woman who is trying to break codes of femininity and be a very serious and efficient person who transforms the world. I know that she has real body image issues. I think that secretly, these issues obsess her.

Memoirs of a (Sorta) Ex-Shaver

CAROLYN MACKLER

Carolyn Mackler, excerpt from "Memoirs of a (Sorta) Ex-Shaver," in Ophira Edut, ed., *Adios, Barbie: Young Women Write about Body Image and Identity*, Seattle, Washington: Seal Press, 1998. Reprinted by permission.

During the winter of seventh grade, the other girls in my gym class suddenly had legs as smooth as an infant and I celebrated the birth of every new underarm hair by grabbing a pair of scissors and trimming it down. Feeling inexplicably weird about the soft blond peach fuzz coating my legs, I pounded my mom with questions about shaving: "When could I? How do you? Could I get my own razor?"

"Wait," she cautioned. "Shave once and you'll have black stubble for the rest of your life."

Heeding no warning, I crouched in the tub with a bottle of Johnson & Johnson's baby oil and my dad's old black Gillette. I was focused, driven. Through hell or greasy water, I would have smooth legs. This experimental style (which resulted in awful itching) was eventually eclipsed by more conventional methods: my own pastel disposable ten-pack, a can of Barbosal shaving cream, and, a few hours later, a smear of Nivea cream to ease chafing. When I shaved at night, I would lie in bed rejoicing in gloriously silky legs, feeling like a real woman.

Oh, I was quite the shaver. I indulged daily, careful not to omit a patch, not even down near my ankles. I bent my knees to scrape them clean and only rarely sliced off some skin in that difficult place in the front where the bone touches so close to the surface. An impressed family friend once joked she would hire me to shave her legs. The guys at school routinely swiped their hands across girls' legs to patrol their shaving prowess and then taunt them if they were slacking off. If I were running late, I'd protect myself by faux shaving—just doing the strip between the bottom of my jeans and the top of my cotton socks.

And here I lived, in this world of plastic legs, where moms and daughters, teachers and coaches, shaved without a bat of the eye. It was all any of us saw; every woman had smooth legs. It was hygienic, like brushing your teeth or clipping your toenails. I tremble to think of what would have happened if I, a vaguely insecure, overly tall, sixteen-year-old, had paraded into homeroom one morning sporting furry legs and an ample bush under each arm. In a town of conformity (where the gossip of the school was that Marta dared to have "flat hair"—meaning no perm, no hairspray, no poofed bangs—this would have been instant death by humiliation.

Desperately suffocated by this clone-ishness (but seeing no way out from within), I jetted off to college at eighteen, with aspirations of hobnobbing among the potpourri of people boasted on the promotional fliers. I imagined a borderless territory for etching out exactly who one was, in the absence of relentless peer police. Granted, things were different. The word was that the college years were a time to get all the nose rings, crimson hair, and bottomed-out Birkenstocks out of your system, to quick-get-it-over-with and dabble in bisexuality and menages á trois (or at least talk about it), because you'd probably never get another go. So the parameters of conformity had widened, but ultimately, people still navigated within the confines of what was cool and acceptable. And other than on those marginal take-no-shit women, leg and armpit hair was still uncool. Shaving was still the undisputed norm. And the guys were still on hand to check for stubble.

The summer after my sophomore year, something happened that rocked my closely shaven world forever. I took a month-long mountain trek, and with only enough space for essentials, no forecast of running water, and no one to impress, I left my razor on the shower ledge at home. And for the first time since I had any hair to speak of, my leg and underarm hair began to grow. And grow. And grow. And the strangest thing was that I actually liked it. Not only did it feel good to be free of that constant bristle, it looked healthy and fuzzy and strong—somehow the way a woman's leg should look, not all bald and vulnerable like a little girl's. On the other hand, it felt so bizarre and unfamiliar, like I was this androgynous Bigfoot with hairy legs and pits. The second I reemerged into civilization, I shaved away the evidence, but my perceptions had been altered. In other words, I had dipped my hand in the cookie jar and I liked what I tasted.

In the midst of all this, I had been wading through months of dorm-room body-image rap sessions. It was becoming painfully clear that in our high-powered, image-focused environment, eating disorders ran rampant. To be young and white and female was to have "body issues," as we tenderly referred to them. We all had been afflicted by the bug, in varying ways. We freaked out about our bodies. We paid homage to the Stairmaster and hated it. We opted for salad bar, no dressing, instead of cheesy dining hall pizza. We gained the freshman fifteen and struggled to lose the sophomore twenty or thirty. Analyzing it ad nauseam was our way of reacting, fighting back, and learning to overcome this pressure for physical perfection. Meanwhile, as we shaved/plucked/waxed our body hair away, a dialogue on body hair lay dormant. We didn't see anything political in it.

But isn't body hair yet another image issue dumped in the exhausted laps of women? My mind begins to reel when I ponder the whole de-hairing ordeal:

Eyebrows: Pluck into symmetrical arches, or at least interrupt the unibrow over the bridge of the nose.

Moustache (more genteely referred to as upper lip hair): Bleach, wax, or zap it with electrolysis.

Chin hair: Tweeze out ASAP, even if it means using the rearview mirror at an intersection.

Random very long arm hairs: Yank.

Rest of arm hair: Bleach if too dark.

Nipple hair: Tweeze or fry with electrolysis.

Underarm hair: Shave, of course.

"Bikini line" hair (deemed so vile, only a euphemism can be used): Shave (and get a lovely rash), fantasize about being able to afford electrolysis, wear granny-style skirted bathing suits or shorts to the beach.

Leg hair: See Underarm hair.

Toe hair: Pull out while talking on the phone—owww!

Sound familiar? Women's body hair is apparently so dirty, gross, and vulgar that it elicits queasiness in people. It's "excess," meaning it shouldn't be there in the first place. But it is. I'll bypass lugging down the hair-as-fur-for-warmth path, because clothes do that trick—but hair has always been there, and it will always be there. It's easy to forget that women have hairy legs and armpits because we never see them in their natural state. In this society, our eyes have actually been retrained to believe that a woman doesn't have body hair. Our memory omits the razors, waxes, creams, and bleaches that went into making her hairless. In fact, we expect a woman to have smooth legs et cetera and are surprised and often repulsed if she doesn't.

Why has body hair become such a nemesis for women? It poses no health risks. It is not hygienic to remove; it is not cleansing to shave. Rather, the complications arise during the eradication: cuts, infections, rashes, ingrown hairs, dry skin, burning. Is this hairless ideal yet another variation on the tune of "Let's take the best (boobs, curves in some places, hair in very few places) and leave the rest (hips, curves in other places, hair in *lots* of other places)"? Or is it a "Let's make women look like eight-year-olds so we can treat them as such"? Or is it a "If women can fill up their extra hours shaving and obsessing about their bodies then they won't have spare time to plot a world takeover"? Or maybe it's a "Women are *so* grossly overpaid and just don't spend enough on pads, tampons, pantyliners, Ibuprofen, shampoos, conditioners, deodorants, that we should coax them to buy razors, waxes, creams, and bleaches"? Aha, it's probably a "How about setting another unattainable ideal for women so they will always fall short of the mark." I mean, what are women if they're not feeling insecure about something or another?

Chewing on all these questions, I returned to campus in the fall and began to test-drive not shaving. I would make a firm decision to quit cold turkey, toss all my razors, and let the hair do its thing. For the first few weeks, I could pass on the bad shaver–stubble ticket. Okay, fine. But after a month or so, I found myself eager to answer a question in class, yet halted in my tracks by the horror of exposing my tank-topped hairy underarms to the cute guy across from me! Ay! I would settle for wagging my hand around on my desk and vow to stick to T-shirts from then on. But I love tank tops! And here began the eternal debate: Should I shave or should I let it go and feel awkward?

I've finally hit a point where I can hold out through fall, a hairy winter, and well into spring. But come summer (lying on bikini-laden beaches, going to the office in a sleeveless dress without stockings, riding a crowded subway and having to reach up to grip the handrail), I start losing steam. At crunchy folk festivals I'm a card-carrying member, but traipsing to a corporate office in midtown Manhattan? Short of bundling up in wool tights and turtlenecks in 90-degree weather, I feel awfully strange about having hairy legs. I start out by re-hearsing witty comebacks. I feel bold and strong for about a day and a half. Then I invent outfits to disguise my hairy legs and underarms. Then the debate rekindles. Finally, I lose my chutzpah and shave in defeat.

It's throwing in the towel on all accounts: Besides the strength I derive from rebelling against yet another implicit body pressure, hair feels good. Who could have ever imagined the erotic potential in riding a bike or swimming with hairy legs? The breeze ruffles it, the water swishes through it, wow! And sex? Ever sent someone flying out of bed by rubbing your bristly legs against them? Quite the opposite with hairy legs, as it is ultra-stimulating to entwine your furry legs with your lover's. This completely uncharted aphrodisiac is scarily reminiscent of women not being encouraged to experience full sexual pleasure (guys get the hairy leg turn-on). Add to that, body hair looks incredibly sexy and healthy. We're just not used to seeing it on women.

What body hair needs is more visibility. It needs a publicity agent and a marketing campaign. It needs models and actresses to flounce around with hairy legs and pits. When those trailblazing, unshaven singers and songwriters like Ani DiFranco and Dar Williams stomp onto stage, it sends a loud and clear holler into the hairless vacuum. It propels us to see it, to think about it, to actually make the connection that this is a real woman, not the reverse. It cracks open a door that will eventually lead to women having the choice (not the compulsory burden) of whether they want to shave. Maybe someday I'll become a poster child for body hair. For now, I'm just revving up to go an entire summer without shaving, to storm the office in a sundress and sandals, to wear whatever the hell I want to the beach, to not feel ashamed to show my hairy armpits to the world. Every summer I get a little closer. Maybe this time I'll make it.

Browbeating

HAGAR SCHER

Hagar Scher, "Browbeating," *Ms.* magazine, July/August 1998. Reprinted by permission.

While most people barely bat an eyelash at the "news" that hard-core plucking is out for now and big eyebrows in, I confess that I'm absolutely thrilled. This trend makes my heart expand, my fist clench, my mind yell Woman Power! The untamed brows du jour are strong and bold. They remind me of my personal superheroes. Frida Kahlo and Golda Meir, though otherwise unrelated, share the fuzzy-brow bond. Their unwieldy forehead locks stand for what has always inspired me—the courage to live outside the lines and march to an original, booming drumbeat. Respect my eyebrows, respect me.

More than twenty-five years ago in this magazine, writers Harriet Lyons and Rebecca Rosenblatt argued that removing any sort of body hair says that "the real woman is too much." Let it be said that I am not towing such a fuzzy-equals-feminist line, but I do have a knee-jerk aversion to plucking, even though some of my best friends are devotees. As I recently discovered, my dislike of skinny eyebrows stems from personal, emotional, and, well, fuzzy reasons.

A few months ago, I was feeling really low (a dreaded combination of writer's block, winter blahs, and unwashed-dish syndrome). In one of those moments when core beliefs are abandoned for petty concerns, I went to the drugstore to buy myself some tweezers. I was convinced that taming my Oscaresque (as in *Sesame Street*) brows would help me get it together. Poised to do the deed, I suddenly lost my resolve. Ten little hairs lay sink-side. Yet already I felt like Samson. I was scared that by losing my muss I might also lose my muscle. Once I plucked, might I not feel the need to mince words, bite my tongue, make nice with the world?

My big brows are, undoubtedly, an element of my Middle Eastern heritage, like my poor table manners and my low bullshit threshold. Like straightening kinky hair or dying dark locks blond, going for the minibrow look can be an attempt to hide one's ethnicity.

If the eyes are the windows to the soul, then the eyebrows are, at different times, the shield, the curtain, the dark cloud. Evolutionarily speaking, those hairs are there to stop sweat from irritating our peepers, and depleting them plays into the idea that women don't pounce, kick, compete—or perspire. Metaphorically speaking, they're even more commanding. Think Einstein. Maxibrows like his connote deep thought and determination. When thick eyebrows come together, they can express disgust and rage. Genius, drive, anger—misogynistically speaking, these are unfeminine traits. Thin, immobile brows seem less threatening. As a makeup artist would say, they open up the eyes and beckon, "Come on in. It's safe in here."

Ed Christie, art director of the *Sesame Street* Muppets, regretfully admits that despite the show's egalitarian spirit, eyebrows are used to quickly identify whether an "abstract" critter is female or male. Whereas girl puppets have felt brows that give them "a pencil-line, manicured look that prettifies," manly puppets like Oscar, the Count, and Bert have prominent ones that shout "eccentric, wily, wise, Merlin-like, very intellectual," and also "wild man, Neanderthal, untamed spirit."

So did Frida Kahlo's, but I'm pretty sure she heard that nagging voice asking, "Why don't you do something about those things?" I imagine her at a New York City cocktail party, suffering some clueless guy hitting on her with "You've got a pretty face. If you did something about that unibrow, you'd be a knockout." Kahlo probably had her private moments of self-doubt when she reached for Diego's nose-hair clippers. But in the end, those dramatic brows were a constant in her life, a reminder, perhaps, of who she was. They made her appear moody, remote, unapologetically artistic.

Golda Meir, my grandpa once told me, was unapologetic in every way. They were members of the Israeli parliament together and although they were at odds politically, he was awed by her. A peacenik like him, I nonetheless am drawn to Meir because of her unflinching resolve, her sharp tongue, her ability to command the attention of a group of men steeped in macho Mediterranean idealism. When I think of Golda, I see two messy brows that sit above two piercing eyes, sending a message: *You'll have to look beneath these furry beasts to find me.*

A few weeks after my near-pluck experience, I flew to London to be with my mother. It was only our second chunk of together-time since she'd been diagnosed with colon cancer last summer. Apart from the bulging red scar that cut from her pubic mound to her chest, she seemed the same to me: calm, brilliant, charming, warm, honest, goofy, with a refreshing disregard for what other people think. One thing was new to me, though. As weird as it seems, I had never before noticed how amazingly bushy my mother's eyebrows are, stray hairs jumping out every which way. In my vision, tousled brows connote a productive life—like my mother's—in which trivial details fall by the wayside and societal constraints play second fiddle to self-realization. An existence like the one I aspire to.

Dreading It . . . Or How I Learned to Stop Fighting My Hair and Love My Nappy Roots

VERONICA CHAMBERS

Veronica Chambers, "Dreading It . . . Roots," *Vogue*, June 1999, excerpted from Sharon Sloan Fiffer and Steve Fiffer, eds., in *Body*, Austin, Texas: Bard Press, 1999. Reprinted by permission.

There are two relationships I have with the outside world—one is with my hair, and the other is with the rest of me. Sure, I have concerns and points of pride with my body. I like the curve of my butt but dislike my powerhouse thighs. My nose suited me fine for the past 28 years. Then last week, for some strange reason, my nose seemed too big and I started to wonder about a nose job. My breasts, once considered too small, have been proclaimed perfect so often that not only am I starting to believe the hype but I'm booking my next vacation to a topless resort in Greece. But my hair. Oh, my hair.

I have reddish-brown dreadlocks that fall just below shoulder length. I like my hair—a lot. But over the past eight years that I have worn dreadlocks, my hair has conferred upon me the following roles: rebel child, Rasta mama, Nubian princess, drug dealer, unemployed artist, rock star, world-famous comedienne, and nature chick. None of which is really true. It has occurred to me on more than one occasion that my hair is a whole lot more interesting than I am.

Because I am a black woman, I have always had a complicated relationship with my hair. For those who don't know the history, here's a quick primer on the politics of hair and beauty aesthetics in the black community, vis-á-vis race and class in the late twentieth century. "Good" hair is straight and, preferably, long. Think Naomi Campbell. Think Whitney Houston. For that matter, think RuPaul. "Bad" hair is thick and coarse, aka "nappy," and often short. Think Buckwheat of the *Little Rascals*. Not the more recent, politically correct version, but the old one, in which Buckwheat looked like Don King's grandson.

Understand that these are stereotypes: broad and imprecise. Some will say that "good" hair versus "bad" hair is outdated. And it's true, it's much less prevalent than it was in the seventies, when I was growing up. Sometimes I see little girls, with their hair in braids and Senegalese twists, sporting cute little T-shirts that read Happy to Be Nappy and I get teary-eyed. I was born in the sandwich generation between Black Power afros of the sixties and the blue contact lenses and weaves of the eighties. In my childhood, no one seemed very happy to be nappy at all.

I knew from the age of four that I had "bad" hair because my relatives and family friends discussed my hair with all the gravity that one might use to discuss a rare blood disease. "Something must be done," they would cluck sadly. "I think I know someone," an aunt would murmur. Some of my earliest memories are of Brooklyn apartments where women did hair for extra money. These makeshift beauty parlors were lively and loud, the air thick with the smell of lye from harsh relaxer, the smell of hair burning as the hot straightening comb did its job. To this day, the sound of a hot comb crackling as it makes its way through a thick head of hair makes me feel at home; the smell of hair burning is the smell of black beauty emerging like a phoenix from metaphorical ashes: transformation.

My hair was so thick that the perms never lasted through the end of the month. Hairdressers despaired like cowardly lion tamers at the thought of training my kinky hair. "This is some hard hair," they would say. As a child, I knew that I was not beautiful and I blamed it on my hair.

The night I began to twist my hair into dreads, I was nineteen years old and a junior in college. It was New Year's Eve, and the boy that I had longed for had not called. "We'll all meet at a club," he had said. "I'll call and tell you where." But the phone never rang. A few months before, Alice Walker had appeared on the cover of *Essence*, her locks flowing with all the majesty of a Southern American Cleopatra. I was inspired. It was my family's superstition that the hours between New Year's Eve and New Year's Day were the time to cast spells. "However New Year's catches you is how you'll spend the year," my mother reminded me my whole life long. We spent the days before New Year's cleaning our room, watching as our mother put clean sheets on the bed and stocked the house with groceries. On New Year's Eve, my mother tucked dollar bills into my training bra and into my brother's pants pocket so that the New Year would find us flush. The important thing on New Year's Eve was to set the stage, to make sure you kept close everything you needed and wanted.

Jilted on New Year's Eve, I decided to use the hours that remained to transform myself into the vision that I'd seen on the cover of *Essence*. Unsure of how to begin, I washed my hair, carefully and lovingly. I dried it with a towel, then opened a jar of hair grease. Using a comb to part the sections, I began to twist each section into baby dreads. My hair, at the time, couldn't have been longer than an inch. I twisted for two hours, and in the end was far from smitten with what I saw—my full cheeks dominated my face, now that my hair lay in flat twists around my head. I did not look like the African goddess that I had imagined, but it was a start. I emerged from the bathroom and ran into my Aunt Diana, whose headful of luxuriously long, straight black hair always reminded me of Diahann Carroll on *Dynasty*. "Well, Vickie," she said, shaking her head. "Well, well." I knew that night my life would begin to change. I started my dreadlocks and I began the process of seeing beauty where no one had ever seen beauty before. Like Rapunzel, I grew my hair and it freed me, not only from perms that could never quite tame my kinky hair down but from a past in which my crowning glory was anything but.

There are, of course, those who see my hair and still consider it "bad." I have been asked by more than one potential suitor if I had pictures of myself before "you did that to your hair." One friend was so insistent that I must have been prettier without dreadlocks that I wore a wig to meet him one day. Not only did he not like me in the straight black bob that I wore, he didn't recognize me. "I get it," he said. "Those dreads are really you." I have occasionally thought that I carry all of my personality around on my head. A failure at small talk and countless other social graces, I sometimes walk into a cocktail party and let my hair do the talking for me. I stroll through the room, silently, and watch my hair tell white lies. In literary circles, my hair brands me as "interesting, adventurous." In black middle-class circles, my hair brands me as "rebellious" or "Afro-centric." In predominantly white circles, my hair doubles my level of exotica. My hair says, "Unlike the black woman who reads you the evening news, I'm not even trying to blend in."

That said, it is important to remember that at

the end of the day, my hair is just hair. "Do you think this could work out?" a man said to me recently. Mind you, it was only our second date and I was pretty convinced that I didn't want there to be a third. "What do you mean?" I asked him, sweetly, even dumbly. "I'm very traditional and you're so wild," he said, reaching out for my hair. "I'm not wild. You only think I'm wild," I wanted to scream. For those who are ignorant enough to think that they can read hair follicles like tea leaves, my hair says a lot of things that it doesn't mean. Taken to the extreme, my hair says that I am a pot-smoking Rastafarian wannabe who in her off-hours strolls through her house in an African dashiki, lighting incense and listening to Bob Marley.

I have been asked to score or smoke pot so often that it doesn't even faze me anymore. Once after a dinner party in Beverly Hills, a white colleague of mine lit up a joint. Everyone at the table passed and when I passed too, the man proceeded to cajole me relentlessly. "Come on," he kept saying. "Of all people, I thought you'd indulge." I shrugged and said nothing. As we left the party for the night, he kissed me good-bye. "Boy, you were a disappointment," he said as if I had been a bad lay. But I guess I had denied him a certain sort of pleasure. It must have been his dream to smoke a big, fat spliff with a real, live Rastafarian.

Similarly, it's such hair judgments that make me a magnet for airport security. I loathe connecting international flights in Miami and London, for I am sure to be stopped and stopped again. On a recent trip from Panama, I was stopped by five officers in one hour; each took his time poking through my suitcases. Finally, imprudently, I let the last officer have it. "I know what this is," I told him. "This is harassment. And it's because of my hair." He didn't even blink an eye. "We stopped them too," he said, pointing to a group of white missionaries. "Nothing wrong with their hair." In the Bahamas, a friend and I weren't allowed into a local nightclub because, as the bouncer pointed

out, the sign said No Jeans. No Sneakers. No Dreadlocks. I would have laughed if I didn't want to cry. You can change what you're wearing. How do you change the hair on your head? And why should you have to?

I have thought, intermittently, of changing my hairstyle. My hair is too big for me to wear hats, and I sometimes envy women with close-cropped cuts and stylish headgear. The other night, I watched one of my favorite movies, *La Femme Nikita*, and I admired Nikita's no-nonsense bob. "I couldn't be a female assassin with hair like this!" I said, jumping up out of my chair. Even pulled back, my hair is too voluminous to be stark. Then I remembered how, in the movie *Foxy Brown*, Pam Grier pulls a gun out of her Afro, and I was comforted that should I choose the career path of professional ass-kicker, my hair would not be an obstacle. Once, after the end of a great love affair, I watched a man cut all of his dreadlocks off and then burn them in the backyard. This is perhaps the only reason I would ever cut my hair. After all, a broken heart is what started this journey of twisting hair. A broken heart may find me at a new hair road. Because I do not cut my hair, I carry nine years of history on my head. One day, I may tire of this history and start anew. But one thing is for sure, whatever style I wear my hair in, I will live happily—and nappily—ever after.

BREASTS

The Anatomy of Your Breasts

MARVIN S. EIGER AND SALLY WENDKOS OLDS

Marvin S. Eiger and Sally Wendkos Olds, excerpt from *The Complete Book of Breastfeeding*, 3d ed., New York: Workman, 1999. Originally published in 1972. Reprinted by permission.

No matter what the size and shape of your breasts, you can have a gratifying breast-feeding experience. Whether your breasts are broad or narrow, high or sloping, small or large, you can happily nurse your baby. Just as women differ in height, general body build, and facial characteristics, they vary considerably with regard to the size and shape of their breasts. Furthermore, most women have one breast that's larger than the other. None of these characteristics are important for feeding a baby.

This is because the milk-producing glands are just one of the four types of tissue that make up the breasts. These four types are the *glands* that secrete milk, the *ducts* that carry it, the *connective tissue* that supports and attaches the breasts to the muscles of the chest, and the *fatty tissue* that encases and protects these other structures.

The size of your breasts is determined by the amount of fatty tissue they contain, and since the only purpose of this tissue is to encase and protect the more functional elements, it has no bearing at all on your ability to produce and give milk. You can be an excellent breast-feeder no matter what the size or shape of your breasts.

THE NIPPLE

Let's look at the breasts with a baby's-eye view. The nipple is the handle by which the infant grabs hold of the breast and also the spout through which she receives her milk.

The size of the nipple is usually as unimportant for nursing as is the size of the breast itself. Nipples come in different shapes. They are cylindrical in some women and conical in others.

The nipples of some women look flat or folded in and do not become erect when cold or when stimulated. Most often, however, by the end of pregnancy such "pseudo-inverted" nipples protrude normally and come out fully when the baby starts to suckle. In very rare cases, a woman has truly inverted nipples, which do not protrude enough for the baby's mouth to grasp them and which do not protrude with the baby's suckling. Fortunately, this condition is almost always correctable during pregnancy.

You have probably noticed that your nipples become erect when they're cold or when you become sexually excited. The erect nipple becomes two to three times longer than in its softer state. The same thing will happen when your baby nurses.

Each of your nipples has fifteen to twenty tiny openings through which milk is excreted. As the nursing baby stimulates the many nerve endings in the nipple, this causes uterine contractions that help return the uterus to its prepregnancy size.

THE AREOLA

Surrounding the nipple is a darker-colored circle called the *areola*. In most women the areola is between one and two inches in diameter, but it can be considerably larger. The areola and nipple are darker than the rest of the breast, ranging from a light pink in very fair-skinned women to a very dark brown in others.

The areolar pigmentation deepens in pregnancy and remains darker during lactation, after which the color fades somewhat; it never reverts, however, to the lighter shade it was before pregnancy. (This is one way doctors sometimes determine whether a woman has ever borne a child.) The darker color of the areola may be some sort of visual signal to newborns, since they must close their mouths upon the areola, not upon the nipple alone, if they are to obtain milk.

You may have noticed little bumps on your areola. These are called *Montgomery's glands*. They become enlarged and quite noticeable during pregnancy and lactation, because they secrete a substance that cleanses, lubricates, and protects the nipple during nursing. The antibacterial properties in this substance also help to prevent infection in both mother and baby. After lactation, these glands recede to their former unobtrusive state.

HOW YOUR BODY MAKES MILK

Directly beneath and behind your areola is a group

of *milk pools* (known scientifically as *lactiferous sinuses*). These pools are widened parts of the milk-carrying canals (*lactiferous ducts*), which transport the milk from the place in the breast where it is made to the nipples, where your baby can obtain it.

Each of your breasts has from fifteen to twenty ducts, each of which ends at the tip of the nipple. These ducts branch off into smaller canals within the breast toward the chest wall; these canals are called *ductules*. At the end of each ductule is a grapelike cluster of tiny rounded sacs called *alveoli*. The milk is made in these alveoli. Each cluster of alveoli is referred to as a *lobule* (a small rounded complex); a cluster of lobules is called a *lobe*. The lobes, each of which is a miniature gland, are situated at the base of the breast next to the chest wall. There are from fifteen to twenty lobes in each breast, each lobe connected to one duct, each duct emptying into one nipple opening, or milk pore.

Both the ducts and the alveoli are covered with smooth muscle cells. Under the influence of the hormone *oxytocin* (more later about this important hormone), these smooth muscle cells squeeze the milk out from the alveoli into the duct system. Then the cells in the alveoli burst and extrude fat cells to form the *hind milk* (the fatty milk released at the end of a feeding session).

THE SUPPORTING STRUCTURE

In some cultures, women deliberately pull at their breasts to make them longer so that it will be easier to nurse a baby strapped to their backs. Since this is probably not your aim, you'll want to give your breasts as much support as possible.

Nature provides some support—through the muscles attached to the ribs, the collarbone, and the bones of the upper arm near the shoulder. You can help Mother Nature along by wearing a good, supportive bra, even during sleep, during the latter part of your pregnancy and during lactation.

Although wearing a bra or going without one has no effect at all upon the breast-feeding function, the force of gravity will tend to pull down the heavier breasts of the pregnant or nursing woman. A supportive bra helps to prevent undue stretching of the suspensory ligaments of the upper part of the breast. Some doctors feel that a woman whose breasts are wide at the base will retain her figure whether or not she wears a bra.

THE LET-DOWN REFLEX: HOW YOUR BABY GETS YOUR MILK

When your *let-down reflex* is operating well, you are overjoyed, not "let down" in the sense of feeling disappointed. Also known as the *milk-ejection reflex* (*MER*) and, in England, the "draught" (pronounced "draft"), the let-down reflex lets down your milk from your breast to your baby. The let-down reflex is automatic, and in almost all cases it does operate well, as it has for millions of years for almost all women (see below).

In the early stage of lactation, it takes anywhere form several seconds to several minutes of your baby's suckling to produce a let-down reflex. After lactation is well established, you may find that hearing your baby cry or even just thinking about your baby will bring it on. . . .

As your baby suckles, she stimulates the nerve endings in your nipples, which then send signals to your pituitary gland, directing it to produce more of the hormone prolactin. The prolactin stimulates the alveoli to produce milk. As long as your breasts are suckled or otherwise stimulated (as with a breast pump or with manual manipulation), they will continue to make milk.

Your baby's suckling also causes your pituitary to release oxytocin, another very important hormone for lactation. Oxytocin travels through your bloodstream to your breast, where it causes the smooth muscle cells surrounding the alveoli to contract. As they contract, they squeeze the milk from the alveoli into the ducts. The walls of the ducts also contract, sending the milk out to the milk pools beneath the areolae.

While prolactin makes the milk, oxytocin makes

it available to your baby. Animal research suggests that oxytocin also plays a part in stimulating the release of prolactin. In addition, oxytocin released into the brain promotes calming and positive social behaviors. Oxytocin has been called "the quintessential mammalian hormone," "the satis-factional hormone," and the "hormone of love." Besides its role in fostering bonds between parents and offspring, it also causes the uterus to contract during childbirth, orgasm, and lactation.

The Renaissance artist Jacopo Tintoretto portrayed a beautiful representation of the let-down reflex in his work *The Origin of the Milky Way*. The painting tells the story of Hercules, Zeus's son by a mortal woman, whom Zeus put to the breast of the sleeping goddess Hera to make him immortal. After the infant had stopped drinking of Hera's milk, the milk continued to flow from the goddess's breasts. Some went up into the sky, forming the galaxy, and the rest dropped on the ground, forming a garden of lilies.

The British scientist S. J. Folley points out that this picture illustrates two important attributes of the let-down reflex: first, that the stimulus of suck-ling creates an increased pressure of the milk inside the breasts, causing it to spurt from the nipples, and second, that even though only one breast may be suckled, milk will flow from both.

Although the let-down reflex operates like clock-work in almost all women, occasionally some women need a little help to "oil the mechanism." Problems with let-down can usually be resolved quite easily. The let-down reflex has a strong psychological basis. The pituitary gland, which controls the release of oxytocin, is itself controlled by the *hypothalamus*. This walnut-sized organ in the brain is often referred to as the "seat of emotion," since it receives messages about the individual's psychological state and, acting on these messages, sends its own orders to the glands, translating emotions into physiological re-actions. The emotions, therefore, exert a powerful influence on such hormone-regulated functions as the menstrual cycle, childbirth, and lactation.

When you have the confidence that you will have milk for your baby, even major stresses like war or natural disasters will not dam up the flow. But when you live in a society like ours, in which women often worry about their ability to provide milk, the slightest of emotions can interfere with your milk production. Pain, embarrassment, fear, fatigue, illness, or distraction can inhibit the let-down reflex and hold your milk back from your baby. If your nipples hurt you, your let-down may not work right. If you are distressed by the dis-paraging remarks of relatives and friends, your let-down may let you down. If you overtire yourself, don't eat properly, or don't respect your own needs for privacy and for relaxation, your let-down reflex may be affected.

SIGNS OF AN ACTIVE LET-DOWN REFLEX

Some of the most common signs that your let-down reflex is functioning are:

➤ A tingling sensation in your breasts
➤ A feeling of warmth and/or fullness in your breasts
➤ Dripping of milk before your baby starts to nurse
➤ Release of milk from the nipple other than the one your baby is suckling
➤ Cramps caused by the contractions of your uterus
➤ The relief of nipple or breast discomfort as your baby nurses

Some women with very powerful let-down do not experience many of these sensations, and some feel a brief period of pain in the early days when their milk lets down. Another way to check your let-down reflex is to look at your baby for signs of active swallowing; if she's swallowing, you're getting milk to her!

The Bra Story

LORI BARER

©1999 by Lori Barer. Original for this publication.

Bra, aka brassiere, undergarment, over-the-shoulder-boulder-holder, and pick-me-upper. Lingerie companies make them, we wear them. Since approximately 1913, bras have been marketed and sold in the United States; before this time "there was absolutely no interest in [the] uplift [of breasts]." Today, women of all ages, myself included, consider the bra an essential item in our wardrobe. As I lay awake each morning deciding what outfit I should pick out for the day, I cease to ponder whether or not I should wear a bra. I simply step out of bed, brush my teeth, and turn directly toward my underwear drawer. To rid myself of this unfathomably uncomfortable norm I call a "bra" was my idea of fun (or so I thought).

I woke up Friday, February 5, with butterflies in my stomach; I couldn't move. I did not want to get out of bed, for today was my big day. I wore a tight shirt with a sweater over it, no bra. From the moment I stepped out of my room until the moment I reached it again, with all intentions of putting my bra on, I was miserable. I felt ugly, fat, weird, and all together brutish. There was not one point in the day in which I felt secure and proud that I was defying a societal norm; it was horrifying. No one said a word about my hanging breasts. Not one remark from my boyfriend, nor my roommates, nor strangers. I was shocked. What I did get were stares. All day long people stared at me, as if there was something to stare at; perhaps they thought I just had low-hanging breasts and I was, in fact, wearing a bra—what a stigma I might then have.

My boyfriend was the first to see me. He stared, he literally stared at my breasts while he spoke to me. No eye contact, no embarrassment that he wasn't looking at some other part of my body, he spoke directly to them. He was very, very confused. He didn't know whether I was wearing a bra and it for some reason or other wasn't "working" or if, heaven forbid, I didn't have one on. When he finally realized that there was just no way I was wearing one, he was almost embarrassed for me, he didn't know how to react, and never brought it up. My roommates all had the same reaction, they simply stared at my chest, then looked up at my face and down again to perhaps ponder whether my breasts had always been near my ankles or perchance gravity was beginning to take its toll.

When I finally ventured outside of my house where I was more likely to encounter people I didn't know (I went to several places, the pharmacy, the food store), I was hoping to receive a different reaction. I don't know what I was looking for, I think I almost hoped someone would scream out "*Look at Her Sagging Breasts!*" so that this experiment I had planned for myself would, in fact, be worthwhile. They didn't. Again, no one said anything. They just looked . . . at my breasts. People commonly look at my breasts, this has been something I have had to deal with my entire postpubescent life, as I have large breasts and people notice. The body of a woman was nearly exactly that of my own as a peripubescent thirteen-year-old, where full shapely breasts smothered my tiny torso and often seemed to block my innocent face. To have this body as a young girl meant having the repercussions that went along with it. This meant my eighth grade English teacher, who couldn't keep his eyes to himself. He often sent girls to the nurse's office because he said he could see their bra strap. He was known to seat the prettiest, shapeliest girls in the front and those less pleasing to the eye in the rear of the classroom. I still had my prepubescent figure and had gained my large breasts quickly and noticeably, putting me at center stage. What it was at this point in my life to have a female's body was to be stared at, to have all eyes on my chest, to have to go home and tell my mother, and my father, and ultimately the principal, that my teacher couldn't stop staring at my breasts. In summation, this meant sending my mother in a rage to my middle school to verbally beat the living shit out of this man. It also meant my embarrassment; telling the other children why I couldn't be in his class anymore, why I had to rearrange my schedule in the middle of the school year to get away from this very sick man.

This staring was different though. People were staring in disgust. It was as if they could not believe that a "normal" looking, well-dressed woman would go out of the house like this. I was mortified and saddened by what I thought could have been a truly liberating feminist experience turning into one that was actually quite shameful. I'm disappointed in myself, after studying gender and women for so long, for still succumbing to societal pressures of bodily norms in accordance with gender.

Gender on a whole is socially constructed. This means that one is not born with gender; the individual's particular society molds gender and thus molds human beings to act or not act with certain gender-esque attributes. In our culture, for instance, people born with penises are acculturated to be aggressive and dominating—they should wear pants and suits and ties. On the other hand, people born with vaginas are shaped to be sensitive and emotional, to wear jewelry and high heels, and most certainly a bra. Unfortunately, this dichotomy of gender should look more like a continuum, but it does not. This therefore means that an individual is either "feminine" or "masculine," a "man" or a "woman." There are no in-betweens and there will be no crossing of boundaries. The "experiment" that I undertook did exactly that, I crossed the boundary. Wearing a bra in our society is distinctly feminine. This does not hold true for all societies and certainly not for everyone living in ours, but for the most part, it is upheld.

My rebellion against this particular aspect of gender norming was wildly successful. It showed that while the practice of wearing a bra is not "natural," we need to abide by it in order to be accepted within society. It also showed that this gendered bodily practice played an enormous role in self-concept. I have previously discussed how my self-image took a dramatic turn for the worse and my strength and power as an outspoken feminist was muted. While my sex was not altered, I was clearly less feminine. In the study "What is Beautiful is Good," it is concluded that ". . . attractive . . . persons are likely to secure more prestigious jobs than those of lesser attractiveness, as well as experiencing happier marriages, being better parents, and enjoying more fulfilling social and occupational lives."[1] This exemplifies the notion that my unattractiveness as a woman led to perceptions of me by others who perhaps thought the aforementioned conclusion. I was somehow not worthy of a prestigious job or a happy marriage, I was strange. Over time, our society has come to many conclusions about what is acceptable and unacceptable. Somehow, sagging breasts were seen to be unacceptable (most likely via media messages of WonderBras and Miracle Bras), thus my dissociation from society.

In actuality, we can all survive without wearing a bra ever again. If we raised our daughters without bras, they would be just as healthy as we are now (if not healthier according to new studies of a link between wearing bras and breast cancer). Therefore, there is nothing natural about the practice. What is natural, though, are the emotions felt from societies' reactions to breaking these gendered norms. To ostracize and isolate someone based upon a physical appearance, a way of dress, is abhorrent. The emotions felt now make the act of simply wearing something like a bra mandatory. I learned that it is perhaps a good idea to walk in the life of someone who does not abide by gender rules, if only for a day.

The kind of person that walks into a store, and you can't tell their sex, and it bothers you; and you might go home and think about that person all night, and wish you knew whether they were a man or a woman (because they could never be neither), but you would never think about why it matters in the first place, nor how any of those "signs" that you were looking for were ever construed. There is nothing natural about gender, thus nothing instinctive about gender norms.

NOTE

1. K. Dion, E. Berscheid, and E. Walster, "What is Beautiful is Good," *Journal of Personality and Social Psychology* 24, no. 3:285–290.

Breast Reduction

MARTA DRURY

I wish I had had my breast reduction surgery when I was sixteen years old. In every photograph of me from the age of eleven on, I am wearing an oversized jacket or cardigan—even in the Badlands of South Dakota in sweltering midsummer heat—standing with my arms crossed over my chest. When I graduated from high school, I wore a size 42DD bra. Now I wear a 38B.

Thirty-one years later, when I was forty-seven, I was finally ready for the surgery. My mother had recently died, so there was no fear of "offending" her, and I could afford it; I thought it would be considered a "cosmetic" procedure and therefore not covered by insurance, but as it turned out, I was wrong. The surgery would be covered because I had all the classic problems associated with large breasts: forward neck, indentations in my shoulders from the weight of my breasts, tingling and numbness in my arms and hands, and recurring rashes and infections under my breasts.

None of my friends had had breast reduction surgery—or at least none who had talked about it—so I had to do my own research. I interviewed four surgeons. One doctor spent an hour and a half showing me photos and examining me before he told me he wouldn't consider operating unless I lost fifty pounds. But then I met a female surgeon who told me that she liked doing the breast reduction surgery because she had never had a patient who wasn't happy with the results.

Breast reduction surgery is a major operation. It is performed under general anesthesia and requires an overnight stay in the hospital. I have a low tolerance for physical pain, but from the moment I awoke, whatever discomfort I experienced from the incisions and drainage tubes was overshadowed by my delight. I had what I wanted: reasonably sized breasts that looked good. I came through the surgery without any complications, and eventually the sensation in my nipples returned. (I understand that some women lose it.)

Now, nine years later, I have only the scars to remind me of the surgery, and I rather like them—they are like bridges to my past. I feel taller and lighter than before, and finding clothes that fit is no longer a problem. This surgery enabled me to start the process of accepting my body as it is. My only regret is that I didn't do it when I was sixteen.

VAGINA

Breakthrough Against Female Genital Mutilation

NOY THRUPKAEW

Noy Thrupkaew, "Senegalese Women Win Ban on Female Genital Cutting," *Sojourner,* March 1999. Reprinted by permission.

In response to a nationwide campaign led by a Senegalese women's group, the Parliament of Senegal banned female circumcision/female genital mutilation (FC/FGM) on January 15. Senegal joins Burkina Faso, Central African Republic, Djibouti, Ghana, Guinea, Togo, and Egypt in their ban on FC/FGM. The success of the Senegalese women's campaign, a grassroots community-based effort, marks a turning point in increasingly global efforts to eradicate FC/FGM. Tactics previously used in attempts to abolish the practice have ranged from government-led top-down legislation to Western imposition—methods that have not been as effective in promoting widespread change. Increased international pressure to ban female genital cutting—in part due to high-profile cases of women seeking political asylum to escape FC/FGM—has also contributed to recent bans on the practice.

The punishment for anyone "having violated or attempting to violate the physical integrity of the genital organs of a person of the female sex" is six months to five years of imprisonment, according to Article 299 of Senegalese law. The amendment covers all forms of FC/FGM, and men or women who provoke or demand that FC/FGM be performed are sentenced to the same punishment as those who cut young women's genitalia. The maximum penalty is applied to members of the medical or paramedical fields who condone or perform the practice. If a woman dies from her FC/FGM injuries, those found guilty of her death are sentenced to forced labor for life.

While the terms "female circumcision" and "female genital mutilation" are sometimes used interchangeably, each has distinct and powerful political connotations. "Some African people think that the term FGM attacks their culture and tradition, but by labeling it 'female circumcision,' you are making it sound equal in severity to male circumcision . . . you are making it more acceptable," said Rana Badri of Equality Now, a New York–based group that advocates for women's human rights domestically and internationally. Badri, who is the FGM Eradication Campaign director of Equality Now, which publishes an FGM-awareness publication entitled *Awaken,* added that "the term 'Female Genital Mutilation' brings out the ugliness and the severe damage that the practice does to women." The World Health Organization (WHO) calls the practice "FGM" as well.

Seble W. Argaw, women's human rights activist and member of the Boston-based Ethiopian Adbar Women's Alliance, noted, however, that practitioners of female genital cutting who see "FGM" as a foreign label, "can think to themselves—'I don't do that'—and then they dismiss the whole idea." By speaking about FGM in terms of its traditional cultural name, "female circumcision," Argaw seeks to encourage its eradication through "education and persuasion."

Though performed primarily by the Muslim populations in the Middle East and Africa, FC/FGM knows no boundaries of religion or class. In Mali, for example, where an estimated 93 percent of the female population has undergone FC/FGM,

85 percent of the female Christian population has also had FC/FGM performed on them. WHO estimates that 130 million women have been subjected to FC/FGM and each year, 2 million young women, girls, and infants undergo the ritual of genital cutting. While Egypt, Ethiopia, Kenya, Nigeria, Somalia, and the Sudan account for approximately 75 percent of FC/FGM cases, FC/FGM is also performed in Indonesia, Malaysia, Pakistan, and India. Genital cutting practices range in severity. In Senegal, practitioners generally remove the clitoris and part of the external and internal genital folds, and some may also loosely stitch the parts of the wound together.

GRASSROOTS GROUP TOSTAN BREAKS NEW GROUND

The Senegalese women's group Tostan is remarkable not only for its success in convincing the Senegalese government to pass legislation banning FC/FGM but also—more importantly—for mobilizing widespread community support for the ban. Based in the village of Malicounda Bambara, Tostan—which means "breakthrough" in Wolof, the native language of Senegal—did not originally focus on FC/FGM issues. Begun by Molly Melching, a US citizen who had lived in Senegal for over twenty years, and supported by UNICEF, the government of Senegal, and the American Jewish World Service, the group initially worked on literacy, women's health, and human rights. After discussions about how to improve prenatal health, women in the group became aware that many Senegalese women's health problems were a direct result of their past FC/FGM.

The women of Tostan then embarked on a villagewide campaign to persuade husbands, village elders, and religious leaders to commit themselves to abolishing the practice. By enlisting men in their cause, the women gave their message more weight and legitimacy within traditional village social structures. As Ethiopian Adbar Women's Alliance member Argaw notes, "You have to visualize the whole pattern, how it works. The men are thought of as the defenders of the nation, the breadwinners. The women are not in the same position as in the West." To bring about change in this society, "You must convince the men, the village elders."

As a result of Tostan's successful organizing, no FC/FGM took place in Malicounda in 1997. Tostan members spoke to a group of twenty Senegalese journalists, and the press coverage led to the first national discussion on FC/FGM. Bolstered by the support of Senegalese President Abdou Diouf, the campaign quickly spread to other villages in Senegal. The women of Nigeria Bambara followed the lead of the Malicounda Bambara women and renounced the practice of FC/FGM within their village.

Male and/or religious spokesmen came to the forefront of the anti-FGM movement when the village of Ker Simbara decided to consult the members of their extended family over a communal decision to ban FC/FGM. Two Bambara men, Cheikh Traore (a Tostan facilitator) and Demba Diaware (an imam or religious leader and former Tostan participant) traveled to the outlying regions where the Der Simbara kin live, and discussed FC/FGM with the villagers. The outlying villages then formulated the Diabougou Declaration, abolishing the practice of FC/FGM and leading a total of 8,000 villagers into the forefront of the FC/FGM eradication movement.

Thirteen members of the Tostan program spoke about their experiences with FC/FGM before deputies of the Senegalese parliament of January 12, 1999, the first time a group of villagers has testified before the National Assembly. They strongly urged the Assembly to pass the law, but recommended that the legislation be tempered with measures that allow for FC/FGM education programs to ease the transition. Most of the members of the assembly supported the eradication of FC/FGM, but based on the testimony of villages of the Diabougou Declaration, attempted to request a delay for the enforcement of the law. Many members were concerned that repressive measures

would cause a flurry of FC/FGM activity nationwide, a fear backed up by the actions of at least one village. At the end of December 1998, 120 girls in the Kedougou village were cut by one person, wielding one knife, perhaps in anticipation of the ban. The National Assembly is still conferring over the best way to implement and enforce the law.

NEW MODELS, OLD PROBLEMS

Many activists say that Tostan provides a critical new model for fighting FC/FGM. By beginning with a broad examination of the totality of women's lives, Tostan opened up a forum for women to discover for themselves the far-reaching effects of their past FC/FGM. Argaw commented that native women's leadership in such campaigns was essential, adding, "A grassroots approach is very important." After Senegal's ban was announced, Carol Bellamy, executive director of UNICEF, also commented on the grassroots, women-led campaign. She told the *New York Times* that, "The work of African grassroots organizations seems increasingly to demonstrate that most women would not accept female genital mutilation as a part of tradition if they had the power to change their fate."

Badri noted that the Tostan campaign differs from earlier FC/FGM eradication efforts that tended to focus on ideological opposition to genital cutting. She said that Tostan has shown that "the only way to stop the practice is to raise awareness of the [health] side effects. There is a shift in approach and strategy."

Both Argaw and Badri stressed that organizing against FC/FGM is complicated because the practice is viewed in countries that practice it as a sacred religious ritual or age-old cultural tradition. Reluctant to abandon the practice in the face of increasing Westernization, male and female practitioners defend the tradition as part of their culture. The context behind FC/FGM is further complicated by political and ethnic divisions. Some ethnic groups practice it, and others have no history of the tradition. As so many regions of

Africa depend on a delicate balance between such groups, potentially divisive issues such as FC/FGM do not enter public debate.

Western anti-FC/FGM movements are often perceived as heavy-handed colonialist interference. According to Badri, "Some efforts were unsuccessful because they attempted to impose drastic changes upon the natives." Argaw concurred, stating, "Sometimes people feel defensive, like Westerners are looking down on or putting down their culture. Some people feel that Westerners also do strange things—breast implants, plastic surgery. They feel it's an assault on the culture. So there's a conflict within the immigrant community here too." Immigrants in the United States who turn against FC/FGM practice are often viewed as "agents of Westernization" who have betrayed their native culture.

Some human rights groups have proposed that Western governments link foreign aid negotiations with abolishment of FC/FGM, but this approach seems counterproductive and ultimately unjust to many grassroots activists. Similarly, repressive, top-down government measures often result in frantic outbursts of FC/FGM activity. The governments of Egypt and Sudan placed bans of FC/FGM but did not meet with much success. In contrast to the current situation in Senegal, the anti-FC/FGM movement in Egypt and the Sudan had not gained sufficient popular momentum before the bans were implemented, "and huge numbers of young girls are still initiated into the painful reality of living with FC/FGM in these countries."

INCREASING WESTERN AWARENESS OF FC/FGM

While much work remains to be done to improve working relations between Westerners and native FC/FGM eradication activists, increased Western awareness has aided the movement greatly. The efforts of grassroots organizations and the increase in Western scrutiny have created an environment that encourages governments to address FC/FGM through education and legislation.

US awareness of FC/FGM issues has grown as immigrants from practicing countries arrived in the United States in increasing numbers. As doctors and other health care providers began to encounter women whose genitals had been cut, "a need emerged to develop policies to address the most appropriate way to respond to the needs of circumcised women," Badri explained. Unaware of the cultural differences between the United States and their respective homelands, "immigrants would go to the hospitals to have their girls circumcised," she said.

Western media coverage of FC/FGM has also intensified in the past ten years. In 1992, prominent author Alice Walker wrote a fiction book on FC/FGM, entitled *Possessing the Secret of Joy,* and followed that book with a nonfiction account of research into FC/FGM. Of these books, Badri remarked, "They help raise the awareness of the American community, draw attention to circumcised women's needs, help mobilize activities." Argaw expressed another opinion, stating that the books are "good and bad, in a sense. Good because it publicizes FGM, so more people will be aware. On the other hand, it might create a backlash against perceived Westernization. People say it didn't come from the inside. But it's definitely a start."

The case of Fauziya Kassindja also brought FC/FGM practices into the international spotlight. In December of 1994, Kassindja fled to the United States from Togo after learning that her husband-to-be had demanded that she undergo FC/FGM as a prerequisite to marriage. She was imprisoned after US immigration judge Donald V. Ferlise dismissed her case, stating that her story lacked "rationality and internal consistency." She was subsequently placed in the Esmor Detention Center in Elizabeth, New Jersey—shackled and in an isolation cell.

After a cousin enlisted the aid of law student Layli Miller Bashir, Kassindja's case began to gain momentum. Equality Now began a letter-writing campaign to the US Justice Department, and Karen Musal, law professor and acting head of American

University's International Human Rights Clinic, handled Kassindja's appeal. On April 5, 1996, the Justice Department filed a thirty-six-page brief supporting her continued incarceration. But the *New York Times* ran an article on her case on April 15, 1996, and she was freed nine days later. In June 1996, the Board of Immigration Appeals, the highest administrative tribunal in the US immigration system, overturned Ferlise's ruling and granted Kassindja asylum.

Delacorte Press signed Kassindja to a book contract—*Do They Hear You When You Cry?*—which focused on both Kassindja's experiences with FC/FGM and her incarceration in the United States.

FUTURE CAMPAIGNS: HOLISTIC APPROACHES TO HUMAN RIGHTS

Argaw advocates a holistic approach toward organizing against genital cutting, based around the internal energy of grassroots initiatives run by native women. Badri agrees, adding that for all determination and vision that these women's groups exhibit, they still need the support of women worldwide. Badri declared, "People should recognize that FC/FGM is a violation of women's reproductive rights." Bellamy of UNICEF also commented, "Women around the world who have the courage to take a stand on female genital mutilation need sustained international support in order to convince their societies to move away from this horrendous practice."

As for how Western feminists can be most helpful, Argaw urged greater involvement in "the big picture of human rights and conditions," saying that only after people "have enough to survive, food on the table," can they begin to talk about FC/FGM. She said, "Western women should work with the grassroots organizations on broad issues like nutrition, motherhood, opening hospital branches." Africans often become defensive about the Western attention to FGM, thinking that "all the American women talk about circumcision

when so many other issues are not addressed as a whole. This is not the only thing that happens to women." She added, "It's part of the whole picture of oppression."

THE HISTORY AND PRACTICE OF FC/FGM

The practice of FC/FGM ranges in severity from region to region. As classified by the World Health Organization (WHO), type 1 refers to genital cutting where only the prepuce (skin of the clitoris), and/or parts of the clitoris are removed. Type 2 FC/FGM involves the excision of the clitoris with partial or total excision of the labia minora. Type 3, infibulation, accounts for approximately 15 percent of FC/FGM. Infibulation encompasses the excision of part or all of the external genitalia. The incision is then stitched together, leaving a matchstick-sized opening for urine and menstrual blood to pass out of the body. Most often, countries in the Horn of Africa—Djibouti, Somalia, the Sudan, and parts of Ethiopia—practice infibulation. Type 4 involves a whole host of genital mutilation, ranging from the piercing or burning of the clitoris, scraping or cutting of the vagina, or the insertion of corrosive substances or herbs into the vagina to cause bleeding or to narrow or tighten it.

In all of its forms, FC/FGM affects normal bodily functions, often causing difficult childbirth, hemorrhaging, infection, and sometimes death. Often performed under unsanitary conditions with crude, unsterilized tools such as old razor blades, FC/FGM also severely limits sexual sensation, and subjects women to a host of other long-term physical and mental health complications. Traditional practitioners, usually elderly women who have inherited their role... from their families, often lack medical training and do not have the resources to effectively address medical complications that can arise from FC/FGM. Wealthier families can turn to health care professionals, who can—in many ways—do even greater damage by "medicalizing" and legitimizing the practice of FC/FGM.

The practice of FC/FGM is deeply embedded within cultural traditions. Many practitioners believe that Islam mandates FC/FGM, while others believe in the sanctity of cultural traditions and the rule of their forefathers' way of life. As the WHO FC/FGM Web site notes, "Some Muslim communities . . . practice FGM in the genuine belief that it is demanded by the Islamic faith." As they also note, however, "the practice predates Islam." In a ruling upholding a ban of FC/FGM, the Egyptian Supreme Court recently ruled that FC/FGM had no place in the Islamic religion.

Often performed as part of a woman's coming-of-age ceremony, or prior to her marriage, FC/FGM is traditionally thought to signal a woman's arrival as a full, mature member of her community. But as the age of the FC/FGM inductees drops every year, WHO argues that FC/FGM's connection to coming-of-age rituals is growing more tenuous. In much of Ethiopia, for example, FC/FGM is performed "very early in childhood, perhaps forty days after birth," according to Seble W. Argaw of the Ethiopian Adbar Women's Alliance. "It's done so early, you wouldn't know you had it. You don't know if your future sickness comes from that or not."

Issues of control of women's sexuality are also deeply intertwined with the tradition of FC/FGM. Rana Badri, director of the FGM Eradication Campaign of Equality Now, told *Sojourner*, "the reason why people practice this is to curb women's sexual behavior." The WHO FGM home page also states that FC/FGM is thought to "maintain chastity and virginity before marriage and fidelity during marriage, and increase male sexual pleasure." Some men say the artificial tightness of infibulation enhances their pleasure. Others find the smooth scar aesthetically pleasing. But the scar ultimately serves as a chastity belt of a women's own flesh, deadening her sexual pleasure, or even causing severe pain during intercourse.

Badri continued, "Some people think a woman's clitoris has a poisonous discharge, so by removing it, they are protecting her husband and child." An uncut woman is often perceived as unclean, or oversexed, selfishly seeking out her sexual pleasure despite the shame it would bring upon her husband or male relatives. Traditional practitioners of FC/FGM argue that it serves as a manmade safeguard against the social disorder that women's infidelity or sexual promiscuity can cause. In this way, FC/FGM is thought to maintain "social integration and the maintenance of social cohesion," according to WHO.

Intact women are often mocked and ostracized, and their fathers may be forbidden from speaking at village meetings. Men's power and status seem inversely linked to women's sexual freedom—the men gain more respect when the women's power or sexuality is curtailed, or brought in line with social norms. In this way, FC/FGM becomes a powerful indicator of men's status as well. They are rendered socially and politically impotent if their female relatives remain intact. Men often, therefore, put pressure on the women around them to submit to FC/FGM in order to regain or increase their political power.

As for its part in the commodification of women, FC/FGM serves as a status marker of a woman's marriage and social standing and a physical indicator of her future economic well-being. According to WHO, some practitioners believe FC/FGM enhances fertility and promotes child survival—without this ritual, a woman can lose valuable status because she may be perceived as potentially sterile. Because many men perceive intact women as damaged, or flawed, it becomes difficult for these women to marry and gain economic stability. Their families often cannot afford to support them, and the women are left with no choice but to undergo FC/FGM. During the ritual, a young woman's sexual status is also established—if the woman is a virgin, she can earn a larger dowry and her family is honored. According to folklore, nonvirgins bleed profusely during the cutting, while virgins do not. After the ritual cutting, the young woman is feted by hundreds of family members who feast and celebrate for days, and many young girls look forward to the day they will be so honored.

CHAPTER 19

Sexually Transmitted Infections

IT IS ESTIMATED THAT during World War I, thirty thousand women were taken into custody and tested for sexually transmitted infections (STIs). Those who tested positive—around fifteen thousand women—were held without formal charges and "treated" against their will.

The ostensible reason for violating these women's civil rights was protecting soldiers against the various plagues that they could be infected with so that they were able to keep performing their military duties to the best of their abilities. The fact that soldiers were treated as victims and their sexual partners criminals was not explained. This sad, little-known history is the subject of Michael Lowenthal's beautiful novel *Charity Girl*, and it highlights one incident in the difficult history of women and sexually transmitted infections.

In the second half of the twentieth century, hormonal contraception made preventing pregnancy easier, but it made sexual infection more likely as barrier methods like condoms and diaphragms fell into disuse. Condoms had a revival after the emergence of AIDS in the 1980s, although today, rising rates of chlamydia and gonorrhea make reeducating young people about the importance of barrier protection all the more necessary.

Women have always faced discrimination for having sexually transmitted infections. The challenge of the women's health movement as we enter the new millennium remains raising awareness and educating women about prevention and treatment.

Jane Fowler writes about the reality of living with HIV in the long term. As a woman who caught the infection from a lover in her midfifties, Fowler is now in her seventies and fighting to raise awareness about the unique needs of older patients. She cautions aging women to realize that you are never too old to need sexual protection. Efforts like hers not only save lives, they help to make things easier for women who are living with the infection by dispelling stereotypes of what an HIV patient looks like.

Even as new scientific advances bring hope for the prevention and treatment of certain STIs, old attitudes are holding back real progress. A particularly complicated and compelling example of this is the debate over the so-called "cervical cancer" vaccine, Gardasil. The vaccine actually works to combat certain strains of Human Papilloma Virus (HPV). This virus—frequently transmitted through sexual contact—is incredibly common in the US population. It is estimated that close to 50 percent of college students carry antibodies, meaning they have come in contact with, and potentially fought off, the virus. Those who do contract the virus have a greater risk of developing this horrible cancer.

When George Papinicaloau, a Greek-American doctor, developed the Pap smear in the late 1920s, he changed cervical cancer from an always-fatal diagnosis to a more predictable ailment. The screening test—now common—has saved countless lives. It was withheld for decades for political reasons, among them the fact that it could be taken and analyzed by nondoctors, seemingly making a significant crack in physician dominance of medical care.

Today we face the opposite problem with Gardasil. Rather than withholding a possibly life-saving preventative method, the promising vaccine is being rushed to market and pushed on girls. The major trials on Gardasil were conducted on less than twenty thousand, and results were favorable. Many states tried (and in most cases, at least initially, have failed) to make the vaccine mandatory for girls of eleven and twelve, only about 1,100 of whom were included in the trials. The hope is to act preventively before the girls become sexually active. I feel that while such efforts may be well-intentioned on the part of many doctors, activists, and parents, they are misguided.

First, very few girls this young were included in the trials, and there is no way to know how it might adversely affect them. Second, long-term data on the effects of the vaccine on health isn't yet available—a dubious situation to live with when you are making a medical procedure mandatory. Third, the vaccine is only good for a certain number of years, and initiating it at such a young age may not be the best way to prevent disease in young women who delay sexual activity until later.

HPV vaccination was finally approved in the United States for use in boys several years after the shot was given a green light for girls. Vaccine makers decided not to market the shot to male populations, and women's and family health groups continue to ask hard questions about the safety and usefulness of the HPV vaccination in young people.

It is worth asking why the Pap smear was withheld and Gardasil marketed so hastily. The answer probably has less to do with lessons learned and more to with the fact that Pap smears threatened to take power out of doctors' hands while Gardasil promises to put lots of money into the pockets of drug companies.

Charity Girl

MICHAEL LOWENTHAL

Michael Lowenthal, excerpt from *Charity Girl*, New York: Houghton Mifflin, 2007. Reprinted by permission.

Michael Lowenthal performs an invaluable service for women by remembering and reconstructing a shameful episode in the history of American policy toward its female citizens. During World War I, nearly fifteen thousand women, mostly poor and immigrant women, were indefinitely held without formal charges and forced to undergo medical treatments simply because they were identified as having sexually transmitted diseases. Lowenthal imagines the story of Frieda, who after a tryst with a young soldier finds herself sick and imprisoned with no idea when she will be released. This important chapter in American history is revived and preserved in this powerful book.

Mrs. Digges instructed Frieda not to "void" herself, since doing so might thwart the doctor's findings. The holding of her water all these hours since waking up, joined with fear, has turned her bladder into a bomb.

She sits in a chair outside the treatment room door, waiting for Flossie to come out. A shelf holds teetering stacks of leaflets: "The Soldier, Uncle Sam, and You"; "The Nation's Call to Young Girls." Queasy, she picks up a leaflet and reads. The need to pee goads her thumping heart.

DO YOUR BIT TO KEEP HIM FIT

Women have believed that:

➤ They should know little of sex matters— and never discuss them.
➤ A young man's "wild oats" should be forgiven; a woman's, never.

Women know today that:

➤ There is danger to themselves and to their children in irregular sexual relations because of the probability of venereal infection.
➤ They are responsible for their acts not only to themselves, but to their community, their country, and their future; and that "desire" is a fatal excuse.
➤ Social and industrial inefficiency result from the selfish indulgence of an appetite. We scorn the glutton; we are beginning to exercise social control over the alcoholic; we must now control venereal diseases.

Women's duty is to:

➤ Refuse to be ignorant and to raise their moral standards.
➤ Believe that men and boys with whom they associate can and will lead clean lives.
➤ Help their communities to close evil resorts and to organize in stamping out disease and delinquency, thereby aiding the government in saving our country from the gravest menace.

Scanning through the words leaves Frieda feeling scummy. The leaflet sounds like Mama (if Mama could speak good English): *desire kills, appetite is evil.* Mrs. Sprague, too, thinks Frieda, and now Mrs. Digges . . . all these people, cinched up tight, terrified of wanting. Were they born that way, or have all of them sustained some awful blow that changed them into quavering prigs? (*Waiting for you, Shaynah, if you ever change your mind. Waiting with all my love —Leo.*) What if the Home—being here—is the blow that will change Frieda? Get me out, oh get me out, she prays.

Flossie scuffs from the treatment room: pale, her sass drained.

"Next," comes a voice from inside.

"How . . . ?" Frieda starts to ask, but Flossie bows her head.

Frieda weakly rises, feels faint, sits back down. Her throat balks at a rising up of acid.

"Next!"

She tries again and this time stands.

"Come in," says a man in a shabby white smock, the cuffs of which appear freshly spattered. Greeting her, he doesn't bother looking at her face—just her trunk, as if assessing livestock. "This shouldn't take long. I'm Dr. Slocum." The bags beneath his eyes are the color of liverwurst. Big ears, a bald pate that scatters light. Frieda suffers another surge of acid.

"Boldt's table, as usual. Dorsal position."

He addresses a man Frieda didn't note until now, standing, like a butler, to the side.

"Stirrups?"

The doctor nods. "Yes, of course. I'll be right back." At the door he adds, "Oh—and this is Miller. Medical student from the Boston University. His practicum."

Frieda and the student are left alone.

The room is too cold. Her fingers shake.

Backed against the wall, as if facing a firing squad, Miller says, "Could you please loosen your clothing? Corset, waistband—anything constrictive."

It sounds as if he's reading from a textbook. Can't he see she wears nothing but her denim frock? She stands there. She can't calm her fingers.

"On the table, then?" He points to a white contraption with metal bracing and a smudgy glass top. "You . . . you don't have to remove . . . we'll make arrangements."

The suggestion of apology allows her to obey. Tremulous, she scoots onto the table.

Miller's left eye wavers on the verge of being crossed, which gives him an air of inquisitive concentration. He reminds her of someone—his strickenness, his absorption—but she can't put her thumb on just whom.

"Lie back, that's right. Knees up high." He covers her with a flimsy cotton sheet. "And the frock." He pushes the fabric above her waist.

Glass against bare skin, shocking chill. She fears she'll stick to the sting of it, as to ice.

Miller guides her left heel, then her right into the stirrups, and turns a crank to force her feet apart. She's open. She's a hole. A running sore.

With a squeaky snap of rubber, Dr. Slocum walks back in, pulling two gray gloves onto his hands. (The rubber's smell: powdery, neutered.) He peers between her legs, and says, "Wider."

Fumbling, the medical student readjusts the stirrups. He, too, snaps on a pair of gloves.

"Typically," says the doctor, looking absently at Miller, "you'd obtain a patient history before beginning. But the girls here tend to be unforthcoming."

Above her knees, Frieda catches a glimpse of the doctor's nose: bulbous, riddled with burst vessels.

"And," he adds, "we can fairly well surmise the story, can't we? Especially with a girl of this one's race."

Miller's left eye quivers. He says, "Sir?"

"She's a Jewess, if I'm not mistaken, no?"

"Yes, sir. I believe so, sir. She is."

"Well, it's the Jew traders—the Jews and the Italians—who run the rings. And the girls they traffic are most often their own."

Miller mumbles, "I . . . Do you know I'm Jewish, too?"

"That so? Name like Miller? Wouldn't have

thought." In his voice, not a note of discomposure. "Didn't you tell me you were from the Middle West?"

"Yes, sir. Not far from Kansas City."

"Kansas? Didn't know they had Jews there. Well, be that as it may, let's get to business. Visual exam, smears, draw blood from the Wassermann. If you will now, Miller, aim that light."

Frieda flinches, tries to shut her legs; the cold stirrups clamp her heels in place. What will the doctor see? What will Miller? ("Guts, that's what. The parts you throw away.") She stares up at the ceiling, its pattern of pressed tin: a jumble of infinitely joined vines.

"Note all this clitoral irritation," says the doctor. "Habitual self-abuse, it seems clear. We see evidence of delinquency here . . . and also here. The hymen is predictably destroyed. By this trauma—see it?— we can estimate the latest indiscretion. Less than forty-eight hours ago, I'd venture."

The vines could be ivy, maybe grape. Each curling stem joins with another, with another . . . impossibly, as plants might grow in heaven. She smells the lush green blast of such a place.

". . . the difference from a common leukorrhea?"

"Difficult, yes, admittedly," says the doctor. "The inflammation is strong presumptive evidence. More so if the canal is patulous."

"And could this chancre here have been syphilitic?"

"We'll see when the Wassermann is done. Feel the glands here at the groin—see how hard? I'm guessing yes."

Glove against her ankle. Whisk of skin.

Clamminess: Did they wet her? Did she leak?

". . . and swab up some of this gleety discharge," Dr. Slocum is saying. "So if you'll label those glass slides. Numbers one and two, 'vulva'; three and four, 'urethra'; five and six, 'glands of Skene'—"

A telephone bell overpowers his voice.

"Oh, of all times! Could you answer that, Miller? I'll get the alcohol flame lit."

Frieda's muscles clench. She shuts her eyes.

She listens to the hurry of Miller's footsteps in

the hall, an overeager greeting, a brief pause. "I'm sorry, no, he's with a patient now . . . Oh, yes, ma'am. Right away, Mrs. Slocum."

Then it's the doctor's departing footsteps, and his voice, airy and stiff, like beaten egg whites: "It's wartime, darling. These things are hard to come by . . . You really can't make do with molasses? . . . Oh, don't fret me to death! I'll try my best to find some."

Frieda opens her eyes to see Miller, standing tall, but peeking down between her knees with a look of squeamish thrill. She remembers now the boy he makes her think of—in shul, when she was twelve, Morris Berman. The morning of Morris's bar mitzvah. A wispy kit, not more than four feet ten and ninety pounds, his arms shook when he went to lift the Torah.

Raising it, he saw her, and she held his gaze and smiled, and suddenly his forearms turned to steel. *As I hold this, now,* he seemed to say, *I could hold you. We'd grow old together, hand in hand.* She lifted her arms, too, as if to hug him across space, hugging the future that lay before them both.

"I do, too, darling," comes Dr. Slocum's voice. "All right, then. Soon as I can. So long."

Who would want to grow old with Frieda anymore? Not Morris Berman. Not Miller—who looks up now and sees that Frieda's caught him. He inhales with inscrutable vehemence: ashamed of himself, or of her, maybe both. "I beg," he starts to say just as the doctor strides back in, laughing about his wife's endearing spoiledness.

"Won't settle for less than perfect, that one. Which I guess must speak fairly well of me!" Dr. Slocum chortles overloudly. "Now, where were we? Ah, yes, the smears. Miller, take one of those applicators and sterilize it in the flame. Ten, fifteen seconds does the trick. Good, then the cotton. And in we go . . ." The steel swab penetrates. Frieda stares up: vines upon vines, an endless knot.

She finds the girls working hard at hospital gowns again, the cloth cut from pigeon blue bolts. The clatter of stitching needles sounds like rodents running wild. Bobbins whiz, treadles clack and hum.

The workshop must have been the bordello's poshest suite. The wallpaper—repeated images of mating birds and bees—is yellow with smoke stains toward the ceiling. On a chandelier, glitz competes with dust. Frieda takes the Singer next to Yetta's.

"Hope it wasn't *too* bad?" Yetta offers.

Frieda can't quite find the voice to answer.

"Gets easier," Yetta says. "First time's worst."

Sexually Transmitted Diseases on College Campuses

LORI BARER

In sharp contrast to the steady decline of teenage pregnancy, the epidemic of sexually transmitted diseases (STDs) in young adults is increasing at an alarming rate. Each year, approximately 15.3 million new cases of sexually transmitted diseases are contracted with 65 percent of those cases affecting people under the age of twenty-five. With so many young people affected, college campuses are virtually swarming with infection. For many, college is a time of self-discovery and exploration. As the first time away from home, inhibitions are often silenced under the deafening sounds of fraternity music and drowned in cheap beer. Young adults awaken in unknown dormitory rooms with little or no recollection of the night before, not to mention the person beside them.

Young women have become at particular risk for STDs as date rape drugs become ever more popular. College parties have become sites of these drugs, such as rohypnol and gamma-hydroxy butyrate, which foster the STD epidemic with the incidence of unconsensual, and often unprotected, sex. While date rape does not account for an enormous portion of STD infections, date rape drugs are being used more and more frequently which only increases the number of young women unknowingly infected.

Forty-six percent of female college students are now infected with human papilloma virus (HPV), the same virus that causes both genital warts and cervical cancer. Many of these women will now be plagued with one or both of these ailments for the rest of their lives. Generally, women suffer greater consequences of STDs than men, in part because the infections are so often asymptomatic that care isn't sought until serious complications have developed. These complications may be of great emotional, physical, and monetary cost to the women. The societal cost of these ailments is also huge, costing taxpayers billions of dollars. In 1994 sexually transmitted diseases and their complications, not including HIV, cost the United States almost $10 billion.

Meanwhile, colleges around the country are failing to provide adequate knowledge and distribution of barrier contraception, the only reliable method for preventing STDs. Health care professionals at many colleges and universities may be too quick to prescribe birth control pills. While the pills are one of the most reliable birth control methods when used correctly, they do not provide any protection against STDs. Birth control pills, if prescribed at all, should be meant for women in monogamous relationships that have been tested (along with their partner) for sexually transmitted diseases. Instead, they are handed out faster than fliers on central campus: young people are not being careful enough.

At the University of Michigan in Ann Arbor, condoms are freely displayed throughout the University Health Services. Students are encouraged to take as many, as often, as they want. If a woman does decide she would like to use birth control pills, she must first watch a video explaining the seriousness of the pills. Then, she is given a gynecological examination, after which she can discuss the various options of birth control and the preferred options that she is interested in using with her doctor. Unless there are no medical concerns, the clinician will at that point normally prescribe the requested method. The woman is instructed to wait until the Sunday after her next period before starting the birth control pills. The women usually then have ample time to decide if the pill is the appropriate form of contraception for them. By making the birth control pills more difficult to attain, the spread of STDs is combatted at a faster rate.

Many parents feel that, even at the college level, handing out condoms promotes sexual promiscuity. Although many studies have been performed to prove this correlation, they have never been successful. However, universities often hear only the sound of crisp dollar bills, and since tuition is coming from Mom and Dad, so are the university's policies. Now we have created an environment where it is easier, and perhaps much less embarrassing, to offer medication that could very well be harmful to your health, than it would be to make free condoms available at the health clinic. We have also created a lot of new STDs, wasted a lot of money and left a lot of parents wishing their children had used protection.

A Circle of Women

TARA GREENWAY

Tara Greenway, excerpt from *A Circle of Women*, 1998. Reprinted by permission.

A circle of women gather in a public high school room in Manhattan every fourth Tuesday evening of the month. We are young, old, and in between; businesswomen and homemakers; single, married, and divorced; mothers and club hoppers. We talk, almost exclusively, about our vaginas.

We are not a consciousness-raising feminist group. We are not in the room to get in touch with our sexual selves. We are here to talk about our pain—our doctors, our drugs, our herbal remedies, our methods of managing or avoiding sex. We are here to confirm that our pain is not in our imaginations. We are here to pull each other through our pain.

For a roomful of women talking about pain, we are having a really great time. We do not have to explain that although our vaginas hurt like the devil almost all the time and have for the past year or five years or ten years, we are still attractive and sexual women. We talk about our doctors' or our lovers' ignorant reactions to our pain, and we laugh uproariously, because when we come to this circle, the whole thing is suddenly . . . hilarious. When a new woman comes, we let her speak first. We just say, "Tell us your story." Her eyes widen, and she looks a little pale. She begins hesitantly:

"It started when I was twenty-six. There was this burning and stinging down there. I went to the gynecologist; he said I probably had a yeast infection. He gave me Monostat. I used it up, but the burning got worse. My boyfriend and I were really in love, and before all this, we had sex, like, all the time. But after this started, we'd try to have sex, and there was this incredible pain, like . . . like a knife going up me."

"And the rest of the time it felt like squatting over a blowtorch?" someone asks helpfully.

"Yes!" the new woman says, perking up a little. "I kept changing doctors because the second or third time I'd go in and say it was worse, not better, the gynecologist would always get really mad at me. He'd say, 'Well, if you won't respond to the treatment there's really nothing I can do.'"

"How about, 'You'll just have to learn to live with the pain'?" someone interjects.

By now the new girl's eyes are flashing and her cheeks are pink. "Yeah! One said that to me! And they would run all kinds of tests, for yeast, HIV, AIDS, herpes, and they'd all be negative, and they'd say, 'There's absolutely nothing wrong with you, dear. . . .'"

Five or six voices complete the infamous sentence with her: "It's all in your head!"

Chuckles of recognition ripple through the circle, and someone asks, "So who finally diagnosed you?"

"No one. I was searching the Internet one day, and I came across all this stuff about vaginal pain.

I found you guys, and I came tonight. Do you know what's wrong with me?"

We have good news and bad news for the new woman. The bad news is she almost certainly has vulvar vestibulitis. When you are finally told that you have this incurable disease, the first feeling you have is relief. It has a name. Only later do you think, Oh, no. What am I going to do? But then there's more good news. There are many treatments for vestibulitis (although they are not cures). Everyone's symptoms and responses vary, and you have to work through each treatment by trial and error, but eventually one of them will probably work for you.

From the time vulvar pain, and the resulting excruciating intercourse, was documented in ancient Egypt through Freud's theories, the medical community has rushed to the curious conclusion that if women complain of pain during sexual intercourse, they are emotionally disturbed. Finally, in 1983, vulvodynia was defined by the International Society for the Study of Vulvar Diseases as "chronic painful vulvar discomfort." (Vulvar vestibulitis is one type of vulvodynia.) Vestibulitis is not an easy diagnosis, since frequently it has no visible symptoms—although often there is significant red inflammation of the vulva.

Vulvar vestibulitis has the reputation of being a "rare" condition, and the commonly reported statistic is that it affects 1 percent of women. However, in a study by Dr. Martha Goetsch in 1990, 37 percent of women visiting gynecologists had some vulvar pain and 15 percent had vulvar vestibulitis. In our monthly meetings we have noted that there are more women with vestibulitis than there are with breast cancer—and breast cancer has a postage stamp!

Even when a doctor knows it is a physical problem, not a psychosomatic one, he or she often will tell a patient that the only treatment for the condition is surgery, but there are dozens of documented treatments that must be tried first. Treatments include blocking the pain with drugs such as tricyclic antidepressants like Elavil and anticonvulsants like Neurontin. Biofeedback, which involves inserting a sensor into the vagina and doing pelvic floor rehabilitation exercises, has helped many women. The low-oxalate calcium citrate diet and the no-yeast diet have also proved helpful. Many have found relief taking combinations of herbs recommended by herbalists and naturopathic-homeopathic doctors, and others find acupuncture valuable. Interferon injected into trigger points is another treatment, as is physical therapy including myofascial release. Some treatments that have proven to do more harm than good are laser surgery, topical or oral antibiotics, and topical steroids. Vestibulectomy (a surgery performed by scalpel, not by laser) has been successful for some women.

Although these treatments are effective in varying degrees, most people with vestibulitis are still living with some pain, and some have found no relief at all. The condition desperately needs the attention of the medical community; it needs funding for research and publicity. Physicians could tell patients about the fact that antibiotics kill off "good bacteria" along with "bad bacteria" and recommend taking acidophillus to replenish the system's natural flora while on antibiotics. Gynecologists could learn that if a woman says her burning is worse after taking Monostat, they should not just ignore her feedback and prescribe more.

What can we do when we sit in overwhelming pain as the fifth doctor in a row looks us straight in the eye and says, "It's all in your head"? For now, we can join together. We can believe each other. We can become members of the nationwide grassroots organizations started by women with vestibulitis—the National Vulvodynia Association and the Vulvar Pain Foundation. We can be part of a "virtual support group" on the Internet, where there are hundreds of articles and many Web pages, including an e-mail list. For now, we can be one of a circle of women meeting across the nation, telling each other of medications and herbs and doctors; sharing our pain and our vagina stories; reminding each other of our grace, our humor, our strength, our hope.

And for Breast-feeding, Too, the Band Played On

EDITH WHITE

Edith White, adapted from *Breastfeeding and HIV/AIDS: The Research, the Politics, the Women's Responses*, North Carolina: McFarland & Co., 1999. Reprinted by permission.

In 1989 the prestigious *New England Journal of Medicine* reported that 83 percent of the babies who were breastfed by HIV-positive French mothers became HIV-infected, compared to only 25 percent of the bottle-fed babies. Numerous reports from other countries confirmed that while HIV-positive women can transmit the virus to their babies before or during birth, breast-feeding significantly increases the risk. The information about breast-feeding and HIV, however, has been downplayed by the leading health agencies, for fear that the information would hurt campaigns to promote breast-feeding for all its benefits to HIV-negative mother-baby pairs. Like Randy Shilts's 1987 book *And The Band Played On,* this section chronicles delays and failures on the part of leading health agencies to respond to the threat of HIV.

African delegates to the May 1997 World Health Assembly expressed their unhappiness at not having been informed about breast-feeding and HIV. Dr. Timothy Stamps, Zimbabwe's Minister of Health and Child Welfare, made a joint presentation on behalf of the African countries. Dr. Stamps had long been a harsh critic of the formula companies for their unethical marketing of formula in areas where clean water is lacking. Now Dr. Stamps was critical of UNICEF and the World Health Organization (WHO). He asked: "Are we to accept that our children's survival should be compromised by the risk of infant AIDS in the cruelest sense through the promotion of unlimited, unmodified, and unchallenged breast-feeding policies?"

The silence about HIV and breast-feeding was

not limited to Africa. Most people in industrialized countries still do not know that breast-feeding can readily transmit HIV. Either the primary research articles about HIV and breast-feeding were not discussed, or the findings were given a better spin when they were mentioned in secondary sources. Looking back now at some of the reports from the 1980s and 1990s gives an overview of what the international agencies were saying about breast-feeding and HIV. Annually published reports such as UNICEF's *State of the World's Children* are particularly revealing.

The early 1980s were the highpoint in worldwide breast-feeding promotion efforts. The 1982–83 *State of the World's Children* announced that breast-feeding was to be one-fourth of a children's survival revolution—one-fourth of a world revolution being a huge undertaking. But between 1983 and 1987 less and less emphasis was placed on breast-feeding. The 1987 report hardly mentioned breast-feeding.

UNICEF and WHO never discussed why they placed less emphasis on breast-feeding. But others have. Director of the Human Lactation Center Dr. Dana Raphael suggested that UNICEF de-emphasized breast-feeding because of HIV. Leading AIDS researchers Dr. Sophie Le Coeur and Dr. Marc Lallemant suggested that WHO saw doubts about the safety of breast-feeding and HIV as a threat to years of prevention efforts. Dr. Susan E. Holck, a WHO expert on breast-feeding, said that she was "struck by how much denial there was around 1990 of the evidence we had that HIV could be transmitted through breast-feeding." Much of the denial, she claimed, "undoubtedly was fed by people who had invested so much in promoting breast-feeding and feared what confirmation of that transmission might do to the gains that were made in breast-feeding."

The initial de-emphasis on breast-feeding happened just after HIV transmission through breast milk was first reported in the medical journals. Nor was there much by way of solace in other scientific reports. Researchers already knew that maternal milk was a major mode of transmission for many animal retroviruses. They knew that breast milk was a major mode of transmission for the first recognized human retrovirus, HTLV-I. Researchers, moreover, had already confirmed that HIV was a retrovirus. In the mid to late 1980s, some hoped that the antibodies in breast milk would protect babies, even though antibodies generally do not stop milk-born transmission of other retroviruses. Also, by the end of 1986, people realized the magnitude of the epidemic in Africa. In short, there was good reason to worry.

It is understandable that UNICEF's strongest promotion of breast-feeding slacked off between 1983 and 1987. Those who had the benefit of scientific advisors must have recognized that HIV transmission via breast milk was a potentially huge problem. If there was any doubt that HIV/AIDS could devastate breast-feeding programs, it was soon shattered by the early reports from Africa. Take for example the scene in 1988. The report had just come in from Kinshasa, capital city of Zaire (now renamed Democratic Republic of Congo). A radio broadcaster pointed out the connection between breast-feeding and AIDS. There was an immediate 30 percent drop in breast-feeding initiation rates. That 30 percent drop must have been the most unwelcome news to those who were trying to restore exclusive breast-feeding. And this was just one of many radio reports in Africa, where people get much of their news from radio and by word of mouth.

In 1987 the WHO issued a statement about HIV and infant feeding. It noted that there was insufficient evidence to conclude that breast-feeding was a significant source of HIV transmission, and that in developing countries, breast-feeding was a life-saving intervention. Therefore HIV-positive women should still breast-feed.

The 1988 *State of the World's Children* said that HIV could threaten breast-feeding if misinformation was allowed to affect breast-feeding programs. This report stated that it is theoretically possible that breast-feeding can transmit the AIDS virus and "worldwide there are two cases where this is thought to have happened." It is not clear which are the "two" cases acknowledged in this 1988 report, even if one counts only the reports already published in the medical journals.

LESS AND LESS TALK ABOUT HIV AND BREAST-FEEDING

The 1989, 1990, and 1991 *State of the World's Children* reports each had a full-page panel devoted to AIDS. The 1989 report insisted that "breast-feeding is not a significant means of transmitting AIDS," though it cited no research that corroborated its position. On the contrary, reports published in leading medical journals such as the *Lancet* and Blanche's report in the *New England Journal of Medicine* had already suggested that breast-feeding was a very significant means of transmission. In the Italian Multicenter Study, of sixty-five babies who were breast-fed by HIV-positive mothers, forty-six became HIV-infected.

UNICEF's 1990 and 1991 full-panel reports on AIDS completely omitted any reference to breast-feeding and AIDS. The 1992 *State of the World's Children* report had only one sentence about mother-to-child transmission; it stated that one million children have been "born HIV-positive." Later *State of the World's Children* reports also failed to address the emerging picture of HIV transmission through breast-feeding, even though the medical journals and conferences were continuing to make significant announcements. The large European Collaborative Study, for example, reported in 1991 that 32 percent of babies breast-fed by HIV-positive mothers became infected, compared to only 12 percent of bottle-fed babies.

In 1991 Baker reported that women in Zambia knew that breast-feeding can transmit HIV and many were afraid to breast-feed. Further, health workers in Zambia were accusing authorities of having a double standard for infant feeding in developed and developing countries.

UNICEF's 1992 and 1993 reports did not even mention breast-feeding and HIV. In 1993, UNICEF published a lengthy booklet, "AIDS: The Second Decade," in which UNICEF executive director James Grant described in detail efforts to reduce HIV infections among adults and adolescents. But this report from a children's organization did not discuss how children become HIV-infected. The one relevant sentence in the long report fails to clarify the role of breast-feeding and HIV: "Approximately one of three children born to these women is HIV-infected."

In 1993, the WHO published a book called *Breast-feeding: The Technical Basis and Recommendations for Action*. The book referred to discussions about research on the possible transmission of HIV through breast milk as belonging under the category of spreading false rumors.

UNICEF's 1994 report acknowledged that AIDS was reversing hard-won gains in child mortality, but never discussed the ways by which children get AIDS. It said that children are "born with the virus." The 1995 report mentioned very briefly that HIV was known to have been transmitted in breast milk in some instances.

UNICEF's 1996 report mentioned HIV/AIDS very briefly, noting only that children become orphaned when their parents die of AIDS. The report never mentioned that children become HIV-infected. The report also discussed the under-five mortality rate (the rate of child mortality for children up to their fifth birthday). It said that this rate "appears to have increased in several countries, including Madagascar, Zambia and Zimbabwe." It never said why.

UNICEF's 1996 *Promise and Progress: Achieving Goals for Children* also noted that the under-five mortality rates were up in some areas, but it too failed to explain why. UNICEF, however, did make a recommendation: the countries should readjust their mortality targets.

UNICEF's 1997 report mentioned HIV/AIDS very briefly, and then only to note that the epidemic had pushed more children into the labor market because their parents died. Even though AIDS was the leading cause of death for children in a growing number of countries, the report never mentioned AIDS in children.

UNAIDS (1997) noted that, in Namibia, HIV caused nearly twice as many deaths across all ages as malaria, the next most common killer. In the trading centers of Uganda, nearly nine out of ten deaths are related to AIDS. A report in conjunction with the 1996 International Conference on AIDS noted that AIDS may increase child mortality rates in Zambia nearly threefold by the year 2010.

In 1997 WHO issued a fact sheet called "Reducing Mortality from Major Childhood Killer Diseases." It never even mentioned HIV/AIDS. The section about major childhood killer diseases in Zambia did not mention AIDS, although AIDS is the leading cause of childhood death in Zambia.

Finally, in 1998, UNICEF's *State of the World's Children* report had a section on breast milk and transmission of HIV. It made many of the same recommendations as UNAIDS, suggesting, for instance, that voluntary testing and counseling be made more accessible. It stated that if an HIV-positive mother has access to adequate breast milk substitutes that she can prepare safely, she should consider this, wet-nursing, or heat treatment of expressed breast milk.

COMMENTARIES

Various commentators have offered opinions on the responses of the international health agencies. Nicholas Eberstadt, a researcher with the Harvard Center for Population and Development Studies, opined that UNICEF's "blinding ideology" to promoting breast-feeding and boycotting Nestle's had left it particularly ill-equipped to deal with HIV transmission through breast-feeding: "You can think of UNICEF's medical obtuseness as a cruel manifestation of bureaucratic inefficiency, a product of blinding ideology, a simple human tragedy, or some combination of the three."

Elliott Abrams, who had been US assistant secretary of state for international organizations, also accused UNICEF of being addicted to the ideology of breast-feeding, declaring that UNICEF was in a state of denial.

Zambian gynecologist Mavis Sianga was critical of the prohibition of free formula for babies of HIV-infected mothers. "It is rather unfair that women in developing countries must risk passing on the infection just because WHO and UNICEF want to keep their programs flying." She feels that a policy of not helping HIV-infected women to formula-feed has chauvinistic overtones. Men are given free condoms, but when it comes to a woman wanting to protect her baby, it is "suddenly political, it is cultural, it is expensive, it is impossible. What nonsense is this?" asks Geloo.

UNAIDS, WHO, and UNICEF no longer recommend that HIV-positive women in developing countries should breast-feed. Instead, they recommended that all women be allowed to make an informed choice about how they feed their babies. Most women, however, are still not given any information about HIV.

While UNICEF announced in March 1998 that it would begin pilot projects to distribute generic infant formula to babies of HIV-positive mothers, no HIV-positive mothers had been given any formula as of May 1999. For breast-feeding, the band still seems to be playing on.

Midlife and Older Women Living with HIV/AIDS

JANE P. FOWLER

Jane P. Fowler, "Aging and HIV/AIDS," 2008. Original for this publication.

It was an unexpected letter I opened in January 1991, alone in my Kansas City, Missouri, apartment, that profoundly changed my course in life, transforming me from professional journalist—an interviewer—into media interviewee, from private person to public activist.

Today, because of those contents, I am a seventy-two-year-old HIV/AIDS prevention educator, speaking in venues across the United States, even internationally, urging diverse populations, particularly middle-aged and older women, to recognize that this sexually transmitted virus does not discriminate, but can infect anyone.

The letter, from a health insurer to which I had applied for new coverage, announced I had been rejected because of a "significant blood abnormality," revealed in a routine test. Shaken by the startling news, I telephoned the underwriter who signed the letter. "What is the 'significant abnormality?'" I inquired. Her curt reply: "I'm sorry, that's confidential. Only a doctor can tell you."

Within hours, I was in the office of my family practitioner, who looked troubled as she referred to a fax and said, "Jane, this insurance company claims you've tested positive for HIV." Stunned, I had a second test two days later, convinced there had been an error.

Then I waited two weeks—the most agonizing two weeks of my life—but those results only confirmed the presence of HIV.

My family and the few friends I told were shocked, because I didn't fit an HIV stereotype. I was not a gay man, I had never been an injecting drug user, nor had I ever had a blood transfusion. I was, at the time of diagnosis, a fifty-five-year-old career woman, who after graduating from the University of Kansas journalism school, spent fifteen years as a reporter and feature writer for *The Kansas City Star*, next was an associate editor of *Bon Appetit* magazine, then continued as a freelance writer for another two decades.

I had lived a conventional, traditional lifestyle. I had been a virgin on my wedding night in 1959, and remained monogamous during twenty-three years of marriage. But, in the early 1980s, I was divorced—not by choice—and was dating again for the first time in a quarter century.

I didn't consider myself promiscuous. I didn't frequent singles bars, I went out with men my age, who, like myself, had been married and were divorced. In those days, I knew little about HIV/AIDS, only that a mysterious, fatal ailment was affecting the gay community. What did heterosexuals have to fear? I didn't know I would put myself at risk by engaging in unprotected sex (that's right: no condom, because I knew I couldn't get pregnant) with an attractive, intelligent man of many interests, who had been a close friend my entire adult life.

But what happened to me at age fifty at the end of 1985—I later learned—was infection with HIV.

Upon receiving my diagnosis and determining the infection date, I retreated from public life, calling myself "retired." I told the small circle of friends who knew my condition that I would withdraw and live quietly, in order to reduce stress and protect my health as long as possible.

But that was a lie. The truth was that I needed to keep my HIV secret: after all, an old lady can't have a stigmatizing sexually transmitted disease, right? During four years of semi-isolation, I spent time only with my family—my parents and my adult son, Stephen, and his fiancée—and those friends in the "loop," who sustained me with their compassion.

Then, in 1995, I was motivated to break my silence, speak out, and preach prevention. Encouraged by family, friends, and my physician, I decided to stand up and say: "Look at this old wrinkled, jowly face. This is another face of HIV. It's not who you are, or how old you are, but what you do and don't do in regard to transmission of the virus."

Twelve years have passed (during which my health has remained strong), and I have given more than a thousand presentations to audiences of all ages in a variety of settings. After seven years of leadership in the National Association on HIV Over Fifty, I stepped down in 2002 to found the national HIV Wisdom for Older Women program, based in the Kansas City area.

Since my diagnosis, my goal in life has changed. I am now committed to helping women remain free of HIV by confessing to the mistake I made twenty-plus years ago, when I didn't know the necessity of practicing "safe sex." I don't ask for sympathy or pity because of my infection, only that people assist me in my campaign to educate.

My role as a spokeswoman for the older generation has attracted the attention of the national print and electronic media and resulted in my story being told in major US markets (including the *Oprah Winfrey Show* and National Public Radio). This has enabled me to reach incalculable numbers who might otherwise remain uninformed about HIV transmission and prevention.

The stigma of ageism shows up in the lack of prevention endeavors: common thinking is that Granny should not be out there, screwing around. Yet, "senior" women are sexually active, and this fact needs to be acknowledged, especially by health care and social service providers to the aging community.

I continually remind everyone that HIV is a disease that can be prevented, and that "you never know the sexual history of anybody but yourself." I want women, especially vulnerable or naïve older women coming out of long-term relationships that have ended due to death or divorce, to understand what's out there today.

It's been reported that singles in the fifty-five-to-sixty-four age bracket represent one of the fastest growing segments of the dating services industry. This is another reason for women to remember that if they are not in a mutually monogamous relationship, they must practice safe sex. "If a partner won't use protection," I say, "find another partner."

Breaking the Walls of Silence: AIDS and Women in a Maximum State Prison

AIDS COUNSELING AND EDUCATION PROGRAM, BEDFORD HILLS CORRECTIONAL FACILITY

AIDS Counseling and Education Program, Bedford Hills Correctional Facility, excerpt from *Breaking the Walls of Silence: AIDS and Women in a New York State Maximum State Prison*, Woodstock, New York: Overlook Press, 1998. Reprinted by permission.

I often ask myself how it is I came to be open about my status. For me, AIDS had been one of my best-kept secrets. . . . I could not bring myself to say it out loud. As if not saying it would make it go away. . . .

Somewhere behind the prison wall in Bedford Hills, a movement or community was being built. It was a diverse group of women teaming together to meet the needs and fears. . . . [They] believed that none of their peers should be discriminated against, isolated, or treated cruelly merely because they were ill. . . . They managed to build a community of women: black, white, hispanic, learned, illiterate, robbers, murderers, forgers, rich, poor, Christian, Muslim, Jewish, bisexual, gay, heterosexual—all putting aside their differences and egos for a collective cause. . . . Right before me lay a model of how we, as a whole, needed to combat all the issues AIDS brought and we were building it from behind a wall, from prison. We were the community that no one thought would help itself. . . .

AIDS IN PRISON

AIDS is the leading cause of death in prison in New York State prisons . . . [A]n estimated 17 to 20 percent of the 63,000 inmates in the Department of Correctional Services are infected with HIV; 8,000 have been definitely identified as HIV-positive. . . . In [a] recent blind study of incoming inmates in New York State Correctional Facilities, the rate of HIV infection among women was twice that of men, 20.3 percent compared with 11.5 percent.

HOW AIDS COUNSELING AND EDUCATION PROGRAM (ACE) WAS CONCEIVED

We really didn't know a lot . . . Some of us leaned toward wanting the administration to be better about isolating people; others were concerned about supporting people who got sick. But the one thing we all shared was that we knew that our greatest enemy was fear and ignorance . . . We asked such things as was the laundry separated. There's a laundry where everyone sends their clothes to be washed. Although the clothes are in individual laundry bags, they are all washed together in one machine. One of the fears raised at the meeting was that maybe AIDS spread from clothes to clothes and what could be done about that?

THE BIRTH OF ACE

When Blackie first moved onto the floor, she could leave her cigarettes on a table and no one would touch them. And you know in here, people take things that are left around, especially cigarettes—you can't ever forget a pack of cigarettes on a table because it won't be there when you go back for it. Then one day, Blackie came into the meeting so happy and told us, "They stole my cigarettes, they stole my cigarettes." She was so happy that now she was being treated like everyone else.

Women's Health Care in Prison

CASSANDRA SHAYLOR

© 1999 by Cassandra Shaylor. Reprinted by permission.

Sherrie C. is a forty-one-year-old African-American woman who discovered a lump in her breast while in prison in 1984. Despite repeated requests for treatment, prison staff failed to diagnose her for ten years. By that point, the lump was visible through her clothes and the cancer had spread to her other breast and uterus. As a result of this medical neglect, Sherrie was forced to have a double mastectomy and a total hysterectomy. She has received no follow-up care and no pain medication.

Sherrie's story is not unique. Across the country women in prison face tremendous barriers to adequate health care and report a systematic pattern of medical neglect. Women's specific health needs, including routine gynecological care, are largely ignored. Serious illnesses, like Sherrie's cancer, often develop because prison officials fail to respond to complaints early. Pregnant women receive substandard prenatal care, and as a result experience avoidable complications and a high number of miscarriages; in many jurisdictions they are forced to give birth in shackles. Women do not receive regular treatment for chronic health problems like diabetes and heart disease,

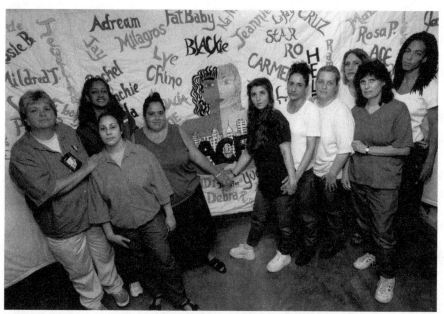

Members of the ACE staff at Bedford Hills Correctional Facility. [Carol Halebian]

which often leads to serious complications and sometimes death. Prison officials are generally unwilling to address the spread and treatment of diseases like hepatitis and HIV, and as a result are creating a public health crisis inside prisons.

The number of women affected by this medical mistreatment is growing rapidly. In this "tough on crime" political climate, with its increasing reliance on imprisonment as the catch-all solution to a wide range of social problems, women are the fastest growing population of people in prison. There are now approximately 150,000 women in prisons and jails in the US, compared to 10,000 only twenty years ago. More than 80 percent are serving time for nonviolent, property- or drug-related crimes. Women of color are disproportionately represented in prison systems across the nation, comprising more than 60 percent of imprisoned women. As a result, a large number of the women who will suffer as a result of inadequate medical care will be women of color.

All of the problems confronting women generally are exacerbated by the prison system, which often fails to acknowledge even women's fundamental humanity. While women in general often feel alienated and infantilized by the medical care system, these feelings are even more profound in women in prison. While women on the outside (may) have a choice about their health care provider, women in prison do not. Furthermore, they are dependent on mostly male correctional officers for access to medical staff; these guards frequently disbelieve the women's assessments of their own health and accuse them of malingering. In addition, women prisoners often face sexual harassment and abuse by medical staff.

Mental health treatment inside is equally appalling; women are consistently overmedicated and ignored. Increasingly women are being confined for extended periods, sometimes for years, in solitary confinement, which often results in severe mental deterioration. Women prisoners are rarely provided any type of therapeutic counseling, though more than 60 percent have experienced some form of sexual or physical abuse at some point in their lives. They often report that the misogyny and abuse of the prison system amounts to a re-experience of that past trauma. In order for women's health care in prison to be adequately addressed, our definition of health must also include mental health and freedom from physical intimidation and violence.

People on the outside can provide vital links to women in prison. We can: provide information about women's health to prisoners; build grassroots campaigns to educate our communities about conditions inside; advocate for women's access to health care through legislatures and courts; and build coalitions with health care providers, student groups, women's groups, and human rights organizations to fight for women's rights to adequate health care, bodily integrity, and human dignity.

CHAPTER 20

Chronic Illness

IT IS HEART-WRENCHING to read the novelist Fanny Burney describe her 1811 mastectomy, conducted before anesthetic was available. In a letter to her sister, Burney relays a conversation before the procedure with her doctor. She tried to explain to him why the surgery bothered her so much: "Can You, I cried, feel for an operation that, to You, must seem so trivial?" Her fears proved well founded when, while she was being restrained before the cutting began, she realized that the doctor intended to remove her entire breast, not just the small point where she felt pain. She argued with him, but to no avail. Of the pain of the operation Burney wrote, "I began a scream that lasted unremittingly during the whole time of the incision—& I almost marvel that it rings not in my Ears still! So excruciating was the agony." Burney noted the lingering physical and psychological trauma that accompanied her ordeal, writing that even nine months later she still relived the experience and felt lingering pain.

Few women's health issues have received so much media attention in recent years as breast cancer research, prevention, and treatment. Pink ribbons (and products) line store walls and promise to help, in time, to find a cure for this dreadful disease.

It's hard to believe now, as we look at the massive scale of fund-raising and public awareness campaigns around breast cancer, that activism on this issue started small, with the work of a few radical women.

Terese Lasser was forty-eight years, in 1952 when her doctor scheduled her for a biopsy following the discovery of a lump in her breast. The wife of a noted tax expert, J. K. Lasser, Terese was used to being involved in making important decisions, helping her husband with the writing of his best seller, *Your Income Tax*. She didn't worry about the biopsy, and didn't even mention it to her husband. Imagine her shock upon waking after the procedure to discover that her entire right breast had been removed. The psychological damage of such a huge decision being made without her involvement was compounded by a total lack of resources for women who had undergone mastectomy. Lasser was radicalized, and began her own efforts to help women in her situation.

While recovering from the removal of her breast, Lasser came to believe that certain exercises were helpful in healing the muscles after the trauma of surgery. She began her activism by entering the hospital rooms of friends who had undergone mastectomy, often only hours after surgery, and urging them to get out of bed and begin exercising. Such action led to the publication of a manual and the founding of the group "Reach to Recovery."

Rose Kushner was another woman whose activism began after she received a diagnosis of breast cancer. At the time a procedure called the Halstead radical mastectomy was standard practice. Rose believed that lumpectomy—a far less dangerous, less invasive procedure—was better for many women, despite conventional medical wisdom. She persuaded President Jimmy Carter and the National Institutes of Health to get behind massive clinical trials to determine if the radical mastectomy—automatic treatment at the time— actually saved more lives than the less extreme operation. Rose won. Lumpectomy won. And even old-fashioned breast doctors took off their hats to Rose and agreed that the Halstead radical mastectomy was "the greatest standardized surgical error of the twentieth century."

Today, despite extensive activism, we are still waiting for a cure for the cancer that most commonly afflicts female patients. Dr. Susan Love is one of the people actively engaged in trying to find preventative measures and a cure. Her groundbreaking *Breast Book* has helped millions of women and her research continues to provide hope for the future.

Excellent activist groups continue to raise awareness about the disease and work for better preventative methods as well as treatments. In particular, Breast Cancer Action remains the only national breast cancer organization that won't accept money from the drug or cancer treatment companies, or any corporation that pollutes the environment. Headed by Barbara Brenner, a former corporate lawyer and breast cancer survivor, the organization has over 16,000 members throughout the United States (www.bcaction.org).

The Oral History of Rose Kushner

INTERVIEW BY ANNE S. KASPER

Anne Kasper, excerpt from "The Oral History of Rose Kushner," for the Schlesinger Library of Women's History, Radcliffe College, April 1983.

RK: My major interest since 1979 when I was on the NIH Consensus Development Conference that recommended the two-stage proceeding . . . has been to do something in that period between the biopsy and mastectomy or whatever is done—I call it the definitive treatment—to tell women about the availability of options in primary treatment.

The big area where there is a huge information gap is in the newly diagnosed woman. Now let me add that it's also the newly diagnosed cancer patient, period. But I am sticking to breast cancer because that is, as they told me on the board, my "organ site." So, I see no point in giving a woman two weeks between diagnosis and treatment if all she is going to during those two weeks is sit and sweat.

And I consider and have always considered the giving of information to be the first step of rehabilitation. I do think the first thing that any agency or individual can do to help newly diagnosed women is to immediately inundate them with things to do—go to the library, read this or that, and let them know—not just think—that they have a finger in choosing their own destinies.

They've got to know. I will refer women to the National Cancer Institute if they are local, where they are doing clinical trials on comparing mastectomy with lumpectomy and radiation because I think that the people there give the most even-handed, balanced presentation of the risks and benefits, the advantages and disadvantages of both forms of treatment. Out in the real world, if a woman goes to a radiation therapist, no matter how much that person may want to be objective, there will be a bias toward radiation therapy and away from surgery. And the same is true of surgeons; no matter how fair they might try to be, they'll be biased in favor of mastectomy because that's what they were trained to do.

And there are disadvantages and risks attached to radiation therapy and these are rarely spelled out—I'm not talking about the long-term risks of radiation. I'm talking about having to take five days off from work to run to the hospital every day for treatment. Not all women can do that or are temperamentally suited to do that. I don't think I could. Of course, there is the worry about the side effects of radiation: burnt lungs, burnt heart, lymphaedema as a result of the radiation burning off the capillaries, and so on.

AK: Go back to the beginning of the Breast Cancer Advisory Center. When that started, how it started, who are the women that you've served in the past, who are you serving now, the mechanics of doing it . . .

RK: The Breast Cancer Advisory Center was officially incorporated in late 1974, but it did not get rolling until September 1975, when my first book, *Breast Cancer,* was published. It was going to be temporary but it didn't turn out that way. The first people who contacted me were people who heard about the center as I went around promoting the book. Harcourt, Brace, Jovanovich sent me to sixteen cities and I had enormous amounts of media coverage—radio, magazines, and newspapers. I never really appreciated their efforts probably until I got hung up with other publishers. And I would always put out the number. At that time, there was no working cancer information center. So, at that time, the Breast Cancer Advisory Center was the only place anybody had to go.

Dr. Susan Love

INTERVIEW BY TANIA KETENJIAN

Susan Love, M.D. is the author of *Dr. Susan Love's Breast Book* and *Dr. Susan Love's Hormone Book.* This interview was conducted in April 1999.

TK: Rose Kushner was a major pioneer for breast cancer. How did she influence you?

SL: Rose Kushner was one of the first real breast cancer activists. She didn't stop at being dissatisfied with her own treatment. She continued to lobby and advocate until things were changed for everybody. I think there are greater things than just your personal issues. One person actually *can* change how a disease is approached. And Rose worked pretty much by herself. She inspired a lot of people. She didn't have a huge grassroots organization behind her, and she did great. So I think her chutzpah was a great example of what one person can do.

TK: Who else was a great influence on you?

SL: Eleanor Roosevelt [laughs]. She's another example of how you really can make a difference on a broader stage if you just try. People like Mary Howell and Barbara Seaman. Both were among the very early workers looking at health and women, who said, "Wait a minute, we don't just have to do what doctors say we have to do. We can actually take some action ourselves and change the way things are done." They were a strong influence. I was coming up through medical school at that time to residency, where I would get just the opposite message crammed into my head. Internship and residency and even medical school are a little bit like a cult. You're sleep-deprived and overworked, and then they're giving you all these messages, so it's very important to have a countermessage out there. For me it was people like those at *Our Bodies, Ourselves,* people like Mary Howell, people like Barbara Seaman, who changed the balance.

TK: Dr. Mary Howell declined cancer treatment because she didn't want to destroy the quality of her life at that time. What do you think of that?

SL: Oh, I think she was a smart person. She knew

a lot about what therapy—as far as we could tell—could do, and she was a grown-up, and I think you have to let grown-ups make their own decisions. We don't cure all breast cancers, and we do indeed spend a lot of energy and time giving people treatment that destroys their lives and the lives of the people close to them. She wasn't being totally crazy. According to the data, we have about twelve thousand bone marrow transplants per year in this country, and there is no evidence that they work. She knew that once you get sucked into the medical system, you're going to get lots of treatment, and it may or may not be worth doing. Now the other side of the question—and I don't know the answer, because I didn't take care of her—involves whether she was really in a situation where nothing would work. That's hard to know, and it's hard to dispute, too. In the long run I give her credit for being honest and making the decisions that were good for her.

TK: I understand you were in a convent. Then, after medical school, you became a general surgeon, and then you focused on breast surgery. How did that whole process happen?

SL: Well, even when I was in the convent, which wasn't for a huge amount of time, I was still planning on becoming a doctor. So that part was pretty firm in my mind. But then I went to medical school and decided that what I liked best was surgery. At that time there were still quotas for women. It was ten percent where I went to school, but five percent at other New York schools, and many of the schools that I applied to said, "Sorry, we're not interested." The amazing thing to me is that I didn't think that was abnormal. I just said, "Oh well." It never occurred to me that that wasn't fair and they shouldn't be allowed to do it.

When I was in the middle of medical school things opened up. But there were very few women applying, so the process turned around in our favor. I went to Harvard Medical School and trained in surgery at Beth Israel, which is one of Harvard's hospitals, and I was the second woman in my program. When I was finishing I said, "I am not going to do breast surgery," because in those days people who did breast surgery were basically old and tapering down—they just were not very capable. But very soon I went into practice and started being sent patients who had breast problems—they weren't going to send me male patients, God forbid. It was still very strange to have a woman surgeon—it was considered very brave to be a patient with a female surgeon. But it became very clear to me [that these women with breast cancer] were not being treated very well and that I had much more to offer. I could really change their thinking, since the way you think about your breast is a lot different from the way you think about your gallbladder. At the time people said, "Oh, you can never make a living as a breast surgeon, there's not enough work, blah, blah, blah." Of course none of that was true, and before I knew it I became part of a mission. And here I am, still doing it, still on a mission.

TK: Do you see yourself as an activist?

SL: Oh there's no question that I have been an activist from the beginning. When I was first going into practice, there was good randomized, controlled data about radiation being as good as mastectomies, and yet surgeons were offering mastectomies as the only option. So the first thing I did was start yelling and screaming about that. It became clear to me that doctors were not talking to women and not giving them the information they needed to make their own decisions about breast cancer, so I wrote my book about breast cancer, and it did very well. But doctors believed that you shouldn't share information with the public, God forbid, they might find out we don't know everything.

Then, as I was doing my book tour, it became very clear that the moment had arrived to politicize breast cancer. The AIDS movement, which had been around for a couple of years, was the model for people with a disease lobbying for greater medical information. Three or four groups popped up, almost like spontaneous combustion, in different parts of the United States: Berkeley, California, Cambridge, Massachusetts, Washington DC. I thought, "Boy, somebody's gotta pull this all together, it's really the moment to be doing it." Then I was in Salt Lake City giving a talk to about six hundred people in the middle of the day, middle of the week, mostly older women who were not working. I was looking for a laugh in a long talk about breast cancer, and I said, "I don't know what it's going to take to eradicate breast cancer, but maybe we need to march topless on the White House." The image of George Bush dealing with all those topless women was a great one, and everybody laughed. But then I thought, "If they're ready to march on the White House in Salt Lake City, Utah, the time has come to really politicize the issue."

So I went back home and called a couple of people. Within a year we had the National Breast Cancer Coalition. Within a couple of years we not only increased the funding for breast cancer, but made sure that people with breast cancer were involved in the decision-making at all levels, how the money is spent. We really changed the landscape. Now you won't see a medical program or a conference that does not include sympathy for a layperson's needs. So am I an activist? Yeah, a troublemaker.

TK: What are some of the greatest misconceptions about breast cancer?

SL: One is that if it's not in your family, you're not going to get it. Only 5 percent of women with breast cancer have a history of it in their family. People think somehow they are immune because it's not in their family. Another is that if you're diagnosed with breast cancer, you have to have surgery, something has to be done, it's an emergency. The truth is that most breast cancers have been there eight to ten years, and if you're doing something this week or next week, it really isn't a critical factor. Those two are big ones. Another one is that coffee has something to do with lumpy breasts or cancer. That was disproved a long time ago.

TK: For 70 percent of women with breast cancer the cause is unknown.

SL: Right.

TK: What do you think causes it?

SL: Well, I think we know some of the reasons. We're awash in hormones in our society, whether environmental hormones from pesticides or all the drugs we take. Think about what we do to women these days. We start out taking birth control pills early on and take them until we're ready to get pregnant. By then we need fertility drugs—and God knows how bad they are—and next we go on postmenopausal hormones until we die. What is this doing to and saying about women's bodies? Some very provocative recent studies show that women who take birth control pills and then take HRT have a much higher risk of breast cancer. We're just pumping up our bodies with these hormones, with this notion that we need high-level hormones to be healthy. But the data for that are really not very strong.

Diet, exercise, lifestyle changes probably do have something to do with breast cancer. We don't know exactly what, but we know that in Japan there are very low percentages of women with breast cancer, and when Japanese women emigrate to this country, their breast cancer rates increase significantly, and so do their daughters'. What is the reason for that? Lifestyle, diet—right now the "in" thing is soy. We don't know exactly what the reason is, but it's something we need to investigate because not enough has been established. Breast cancer is much more common among women at a high socioeconomic level than among poor women. It's higher in white women than in black women. That speaks to something environmental or genetic.

TK: Some people were very disturbed by how your hormone book was treated. Do you feel your books accomplished what you wanted them to?

SL: Well, the breast book certainly accomplished what I wanted it to. In fact, I'm now working on the third edition. It's a heavy thing. It's the bible on breasts, and I feel a greater responsibility to make sure everything is right. But I think the hormone book touched a nerve, and if you're going to touch a nerve, you have to put up with the consequences. I think there's no question that the way we have prescribed HRT in this country for menopause is short-sighted and not based on a lot of data. When you point that out to people, it's like saying the emperor has no clothes. They get very defensive because they know at some level that there really isn't that much data, yet here they've been pushing the treatment.

I feel that the way that book was treated shows that this really is an area we need to shine some more light into. The data are not as strong as people would like, and since the book came out, that's become obvious. The first study on HRT and heart disease showed no benefit. So all these people who said, "Oh well, it reduces heart disease by fifty percent and that trumps breasts cancer" are now saying, "Oops, no benefits. What does that mean?" and going back to the drawing board. I think my book and other books played a role in this, they've made people say, "Well, you know, she's right, we don't have all that data," and maybe they don't come on quite as strong as they did before.

People who are very quick to believe in science and some popular notions tend to forget that we don't have the data to support HRT. Observational data are very good for generating hypotheses. So we compare the women who are not on HRT to the women who are on HRT, and indeed the women who are on it have 50 percent less heart disease. But they also are women at higher socioeconomic levels, so they go to the doctor more often, they exercise more often, they are more likely to treat their high blood pressure. The question is not so much, "Do hormones make you healthy?" The question is, "Do healthy women need hormones?" Until you do a study with a good number of couch potatoes in each group, you won't be able to answer that. What happened

was that we took that kind of data, which is nice and interesting, but only enough to say, "Gee, we really ought to look into this," and we extrapolated from that as if it meant that HRT worked, and you can't say that. It's like saying lung cancer is more common among people who carry cigarette lighters in their pocket. That's probably true, but you can't then assume that cigarette lighters cause lung cancer, and reducing the use of cigarette lighters is not necessarily going to reduce the rates of lung cancer.

People start believing all this observational data, not questioning it, and before you know it they forget that they actually haven't proven what they're saying. My job is to be the annoying kid who says, "Hey, the emperor has no clothes." I think that's an important job. But if you do that, you can't expect people to love you because they don't like having it pointed out to them; it makes them feel like fools. So I was not surprised by the reception the hormone book got. I would have been surprised if people had embraced it as a great thing. When the breast book first came out, it wasn't embraced either. I'll be interested to see the data becoming clearer over the next few years. Already my points are being validated. I don't care if I get credit for it, but it does make me feel like I at least contributed to asking questions.

TK: You have accomplished so many things, and these books are just an example of that. What are some of them?

SL: We made a model of how to treat breast cancer at UCLA. It says we need a multidisciplinary approach: patients need to see the medical oncologist, plastic surgeon, and mental health specialist. In the way we used to do it, you'd see a surgeon, be diagnosed, be sent to an oncologist and then to a radiation therapist, but none of them ever talked to the others, there was no coordination. At UCLA people were seen by a panel all at once, and it was done for the convenience of the woman rather than the physician. Everybody sat down together with the slides and the mammograms, reviewed the case, decided what to do, and then as a team took care of the patient. That model and variations of it have been picked up in many places around the country. It's now considered the way that women with breast cancer should be treated. They're not always treated that way, but it's certainly the model, and that was one of the major contributions. The whole concept that women have the right to information, second opinions, and all that didn't exist before.

Some of these things are not uniquely mine. What happened was that I said a combination of my ideas and things that various other people had said in a loud voice. Other people—and this goes full circle to what you asked about Rose Kushner—may be saying and doing the same things. But having the chutzpah or whatever to say it out loud, to publish it, to say it in a bigger forum is what I think helps to get things changed. When I was doing the hormone book, I interviewed some of the people who were doing all the science—Deborah Gren, Elizabeth Barrett-Connor. Elizabeth said, "I'm so glad you're doing this. Somebody has to do it, and I don't want to have to do the talk shows and all that stuff." Deborah said, "I don't want to have to answer all the patients' questions that will come up, but I'm glad you're doing it, because somebody needs to." It wasn't always me who came up with these ideas, but maybe it was me who was brazen enough to talk about it out loud.

TK: What are some things other activists are doing now that are helpful?

SL: They're still questioning, and there was no questioning before we started the coalition. People running a group like the Breast Cancer Coalition had to be activists. Having providers like myself do it would just be continuing the traditional model like the American Cancer Society, which is run by doctors, or the American Heart Association, which is run by doctors, and that really was not what we wanted to be. Fran Visco, an attorney and the head of the National Breast Cancer Coalition,

Pat Barr, who is in Vermont, and some of the other advocates against breast cancer are taking things well beyond what I could have possibly done myself. That has been critical if we're going to be successful. I'm sort of a catalyst. The coalition turned out fantastically well, which I attribute to all the activists who were in involved in it. The National Women's Health Network, Cindy Pearson, and that group, in spite of changing winds in popularity and everything else, have continued to be a voice for women against all the forces that are trying to diminish the influence of the women's health movement—against hospitals, against the FDA. These advocates for women started out being enormously popular and now are considered to be a more of a radical fringe. Yet they have enormous power because they are always there and they're always willing to step up to the plate. That is really crucial in how things have evolved.

TK: What projects are you working on now?

SL: Right now I'm eradicating breast cancer [laughs]. That's the plan. I'm not seeing patients, I'm doing research. I founded a startup company to commercialize my research because doing it in the academic setting just didn't work. There's not enough money, and it's too hard to get the money that there is. It takes too long and they don't like innovation, they just want to do the same old thing. So I have fifteen employees in Menlo Park, a kind of venture capital company. We have a new device that we hope is going to be a Pap smear for breast cancer so that you can find it really fast, and that will make a difference.

TK: Do you agree that many changes have happened in the last twenty years in the field of breast cancer?

SL: Yes and no. I think we are actually on the verge of the real changes. The changes that have happened up to now are changes in the quality of people's lives. Certainly doing lumpectomy and radiation instead of mastectomy, doing reconstruction immediately instead of delaying it, and being able to give chemotherapy without destroying people's lives in the process are major changes. But we really have to reduce mortality. The first year there was any decrease in mortality was 1998, and it was only about one to two percent. That's good, but far from perfect. My real concern is that we haven't found the Big Cure.

But I think we're on the verge of some major paradigm shifts that will lead us toward that. Right now, we're at a crossroads. We've treated breast cancer as if it were a foreign invader and our job was to kill every cancer cell, stamp it out. Chemotherapy, bone marrow transplants, all of that is based on that idea of a bigger, stronger, harder attack—kill every cell. What we're starting to learn is that killing every cell may not be necessary. We may be able to reverse the cancer, we may be able to control it, sort of like mental health. These are not foreign invaders, they're just cells that are going kind of crazy. If they've gone too far psychotic, we may not be able to intervene, but otherwise we probably can reverse the process and rehabilitate them. That's really where people are moving at the moment in terms of treatment and perception, and some of the new biological treatments are opening that door.

The flip side of that is the part I am working on, which goes along both with identifying the chain of causation for breast cancer and with some prevention tactics. I don't think we're quite there yet—I'm not sure tamoxifen is the right drug for prevention—but I think the paradigm will be prediction and prevention rather than diagnosis and treatment—that is, being able to figure out at a much earlier stage who is going to get the disease and then reverse it so that they never get it, much as we do with Pap smears. If you're getting regular Pap smears, it's rare to get cervical cancer. We discover it in an early stage and then we do something to fix it. I think that's where we're heading. Those two changes are going to make an amazing difference, so that the next generation just won't know breast cancer.

Stolen Conflicts: A Feminist Revisioning

SHARON BATT

Sharon Batt, adapted from *Patient No More: The Politics of Breast Cancer*, Charlottetown, Canada: Gynergy Books/Ragweed Press, 1994.

When I was undergoing treatment for cancer, I often felt disconnected from the medical proceedings. What impressed me about AIDS activists was precisely their personal involvement in the public process. They refused to parcel AIDS into public and private components. When I decided myself to speak out publicly, in a newspaper article, the process was exhilarating. I felt engaged in a personally meaningful struggle, not just as a "woman fighting cancer" but as a citizen taking part in a larger societal battle with the disease.

In the past ten years, increasing numbers of women have decided to "go public" about having breast cancer. Often, they describe their encounter with the medical system in terms of estrangement. They liken medical treatment to being on a conveyer belt. They seek vital information in vain. They don't understand what the doctor is talking about. When they try to articulate their fears, those around them urge a "chin up" attitude.

BREAST CANCER AS PROPERTY

The cancer patient's alienation can be framed in personal terms—you are in shock, facing a new situation, terrified of death—but this is a too-easy out. Of course every woman with breast cancer suffers personal trauma. But equally important, the institutionalization of our "problem" distances us from our lived reality. The state system, designed to "control" cancer, in reality controls the woman—and particularly her conflict with cancer—more effectively than it controls the disease. We are labelled "patients." We are thrust ("no time to waste!") into a medical system governed by undisclosed rules. Here, "compliance" gains approval. Physicians speak to us in the private jargon of medical science, or with an infantalizing "there, there dear" paternalism. "Recovery" programs encourage us to "look normal" and "get on with life." Soon charities descend, urging us to "fight cancer with a checkup and a check." The money goes into "support" programs in which we have no say, or to researchers studying questions unrelated to our own.

From the moment of diagnosis, we are protagonists in a drama which may end in our death. If ever we should feel fully engaged, it is now.

BREAST CANCER TURFS

We live in a society that values expertise. In every sphere, we divide the world into professionals and the lay public. Professionals engage in the work of problem-solving in their own sphere. They own those problems. If we challenge the strict separation of breast cancer into public and private property, we are saying professionals will have to cede some of their ownership of the disease.

As a property, breast cancer is vast. No one agency lays claim to the whole. In the past century, various groups have divided up the turf and set mutually agreed-on boundaries. Treatment is one parcel and the main owners are oncologists. Research is another parcel. Medical researchers stake the largest claim here. Fundraising is a third parcel, owned by the cancer charities and the state. A fourth large chunk, encompassing support and educational services, is owned largely by the cancer charities. The private anguish of breast cancer is a separate turf. That belongs to the woman with the disease and her loved ones.

In the analysis that follows, I examine each of four public turfs to see how the present owners gained title and what the conflict means to them. I examine the reasons activists have ventured onto each section of public property and the reaction they have met on arrival.

THE TREATMENT TURF

A study of oncologists at Harvard teaching hospitals explored the reasons why these physicians chose oncology. The researchers found that the physicians described their commitment to the field in terms of "challenge." A radiation oncologist said, "We have a superb program . . . it is dangerous . . . we are right up to what we can get away with. It's exciting. . . ." Another, a medical oncologist, explained, ". . . I didn't want to deal with zits. Or people who couldn't sleep, or have low back pain and are depressed. *Everyone who walks into my office might die.* And although I don't wish them all to die, I . . . get more of a buzz out of dealing with something."

Women with breast cancer have entered the treatment turf largely because they question the current treatments. Many are angry to learn that punishing treatments which had been promoted as cures have uncertain and limited benefits. They are shocked to discover how little mortality rates have changed in fifty years. They wonder if other treatments, particularly less toxic ones, might not be just as beneficial as the "slash/burn/poison" trilogy—or more so. Women also seek to expand the definition of treatment into the psycho-social sphere. Medical treatments don't begin to address our subjective experience of cancer, which reaches to every area of our lives.

Women with breast cancer want more than the much-touted partnership of shared decision-making in medical treatments. This would be relatively easy to negotiate. The more contentious ownership questions involve redefining the treatment terrain—moving the boundaries beyond the medical. Oncologists resist because their primacy in the treatment struggle is questioned.

THE RESEARCH TURF

Researchers own the enigma of breast cancer. As custodians of the intellectual conflict with the disease, they engage in the search for understanding that could eventually solve the puzzle. In this struggle with the unknown, they define what questions are important.

In the researcher-driven process, scientific peer review panels explicitly exclude members of the public. A place on the research turf, however, is one of the demands advocates have pressed hardest for. As with treatment, women with breast cancer seek involvement on a changed turf, not the one that currently exists. We ask different questions.

In San Francisco, the group Breast Cancer Action has lobbied for advocacy representatives on breast cancer research committees at all levels. Their goal was "a say in the research process based upon the real-life experience of people living with cancer." They were determined to be engaged in the process, ideally in a collaborative relationship with scientists. "We can be adversaries or partners in accelerating research," they said. "We would prefer to be partners." After eight months of negotiations with the head of the local cancer center, the activists had the beginnings of a working partnership. Dr. Craig Henderson, who described the women as "surprisingly intelligent, bright, and verbal," granted a seat for an activist on scientific committees, review of grant proposals for new projects, and input into the research process for large clinical trials groups.

Despite such concessions, many researchers still oppose patients' participation in the research arena, even though breast cancer activists have dramatically increased the amount of money available for breast cancer research. The nub of the resistance is our wish to redefine the puzzle.

THE FUNDRAISING TURF

Cancer fundraising was first "owned" by the American Society for the Control of Cancer (ASCC), precursor of the American Cancer Society. ASCC founders were progressive-thinking physicians and wealthy women in the New York area. From 1913 until the mid-1940s, the ASCC was a relatively small charity that raised most of its money through rich local benefactors.

The first cancer fundraising turf war took place in the mid-1940s when Mary Lasker took over the ASCC and transformed it into the American Cancer Society (ACS). Lasker was the wife of advertising tycoon Albert Lasker who pioneered a campaign urging women to smoke using the slogan, "Reach for a Lucky Instead of a Sweet." She added leading businessmen to the board and applied corporate advertising and fundraising techniques to cancer charity work. Lasker also cultivated links with influential federal politicians and drove the lobby to expand the funded National Cancer Institute (NCI) into a major research institute.

When the tax-funded NCI began to boom in the late 1940s, ACS leaders worried that the American public would let their donations flag. The two agencies agreed to divide the turf: the NCI would use its funds, raised from taxes, for research; the donations-dependent ACS would have jurisdiction over services and education. The plan worked. In the postwar years, the budgets of both organizations expanded exponentially. The public has had scant say in how these funds are disbursed.

In a few short years, breast cancer advocacy has radically transformed cancer fundraising. In late 1992, advocacy pressure sprang $214 million in earmarked breast cancer funds from the American defense budget. Rather than welcoming the new money, however, researchers responded anxiously. Typical was a breast cancer researcher at the Mayo Clinic in Rochester, Minnesota, who complained the increase in funds was "very politically motivated."

In fact, politics are hardly new to research fundraising. The NCI was born of assiduous lobbying by the cancer research community. The difference in this case was that breast cancer activists took the bows and demanded a say in how the monies would be spent.

In many communities, women with breast cancer have formed small grassroots self-help groups which raise funds to finance their own activities. Often the incentive for forming these groups is the women's dissatisfaction with Cancer Society services.

THE SUPPORT AND INFORMATION TURF

Charities have also owned breast cancer support and information services. These activities have long emphasized the importance of early detection and prompt medical care. Appeals for funds are effective because the public backs these goals.

The educational messages of the cancer charities reflect the views of physicians rather than patients. Established services don't begin to meet the emotional and informational needs of women with breast cancer. Services may even aggravate, not alleviate, patients' problems. The late Jackie Winnow, who was diagnosed with breast cancer in 1985, described a seven-week ACS support group she attended as "very controlled." At one point, she recalled, "somebody had a lot of complaints about a doctor and I wanted to know who that doctor was. The social worker said, 'You can't ask that question because it's not an objective response.' I was horrified." The incident catalyzed Winnow to start a Women's Cancer Resource Center in San Francisco.

Support turf owners may respond to survivor-run support services by trying to absorb them. Women should be cautious of agreeing to such takeovers in the area of support, says Monique Bégin, for many years Canada's minister of health. Government bureaucracies try to absorb these initiatives into their ways of doing things and, in doing so, may kill what is so special about them, notes Bégin. "While this may be the price of success, it must be opposed."

THE PRIVATE TURF

In the established order, the personal anguish of breast cancer is women's private domain. Paradoxically, the taboos against exposing the lived experience of breast cancer disengage us from our feelings.

Audre Lorde wrote forcibly about the politics of silence. What is important to me, Lorde said, "must be spoken, made verbal and shared." In the harsh light of self-examination following her first breast biopsy, Lorde saw what she regretted most in her life: the occasions when, out of fear, she silenced thoughts she wanted to speak. Her understanding that the ultimate silence—death— might come sooner than expected pushed her to another realization: silence would not protect her from dying. Silence isolated her; speaking her beliefs brought her into contact with women who had the same fears and sparked a collective, strengthening examination of the issues.

Psychologist Ross Gray, an advocate of patients' participation on policy planning committees, surveyed health care professionals' attitudes to having people with cancer sit with them around the board room table. Professionals in the cancer community, he found, resist having people with cancer on their committees because patients raise personal, emotional issues that medical professionals and administrators would rather not discuss. No wonder the medical system deals poorly with our emotional trauma! Removing the artificial barrier between public and private spheres can only improve this glaring weakness in the system.

PATIENT NO MORE

Masculine values define oncology. Characteristics of the field are specialization, hierarchical power structures, heroic intervention, rational-scientific thinking, and high-tech methods of treatment and diagnosis. The popular war metaphor used to describe the fight against cancer creates a military climate that further valorizes macho behavior. From diagnosis to death, oncology veers to the highest cost and the riskiest heroics. Even when the cancer strikes a female organ, male ownership of the struggle seems almost mandatory.

As more women with breast cancer find their voices, the clash between the masculine ideology of the owners and the feminist values of the owned is increasingly obvious. One example is the activist opposition to experiments in hormone manipulation. Another is the pressure for preventive research into environmental toxins. A third is the interest in "soft" alternative treatments that enhance the woman's sense of well-being and control. Women with breast cancer are bargaining for noninterventionist, preventive, and low-tech solutions.

We are saying: it's our conflict. We want it back.

POSTSCRIPT TO A DECADE OF ACTIVISM

The breast cancer movement had, and still has, a radical core. Many of the women who spoke out at the beginning had been involved in activist politics before their diagnosis and I continue to meet politicized women with breast cancer who bring a mature feminist outlook to their current activism. Yet fundamental change remains elusive. One explanation is that many women who wrote and spoke and lobbied had no political analysis. They just had breast cancer. These women were co-opted very early on by vested interests who saw the harnessing of women's energy as a way to leverage more research funds, and to promote mammography, treatments, and genetic testing. Establishment and corporate-sponsored vehicles like National Breast Cancer Awareness Month and the shower card brigade already existed when the movement was defined in the early 1990s. They very quickly got bigger and slicker. By sheer force of marketing, they soon shaped the movement in their own image. With the vast majority of the medical community onside, it wasn't difficult to persuade most women in search of direction that wearing a pink ribbon, handing out shower cards, and Running for The Cure were ways to bring about change. The simplistic idea that breast cancer was an underfunded area of research had enough of a feminist ring that a lot of women bought it without question, along with the corollary that lobbying for more funds would soon turn things around. What about the radicals? A lot of them died. It's easy to underestimate the impact

of death as a looming presence for women with breast cancer, compared to, say, women dealing with the birth control issue who had their health and their whole productive lives ahead of them. With breast cancer, you get a group together and within a few years someone will develop metastasis. Some women get scared and pull back. Others become caregivers to the dying women. When she dies, the mourning process changes the energy of the group. And if she was the group's leader, well, she's gone. Do you regroup, or do people go back to their families and jobs? I believe we're in for a long struggle, with a lot of redefining of issues and factions within the broad movement, like the women's movement itself. Eventually, people will have to question the adequacy of shower cards and fund-raising runs. There will be a defining book or a medical scandal or a critical mass of savvy women and we'll have a second wave.

Fighting the "War" on Breast Cancer: How a Metaphor Has Shaped the Debate on Early Detection and Treatment

BARRON H. LERNER

Barron H. Lerner, adapted from earlier versions that first appeared in *Annals of Internal Medicine*, July 1, 1998, and *The Journal of the College of Physicians and Surgeons of Columbia University*, Winter 1999. Reprinted by permission.

More than twenty years ago, Susan Sontag argued that metaphors interfere with how American society understands and responds to diseases such as cancer. In the case of breast cancer, "war" has been the dominant metaphor, implying that the disease is an actual enemy to be vanquished on a medical battlefield.

Military language has revealed the fierce determination of anticancer organizations, such as the American Cancer Society and the National Cancer Institute, to lower mortality from the disease. The notion of fighting breast cancer has also held great personal appeal for many women with this dreaded disease. But the use of war metaphors also points out how physicians and activists involved in the war effort have at times oversold the value of available screening and treatment modalities.

Although Richard Nixon formally initiated the US government's war on cancer in 1971, that war had been raging since at least 1936 when anticancer activists formed the Women's Field Army. The Army's "war cry" was for "trench warfare with a vengeance against a ruthless killer"—cancer. Since then, it has been almost impossible to discuss breast cancer without using military terminology.

By 1950, the standard strategy for breast cancer was early detection of cancerous lumps, followed by an extensive, deforming surgical procedure known as the radical mastectomy. The operation removed not only the cancerous breast but the underarm lymph nodes and both chest wall muscles on the affected side. By the early 1950s, a small group of physicians and statisticians began to question the value of early detection, and the universal need for radical mastectomies. These critics pointed to data that showed no consistent association between a delayed diagnosis and the extent of the cancer or between the size of the primary lesion and the cancer's spread to other sites. They also noted the failure of radical mastectomies to reduce national mortality rates. They proposed an alternative model of "biological predeterminism," which attributed the fate of patients more to biological factors, such as tumor virulence and immune response, than to early detection.

The data were ambiguous, pointing definitively in neither direction. But the scientific debate reflected none of that. The vitriolic tone of the discussion bespoke an unwillingness to analyze a thorny problem in a rational manner. Limited warfare held little appeal.

Physicians had long identified breast lesions resembling cancer that had not invaded the underlying breast tissue. By the 1930s, pathologists, believing that such lesions were "precancers," began to term them ductal or lobular "carcinoma in situ." Carcinoma in situ raised two questions: (1) Were such lesions inevitably precancerous? and (2) Did detection mandate mastectomy?

A few surgeons favored a conservative approach, advising only observation. However, most physicians, using familiar military metaphors, essentially equated breast cancer predisposition with the actual disease. Viewing lobular carcinoma in situ as a "powder keg," surgeons generally recommended mastectomy.

Treatment of the lobular carcinoma in one breast led to scrutiny of the other breast. Studies had reported that women with lesions of one breast developed cancer in the other breast in as many as 25 percent of cases. Mammography was most often used to find such lesions, but some surgeons recommended a more aggressive approach: random biopsy of the second breast. Such biopsies were of high yield, generating cancer or carcinoma in situ up to 59 percent of the time. In such cases, mastectomy of the second breast usually followed.

Some surgeons pushed early detection and treatment even further. Fearing that biopsies would miss existing lesions, they performed routine prophylactic removal of the second breast in women diagnosed with lobular carcinoma in situ. The war on breast cancer may have reached its pinnacle when a marker of possible future cancer in one breast became a rationale for bilateral prophylactic mastectomy in women without other risk factors.

By the mid-1970s, the use of mastectomy for lobular carcinoma in situ was being challenged. Physicians increasingly concluded that most women treated only with lumpectomy never developed breast cancer, and those who did often developed ductal carcinomas, which could not have emanated from the lobular lesions. Meanwhile, extensive controlled trials demonstrated, as the predeterminists had claimed, that radical mastectomy was almost never necessary for the treatment of actual breast cancer.

In January 1997, angry debate about early detection of breast cancer broke out once again when an NIH panel decided not to recommend routine screening mammograms for women forty to forty-nine years of age. The debate had little to do with the scientific value of mammography; it has been claimed that there was broad agreement on what the data showed. Instead, the antagonism stemmed from political, economic, and legal concerns. Interest groups, ranging from cancer activists to radiologists to the US Senate, had again proven unwilling to declare a truce and discuss the pros and cons of breast cancer screening in a dispassionate manner. As a result, physicians and patients were left without adequate guideposts for applying early detection to clinical practice.

The next front in the war against breast cancer will be the "genetic battlefield." Tests identifying BRCA1 and BRCA2 genetic mutations, which are already being termed "time bombs," represent a powerful new method for obtaining early information about potential breast cancers. Healthy women who test positive for the BRCA1 or BRCA2 genetic marker are at very high risk for the disease. In order to decrease their likelihood of developing breast cancer, some women are choosing to have bilateral prophylactic mastectomy.

Lacking knowledge about the actual value of genetic testing, history warns us not to conflate the *ability* to find these markers with the *need* to find and act on them. In the past, at least, an "all or nothing" wartime mentality has encouraged aggressive intervention for such ambiguous lesions. While prophylactic mastectomy may be the correct choice for some women, careful counseling about the limitations of the operation remains mandatory.

Anne S. Kasper

INTERVIEW BY TANIA KETENJIAN

Anne S. Kasper, PhD is a senior research scientist at the Center for Research on Women and Gender at the University of Illinois at Chicago and the coeditor of *Breast Cancer:*
Society Constructs an Epidemic. This interview was conducted in April 1999.

TK: In Rose Kushner's book entitled *Why Me?*, she raises some serious issues about breast cancer and its effects on feminine identity. How do you think these issues manifested in her? How did her cancer affect her identity as a woman and as a person?

AK: Having breast cancer totally fired her up to be a public advocate on behalf of women with breast cancer and, in fact, I think it's reasonable to say that she was the first breast cancer advocate.

TK: After her mastectomy, Rose decided to get breast implants, and unfortunately they burst. What do you think led her to make that decision?

AK: Don't forget that at the time that Rose Kushner had breast cancer, and it's still true today, physicians would tell women that they really wouldn't be able to recover, appropriately return to normal, feel like themselves as women, so forth and so on, without breast reconstruction or breast implants. Although we know that it's not part of breast cancer treatment per se, it's often billed as such and it was probably even more so when Rose was diagnosed. Also, don't forget that these were basically prefeminist days when not only women took seriously everything their doctors told them, but a lot of women were still subjected to pretty precise oppressive and finite definitions of what it meant to be a woman. Today, it's a different story. There are lots of ways to be a woman. Even though doctors today will frequently tell women that they must have breast implants or breast reconstruction to return to normal or feel like a woman, a lot of women today have their own definitions about what it means to be a woman and will reject that outright or simply say, "Yeah, sure, I mean I'm interested in breast reconstruction, but that's not what's going to make me feel like a woman again."

TK: How did Rose's personality incorporate itself

into her cause. Did she already have activist tendencies?

AK: Yes, she did. She told me this wonderful story about when she was a little girl, it was during the Depression, and her parents had been small-shop owners in Baltimore and I think they both died within a few years of each other when she was very young and she was sent to live with some aunts. She remembered social workers coming every Saturday with bags of clothing and food for the family because everybody was suffering at the time, unless they were very well-to-do, and Rose Kushner's family was not. She remembered these social workers very vividly, and she said that what she was doing was being a social worker on behalf of breast cancer. For her, it was a way of repaying the care and kindness that she had as a young child from these social workers. Much of what she did was in fact a form of social work in the arena of breast cancer.

TK: You mentioned the reaction of women toward doctors, their seemingly unrelenting trust, prior to the movement. How did Rose Kushner's reactions to doctors reflect the sentiments of the women of her time? She seemed to be constantly challenging her doctors and yet at the same time she did feel a kind of safety with them. . . .

AK: I think you hit the nail on the head. She was very assertive and even aggressive and her feelings were so strong on this subject that even as she put a lot of faith in her doctors—which was pretty much the rule at the time, you don't question your doctors, you put your health in their hands—she was also willing to challenge them up to a point, even challenge prevailing medical notions. That was how she came to fight for other women in the women's health movement around the issue of DES, because she believed that her breast cancer was a direct result of her taking DES when she was pregnant with her children. In the 1940s, 1950s, and 1960s, doctors told women that DES was perfectly safe for use in pregnancy. But Rose came to the conclusion that it was anything but, that in fact it had caused her breast cancer, and this led

to her subsequent role as a breast cancer advocate. So there were lots of places where she stood up and said, "Wait a minute, guys, this isn't right."

A classic example of what we owe her—the one she's best known for—involves the fact that when women receive a biopsy and the diagnosis is positive, they now have the option to go home and think about this and meet with their doctors or read up and become informed and begin to make some choices that are consonant with their needs and desires. Whereas, in the past when women were biopsied and it was positive, right there on the operating room table their breasts were taken off. She said, "This is just appalling. You doctors can't continue doing this kind of thing. Women need to have some say in it. We know that timely breast cancer treatment is important, but there's nothing to indicate that a woman can't go home for a week, two weeks, a month and make decisions that are consonant with her well-being before she has a mastectomy." And we really owe that to Rose Kushner, she made clear not only that it was important for women's well-being, but that it wasn't in any way going to impair their health any further. And it really changed medical practice.

TK: What do you think of early detection claims? Do you think it has improved survival rates?

AK: Well, I certainly don't think it's all that it's been touted to be by any stretch of the imagination and I'm very disturbed that a lot of women think not only that early detection is the be-all and end-all, but also that it's entirely in their hands—that they are somehow responsible for this early detection, and that if they don't find anything and then get breast cancer, it's all their fault. If only they had been more diligent in practicing breast self-examination for however long, they might have found this breast cancer and now they wouldn't be "victimized" by this disease. Another thing that really disturbs me is that we have been so overly diligent about the message of early detection that we have actually cast it as a preventative, so there are women who actually believe that early detection is prevention. And no small wonder—essentially that's the message, hidden or overt, of many of our public education messages about breast cancer. During my research for my current study of poor and low-income women with breast cancer, people in Chicago told me they were really puzzled when they noted a lot of young latina women coming to breast cancer screening clinics or other clinics asking for mammograms. These women were seventeen, eighteen, nineteen. After a while the clinics asked them, "Why are you here? You're basically too young to have breast cancer. Why are you requesting mammograms?" Many of these women were recent immigrants to this country and perhaps they weren't fully acculturated yet. They answered, "We understand that a mammogram prevents breast cancer. I'm here to have my mammogram, so that I won't come down with breast cancer." That's really an overzealous message.

TK: Since we don't know exactly how many women die of breast cancer, can the statistics be accurate?

AK: There are a certain number of women, perhaps older women, who are diagnosed who will not die from breast cancer because, especially in older women, it's much more slow-growing. As a result the curative rate, or the success rate in treating breast cancer, or maybe even preventing it, has been exaggerated. A lot of women who get breast cancer don't get treated or even diagnosed with breast cancer, and they don't die from it, they die of something else—heart attack, stroke, or any other disease. I don't know the accurate statistics in breast cancer and I don't know if anybody does. One thing that concerns me about poor and low-income women is that they present with much more advanced disease and their survival rate is much lower than for low- and middle-class women. I often wonder if there are women out there who literally don't get seen and don't get treated for their breast cancer and who wind up dying of something else. Since an autopsy is never done,

we just don't know if it was breast cancer that killed them or if it was something else. I honestly don't know what the accurate statistics on breast cancer would look like even if we were able to collect them, and I certainly don't think anybody is collecting really accurate ones. I think part of the problem is that the National Cancer Institute has a vested interest in collecting statistics that reflect well on this so-called war on cancer.

TK: Let's talk about the war on cancer. Some say that many latter-day activists don't attribute the fight against cancer to Rose. They attribute their fame and in part the strength of their cause to AIDS groups.

AK: I think the difference is that AIDS had a lot of visibility, in part because at the time there was no chance of a cure—everybody would die—so it had an element of drama that breast cancer and other diseases didn't have. And we mustn't forget that the majority of people with AIDS in the early days were men, and you know men are the power holders. Many who became AIDS activists became easily vocal and powerful because power came naturally to them as men. The breast cancer movement certainly learned something from the AIDS movement, but it also was a natural consequence of the women's health movement that had developed in the late sixties and early seventies, and like a lot of things it just took its time to coalesce. I think we have ignored the fact, to some degree, that Rose Kushner played a pivotal role in the formation of the breast cancer movement. Some attention has been paid to her but certainly not enough. The other problem is that Rose died at a time when there was a mainstream resurgence of the women's health movement. During this so-called rebirth in the early 1990s, when it gained a lot of popularity, a lot of people claimed that they had just simply invented it—the drug companies, high-powered women in Washington, or other people who thought this women's health stuff was their creation. Not only was the previous women's health movement instantly erased, but so was Rose Kushner.

TK: How important was Rose's husband Harvey, not only as a partner but also as an affluent companion who could support her?

AK: Harvey was very supportive of her work with breast cancer; he really stood by her. I imagine it couldn't have always been easy because she ate, slept, drank, breathed the thing.

TK: Can you tell me about your own research?

AK: I have a PhD in sociology and a masters in women's studies, and I've been a member of the women's health movement for more than twenty years. My doctoral dissertation was a study of middle-class women who'd had breast cancer. I wanted to understand how they coped with that diagnosis. My current study, which is funded by a federal agency that's part of the public health service, is a study of poor and low-income women with breast cancer. My basic question is: Is breast cancer different for poor and low-income women than for other women? The unequivical answer is yes, it certainly is. There are lots of social factors in these women's lives which have deep and abiding consequences for their health and their survival from breast cancer.

TK: How do you feel Rose influenced you?

AK: I think there's a little bit of the social worker in me just like there was in Rose. Her passion was very visible and moving, and I think it was infectious. I think my own activism predates knowing Rose, but there's no question that because she lived in the same city—and would drive me crazy with phone calls at midnight—she was influential. I know she had a reputation for being very aggressive and very assertive and she was going to do something about breast cancer if it was the last damn thing she ever did. And in fact she did. She did leave this quite remakable legacy, but while she was alive she was quite rampant about it and I think she infected me with a bit of her passion and her deep concern for women with breast cancer. When I was defending my doctoral dissertation in 1988, at the end I said very nervously to all the professors sitting in the room that I thought breast cancer had such power to it as an issue that soon it would have a political movement of its own, in some degree like the AIDS movement. And I was right. So Rose Kushner was a major influence on me, and I am sure far beyond me.

Women's Hearts at Risk

CHARLOTTE LIBOV

Charlotte Libov, *The Woman's Heart Book*, New York: Plume, 1994. Reprinted by permission.

When I was forty years old, I was stunned to learn I'd been born with a congenital heart defect, a "hole" in my heart. Since I had never heard of women having anything go wrong with their hearts, I was shocked. I learned the hard way that women do indeed develop heart disease. This is true, despite the stubborn myth that women's hearts are immune.

In fact, heart disease is the biggest killer of women. About 235,000 women die annually from heart attacks. When you add in the deaths from all types of heart problems, the figure mushrooms to over half of a million female deaths a year. These statistics not only involve elderly women; an estimated 74,000 women between the ages of forty-five and sixty-four suffer heart attacks annually, according to the American Heart Association. Heart disease is also a major risk factor for stroke, the third leading killer and greatest crippler of women.

But the problem of heart disease in women is one that has been overlooked for years. "Clear evidence exists that women are not being treated aggressively to prevent heart disease," according to a 1999 statement issued by the American Heart Association and the American College of Cardiology.

This myth that "women don't get heart disease" persists among doctors as well. A 1996 Gallup survey found that nearly two-thirds of the internists and family practitioners queried know that there are important differences in the symptoms of heart attacks and in diagnostic tests for women.

Studies were done on the assumption that only men developed heart disease. These included the 1982 Multiple Risk Factor Intervention Trial, aptly dubbed "Mr. Fit," which looked at lifestyle factors related to cholesterol and heart disease. Later, the Physicians Health Study looked at the preventative powers of aspirin on heart disease in male doctors.

GENDER BIAS AND WOMEN'S HEARTS

"Gender bias" refers to the concern that because it is believed that women are less likely to get heart disease, they are less likely to be properly treated.

WHAT IS CORONARY HEART DISEASE?

Although all types of heart problems are encompassed in the umbrella term of "heart disease," it is coronary heart disease that leads most often to heart attack and death. A heart attack is usually the result of a disease process known as atherosclerosis, which causes the coronary arteries to become narrowed and clogged, shutting off the vital blood supply to the heart.

As we age, our risk of heart disease rises. As women, though, we are generally diagnosed with heart disease ten to fifteen years later than men, when we're in our 50s and 60s. This difference, known as "gender protection," is ascribed to estrogen, the so-called female sex hormone.

FAMILY MEDICAL HISTORY

Your risk of heart disease is increased if you have a parent who developed early-onset heart disease. This refers to fathers who developed heart disease before the age of fifty-five or mothers before age sixty-five. The more close relatives you have with early-onset heart disease, the greater the possibility of this genetic link.

RACE Heart disease is the biggest killer of American women, no matter what their race or ethnicity.

However, more African-American women develop it at a younger age, most likely because they develop high blood pressure, diabetes, and high cholesterol earlier as well.

HIGH BLOOD PRESSURE After the age of fifty, women develop high blood pressure, or hypertension, twice as often as do men. High blood pressure usually occurs in the absence of symptoms and can cause damage years before being diagnosed.

DIABETES Diabetes, a metabolic disorder, is a powerful risk factor that erases a woman's normal gender protection, meaning she may develop heart disease earlier. Diabetes also causes neuropathy, a nerve disorder that can mask symptoms of chest pain, so a diabetic may not recognize this key warning sign of an impending heart attack.

HIGH CHOLESTEROL When it comes to coronary heart disease, there are three types of lipoproteins that are emphasized. Low-density lipoprotein, or LDL, cholesterol, is the so-called bad cholesterol that builds up within the walls of coronary arteries. Triglycerides are another important type and contain most of the fats in the blood. These are the two types of lipoproteins that contribute to coronary heart disease. A third type of cholesterol, high-density cholesterol, or HDL cholesterol, is known as good cholesterol because it blocks the accumulation of LDL cholesterol by transferring it away from the arteries.

Prior to menopause, women tend to have high levels of the beneficial HDL, cholesterol, so it's not enough to focus on your total cholesterol number. Women need to have their total cholesterol profile done to compare the ratio of the HDL cholesterol to LDL cholesterol and triglycerides.

Traditionally, cholesterol screening has involved just checking these three lipid levels. However, up to half of those who suffer heart attacks have normal cholesterol levels. Because of this, research is ongoing into more than a dozen more cholesterol patterns to learn how the molecules that make up these cholesterol patterns are arranged. Currently, most interest centers on three patterns: LDL pattern A, lipoprotein (a), and LDL pattern B. If you come from a family with a history of heart disease but not high cholesterol, you might want to ask your doctor about being tested for these additional patterns.

SMOKING Female smokers have nearly double the heart attack rate and are more likely to suffer from advanced heart disease than nonsmokers. Smoking also has been found to contribute to the development of heart disease earlier. Even smoking just four cigarettes a day increases heart disease risk. Also, although oral contraceptives alone do not cause heart attacks in women under the age of thirty-five, they do increase the risk for women over that age.

OBESITY Weighing 20 percent or more than ideal increases the probability of coronary heart disease, although the telling factor seems to be in what manner the excess weight is distributed. The risk is higher for women who are "apple"-shaped, women who accumulate excess weight in their stomach, than for those who are "pear"-shaped and carry the excess weight in their hips.

INACTIVITY In the past, being inactive has been associated with heart disease because, if you're inactive, it is more likely you'll develop other risk factors, such as high blood pressure and diabetes. But studies have found that, even in the absence of these other risk factors, being inactive increases the risk of heart disease.

EMERGING RISK FACTORS

HOMOCYSTEINE Homocysteine, an amino acid in the blood, can build up, damage the coronary arteries, and set the stage for coronary heart disease. Not all studies have linked homocysteine risk with increased heart disease, leading to speculation that the amino acid may not be the risk factor but only a marker —the culprit may possibly be low levels of B vitamins.

There is a blood test you can take to check your homocysteine level, but because all the re-

search isn't yet in, it isn't generally recommended. However, if hyperhomocysteinemia, a rare genetic condition that causes too-high homocysteine levels, runs in your family, or if you have family members who developed heart disease in the absence of other risk factors, ask your doctor about it.

STRESS Exactly how stress harms our coronary arteries isn't fully understood, but it is apparently related to the physiological changes that occur. When we are under stress, our nervous system releases hormones that cause our coronary blood vessels to constrict, and our heart rate to increase and even the cells that line our blood vessels to undergo changes.

DEPRESSION Several studies find that clinical depression, the type of hopeless despair that is impossible to shake, may increase heart disease risk.

HOW WOMEN CAN PREVENT HEART DISEASE

QUIT SMOKING Once you quit smoking, your risk of suffering a heart attack immediately diminishes; some studies show that you can decrease the added risk by up to 70 percent.

LOSE WEIGHT If you're overweight, losing weight will reduce your risk. If you're very overweight, you don't necessarily need to lose all those pounds. Research finds that even a modest weight loss 5 to 10 percent of body weight—can significantly lower your heart disease risk.

EAT SMART The American Heart Association recommends that you get no more than 30 percent of daily calories from fat. Saturated fat, which generally comes from animal products, raises blood cholesterol more than any other type, so you should eat no more than 10 percent within that 30 percent figure. Instead, choose liquid vegetable fats, such olive oil.

The possibility that vitamins may help prevent heart disease is a tantalizing one, and the research involving the antioxidant vitamin E is the most hopeful. But not all the research has been consistent.

EXERCISE REGULARLY Regular exercise, such as brisk walking, aerobics, biking, or other types that raise your heart rate for at least thirty minutes three times a week, helps to prevent heart disease. When you exercise, you burn calories, which helps control weight. This, in turn, helps prevent high blood pressure. Exercise also helps you metabolize glucose more efficiently, reduce the risk of diabetes, and improve cholesterol levels.

CONSIDER HORMONE REPLACEMENT THERAPY Numerous studies demonstrate that women who take estrogen after menopause have about a 40 percent decreased risk of heart disease. Estrogen appears to lower heart disease risk in three ways. First, estrogen modulates the manufacturing of cholesterol in the liver, lowering the amounts of the "bad" LDL cholesterol while boosting the production of plaque-fighting HDL cholesterol by up to 20 percent. In addition, estrogen helps keep the blood vessels smooth, elastic, and flexible. Furthermore, estrogen lowers blood levels of fibrinogen, a substance involved in the formation of blood clots that can cause heart attacks. Most of the studies showing this benefit have been done using estrogen alone, known as estrogen replacement therapy (ERT).

In recent years, a new type of hormone replacement, selective estrogen receptor modulators, or SERMs, has developed. They are designed to protect against osteoporosis and heart disease without increasing cancer risk. The first of these drugs, raloxifene (Evista) was approved in 1996. A 1998 study in the *Journal of the American Medical Association* found that, although raloxifene does increase bone density, its ability to prevent coronary heart disease risk is not as strong.

Although the benefits of estrogen are well-documented, not all the answers are in. Most of the studies have been observational ones, and more randomized studies, where some women are put on hormones and others take a placebo, need to be done. Also, although many doctors advocate hormone replacement therapy, there are also non-drug alternatives to reduce the risk of heart disease, including losing weight, diet, and exercise.

HEART ATTACKS IN WOMEN You're probably aware that chest pain is often a warning sign of an impending heart attack. However, this appears to be less true for women. Although some women do suffer chest pain, it is often more subtle and is better characterized as discomfort. Also, unlike chest pain in men, which is acute, such discomfort in women can last for hours. In addition, women may more typically suffer pain elsewhere, like the jaw, back, or even the stomach, as well as symptoms such as shortness of breath, fatigue or weakness, nausea, dizziness, or indigestion.

DIAGNOSING HEART DISEASE IN WOMEN

When it comes to heart disease, women are at a disadvantage because heart disease is more difficult to diagnose. First, heart disease symptoms in women are more subtle and because, when women are younger, they are more likely than men to experience chest pain from non-heart-related causes, such as muscle pain, gallbladder disease, heartburn, and even anxiety.

Another problem is that the most common test for coronary heart disease, known as exercise stress testing, or sometimes treadmill testing, is more accurate when used on men. In women, however, this test too often results in a "false positive" reading that indicates heart disease is present when none exists.

Although this test is not adequate for screening, there are tests that are used to investigate the possibility of heart disease in women who are experiencing symptoms. One technique is to improve the accuracy of this test by combining it with an imaging agent that also provides pictures of the blood flow to the heart. Another alternative is to combine the exercise stress test with echocardiogram that furnishes ultrasound images of the heart.

Women are not referred as often as men for diagnostic tests. This is a particular concern relating to the test known as cardiac arteriography, or cardiac catheterization. This test is required in deciding such interventional techniques as balloon angioplasty and coronary bypass surgery should be considered.

TREATING HEART DISEASE IN WOMEN

Treating coronary heart disease usually involves ways to widen arteries narrowed by atherosclerosis to result in more blood to the heart and prevent heart attack. The main techniques to do this are percutaneous transluminal coronary angioplasty, commonly known as balloon angioplasty and coronary artery bypass grafting, or bypass surgery. In both of these areas, statistics show that women are far less likely to be offered these treatments.

In balloon angioplasty, a catheter-tipped balloon is used to widen the narrowed coronary arteries. Because this technique can replace the need for open-heart surgery, it's not surprising that it is extremely popular. But, according to the American Heart Association's latest figures, only one-third of the 482,000 angioplasties done annually are performed on women. This may be in part because, years ago, when this technique was first devised, it was riskier in women because the instruments used were too large for a woman's more delicate arteries. However, this is no longer true; studies show this is a safe and effective technique for women. Bypass surgery is open-heart surgery performed to reroute, or "bypass," blood around clogged arteries and improve the supply of blood and oxygen to the heart. According to the American Heart Association's most recent figures, only 29 percent of the 598,000 surgeries were done on women. This may be due to the fact that although bypass surgery is safe and effective, it is riskier for women. This is usually attributed to the fact that women have smaller, delicate arteries that make

the surgery more technically difficult. Minimally invasive bypass surgery, a new technique that minimize the trauma to the body of bypass surgery, is raising great interest. There are two approaches commonly used: port-access coronary artery bypass, also referred to as PACAB or PortCAB, and minimally invasive coronary artery bypass (also called MinCAB). But research needs to be done to learn what extent this will prove as an alternative to traditional bypass surgery. Rarely, the heart is so weakened as to require a heart transplant. Although an estimated 40,000 individuals could benefit from transplants, the most recent figures show that only 2,290 were done and, of those, only about 25 percent were done on women.

The Myth of Osteoporosis

GILLIAN SANSON

Gillian Sanson, excerpt from *The Myth of Osteoporosis*, MCD Century Publications, 2003. Reprinted by permission.

It was 1994, and I was relaxing in my New Zealand home, talking with guests, when my daughter rang from the Auckland Hospital fracture clinic. Camille, who was sixteen, had been having a follow-up visit for a wrist fracture sustained on the ski slopes a few weeks previously—her sixth fracture. It was the normal sort of teenage call: "I won't be home for a while," she said, "I am going into town to meet some friends." She added: "Oh, and by the way, the doctor who looked at my X-ray says that I have the bones of an eighty-year-old."

I was speechless, devastated, and immediately stricken with guilt. I assumed Camille's condition was due to bad mothering, and I immediately started examining how I had raised her. Perhaps her condition arose because of an inadequate vegetarian diet lacking sufficient calcium. Or was it my diet during pregnancy that was at fault? I had always been conscientious about giving my children good food, but maybe I had made some critical mistake. My fears were irrational, of course, but I had many such questions and few answers. I was determined, however, to learn all I could about osteoporosis. That phone call became the impetus for this book.

In the meantime, Camille became justifiably frightened. She was young, alone, and had no context in which to gauge her diagnosis. Believing her fragile bones could not withstand any knocks or pressure, Camille immediately cut back on physical activity—conduct that was contrary to what she ought to have done, yet no such advice was given. (Years later, when I consider the event, I am appalled by the thoughtlessness of how she was told of her condition.)

Camille soon went for a bone densitometry scan, which confirmed that she had very low bone mineral density for her age. Extremely low bone density in young people is a concern because it means they haven't achieved the recognized, normal, healthy peak bone mass to take them through to adulthood and older age when bone density naturally declines and fracture risk increases. Initially, we were told that existing bone mass is like a bank account which can be drawn on. In Camille's case, according to current understanding, she was already in debt.

The family participated in a study at the endocrinology department at Auckland Hospital to determine a genetic risk factor. Measuring the bone densities of the entire extended family revealed that my three siblings, parents, husband, son, daughter, and I have varying degrees of low bone density (BMD), culminating most seriously in my son and daughter. Six of us have osteoporosis, as defined by a BMD of -2.5 standard deviations (SD) below norm or less, and the rest of us have what is called osteopenia, or low bone density, a BMD of -1 SD to -2.5 SDs below the norm. Males and females in the family are similarly afflicted, although none of us has fractured a bone since we were children—with the exception of my mother, who had a wrist fracture in her sixties. Growing up, my sister, brother, and I routinely broke wrists, the occasional digit, leg, or collarbone,

and accepted that this was normal childhood wear and tear. In our small town of 14,000 inhabitants, we rather proudly held the record for the most X-rays at the local hospital. The fracturing eased off as we became adults, and when my children in turn started occasionally breaking their limbs, I stoically assumed the role of fracture-clinic mother, believing this was all a normal part of parenting.

Identifying idiopathic osteoporosis (osteoporosis of unknown origin) in our family raised many questions but provided no answers. Efforts to determine a cause were inconclusive. Blood DNA samples from individuals in the family and other similarly affected families were sent to Oxford, England, to screen for a common genetic factor. Researchers determined that there was a genetic link—though they were unsuccessful in isolating such a gene.

For my children it was difficult to know what actions to take. There wasn't any known treatment for very low bone density in a young person. All the tested, prescribed treatments were for postmenopausal women with low bone density. Hormonal treatments were inappropriate (like other healthy young women, my daughter's estrogen and progesterone levels were normal), and it wasn't clear that nonhormonal treatments would be effective in a person her age. I also remained unconvinced that the recommended drug (a bisphosphonate) would be safe, given the current lack of data on its use in young people.

Some family members had high levels of antibiotics in their blood, which could indicate gluten intolerance or celiac disease. Celiac disease is known to be a "secondary" risk factor for osteoporosis, as it causes the villi (fingerlike projections) in the wall of the small bowel to atrophy or disappear, thereby limiting the absorption of essential minerals. It is believed that maybe 1 in 130 people have this condition, often without realizing it—particularly those of Celtic origin, such as my family. The four of us in my immediate family embarked on a gluten-free diet—one of the recommended treatments for people who have celiac disease. After eighteen months, our bone density remained unchanged.

I began to look deeper into possible causes of osteoporosis, ever conscious that the years when peak bone mass is established in a young person (up to about age twenty) were almost over for my children. Camille's situation was identified as more serious than her brother's. His bone mass was low, though hers was significantly lower. Further, a young female can be at risk for additional bone loss during pregnancy and may lose bone mass more rapidly after menopause.

When I began my research, I quickly learned that members of my family were not the only ones who were worried about their bone health. As a women's health educator, I conduct seminars and workshops in the community to help women manage the menopause transition and stay well in the years to follow. The subject of osteoporosis always surfaced in my classes, evoking feelings of anxiety and fear among many women who were convinced that they were candidates for osteoporosis by virtue of their age alone, once they passed through menopause. For most women, the question was not whether they were at risk for osteoporosis, but what to do about the impending condition. I would later discover that the widespread notion that all women are at risk for osteoporosis is a myth—though not the only one.

In these discussions, hormone replacement therapy (HRT) attracted much attention. For decades, women had taken HRT to relieve symptoms associated with menopause. Increasing numbers of women, however, were also taking HRT to prevent postmenopausal diseases such as heart disease and osteoporosis. Questions arose. Should women take HRT following a diagnosis of low bone density? Would HRT prevent osteoporosis? Was the hormone therapy linked to an increased risk for breast cancer? There seemed to be many information gaps, and women often joked that they felt stuck between a rock and a hard place, that the choices were too difficult. This book, then, is also for women in general who want information

that cuts through much of the anxiety surrounding osteoporosis.

A revelation came in 1999. My son, Jude, was staying in a cabin on a lake in Manitoba, Canada, for a weekend. Among the magazines in the cabin was a 1998 *Homemakers* magazine with a cover article by journalist Elaine Dewar titled "Breaking News—Blowing the Whistle on Osteoporosis." Jude mailed me the article, which called into question the accuracy of bone density testing diagnoses. The article referred to a large Canadian study that found DXA machines using the manufacturers' reference standards for measuring bone density were diagnosing up to three times as many cases of osteoporosis than when a Canadian reference standard was used. The findings were significant: Osteoporosis had come to be defined by low bone density, but, as the Canadian study discovered, DXA manufacturers had not standardized their machines.

Suddenly I realized that every aspect of the disease was up for debate. Was osteoporosis as prevalent as people were being led to believe? Were people being prescribed medication who were not at risk? Was bone density even an accurate predictor of osteoporosis? If low bone density was not necessarily a cause for concern, why were drugs to increase bone density being prescribed so readily? What did this mean for my parents, my sister, my son and daughter? What did it mean for the millions of women who were being tested and told they had the disease? Why was nobody questioning how osteoporosis had gone from being rare to being everywhere?

The more I read, the more I was convinced that women and their doctors were misinformed. I uncovered increasing amounts of evidence that healthy women were being frightened into unnecessary testing, handed questionable diagnoses, and urged to undergo long-term treatments for a disease that they probably didn't have. I discovered that there are many risk factors for osteoporosis in addition to low bone density; and that when osteoporosis is defined as a condition of fragile bones that fracture easily, it is, in fact, a rare disease. I began to feel hope for my children. Maybe their bones were stronger than I thought.

Then one day I had a major breakthrough. I was spending hours each week in the medical school library searching medical journals, unearthing articles, and following any lead, reference, or footnote that would provide further insight into the disease. One article referred to a 1997 report by the British Columbia Office of Health Technology Assessment. The independent, government-funded agency reviewed evidence to determine the effectiveness of bone mineral density testing. The agency reported that BMD testing does not accurately identify women who will go on to fracture as they age—a finding that prompted a Canadian Broadcasting Corporation documentary that alerted the public to what it called "the marketing of fear" to healthy women. The report referred to a study that found that the cracks in Vancouver's sidewalks were a common cause of hip fractures, and that screening large populations of menopausal women for osteoporosis might only prevent between 1 percent and 5 percent of fractures in the elderly. The review raised concerns about overdiagnosis of the disease and overprescribing of medication and addressed the issue of the ineffectiveness of current drug therapies. Similar reviews in countries including the United States, the United Kingdom, France, Sweden, and Australia reached the same conclusions—though the results of these government-funded projects rarely rated a mention in the press. The overriding message remained that BMD testing was a reliable and effective way to diagnose osteoporosis.

My attention moved to the popular treatments for osteoporosis—HRT, bisphosphonates, and the much-heralded prevention strategies of calcium and dairy consumption. There was little evidence to recommend the widely advertised pharmaceuticals or the daily taking of calcium. Coming from a dairy-producing nation that readily accepts the claim that milk consumption results in healthy bones, I was particularly stunned to find that the evidence in favor of dairy just wasn't there. My greatest concern, however, was for the millions of women worldwide who were trustingly undergoing hormone replacement therapy in the belief that it was protecting their bones. There was minimal evidence that HRT prevented fractures, and there was a growing body of evidence that it caused breast cancer and heart disease.

Then in July 2002, the National Institutes of Health released startling findings from its Women's Health Initiative—one of the largest studies of its kind ever undertaken. Researchers announced that HRT use was linked to an increased risk for breast cancer, heart disease, clotting, and stroke.

Many women felt depressed, fearful, and betrayed. Now, many women had to decide which treatment, if any, to undertake. Osteoporosis-preventing drugs such as alendronate (marketed as Fosamax) and raloxifene (Evista) began to fill the void left by HRT. However, questions remain because long-term safety data on these drugs are limited or nonexistent. Preliminary research also indicates that such treatments provide limited benefit.

I encourage women to learn the facts about osteoporosis so that they can see through many of the myths surrounding the disease. I encourage women to question the diagnosis of osteoporosis. Most importantly, I encourage women to investigate all of their options for staying well and maintaining excellent bone health.

CHAPTER 21

Informed Consent, Conflict of Interest, and Pharmaceutical Companies

THE STORY OF PHARMACEUTICAL COMPANIES and their role in American medicine in the second half of the twentieth century is a dramatic one. It has been told and retold recently as more and more people become aware of the potential problems that are created when product makers get too close to doctors and health care professionals, and when those making science, making headlines, and making money get to be the same folks. Like any good drama, this story has heroes and villains, martyrs and converts.

Why do you need to know about drug companies? There are many reasons, but the most important is that they, along with doctors, make up the medical world as we know it. This means that, like it or not, drug makers have an enormous day-to-day impact on the health and well-being of our loved ones. The relationship between drug makers and medical professionals is long and complicated, full of twists and turns, unexpected alliances, and bitter enmities. Understanding both the good and bad things drug companies do is crucial to being a smart patient.

Dr. Marcia Angell is an impressive woman. A former Fullbright Scholar and noted pathologist, she became the first female editor in chief of the *New England Journal of Medicine*. Her tenure in the position was short—she served from 1999 until June 2000. When she left *NEJM*, Angell did not go quietly. In a cutting, angry editorial called "Is Academic Medicine For Sale?," the doctor lambasted journals, researchers, and drug makers alike for a host of financial relationships that she argued were deeply beneficial to all professionals involved, at the high cost of the well-being of patients.

To hear Angell tell it, she *had* to leave the journal—what was the point of giving one's name week after week to a publication that advertised itself as pure science, but was in reality an elaborate public relations vehicle fueled by high hopes and copious drug dollars? An example: When *NEJM* decided to publish an article on antidepressants, no unbiased, qualified people could be found to peer review it. The authors of the article themselves were so embedded with the makers of the products they were testing as to render their work highly suspect: their "ties with companies that make antidepressant drugs were so extensive that it would have used too much space to disclose them fully in the journal."[1] In 2004, Angell published a brilliant, devastating book called *The Truth About the Drug Companies: How They Deceive Us And What To Do About It*, in which she elaborated her argument from her last days at *NEJM*. Her book was followed by several others authored by doctors, journalists, and medical historians. Some looked at case studies while others surveyed the whole system. The conclusion was the same: the relationship between doctors and drug makers needed to change for the good of science, medicine, and patient well-being.

Many young doctors are getting savvy—at a recent medical activism course at Montefiore Medical Center in the Bronx, a group of twenty- and thirty-something medical students debated the merits and drawbacks of accepting free samples of pills from pharmaceutical representatives. Was it an act of social justice, making it possible for doctors to provide free drugs to low-income and uninsured patients? Or was it, regardless of the best physician intentions, the first step on the slippery slope to being a drug company's doctor? Without offering any conclusions, it is fair to say that this conversation is encouraging. It means young doctors are considering the mistakes of the past and thinking creatively about the future.

I've seen again and again over my career the ways in which drug makers can adversely impact patient health, from influencing science (through funding research and offering financial incentives to researchers), doctor education (through freebies and writing that continues medical education), patient education (through sponsoring and buying out consumer advocate groups and patient Web sites) and even freedom of the press.

This last problem I have come to understand personally. When I wrote my first book, *The Doctors' Case Against the Pill*, I was fired from my magazine column at *Ladies' Home Journal*—drug-maker Johnson and Johnson didn't like the questions I raised about some of their most profitable products and they spoke to my employers. They said they'd love to buy some of the biggest ad spots the magazine had to offer—the back cover and the centerfold—for a good chunk of time. They had new baby products they'd love to promote. It meant a huge amount of money for the magazine—more than they could afford to turn down. They had a condition, however. The magazine had this columnist who was saying some terrible things about the pill . . .

I was fired again from *Family Circle* in 1973 after publishing *Free and Female*. My editor assured me this wouldn't happen—they didn't have ads for baby products. He didn't anticipate the importance of advertising dollars from EASY-OFF oven cleaner and other American Home Products wares. American Home Products was a division of Wyeth, the maker of some of the biggest hormone therapy (HT) and estrogen therapy (ET) products I was writing about and criticizing. Again I was fired from *Hadassah Magazine* when I spoke out against major donor Wyeth's big product—Premarin—in my 2003 book *The Greatest Experiment Ever Performed on Women*.

Freedom of speech—medical speech—is a good thing. Whether you agreed with my perspective on the pill, it's hard to argue that the resulting congressional hearings on the safety of the pill and the first patient package inserts weren't good things for patient health.

When medical journals (as has been documented by Angell, among others) and consumer publications allow bad news about drugs to be chilled, they are hurting patient health. Until the professionals change their relationships with pharma, we as patients need to take responsibility for being educated and informed. This is true in our consumption of health information both in the media and from our doctors. Understand that doctors are human. This isn't a bad thing; it simply means that patients have greater responsibility for making smart, independent decisions.

NOTE

1. Marcia Angel, "Is Academic Medicine For Sale?" *JAMA*, vol. 342, no. 20 (May 18, 2000): 1516-1518.

The Amazing Story of DES

BARBARA SEAMAN AND GIDEON SEAMAN

Barbara Seaman and Gideon Seaman, excerpt from *Women and the Crisis in Sex Hormones,* New York: Bantam Books, 1978. Originally published in 1977 by Rawson. Reprinted by permission.

One day, a Virginia woman named Grace M. was reading the newspaper when she noticed an article concerning a drug called DES—diethylstilbestrol, often called simply stilbestrol. The article pointed out a newly discovered danger associated with this drug: The daughters of some of the women who had taken it during their pregnancies had developed vaginal cancer as a result, said the author of the report, Dr. Arthur Herbst.

"I became alarmed and called my doctor immediately," recalls Mrs. M. "I had first taken DES in 1949 when I was pregnant with one daughter, and again in 1955 before the birth of another. So I took both my daughters to the doctor, and from the examinations, Marilyn, the fourteen-year-old, was found to have cancer of the vagina.

"Three weeks later, she had vaginal surgery in New York City. She was four weeks in the hospital. The doctors told me they had gotten all of it, there was no problem, everything was taken care of, this type of cancer rarely ever spreads beyond the female organs.

"And so, reassured, we went back to Virginia. A year later, Marilyn developed cancer of the lung and also three tumors on her trachea and her bronchial tubes. The doctors operated and removed the lung and tumors.

"About four months later, Marilyn started having severe head pains. The cancer had spread into her head. She had whole-head radiation, and from hip radiation she went on to the arms and legs, and eventually she went blind and died, two and a half years after we had discovered the cancer. It is a horrible, terrible thing to watch your child suffer, and eventually, when she dies, you think it is a blessing—the death is far easier to accept than the actual suffering."

Today, Mrs. M.'s other daughter, Patty, who is in her twenties, is under constant care. She is checked every three months because she has adenosis, an abnormal condition in her vaginal tract associated with prenatal exposure to DES and thought to be a precursor of cancer of the vagina.

On December 16, 1975, a twenty-one-year-old woman named Sherry L. spoke on the steps of the Food and Drug Administration in Rockville, Maryland, at a National Women's Health Network memorial service that was held for all the women who have died from unnecessary estrogen products. Sherry herself is a "DES daughter"—like Marilyn M., and *an estimated 1.5 million other young US women.* She has cervical abnormalities that were discovered in a routine checkup at a women's health center and in tests at Massachusetts General Hospital's DES screening program. She has to undergo continual monitoring. Sherry is anxious about the outcome of her life.

"I relieve a lot of my anxiety by working on DES projects, but it's still hard to live with," she says.

Mothers suffer equally. On Long Island, New York, many are active in an organization called DES-Action. This is a group of mothers and daughters who were exposed to the drug and who have banded together for mutual support, advice, and possible action. Similar activist groups are organizing in other areas. DES women in California have prodded the state health department to publish material alerting women and doctors to the dangers of DES, and to offer doctors one-day courses in the use of the colposcope, an instrument that aids in the discovery of vaginal abnormalities. Other women exposed to DES have themselves filed suits against the drug companies who make it—or have joined in filing class action suits.

Why are these tragedies, connected to a relatively small group of people, receiving so much attention? In terms of the population as a whole, the cause of a group of mothers and daughters who, over a 30-year span, were given a drug that proved dangerous to many does not seem of imminent concern to the rest of us.

But these women are not the only ones at risk. Abnormalities are now beginning to show up in some of the sons of women who were given DES during pregnancy. And in spite of the alarming track record of this synthetic hormone in after-the-fact testing, *DES is still being given today in the form of the morning-after pill, a favorite contraceptive handed out at many university health services. It is also being given as a milk suppressant to new mothers* who do not wish to nurse their babies.*

And on top of all that, this known carcinogen *is in the meat we eat.* The fact is that today—man, woman, or child—*we are all chemically medicated to some degree with DES, without our permission and usually without our knowledge.*

MORE NORMAL THAN NORMAL

DES is the grandmother product of all synthetic estrogens, as well as being the loss leader. (Leader to the pharmaceutical industry, loss to the women who have taken it.)

Synthesized by Sir Charles Dodd in England in 1938, it was the first hormone product that was both cheap to manufacture and effective to take by mouth. DES has been defined as a "synthetic compound capable of producing feminizing effects similar to those of the naturally occurring feminizing hormone estrogen." Similar to, but not identical with, as Dodds himself pointed out.

Nearly thirty years later, in 1965, Sir Charles made this comment about his brainchild: "It is interesting . . . to speculate on the difference in attitude toward new drugs 30 years ago and today. Within a few months of the first publication of the synthesis of stilbestrol, the substance was being marketed throughout the world. No long-term toxicity tests on animals such as dogs were ever done with stilbestrol. . . . It is really surprising that we escaped major pharmacological disasters until a few years ago."

THE BOSTON DISEASE: ITS ORIGINS

Paul Rheingold is an attorney specializing in malpractice and drug liability cases. He is planning a class action suit against the drug companies to pay for the health care of the daughters of women who were given DES while they were pregnant. He also handles individual DES lawsuits. "You know," he mused when we interviewed him in 1976, "it's almost like a Boston disease. The closer you get to Boston, the more DES daughters you find, and the farther away you get, the fewer."

He could have said Harvard because, in point of fact, the tragic story of DES begins at Harvard University. The first promoters of DES as a therapy for pregnant women were Dr. George Van Siclen Smith, head of Harvard's gynecology department from 1942 to 1967 and now professor emeritus, and his wife, biochemist Dr. Olive Watkins Smith.

George and Olive Smith married in 1930 when he was a fellow in gynecology at Harvard Medical School, and she was a young PhD out of Radcliffe. Today they are a handsome-enough couple to star in a leisure village advertisement, except that leisure is the one thing they don't have. He is still in private practice, and she performs research—seventy hours per week—at the Fearing Research Laboratory of the Free Hospital for Women in Brookline.

They are tall, the two of them, and blue-eyed. They chuckle a lot together, and they are proud of their grown daughter and son. They also adopt a parental attitude toward the doctors they trained— "our boys"—such as DES investigators Arthur Herbst, Philip Corfman, and John Lewis.

Philip Corfman, of the National Institute of Health's Division of Child Health and Human Development, has given grants for several studies on the aftermath of DES. Dr. George said of Corfman, "He's too young to be an administrator. He was a good resident. We wanted to keep him here."

George and Olive Smith "started right in on the ovary" in 1928, and have been working on it ever since. As Dr. George puts it, "We have just lived ovarian hormones—pituitary and placental—for years and years." The Smiths were among the first to demonstrate how pituitary and ovarian hormones function over the course of the normal menstrual cycle, and, with the help of a tip from their friend Dr. Gregory Pincus, inventor of the birth control pill, were the first to demonstrate estradiol as one of the naturally occurring forms of estrogen.

THE FIRST DES STUDY

From the mid-1930s on, Dr. George and Dr. Olive, together and separately, published many important papers on estrogen excretion in normal pregnancy. It was in 1941, based on their observation of low hormone levels in mothers spontaneously aborting, that they conceived the idea of using the newly developed DES to help pregnancies that seemed threatened by miscarriage. Dr. Olive stated in her landmark report, published in the *American Journal of Obstetrics and Gynecology* in November 1948, "It was found . . . that diethylstilbestrol . . . might theoretically . . . provide an ideal agent for progesterone deficiency in pregnancy."

The report described a study of 632 DES-treated pregnancies, which dated back to 1943. The earliest DES mothers were not all Bostonians, for 117 obstetricians from forty-eight cities and towns in New York, New Jersey, Pennsylvania, the District of Columbia, Illinois, North Carolina, Virginia, Texas, New Mexico, California, and all of the New England states cooperated in the study. Presumably the cooperating doctors gave the pills to pregnant patients who seemed in danger of miscarrying, although possibly some gave them to women who merely had problems with previous pregnancies.

By 1948 the Smiths were convinced that DES could be effective against many complications of pregnancy, including threatened miscarriage and diabetes. In addition, the babies of DES-treated mothers were said to be unusually rugged; the placentas were found to be "grossly more healthy-looking."

THE BIG BOSTON SUCCESS

The following year the Smiths completed their second major study at Boston Lying-In. This study, which had begun in 1947, included 387 women who received DES throughout pregnancy, compared to 550 who did not. All of these women . . . were observed to be having *normal first pregnancies.* Those who did not receive DES got no special treatment, or even a placebo. Women with known illnesses such as diabetes or hypertension were excluded from the study, in spite of the Smith's claims that DES had proved effective in pregnancies threatened by diabetes. Those in the study were all normal and healthy first-time mothers. What was the reason for giving them a powerful drug, except in the name of research? *Yet the women who were given DES were never informed that they were part of a highly controversial experiment.* Some DES mothers recall that they were told the pills were "vitamins."

The Smiths had a dream—a dream of helping women with problem pregnancies achieve motherhood, and then, as their experiment unfolded, a yet more daring dream of making normal pregnancies more normal!

Nowadays, a well-designed drug study must handle both treated and untreated patients in exactly the same way. The untreated patients are given placebos and the same kind of care as the treated. Codes are kept secret so that the doctors and staff (as well as the patients) never know who received the real medication until it's all over.

The regional battle lines concerning DES were drawn on a day in 1949 in Hot Springs, Virginia, at the Seventy-second Annual Meeting of the American Gynecological Society. In general, the New Englanders supported the Smiths—and Harvard—while the Midwesterners did not. Dr. William J. Dieckmann of the University of Chicago and Chicago Lying-In Hospital pointed out that the untreated control group in the Smiths' study was not given a placebo, which he considered essential for scientific accuracy. He proposed a plan for testing DES at Chicago Lying-In, using a placebo as a control.

TROUBLESOME NEWS FROM NEW ORLEANS AND CHICAGO

A New Orleans obstetrician, Dr. John Henry Ferguson of Charity Hospital and Tulane University, also attempted to replicate the Harvard DES work. Like Dieckmann, Ferguson believed that the Smiths had erred in not giving their control patients an inert pill. Alternate pregnant patients at Charity Hospital were given tablets called "white stilbestrol" and "yellow stilbestrol," but only the white ones contained the real stuff.

Ferguson's study was the first to show stilbestrol had no more effect than the placebo. In fact, more DES patients than placebo patients had miscarriages and premature births, while the control group babies (and placentas) were slightly bigger and healthier. The only diabetic patient in the study, a DES mother, lost her baby! Dr. Ferguson had, in the words of one admiring contemporary, "driven a very large nail in the coffin that we will use someday to bury some of the extremely outsized claims for the beneficial effects of stilbestrol."

The Dieckmann Chicago study was begun on September 29, 1950 . . . and completed on November 20, 1952. The DES babies in this study did not do better in any respect. To the contrary: Twice as many of the DES mothers had miscarriages; they had more hypertension . . . and smaller babies

than the mothers on placebos. Dr. Dieckmann and his associates concluded that DES *actually favors premature labor.*

But even more serious in its implications was the testing of DES for carcinogenicity by animal researchers. At the National Cancer Institute, for example, Michael B. Shimkin and Hugh C. Grady dissolved the new DES in sesame oil and fed it to male mice. These mice were of a strain called C_3H, which is so highly susceptible to cancer that most of the virgin females develop breast cancer spontaneously, though the males do not.

The DES males *did.* When the Smiths were conceiving their human experiments, DES had already been proven carcinogenic in mice.

The Smiths were aware of this research, for as Dr. Olive said in 1976, "Before we even started any clinical work at all, we went through all the literature."

"However," said her husband, "you can do all kinds of things to rats and mice by giving them overdoses."

The New Orleans and Chicago reports must have convinced many obstetricians then that there was no value in using DES, though apparently not some of the sons of Harvard. In 1953, when the bad news from Chicago was brought to the Lake Placid meeting, one doctor was quick to quip: "As a former Bostonian, I would be entirely lacking in loyalty if I had not used stilbestrol in my private practice."

THE HERBST REPORT

Back in Boston, while the Lake Placid meeting was taking place, a young New Yorker named Arthur Herbst was graduating *cum laude* from Harvard College, class of '53. Herbst got his MD from Harvard Medical School in 1959, trained in obstetrics and gynecology, and became one of the Smith "boys." In 1966, a fifteen-year-old girl with clear-cell adenocarcinoma of the vagina came to his attention. It was the first time that this type of cancer had ever been seen at Massachusetts General Hospital in any woman under twenty-five.

(Adenocarcinoma is cancer that occurs in *glandular tissue*. In normal women, the vaginal lining has no such tissue, but we now know that the vaginas of most daughters of women who took DES while pregnant, including those who are thus far free from cancer, have many tiny glands.)

Within the next three years, six similar cases of clear-cell adenocarcinoma in young women turned up at Massachusetts General Hospital. The youngest patient was fifteen, the oldest twenty-two. The patients and their mothers were all questioned about possible causes, such as douches, tampons, birth control pills, and sexual activity. "Finally," says Herbst, "*one of the mothers made an intuitive guess that the cause might be the DES she was given in pregnancy.*" The researchers then added prenatal hormones to their list of questions.

And that was the connection. The mothers of the young women with adenocarcinoma had all taken DES while pregnant.

Today George Smith says, sadly: "We've been in on that from the beginning because we're close friends with Dr. Herbst. Of course he felt terrible about it, but a lot is being learned as the result of it, and who could predict thirty years ago that anything like this would develop? I mean, regardless of the rat and mouse work."

Herbst's relationship with the Smiths did not prevent him from publishing his findings in the *New England Journal of Medicine* on April 22, 1971, in an article he authored with Drs. Ulfelder and Poskanzer. At this point, Herbst had examined eight cases of adenocarcinoma in young women. All but one were DES daughters.

The frightening implications of these findings go far beyond DES; for the first time, Herbst showed that estrogen products can be cancer-producing in humans. It had been known since 1896, when surgeons started removing ovaries of breast cancer patients, that hormones—even the hormones produced by a woman's own body—could speed up the growth of an existing malignancy.

It had been known since 1932 that breast cancer could be produced in *male* mice by giving them estrogen injections, that sex hormones could *produce* cancer in laboratory animals, serving as "seed" as well as "fertilizer" in *susceptible* strains.

DES was the first hormone product to be named a human carcinogen. The work of Herbst and his colleagues was a crucial "missing link" concerning estrogens and the *initiation* of cancer in humans, for all estrogens have a similar way of behaving biologically. . . . In 1971, the millions of hormone-using women all over the world should have been warned of the significance of Herbst's DES findings. They should have been warned that estrogens *cause* cancer as well as *help it to grow.*

They were not. Only in 1975, when additional hormone products, such as Premarin and the sequential pill, were also linked to cancer, did the US Food and Drug Administration start to acknowledge that estrogen products must be viewed as a group.

Herbst himself understood the sweeping implications of his 1971 report concerning the DES link among the young women with cancer. In March 1971, the *New England Journal of Medicine* sent galleys of Herbst's article to the FDA. Herbst also shipped the FDA his raw data sheets. Then he waited . . . and waited.

THE GREENWALD REPORT

But while the FDA dallied, health officials of one state—New York—swung promptly into action. Dr. Peter Greenwald, the thirty-four-year-old director of New York's Cancer Control Bureau, was a 1967 graduate of the Harvard School of Public Health. His specialty was epidemiology. He quickly collected data on five young New York women (aged fifteen to nineteen at the time of diagnosis) who had adenocarcinoma of the vagina. Three had died of advanced disease, and two were doing well post-operatively. The mothers of four of the young women had taken DES, and the fifth a series of different estrogens and progesterones.

In Dr. Greenwald's opinion, the symptoms of abnormal pregnancy in some of these mothers had been minimal. One mother had no symptoms, only a history of a previous miscarriage. Greenwald and his colleagues, Drs. J. J. Barlow, P. C. Nasca, and W. S. Burnett, quickly submitted their findings to the *New England Journal of Medicine*, which published them on August 12.

Meanwhile, on June 22, 1971, Dr. Hollis S. Ingraham, New York's Commissioner of Health and Greenwald's boss, sent an individual letter to every physician in his state telling of the Herbst findings and the confirming evidence collected by Greenwald. New York physicians were urged to report all similar cases immediately (Greenwald's phone number was enclosed) and to stop prescribing DES to pregnant women at once. Dr. George Himler, president of the Medical Society of the State of New York, and Dr. Eli Stark, president of the New York State Osteopathic Society, both endorsed Ingraham's appeal.

Though New York saw the situation as urgent, Washington did not. Earlier in June, Ingraham had written a letter to Dr. Charles Edwards, commissioner of the FDA, which said in part: "On the basis of our findings, we are officially notifying all physicians in New York State of the danger of estrogen administration during pregnancy. We also recommend most urgently that the Food and Drug Administration initiate immediate measures to ban the use of synthetic estrogens during pregnancy."

THE FOUNTAIN COMMITTEE

It was *two months* before Commissioner Edwards so much as acknowledged Ingraham's letter. In November, when Congressman L. H. Fountain held a congressional committee hearing on DES, he asked Edwards *why* he had dallied. Edwards said, "Well, I have no response to the delay . . . obviously when I received it, I sent it on to the Bureau of Drugs. I must, however, say that I do not agree with Dr. Ingraham's action. I think he was premature . . . not that his actions are necessarily wrong, but I think he could well have studied it a little bit more than he did."

Herbst had to wait even longer than Ingraham.

The FDA did not get back to him until late October, some seven months after receiving galleys of the "missing link" report. During that seven months, many thousands of pregnant women continued to get DES.

In 1967, the National Academy of Sciences–National Research Council (NAS–NRC) had rated DES *possibly effective* and had sent the FDA the following report:

> The panel feels that estrogens are not harmful in conditions such as threatened abortion, but that their effectiveness can't be documented by literature or its own experience.

This statement gave the FDA a clear mandate, and obligation, in 1968 to prohibit DES in pregnancy cases *unless* the manufacturers came up with new evidence.

Under the circumstances, with the proof of the drug's effectiveness three and a half years overdue, it is astonishing that the FDA did not take action the moment that the Herbst galleys were received.

Let us examine the results of the FDA's inaction: During the 1940s and especially the early 1950s (after the Boston studies had been published, but before they were challenged in Chicago and New Orleans), DES was enormously popular as a pregnancy treatment. It has been estimated that estrogens were prescribed for nearly 6 million pregnant women between 1943 and 1959, resulting in the birth of at least 3 million children who had been exposed *in utero* to estrogens. On the basis of research that has been done on pharmacy records from 1960 to 1970, let's assume that some 30,000 unborn females were exposed to DES in 1971, an average of 2,500 a month. Had the FDA acted decisively upon receiving the Herbst galleys in March, instead of waiting until November, 20,000 young women who are now in danger of developing adenocarcinoma could have been spared.

Don Harper Mills, a physician and lawyer who serves as a medico-legal expert on the editorial board of the *Journal of the American Medical As-*

sociation (JAMA), advises all physicians who have ever used DES in pregnancy to search their records and send a notice to all such patients at their last known address. Few physicians are complying.

Incredibly, not only have a great many doctors failed to notify their patients, but some still prescribe DES for pregnant women.

Neither the drug companies, nor the government, nor any professional medical societies such as the AMA or ACOG have offered to finance the search for and treatment of DES daughters. Who will?

AFTER THE MORNING AFTER

Despite the 1971 bulletin to physicians warning against the use of DES in pregnancy, which Congressman Fountain had wrested out of the FDA in November 1971, DES sales rose by 4 percent in the next nine months! Now that DES had proved carcinogenic in humans, doctors were prescribing it more than ever. The DES market had been salvaged in the nick of time by a new application, the morning-after pill.

THE MICHIGAN HEALTH SERVICE

In the late 1960s, the morning-after pill was being prescribed tentatively by some physicians. But by 1972, an official at the National Institutes of Health announced: "Most university health services are giving the morning-after pill."

How did this happen and why?

Some of the credit must go to the health service at the University of Michigan. On October 25, 1970, just two weeks before the FDA took action *against* DES as a pregnancy booster, *JAMA* published a report on 1,000 women in and around the university who had used it as a morning-after contraceptive. "No pregnancies resulted," according to the author, "and there were no serious adverse reactions"—an amazing statistic considering the fact that no contraceptive, *not even sterilization,* has ever been 100 percent effective in a population of 1,000 people. The report was like a green light to thousands of health service doctors.

THE COWAN STUDY

But something embarrassing happened. Local women in Ann Arbor, who were patients at the student health service, chanced upon the *JAMA* report. They didn't believe it. It didn't fit the facts. A few women who had been given the morning-after pill were pregnant, although they acknowledged it could have been from exposure earlier in the cycle. Other pregnant women treated at the health service had not had any earlier exposure, but were unable to finish the five-day course because the DES pills made them vomit. Then there was a third group: Women who had not had earlier exposure, were not too nauseated to swallow their medication, but were nonetheless . . . pregnant.

But how could the student health service know of these pregnancies when in fact it had *never followed up with most of the DES patients?* The Ann Arbor DES patients were pioneers because, as disbelievers, they performed their own surveys. They continued to monitor the effects of DES, and repeatedly found facts that contradicted those in the *JAMA* report.

On February 27, 1975, Belita Cowan, a health instructor, testified at Senator Kennedy's hearings (the senator broke precedent for congressional health hearings by seeking opinions from patients and consumer advocates, as well as physicians and scientists):

> Last summer, I conducted a survey of over 200 women, ages eighteen to thirty-one, who had taken DES as a morning-after pill in Ann Arbor, Michigan, between 1968 and August of 1974. Twenty-nine percent of my sample stated that they had taken the morning-after pill at least twice within a year's time.
>
> "The study showed that DES is being prescribed with carelessness and casualness. Forty-five percent were not given pelvic or breast exams. Fifty-six percent stated that the doctor did not take a personal and family medical history. Eight women said that they got the morning-after pill not for

themselves but for a friend or roommate. Only 26 percent were followed up to see if they were pregnant.

"The study also revealed that DES is being given to women for whom estrogens are contraindicated. Women who cannot take birth control pills are being given the morning-after pill. They are not aware, nor are they informed, that the morning-after pill is estrogen.

"Fifty-seven percent of the sample were unaware that the morning-after pill did not have FDA approval and that it had not been proven safe and effective.

"Further, the study revealed that many women are not being told of the possible cancerous effects to the fetus if the woman is [already] pregnant. I could not find a single case where a pregnancy test was given prior to and after the DES regimen.

"Six percent of those in the survey stated that they themselves were DES daughters; that is, their mothers took stilbestrol when they were pregnant in the early 1950s. Of all the doctors I interviewed, only one expressed hesitation about giving the morning-after pill to DES daughters. Dr. Ann Pfrender of the University of Michigan Health Services stated that, 'We don't know the effects of the morning-after pill to DES daughters, so I don't give it to them.'

"The most interesting finding of the study is that 24 percent of the women stated that they did not take all ten pills in the series. As one woman put it, 'I got so sick from the first pill that I never took the rest. I couldn't stand to be that ill!' And not surprisingly, 65 percent stated that if they had been fully informed about DES, they would not have taken it [the morning-after pill] in the first place."

SECOND THOUGHTS ABOUT THE MORNING-AFTER PILL

The drug companies themselves are patently uneasy about morning-after DES. As FDA commissioner

Alexander Schmidt admitted in 1975: "DES is a generic drug and is made by many manufacturers, none of whom came forward with data to support the use of DES as a postcoital contraceptive."

They didn't come forward—they backed off!

In the *Physicians' Desk Reference*, 1977 edition, the Eli Lilly Pharmaceutical Company's thousand-word description of its diethylstilbestrol tablets starts out with the warning in oversized capital letters: "THIS DRUG PRODUCT SHOULD NOT BE USED AS A POSTCOITAL CONTRACEPTIVE."

At this writing, the University of Michigan is still using the DES pill, and so are thousands of other health services and private doctors. Doctors, the guardians of health, are prescribing a product for a purpose which its major manufacturer, a frankly profit-making concern, is publicly warning against.

It's Only Once Around the Merry-Go-Round

MARGOT ADLER

Margot Adler, "It's Only Once Around the Merry-Go-Round," *Heretic's Heart: A Journey through Spirit and Revolution*, Boston: Beacon Press, 1997. Reprinted by permission.

My mother, Freyda, has been dead for twenty-five years, but her exuberant energy was so intense that she still receives mail. A skeptic might say that it's the persistence of junk mail in our society that is remarkable, that explains why civil rights groups are still asking her for donations and banks are still offering her credit cards. But as I recently began to go through personal and family documents—journals and letters dating from the 1930s to the 1960s that I'd kept over the years—I came to realize that much of my life has been animated by my mother's persistent spirit, and that she, more than anyone, has a claim on setting and naming the parameters of my political and spiritual journey.

My mother died in January of 1970. She was sixty-one. She had been a heavy smoker who quit too late in life (actually, one of her friends recently hinted to me that she never really quit). Her illness was diagnosed just months after the end of a bitter New York teachers' strike in which my mother, in deep turmoil, had crossed a picket line for the first time in her life—that of her own union—to support a group of black parents. Her illness also happened at a time when she was truly happy and in love, perhaps for the first time. Just a year before her diagnosis, she confided to me that she had finally experienced "going over the rainbow." I always wondered if a small voice inside her said that she came from a suffering people and had no right to such happiness. She developed lung cancer which quickly metastasized to her brain and then her liver. The end was a lingering, unpleasant death that she only partly comprehended.

In the late 1960s, most patients with cancer were not told the truth of their situation. In my mother's case, many doctors, including a psychiatrist, decided that she did not really want to know. Their policy of disguising the truth was taken to such an extreme that when my mother asked to see her medical records, one of her doctors served up a phony piece of official-looking paper that said her tumor was benign. "B-e-n-i-g-n," she told all of her friends, "is the most beautiful word in the English language." And then she could never understand why she wasn't getting better.

Among those of my parents' generation, illness and death were rarely discussed. When I was a teenager my father waited a full week to inform me that my grandmother had died, not wanting to "ruin my vacation." And when my aunt went into the hospital some years later for cancer, I was told "it was a heart problem."

Most of my mother's friends also accepted the wisdom of the time, believing that she either did not want to know or in fact knew everything on some deeper level. At the time I felt intuitively that this policy was hellish, that my mother, a woman who planned so well for everything,

would have despised such paternalism. She would have desired the truth in order to prepare for the end of her life with dignity. But I did not feel I could fight the combined judgment of seven male doctors single-handedly. I acquiesced. And I raged, silently, confused that I, a mere twenty-three-year-old, *knew*, while the most powerful figure in my life was kept from the truth, infantilized. I knew I would never again take a doctor's statement at face value and all institutional documents would remain suspect. For several years after my mother died I would take a longer route to avoid the hospital that had deceived her. And when my mother told me, several months after she'd been told her tumor was benign, "I feel like I am in a dark tunnel, and I can't see the end," I did not find myself reassured that my own silence was right.

How Do You Know It's True?

VICTOR COHN

Victor Cohn, "How Do You Know It's True? Probable Fact and Probable Junk," *NewsBackgrounder*, Los Angeles: Foundation for American Communications, 1994. Reprinted by permission.

A politician says "I don't believe in statistics," then maintains that "most" people or "many" do or think such-and-such. Based on what? A doctor reports a "promising" new treatment. Is the claim justified or based on a biased or unrepresentative sample? A poll says "here's what people think" with a "three point plus or minus margin of error." Believable, when we know polls can be wrong? An environmentalist says a nuclear power plant or toxic dump will cause cancers. An industry spokesman indignantly denies it. Who's right?

What can we believe? What's worth reporting? And the question that must concern us both as reporters and citizens: what's worth doing something about?

Some years ago I set out to try to find some answers, especially answers for a nonmathematician like me, confounded by forbidding formulas. I talked to many statisticians and epidemiologists. I was told that a critical understanding of claims about almost anything requires not so much an understanding of formulas as an understanding of the bases of science and rational evidence. And I found that we reporters could copy the methods of science and try to judge claims of fact, whether by scientists or physicians or others, by the same rules of evidence scientists use. An honest investigator may first form a hypothesis or theory, an attempt to describe truth, then try to disprove it by what is called the null hypothesis: to prove that there is no such truth. To back the hypothesis, a study must reject the null hypothesis. Similarly, a jury is instructed to start with a presumption of innocence and say to the prosecution, prove your case, provide the evidence and disprove innocence. Somewhat similarly, we reporters may say to ourselves, at least, "I don't believe you; show me."

We may ask simple yet revealing questions like:

➤ *How do you know?* Are you just telling us something you "know" or have "observed" or "found to be true?" Or have you done or found any studies or experiments?

➤ *What are your data, your numbers?* Where or how did you get them?

➤ *How sure can you be about them?* What is your degree of certainty or uncertainty by accepted tests? (See "Probability" below.)

➤ *How valid (in science, valid means accurate) are they?* How reliable, which means how reproducible? Have results been fairly consistent from study to study?

We can then go a long way toward discerning the probable facts from the probable junk, a long way toward judging claims and statistics that are thrown at us, by learning six basic concepts that apply to all science, all studies, and virtually all knowledge of society and the universe. Remembering these can teach us to ask, "How do you know?" with a considerable degree of sophistication.

They are:

UNCERTAINTY

All science is almost always uncertain to a degree. Nature is complex, research is difficult, observation is inexact, all studies have flaws, so science is always an evolving story. Almost all anyone can say about the behavior of atoms or cells or human beings or the biosphere is that there is a strong probability that such-and-such is true, and we may know more tomorrow.

This tells us why things so often seem settled one way today and another tomorrow, and why so much is debated, whether the effects of global warming, a pesticide, a high-fat diet, or a medical treatment.

Why so much uncertainty? There are many reasons: lack of funds to do enough research; the expense and difficulty of much research; the ethical obstacles to using human beings as guinea pigs. But a main reason is the lack of long, continuing observations of large populations to track one possible effect or another, observations that would often be perfectly possible.

It is important to tell all this to the public, including our readers, viewers, and listeners, so they will understand why "they" say one thing today, another tomorrow—and how uncertainty need not impede crucial action if society understands and uses these other principles.

PROBABILITY

Scientists live with uncertainty by measuring probability. An accepted numerical express is the *p-value*, determined by a formula that considers the number of subjects or events being compared to decide if a given result could have seemed to occur just by chance, when there actually had been no effect.

A p-value of .05 or less is most often regarded as low or desirable, since it means there are probably only five or fewer chances in 100 that this result could have happened by chance. This value is called *statistical significance.* In judging studies, look for both a p-value and a high confidence level, another measure.

Do not trust a study that is not statistically significant, but know that this may or may not mean *practical* (or in medicine, *clinical*) significance. Nor does it alone mean there is a cause and effect. Association is not causation without further evidence. Remember the rooster who thought his crowing made the sun rise.

The laws of probability and chance tell us to expect some unusual, even impossible-sounding events. Just as a persistent coin tosser would sometime toss heads or tails several times in a row, nature will randomly produce many alarming clusters of cancers or birth defects that have no cause but nature's coin tossing. These produce striking anecdotes and often striking news stories, but they alone do not constitute reliable information that says, "there *is* a cause."

There is something else to remember when someone says, "how do they know this stuff isn't causing harm?" Science cannot prove a negative. No one can prove that little green men from Mars have not visited Earth. The burden of proof should be on those who say something is true.

POWER

Statistically, power means the likelihood of finding something if it's there, say, an increase in cancer in workers exposed to some substance. The greater the number of cases or subjects studied, the greater a conclusion's power and probable truth.

Be wary of studies with only a small number of cases. Sometimes large numbers indeed are needed. The likelihood that a thirty- to thirty-nine-year-old woman will suffer a heart attack while taking an oral contraceptive may be about 1 per 18,000 women per year. To be 95 percent sure of finding at least one such event in a one-year trial, researchers would have to observe 54,000 women. This tells us why we so often learn of a drug's harmful side effects only after it has been studied and approved and is being used by many thousands.

There is also a great problem in trying to identify low-level, yet possibly important risks, whether of air pollution, pesticides, low-level radiation, or some other cause. For lack of power (that is, enough cases), a condition that affects one person in hundreds of thousands may never be recognized or associated with a particular cause. It is probable and perhaps inevitable that a large yet scattered number of environmentally or industrially caused illnesses remain forever undetected as "environmental illnesses," because they remain only a fraction of the vastly greater normal case load.

BIAS

Bias in science means introducing spurious associations and reaching unreliable conclusions by failing to consider other influential factors—confounding variables. Among common biases: failing to take account of age, gender, occupation, nationality, race, income, health, or behaviors like smoking.

For years, older age and smoking were largely ignored variables or factors when scientists considered the ill effects of birth control pills. In occupation studies, the workers exposed to some substance often turn out to be healthier than persons without such exposure. The confounding variable: workers are healthier than the general population with its many unhealthy people.

Polls, political and otherwise, as well as medical and environmental studies, are all subject to sampling bias, since every group studied is only a sample of a larger population, and selecting a sample is never foolproof. If you stood on a street corner and asked people whether they had heart disease, you could throw out the result. Too many of the heart diseased were staying home.

Watch for bias by asking, "Are there any other possible explanations?"

VARIABILITY

A common pitfall of science is that everything measured or studied varies from measurement to measurement. Every human experiment, repeated, has at least slightly (and sometimes markedly) different results. Among reasons: our constantly fluctuating physiologies; common errors or limits in measurement or observation; and biologic variations in the same person, between persons, and between populations. Persons in different parts of the country often react differently to the same conditions, thanks to differences between persons or environments, or thanks to pure chance. This is a common trap for the environmental observer or reporter.

Ask, too, about any association's statistical strength—in other words, the odds. The greater the odds against an association's being a matter of chance, the greater its strength. If a pollutant seems to be causing a 10 percent increase above background, it may or may not be a meaningful association. If a risk is ten times greater—the relative risk in cigarette smokers versus non-smokers—the odds are strong that something is happening.

HIERARCHY OF STUDIES

There is a hierarchy of studies—from the least to the generally most believable, starting with simple anecdotes and going on to more systematic observation or "eyeballing," then proceeding to true experiments, comparing one population or sample with another under controlled or known conditions.

Many epidemiologic and medical studies are retrospective, looking back in time at old records or statistics or memories. This is often necessary. It if often unreliable. Far better is the prospective study that follows a selected population for a long period, sometimes years. The famous Framingham (Massachusetts) study of behaviors and diets that may be associated with heart disease began following more than 6,000 persons in 1948.

When someone tells you, "I've done a study," ask, "What kind? How confident can you be in the results? Were there any possible flaws in the study?"

An honest researcher will almost always report flaws. A dishonest one may claim perfection. All we have said also tells us that a single study rarely proves anything. The most believable studies and observations are those repeated among different populations with much the same result, and supported, if possibly, by animal or other biologic evidence.

Understand rates. There is a wide lack of understanding of the difference between a rate—so many per so many per unit of time—and a mere number. A headline in the *Washington Post* once read, "Airline Accident Rate Is Highest in 13 Years," but the story, like many others misusing the word "rate," merely reported death and crash totals. A correction had to be printed pointing out that the number of accidents per 100,000 departures had been declining year after year.

Similarly, watch risk numbers. Their choice can be someone's decision picked to influence reporters and the public. Someone may use an annual death total, or deaths per thousand or per million, or per thousand persons exposed, or deaths per ton of some substance or per ton released in the air or per facility. There can be lots of choices to make something sound better or worse.

An example. A proposed federal law would have required antipollution devices to remove 98 percent of auto tailpipe emissions, compared with a current 96 percent. Industry called that only a 2 percent increase in removal. Environmentalists called it a 50 percent decline in auto pollution. The solution: report both numbers.

All this says: Look for evidence, including sound statistics, that make a study or indeed any statement of fact supposedly backed by statistics worth reporting. Ask, "How do you know?" and other questions. As a doctor at the National Institutes of Health once said while exhibiting a sophisticated body scanning machine to reporters, "Ask to see the numbers, not just the pretty colors."

Diana Petitti, MD

INTERVIEW BY TANIA KETENJIAN

Diana Petitti, MD, is a practicing epidemiologist and the director of the Research and Evaluation Department at Kaiser Permanente Medical Program in the Southern California region. This interview was conducted in May 1999.

TK: You have long been attempting to help the public distinguish between sound medical studies and those that leap to premature or misleading conclusions.

DP: Yes. I would like people to be more focused on telling the truth about what research says, free of political or commercial biases. I feel that there are many interests that tend to distort the truth to fit both political and financial ends. This is a source of great frustration to me.

TK: What have you done that has caused controversy in the science, health, and pharmaceutical industries?

DP: My research findings have caused controversy because they are not necessarily in the interests of vested groups. Distortions are not limited to the pharmaceutical industry. When people have a bias about a drug or an intervention, they tend to take the data and interpret it selectively for their own purposes, or to attack the person and the data because it doesn't confirm things in their terms.

TK: How should we interpret the contradictory medical information with which we are bombarded?

DP: First of all, people looking at evidence should understand that no single study ever finds the absolute truth, so there's a red light when a single study is interpreted as being definitive. What is truth today may not be all of the truth tomorrow. In thinking about, for example, oral contraceptives and hormone replacement therapy—fields that I work in—in the early '60s, there was a substantial amount of evidence to show that oral contraceptives

used then had a substantially high risk of vascular complications. Now here we are, almost forty years later, and we have new pills and new ways of using oral contraceptives that are safe for most women. There can be problems in using single studies as if those single studies are a definitive answer to a specific question. Take, for example, how the Nurses' Health Study at Harvard and anything that comes out of it is considered to be *the* answer to the question for now and all time. I think that is an oversimplification of the evidence and an unfortunate reliance on a single study.

TK: So how should someone know whether they can really rely on a study? What are the characteristics of a well done study?

DP: Take a topic—for example, does hormone replacement therapy prevent cardiovascular disease—a person who relies on a single study on that topic would really be fooling themselves. I think that when one looks at an individual study and tries to assess its quality, the criteria should be: how well described is the protocol; was this a study that had, depending on the design, a good response rate; has the analysis been conducted appropriately; was there attention to validity and reliability in the primary data collected; have the authors appropriately interpreted the results; and was the study large enough to support whatever conclusions are being made from the data? But again, interpretation of single studies is not really something that concerns me in the science of health today. The problem is more the selection of a single study, and drawing conclusions based on that single study, while ignoring the remainder of the evidence. Even if it is a good study, single studies don't tell the truth.

TK: What answers do we most urgently need?.

DP: I'd like to see us get answers more quickly on some topics where we have fairly definitive evidence for men, but don't have definitive evidence for women. One example is the use of aspirin for the primary prevention of coronary heart disease.

That is a topic where we have a lot of data for men and don't have it for women. I wish we could more quickly get a definitive answer to the question of whether or not hormone replacement is effective as the primary prevention of coronary heart disease. That answer will only come from randomized trials, and we're going to be stuck with no large randomized trials for probably at least another six years.

However, the Heart and Estrogen/Progestin Replacement Study (HERS) has answered one of the questions of hormone replacement therapy and coronary disease for women pretty well. This study was a large—more than 2000 subjects—randomized trial that studied the effect of combined estrogen/progestin replacement therapy on coronary heart disease in women who already had coronary disease. After four years, rates of heart disease and death were identical between the women who took hormone replacement and those who took a placebo.

TK: Can you define a randomized trial?

DP: A randomized trial is a kind of study in which women are assigned to treatment at random . . . that is, by chance. When there is randomization, subjects in the study are identical in all respects other than treatment, and the randomized trial is considered to be the best method for finding out whether drugs and other kinds of medical treatment really work.

TK: The pharmaceutical and medical industries have their own biases and financial needs. How does that affect the work that you do?

DP: The pharmaceutical industry has an enormous amount of money to invest in clinical research and I think that they are, in general, excellent in designing and conducting large-scale randomized trials. The problem is that they are not interested in topics that hold for them no commercial interest. I think the hormone estrogen-progestin replacement study funded by Wyeth-Ayerst (hormone manufacturer–Premarin) is an example of study design being influenced by the company's commercial interest in promoting combination estrogen-progestin replacement therapy. That study should have had an arm that also looked at estrogen alone.

TK: Can you discuss Years of Potential Life Lost—YPLL—and the difference between death of women arising from heart disease, which is more common, versus death arising from breast cancer, where women die at an earlier age?

DP: In the end, it's actually a matter of personal preference more than something that policy makers can dictate. For an individual, it's a question of, "Would I rather get breast cancer when I'm forty in order to prevent heart disease when I'm eighty?" And that is a personal choice. There are a number of measures that attempt to balance adverse effects or positive effects on health at an early-versus-late age and the years of healthy life lost is one of those metrics.

TK: What should a patient know when she is looking into elective drugs? What should she look for; what information should she seek out?

DP: When people are deciding whether or not to do something—to take a drug or make a lifestyle change in order to prevent future death or disability, or to actually prolong healthy life—they have to think very carefully about whether there is an evidence-base for making that lifestyle change or using that drug. When you're healthy and you do something to enhance health, that intervention should be held, both for individuals and for society, to a very high standard of evidence proven to work in randomized group trials. That should be a standard for individuals and for society. Then, beyond that, obviously there are questions of, "Is this convenient for me; how expensive is it; am I likely to be one of those people who will specifically benefit from this?"

TK: How can a patient figure that out?

DP: Scientists and policy makers have an obligation to try and make this information available to people in a form that they can understand. Scientists, funding agencies, and policy makers are obligated to support studies that answer questions definitively and to not promote changes in lifestyle or use of drugs for prevention until they are proven definitively to work.

TK How do you think they can make that happen?

DP: They can get it done through political activism, through organizations like the National Women's Health Network, and through media and the influence of consumers on the media.

TK: What was your experience as an advisor to the Food and Drug Administration?

DP: It was actually fun. I enjoyed participating in the process of deciding what drugs should be allowed onto the market. My experience with the FDA as a member of their advisory committee and as an expert consultant, which I've been doing for almost twenty years now, is that the work done by the FDA is on a very high level scientifically, and that the advisory committee is a group of very hard working people who are doing everything they can to make the right decisions.

TK: So you approve of the way the FDA works?

DP: I like the way the advisory committee that I was on worked; I was impressed with the quality of the work and with the staff.

TK: Do you find that there are some general beliefs about heart disease that are inaccurate and that really need to be changed?

DP: In the last five years there has been a gratifying, increased recognition of the contribution of both heart disease and stroke to morbidity and mortality of women. I do think there had previously been a tendency to think of coronary heart disease in particular as being a disease in men and not a disease in women, so that's been a major change. Because of the promotion of hormone replacement therapy as a way to prevent heart disease, women have in general ignored other things that they might do in order to maximize their cardiovascular health including maintaining ideal body weight, getting screened for cholesterol, and use of cholesterol-lowering drugs if they have high cholesterol. Probably someday, if we have the definitive information, we can start thinking about taking aspirin to prevent heart disease and maybe not taking cancer-causing hormones.

TK: Are cholesterol-lowering drugs effective?

DP: In my opinion, there is convincing data that cholesterol-lowering drugs in people who have elevated cholesterol, and even in people who have only borderline elevated cholesterol, do decrease morbidity and mortality. The data, although very sparse, shows that conclusion also applies to women.

TK: What do you think of estrogen replacement therapy and hormone replacement therapy in relation to heart disease?

DP: In my opinion, we do not have the definitive study showing that either estrogen replacement therapy or hormone replacement therapy is useful for primary prevention of coronary disease in women, and that is an extremely important question. We have a large body of observational data which is sort of consistent but which in my opinion all suffers from the same bias.

TK: What same bias does the body of observational data suffer from?

DP: All observational studies of HRT and cardiovascular disease suffer from the possibility of selection of healthier women and women who follow healthy lifestyles for estrogen use. This has been called "compliance bias"—the observation of lower cardiovascular mortality in men and women who are compliant with taking the medications. Both "prevention bias," the propensity of women who take hormones to be more likely to engage in other behaviors that might prevent cardiovascular disease, and "compliance bias" have been demonstrated empirically. In other words, these biases are not just theoretical.

TK: There seem to be a number of different sorts of biases that can skew test results. Would you expand a little on them?

DP: Bias is a general term that is used to refer to something that distorts the truth. When people who take and don't take a drug differ for reasons other than drug taking, there is the possiblity of bias—distortion of the truth.

Selection bias, prevention bias, and compliance bias are three categories of ways that ERT/HRT users might differ from nonusers and might distort observational studies. Selection bias refers to demographic characteristics such as education and race that differ between users and nonusers. Since education and race are related to heart disease, studies could conclude that ERT/HRT use prevents heart disease when the real reason for the lower risk is factors like race and education.

Prevention bias refers to differences between HRT users and non-users in other preventive interventions and behaviors, for example, exercise or a low fat diet. Since these reduce the risk of heart disease, studies could conclude that ERT/HRT use prevents heart disease when the real reason for the lower risk is more exercise and better diet in ERT/HRT users.

Compliance bias is subtle—it has been shown that people who take their pills, even their placebo pills, are less likely to die of heart disease than people who do not take their pills—even placebo pills. Users of ERT/HRT are all, by definition, pill takers. The lower risk of heart disease in nonexperimental studies of ERT/HRT may be because ERT/HRT users are pill takers—that is, the studies are subject to distortion because of compliance bias.

TK: What made you decide to become an epidemiologist?

DP: I loved statistics and I wanted to be a researcher because, at the time that I was training to be a physician, it was my opinion that much of what we told people to do and not to do was not based on evidence. I wanted to find the answers before I told people what to do with their lives.

TK: What do you feel has changed since you started working as an epidemiologist?

DP: What we tell people to do and the basis of medicine is much more firmly grounded in high quality evidence now than it was twenty-five years ago when I graduated from medical school and decided to become an epidemiologist.

TK: And there are still changes that need to be realized, one of them being that people don't focus so much on one study?

DP: People are no longer focusing so much on one study: studies are bigger, better, and designed correctly. The whole era of the randomized trial is really a phenomenon of the last two decades.

TK: Do you know of any centers or institutions that provide reliable studies in general?

DP: I think that National Institutes of Health–funded studies are very high quality. I have a very hard time finding any randomized trial funded by NIH that is not held to an extremely high standard both in terms of the science and the monitoring of the science, and the publications that come from there. I think we have to be really proud of the industry that we've created through the NIH of getting high quality data.

TK: Of which of your accomplishments are you the most proud?

DP: Well, I am actually proud of my book. I wrote a book entitled *Meta-Analysis, Decision Analysis, and Cost-Effectiveness: Methods for Quantitative Synthesis in Medicine* (New York: Oxford University Press, 1994), which is a methods book about how to synthesize evidence, and the book, which was kind of ahead of its time, has been very successful and very well received. It was a little different than doing an individual study, actually more difficult. I am very pleased with the studies I did on oral contraceptives and vascular disease. I have done quite a lot of work as a member of the World Health Organization's steering committee on reproductive health. I have been on that committee off and on since 1983, and the work that that steering committee oversaw resulted in about 100 different publications related to reproductive health in developing countries. It was a major accomplishment with which my name is not actually associated for anything other than having served on the committee. I am pleased with my membership on the FDA advisory committee because during my tenure, I was on the committee that recommended the approval of emergency contraception and RU-486. Those were incredibly controversial topics for any organization and I think the committee made the right decisions.

TK: What is the most important thing you learned in your work?

DP: The lag time between asking a question and getting an answer is incredibly long and I think that's probably one of the most important things I've learned in the last twenty-five years that I have been working as a researcher: how incredibly long it takes to get an answer. I think the answers to the questions that were posed ten years ago will only be forthcoming in the next five years.

A Different Prescription

ANNE ROCHON FORD

Anne Rochon Ford, *A Different Prescription: Considerations for Women's Health Groups Contemplating Funding from the Pharmaceutical Industry,* Toronto, Canada: Institute for Feminist Legal Studies, 1999. Reprinted by permission.

INTRODUCTION

In Canada over the past ten years, community-based women's health organizations have been experiencing continued government cutbacks.

At the same time, nonprofit organizations in many sectors—not just health—are being strongly encouraged to form "partnerships" with industry. Although it is not always clear exactly what is meant by "partnerships," one thing that is usually implied is the assumption that money should be sought from industry and if money is offered it should not be refused.

For the corporate sector, it is in their best corporate interest to spread some of their wealth and to give generously to community-based organizations and enter into sponsorship arrangements with them.

You may be such an organization struggling with this issue and trying to determine whether you should put your energy into developing such partnerships and, more specifically, whether you should accept money from the pharmaceutical industry.

This booklet may help to shed a little more light on your decision. It has been developed out of strong concerns about the implications of pharmaceutical industry sponsorship of women's health organizations, and what they might mean both to individual groups and to the women's health movement as a whole.

Why just women's health groups? We decided to narrow the focus because women have a particular relationship to pharmaceuticals, which makes some of their issues unique. Women are often the specific target for advertising by pharmaceutical companies, either because of their reproductive needs or because women are most often the ones in their families who make decisions about their family's health care needs. They visit doctors more often than men, either for themselves or for other family members, and therefore are more likely to be prescribed drugs. They are prescribed mood-altering drugs at a higher rate than men. As the sole users of most birth control products—a particularly lucrative market for the pharmaceutical industry—they are often faced with difficult decisions about the safety and efficacy of their choices. As the primary caregivers of sick family members, they are more likely to see the effects—both positive and negative—of other women who have had bad experiences with a particular medication, and are more likely to have read magazine and newspaper articles about medication which has been helpful for particular conditions.

Pharmaceutical companies specifically target women's groups because women's health is becoming increasingly medicalized. It was only a few decades ago that there were no drugs for menopause, menstrual discomforts, irregular menstrual cycles, breast cancer prevention, and fertility problems.

In short, we have a relationship to this issue which is specific to us because we are women. Added to this equation is the fact that drugs and devices that have proven to be harmful to women have appeared on the market in recent decades. Because of the legacy of harmful drugs and devices such as DES, thalidomide, and the Dalkon shield, many North American women in particular have become increasingly wary about the decisions they make in relation to prescription drugs. At the same time, the pharmaceutical industry has increased its efforts to sell its products directly to a public that has become highly dependent on drugs.

A COMMON SCENARIO

A women's health organization in a large Canadian city has been offering useful information and support to women who have been diagnosed with a particular disease or disorder. Users of this service indicate that they are grateful for the help the service offers them in making difficult decisions about treatment options. They appreciate being able to talk to other women with the disease and feel like they can get on with the rest of their lives.

A member of the board of directors of the organization brings a plan to the board and the staff members. She has a good friend who works for drug company X, manufacturers of a drug frequently used by women with this disease. This friend has been telling her that she knows her company would give money to help out the service—they just have to say how much they need. The board member presenting this thinks it is a good idea. The board is divided. Opinions vary widely.

Let's take a closer look at some of the comments made by the board members and staff.

"It's a win-win situation—they get to feel better because they're doing something that makes them look good, and we have money to keep our service running. What can be wrong with that?"

On the surface, this scenario does indeed look like a win-win situation. And some groups will come to the decision to take the money and not only be quite comfortable with that decision but be able to put the money to good use. Their members will benefit and the drug company will be able to say it has done a good deed with their donation.

A representative from a group for women with AIDS who spoke at the panel discussion described their decision to accept pharmaceutical money: The money they have received from the industry has allowed them to offer programs that they feel they could not otherwise offer. She also pointed out that the survival of her group members is partially linked to the drugs they take, so they have always had a close relationship with the drug industry. The money is often used for direct donations to the women in need as opposed to being directly tied to a product line.

On the other hand, others feel that it may look like a win-win situation, but the winning is mostly done by the pharmaceutical company. One panelist, who had canvassed representatives from some of the manufacturers of the most commonly prescribed drugs for women's reproductive conditions, learned that most donations to women's health groups (and other non-profit health organizations) come from the marketing budget of a company. In most cases, donations are linked to a product or product line of that particular company. Therefore, you would not likely see a company which does not manufacture, for example, a fertility medication, giving money to an infertility support group, and similarly, companies which manufacture fertility medication would specifically target infertility groups for their donations.

The industry has much to gain from making such donations and forming such links. First, association with a reputable organization can provide a more credible endorsement of their product than if the promotion were coming directly from the industry (i.e., the goodwill associated with a company's name when they are seen to be making contributions to groups can have a direct impact in the public's mind about the value of their products).

Secondly, if a company is in the prelaunch phase of the introduction of a new drug, they can use the captive audience of the group they have funded to spread awareness among the public about their drug and about the disease that the drug is treating. This awareness will generally not extend to prevention and other forms of treatment, specifically not to other drugs made by competitors. Funding an organization to provide educational outreach about a disease such as osteoporosis serves to raise the general public's awareness of this issue and, importantly for the drug company, of drug treatments which are being developed to treat it.

Finally, if a drug company is seeking approval from regulatory bodies for a drug that they have manufactured, they can use their funded groups to help them argue for the need for approval of this drug.

There is, however, one way in which an industry wins and the recipient of their money can lose: Support from the industry dulls criticism. The National Women's Health Network in the United States, for example, has developed a policy not to take money from the pharmaceutical industry. The main reason they offer is that one of the foundations of their educational work is to encourage women to seek alternatives to pills and surgery in dealing with their health problems, and to look at the social and economic reasons behind much ill health.

"I think we should just take the money wherever we can get it. It's the only way we'll keep this service alive. We can't afford to be purists."

This is a commonly held opinion. Many groups are dealing with the sheer logistics of survival and staying alive, and feel they can't afford to look a gift horse in the mouth.

Although hard to look at, it might be worth asking, "Is this really the *only* way you'll keep this service alive?" Frequently the option of pharmaceutical money comes to groups without a lot of effort. The industry is looking to form partnerships such as this, and in the larger scheme of things, offering money to a community-based women's health organization to keep its doors open represents a drop in the bucket of their profits.

Groups are often surprised when after years of hounding philanthropic organizations and individual donors for money, the offer for money from a pharmaceutical company comes to them almost effortlessly. Understandably, this is enormously appealing to anyone who is sick and tired of trying to raise money. But the question then might be, if this came so effortlessly, is it the only money to be had without much struggle?

You may want to consider the local bank where your group does banking, companies which employ your board members or families of consumers who use your service. Is there a member of your group who knows a wealthy individual dealing with the health problem your group is involved in? One patron can often donate as much as an individual company.

"What do you mean?—'It's dirty money?' Isn't all money dirty money?"

The term "dirty money" has been used to describe money which may have been used for less than honorable purposes. Some people have argued that there is no difference between taking money from the pharmaceutical companies and accepting money from banks, insurance companies, or other large corporations. The argument goes that those companies or financial institutions which may appear to have no strings attached to their money may also be funding practices or carrying out activities, particularly in third world countries, which your group would find ethically questionable.

"Isn't this just free publicity for the company?"

If your organization does choose to accept money from a pharmaceutical company which manufactures a product used by members of your group, it is worth keeping in mind that you are indirectly providing endorsement of that company and their product through your action. It is in the company's best interest to have this endorsement of their product from a non-commercial source.

Similarly, if the company funding you is developing a new product for your user group (e.g., a fertility drug in the case of an infertility group) your group may unwittingly become the focus for promotion of this drug by the company. The group may become a conduit of information for the company to the potential users of the drug. In the case of a drug which is badly needed and has been properly tested, this may not be such a bad thing. In the case of a drug which is simply a copycat of another product on the market, the relationship becomes a little more questionable.

Some groups may be quite comfortable with this while other may not. Each group must come to its own conclusions about what role they may want to play—either directly or indirectly—in promoting a company and its product. Some groups go as far as outright promotion of a product in exchange for funding.

If you are accepting money, you may want to be very clear from the start what the parameters of that relationship are and get it in writing. At a minimum, the company should be made to understand clearly that it cannot directly attempt to influence the advice a group gives its members, nor can it use the members as targets for promotion of their products. This may be easier said than done. You may want to seek legal advice around the wording of your contract or letter of agreement.

"This same company also manufactures pesticides which have been shown to contribute to this disease. Why would we want to endorse that?"

In part from pressure from environmental and health activists, more research is slowly being done into the links between cancer and toxins in the environment, such as pesticides. As women's health groups probe further into this, we have been disturbed to find that sometimes the very companies which are manufacturing cancer therapy are also producing toxic pesticides which may be contributing to cancer in the first place.

For example, Zeneca, the manufacturers of tamoxifen citrate, earn $470 million each year marketing this cancer therapy drug, at the same time as it earns $300 million each year from sales of the carcinogenic herbicide acetochlor.

The women's health movement and more recently the breast cancer movement has long purported prevention as one of the main tenets of its outreach and advocacy efforts. When links are found between potential funders and the causes of the diseases the groups are fighting, this is often a connection many are not prepared to live with.

When considering funding from a pharmaceutical company, it is always helpful to do some background research on the products the company manufacturers and other aspects of their dealings. You may also want to consider a company's employment practices—how it treats its workers, if women have been allowed to advance equitably in the company, and about its practices in Third World countries.

This information is easily found in public libraries, in the company's annual reports, and on the Internet. Doing this kind of research is generally good advice for accepting *any* corporate donations, not just those from pharmaceutical companies, since corporations can often have disparate holdings you are unaware of.

"If we take their money, we're turning our backs on all the women who object to this type of sponsorship, women who feel they've been harmed more than helped by the pharmaceutical industry."

There is no question that many products of the pharmaceutical industry help countless people worldwide to both stay alive and to live a better quality of life. Nevertheless, in its aim to increase its profits, the industry has *also* manufactured products which have seriously harmed many women, usually due to improper initial testing.

It is wise to keep in mind that a decision of whether or not to be involved with the pharmaceutical industry is a decision which is taken within an historical context. The context is one which has a particularly problematic legacy.

"Most women just want the help. They don't really care where the money comes from."

This may be very true for a number of women and for many organizations. Certainly when we are dealing with diseases such as cancer, it is often the case that people will "do anything" to get help or get access to a new treatment, whatever the emotional or financial cost.

Staff members and members of boards have a duty to make fair and ethical decisions on behalf of their members or clients. A group may choose to use this time of decision-making as an opportunity to raise awareness about a number of related issues: (1) the role the pharmaceutical industry plays in our lives and the extent to which we have become a society dependent on pharmaceutical solutions; (2) discuss the level of transparency and accountability in the regulation of drugs by the federal government; or (3) arrange an evening with speakers from women's health organizations who have developed policies on this issue.

There is no one correct prescription for everyone on this issue. Each group must decide for itself which is the best route to go.

"They've told us there are no strings attached to this money and they seem to be willing to stick to that. Their attitude seems to be 'hands off.' Why should we doubt that?"

One women's health organizer, looking at this issue for her organization, commented, "There are strings, but they are strings of gossamer," meaning there are strings but you can't always see them.

It is important to remember that an industry's motivations for giving money to an organization are not philanthropic in nature. They give money to targeted groups in targeted fields that relate to their product lines.

Groups may find themselves in this situation unwittingly. The original overture from a drug company may have come from a perfectly well-intentioned individual who cared about their group. Companies are made up of individuals, and individuals of all companies would like to feel they

work for a business that is a good corporate citizen. As much as companies wish to buy goodwill, staff in drug companies also pressure their employers to make donations to community-based organizations they feel committed to. Although the donation may come from marketing and all that that involves, the original impetus may not.

Similarly, most researchers who work for pharmaceutical companies come directly from university or have been recruited from a research project. Most of them begin their career with good intentions of hoping to "cure" diseases. While the company as an entity is concerned with profit, the individuals lower down the hierarchy are not always so motivated. Contacts between individuals from a pharmaceutical company and a community organization can be made with the best of intentions by the initial individuals. Later the group may be taken by surprise when the company indicates they would like a higher level of public recognition or sponsorship or indicates they don't like the way in which their product or the whole industry is portrayed in the group's literature.

One thing your group can do is talk to other community organizations that have accepted money from or engaged in some sort of partnership with that same company. Find out what their experience has been in working with that company. For example, the Infertility Network (Canada), which has received funds from Organon and Serono, agreed to have their name added to a brochure about infertility produced by Serono. The executive director noted, "This was important to them [the company], but it helped raise our profile and so it suited our purposes to do it." Another group might feel compromised by the same experience. Each organization has their own story to tell.

We can learn from the experience of other organizations who have worked through this issue. The following are some general guidelines culled from the May 1997 panel discussion and from other groups consulted since then about how to proceed when entering into sponsorship agreements with a pharmaceutical company or in accepting money from them.

1. If you are a newly formed group or one that has not yet dealt with this issue, it is probably best to assume that you will be confronted with it at some point. Most groups find it helpful to develop a written policy on the subject and to make the policy known to their members. The policy may be as formal as being a part of your by-laws or, more commonly, a general policy of the organization. Some treat it as a separate policy while others include it as part of their overall policy on corporate donations.

2. Be very clear with newly hired or volunteer fund-raisers what your group's policy is on this issue. Be as specific as possible with anyone doing this work on your behalf (e.g., "We will not consider funds from individual pharmaceutical companies but will consider accepting funds from pharmaceutical organizations." "We will consider all types of funds, regardless of their source." "We will not take money from any organization that manufactures substances that have been linked to cancer." "We will consider money from companies which have made a strong public statement and put money behind the advancement of women," etc.).

3. When dealing with representatives from a pharmaceutical company who may potentially give your group money, you may want to consider, as some groups have, only meeting on your "turf," i.e., not meeting at their offices, and having a policy not to accept free meals or other freebies as part of the discussion. The point is to maintain control of the discussion and not to be beholden to them, whatever your group's decision may be.

4. Be sure that any arrangements entered into with a pharmaceutical company are documented and copies are kept in your files and sent to the donor. These can take the form of a letter of agreement outlining what your terms are (e.g., "We agree to use this money responsibly but/and agree/do not agree to enter into the promotion of company X's product." "We agree/do not agree to carry the company's logo on our printed materi-

als."). Be as clear as possible about your intent. Possibilities left open to interpretation may not always work in your group's best interest.

RESOURCES FOR RESEARCHING SPECIFIC PHARMACEUTICAL COMPANIES

Rachel's Environment and Health Weekly, available electronically or by mail, covers a wide range of environmental and corporate issues. An electronic search will bring up anything they have published on questions relating to the environmental practices of specific corporations. Available from Environmental Research Foundation, PO Box 5036, Annapolis, MD 21043; fax: 410-263-8944; email: erf@rachel.org; Web site: www.monitor.net/rachel.

Multinational Monitor, published ten times a year, tracks corporate activity, especially in the third world, focusing on the export of hazardous substances, worker health and safety, labor union issues, and the environment. To contact: *Multinational Monitor*, PO Box 19405, Washington, DC 20036; email: monitor@essential.org; Web site: www.essential.org/monitor/monitor.html.

IF YOUR GROUP DECIDES TO BECOME INVOLVED WITH THE PHARMACEUTICAL INDUSTRY... David Gilbert, in his paper, "Much to Gain, More to Lose," suggests that there are six questions a group can ask itself when considering this issue: (1) Do we need to accept funding from a company? (2) What do we seek to gain from such an arrangement? (3) What are our views on the use of medicines for the patients we purport to represent—what do the patients think (i.e., attitudes to care and treatment choice issues)? (4) What are our views on the nature of the industry? (5) What are the alternatives to company funding? and (6) What are the risks of such arrangements?

Should Prescription Drugs Be Advertised?

MICHAEL CASTLEMAN AND MARYANN NAPOLI

Michael Castleman, excerpt from "But Wait, There's More," and Maryann Napoli, excerpt from "The Wrong Rx," *MAMM,* October/November 1998. Reprinted by permission.

BUT WAIT, THERE'S MORE

Open newspapers and magazines these days, and you're likely to see ads that were not there a few years ago—ads for prescription drugs. Known as direct-to-consumer advertising, and formerly reserved for medical journals, prescription drug ads now take center stage in magazines such as *Glamour.*

However, you can't just trot down to the pharmacy on your own. You have to ask you doctor for a prescription.

And there's the rub. Many doctors don't want people asking for prescription drugs by name and are calling for restrictions on direct-to-consumer ads. According to a survey of 454 family physicians published in the December 1997 issue of the *Journal of Family Practice* , 71 percent said that TV, radio, and print ads "pressure physicians to use drugs they might not ordinarily use."

Doctors also complain that consumer drug advertising can be misleading; more than 75 percent said so in the *Journal of Family Practice* survey.

Finally, some observers fret that direct-to-consumer ads drive up drug prices. Myra Snyder, executive director of the Center for Healthcare Quality Improvement in San Francisco, contends that drug cost increases are one of the leading causes of medical inflation, and that direct-to-consumer ads fan the flames.

This controversy is not a tempest in a medicine chest. One of the biggest changes in the industry has been direct-to-consumer advertising. The pharmaceutical industry spent just $12.3 million on consumer advertising in 1989. Now it spends an estimated $1 billion a year, an 80-fold increase.

Direct-to-consumer drug advertising does represent a change in our health care culture. And it is difficult for doctors to contend with requests for specific brand-name drugs that might not be best. But doctors are trained to handle some very tough discussions, for example, telling people that they have a terminal illness. Compared with such life-and-death exchanges, it's not all that challenging to say: "No, I don't think that brand is best for you. I'm going to prescribe another."

As for the cost issue, has direct-to-consumer advertising really driven drug prices through the roof? Not according to the Consumer Price Index: Lately, drug-price inflation has been running at a 2.5 to 3.5 percent year, about the same as the overall cost of health care.

It's also a stretch to think that prescription ads seriously mislead the public. We live in a culture absolutely inundated by advertising, and people understand that ads use a germ of truth to spin a web of half-truths.

Direct-to-consumer drug ads are, arguably, less misleading than many other ads. Their information is regulated by the FDA and thus subject to much more government scrutiny. And consumers can't buy prescription drugs without a doctor's approval.

These ads can also alert people that a product exists. Consider the ads for Sporanox, used to treat fungal infections. Millions of Americans have no idea why their toenails are discolored and deformed. Sporanox ads offer an explanation: Hey, what do you know, I have a fungal infection. Maybe I'll get it treated.

Of course, these ads are not an exercise in public health education. They're trying to sell product. Information gleaned from any advertising, not just direct-to-consumer drugs ads, should always be taken with a prudent dose of skepticism.

THE WRONG RX

At first it seemed like a good idea. Advertising prescription drugs directly to consumers would give us some control over our health care. We could learn about a new drug our doctors might not have thought to prescribe, and read about its side effects for ourselves.

As it turns out, the idea was a fantasy.

Advertising is about selling, not about balanced information. It's about creating demand and brand identity for prescription drugs, and it has been part of an enormously successful effort. Americans spent $78.9 billion in 1997 on prescription drugs, up from $37.7 billion in 1990, and the amount is rising at a rate of about 17 percent a year, according to an analysis in the *New England Journal of Medicine*. The pharmaceutical industry allocated $1.3 billion for direct-to-consumer advertising last year, more than the amount devoted to advertising directed at doctors. The doctors, however, were visited in person by drug company representatives at the incredible cost of $5.3 billion for the first eleven months of 1998, according to the *New York Times*.

The ads, of course, promote new drugs. New always means more expensive but not necessarily better. Cheaper and often equally effective alternatives may already be available. For FDA approval, the manufacturer need only prove its drug performed better than a placebo. No head-to-head comparison with an older competing drug is required, no showing of superior efficacy. These "me-too" medications could be a chemical notch or two away from a competitor's drug, without a significant difference in what they do. Think Valium and Librium, Prozac and Soloft, Pravachol and Mevacor—or Coke and Pepsi.

One peril is inappropriate drug choices.

The slick persuasiveness of some ads may also cause consumers to risk serious side effects to achieve a cosmetic result. Novartis Pharmaceuticals, for example, has heavily advertised Lamisil as a remedy for toenail fungus. A course of treatment costs $500 and carries the rare possibility of liver toxicity. Other ads create worry about medical problems that might never occur. "Is it just forgetfulness . . . or is it Alzheimer's disease?" asks

Pfizer's ad for Aricept, a new drug intended to improve cognition, for example.

In the ubiquitous Claritin TV commercials, the name of the drug is used, but not its purpose. By leaving out either the drug name or its purpose, the companies do not have to meet FDA requirements to provide side effect "information. For print ads, these requirements dictate publication of a page of print so fine you need a magnifying glass to read it. What percentage of the participants in trials of the drug benefited from it, and what was the benefit? With rare exceptions, you'll be hard-pressed to find answers to those questions even if you read every tiny word.

If you have any doubts that drug advertising can result in inappropriate drug choices, look at its effect on medical professionals.

Today, an aggressively promoted drug family used to treat hypertension, known as calcium channel blockers (CCBs), stands out as the best documented example of advertising's malevolent influence on physicians. CCBs (like Cardizem, Procardia, and Adalat) should not be the first-choice drug for people with hypertension because the less costly diuretics and beta blockers are the only two drug classes proven to reduce rates of cardiovascular death and heart attack. Over the years, scathing commentaries in medical journals on the underuse of the more effective drugs have failed to put a major dent in the problem. The effect on consumers? An increased risk of death, heart attack, stroke, and cancer, according to several studies on CCBs.

Doctors have at least some education in pharmacology. If they can be dangerously misled, why can't we?

The American Cancer Society: The World's Wealthiest "Nonprofit" Institution

SAM EPSTEIN

Samuel S. Epstein, "American Cancer Society: the World's

Wealthiest 'Nonprofit' Institution," *International Journal of Health Services* 29, no. 3 (1999): 565–578. Reprinted by permission.

The American Cancer Society is fixated on damage control—diagnosis and treatment—with indifference or even hostility to cancer prevention. This myopic mindset is compounded by the interlocking conflicts of interest with the cancer drug, mammography, and other industries. The "nonprofit" status of the Society is in sharp conflict with its high overhead and expenses, excessive reserves of assets, and contributions to political parties.

In 1992, the American Cancer Society Foundation was created to allow the ACS to actively solicit contributions of more than $100,000. A close look at the heavy hitters on the Foundation's board will give an idea of which interests are at play and where the Foundation expects its big contributions to come from. Among them:

➤ David R. Bethune, president of Lederle Laboratories, a division of American Cyanamid, which makes chemical fertilizers and herbicides while transforming itself into a full-fledged pharmaceutical company. In 1988, the company introduced Novatrone, an anticancer drug.

➤ Gordon Binder, CEO of Amgen, the world's foremost biotechnology company, whose success rests almost exlusively on one product, Neupogen, which is administered to chemotherapy patients to stimulate their production of white blood cells.

➤ Diane Disney Miller, daughter of the conservative multimillionaire Walt Disney, who died of lung cancer in 1966.

➤ George Dessert, famous for his former role as censor on the subject of "family values" during the 1970s and 1980s as CEO of CBS.

➤ Alan Gevertzen, chairman of the board at Boeing.

➤ Sumner M. Redstone, chairman of the board at Viacom.

The results of this board's efforts have been a million here, a million there—much of it coming from the very industries instrumental in shaping American Cancer Society policy, or profiting from it.

Of the members of the society's board, about half are clinicians, oncologists, surgeons, radiologists, and basic molecular scientists. The society has close connections to the mammography industry. Promotions of the society continue to lure women of all ages into mammography centers, leading them to believe that mammography is their best hope against breast cancer. These promotions expose premenopausal women to radiation hazards from mammography with little or no evidence of benefits.

Conspicuously absent from the society's National Breast Cancer Awareness month activities every year is any information on environmental and other avoidable causes of breast cancer. This is no accident. Zeneca Pharmaceuticals —the sole manufacturer of tamoxifen, the world's top-selling anticancer and breast cancer "prevention" drug— has been the sole multimillion-dollar funder of National Breast Cancer Awareness Month since its inception in 1984. Imperial Chemical Industries, Zeneca's parent company, manufactures industrial chemicals incriminated as causes of breast cancer. Zeneca profits from treatment of breast cancer, and hopes to profit more from large-scale use of tamoxifen for prevention.

The intimate association between the American Cancer Society and the cancer drug industry is further illustrated by the unbridled aggression that it has directed at potential competitors. Just as Senator Joseph McCarthy had his "blacklist" of suspected communists, the Society maintains a "Committee on Unproven Methods of Cancer Management," which periodically "reviews" unorthodox or alternative therapies. The Committee is comprised of carefully selected proponents of orthodox, expensive, and usually toxic drugs, who naturally oppose cheap, nonpatentable, and minimally toxic alternatives. The committee's statements on "unproven" methods are widely disseminated. Once a clinician becomes associated with "unproven methods," he or she is blackballed by the cancer establishment and funding becomes inaccessible.

HOW TO EVALUATE HEALTH INFORMATION ON THE INTERNET

The Internet is a huge and unwieldy repository of information. With more than 10,000 Web sites offering a wide range of health information, how can consumers be assured of the quality and the context of health information in order to make critical, life-changing decisions? Some questions to assess the content of web sites:

➤ Who operates the Web site? The suffix on the end of the web address provides a big clue: ".edu"—an educational institution; ".com"—a commercial firm; ".gov"—a government site; or ".org"—an organization that is usually nonprofit. A reliable site should list a postal address, an e-mail address, and a phone number.

➤ Is the site operated by an organization or group that you have heard of? Do you know how careful the group is about the quality of information it distributes? This affects the credibility of the site. If you haven't heard of the group before, it doesn't mean the information is not reliable but you should try to corroborate the information through additional sources.

➤ Are there advertisements on the Web site? Some organizations and companies permit advertising by "sponsors" and this may affect the content of the information on the Web site. Organizations may not present all the pros and cons of health issues or treatments if it might undercut a sponsor.

➤ Who wrote the information? Make sure the name of the author, the date it was published or posted, and the credentials and affiliations of the author are listed, and that the research (if mentioned) is cited fully so you can find it.

➤ Is the information presented on more than one site? Does the web site present one aspect of a particular problem or issue? Does the author have a limited point of view? Are there testimonials? If the answer is yes, consider other sites that present different points of view for balance. Do not rely upon only one source. Make sure the in-formation can be corroborated on other Web sites.

➤ How much information should you provide about your condition? The Internet is a transparent way to exchange information between different people whom you do not know. Be cautious about providing personal information over the Net, unless you are clear how that information will be used and interpreted.

➤ A healthy dose of skepticism is appropriate! Focus on the quality and the context of web site information. Stay alert to how Web sites filter information based upon particular points of view of the organization, or the authors, or the funders. For example, if a nonprofit organization's Web site is funded by a pharmaceutical company, the information provided on that site may not be critical of the products made by this company. It is imperative to be careful! Educated consumers can access a wealth of information on the Internet—but need to assess the quality and context of Web sites and make health care decisions in consultation with professionals and other trusted individuals.

CHAPTER 22

End of Life Issues

AS BARBARA SEAMAN AND I SAT in the lobby of the Bethesda, Maryland Marriott waiting for the shuttle to the National Institutes of Health conference on menopause management in March 2005, we weren't talking about the stunning reversal of medical wisdom on midlife health. Instead we talked about the smiling female face on the TVs surrounding us, the woman who was, at that moment, capturing the attention of most of America: Terri Schiavo.

When Schiavo was disconnected from her feeding tubes shortly thereafter and allowed to die after years of unconscious existence, there was hardly a person on any side of the political or religious spectrum who didn't have an opinion about it. For some it was evidence of a culture that didn't place enough value on life, that thought it was free to "play God" and decide what constituted a valuable existence. For others the controversy showed the lengths which certain religious and cultural groups felt free to politicize personal conflicts to demonstrate public agendas. For still others it demonstrated the willful ignoring of end-of-life directives.

Marilyn Webb argues that, among other things, we are having a cultural conversation about new medical technologies that can allow us to prolong life—although not good quality of life—indefinitely. Our social understandings and conclusions simply haven't caught up—or reconciled—with our medical accomplishments. Webb, who cut her activist teeth at the pill hearings in the early 1970s, has become a visible face in the movement to make end-of-life care better.

Among the issues we face are the availability of drugs for pain management, the role of religiously affiliated hospitals in regulating or denying patient wishes not to have life support and other life-prolonging technologies, the ethics of assisted suicide, and more general questions about quality of care and the rights of a patient to die a certain kind of death.

As more women in the second wave of the women's health movement either face issues regarding the care of parents at the end of life or have to make choices about their own deaths, we are joining the heated cultural conversations and bringing the benefit of our years of activism and political consciousnesses to the table. (L.E.)

Out of Pain and Anger

MARILYN WEBB

Marilyn Webb, expanded from "Out of Pain and Anger," *Self*, March 1999. Reprinted by permission.

At the White Hart Inn in Salisbury, Connecticut, a woman my mother's age hangs back from the departing crowd. She whispers to me, still stricken that she could do so little for her husband as he was dying. She felt powerless to get doctors to carry out his medical wishes, even to have them tell him the truth. "He knew he was dying, but he wanted information on what would happen," she said. "His doctors would all look away."

In New York City, another woman says her sister in a nursing home is physically threatened by the staff. If her sister were to go home, her children couldn't afford the help they'd need to give her the proper care. She pleads with me to help her find a good place; she can turn up nothing.

In Florida, a young man is weeping. He still has nightmares about how his partner died writhing in pain, his doctors unwilling, or unable, to give him the narcotic medication he needed. He and his family wonder why. And so do I.

All these people have come to hear talks I have been giving upon the publication of my book, *The Good Death*, a journalist's view, based on more than six years of research and cross-country reporting, of how we die in America. They have also come to tell stories of their own, most of them tales of personal tragedy, pain, and fury. Talking about dying has been like lighting a match in a room filled with gas.

These are tales of ordinary Americans—mothers, fathers, grandparents, children, husbands, wives, sisters, brothers, and lovers—and in them I hear a new kind of anger, the voice of an enormous lack of empowerment in the face of modern medicine, the despair of having failed loved ones at a critical point in life, and not for lack of trying.

This is the terrible atmosphere in which many Americans now die. Yet as these stories have ac-cumulated over the past year I have sensed the birth of a new grassroots movement for change, which in remarkably similar ways has the excite-ment of the early days of the women's movement.

Like that movement, this one is fueled by per-sonal tales that, taken together, paint a much larger political picture. The members of this move-ment do not necessarily agree on how changes should be made, but together they are developing the language, tools, community programs, and networks to change the culture of dying.

The issues are ones of empowerment, the voices of patients and families struggling to change mod-ern dying as natural childbirth has changed modern birth. By and large, this new movement rings out of the passions of women in their role as family caregivers, only now in later stages of life. This movement portends to be just as powerful as that one that went before it, generated often by the very same people, asking the very same questions. Now medicine has changed life at the end of life and this same generation has grown older.

FACING THE EVIDENCE

The way we die today is historically unprecedented, yet dying has changed so fast—in just one genera-tion's time—that it has left us scrambling culturally to catch up. At the turn of the last century we died quickly of infectious or parasitic diseases and there wasn't much doctors could do to postpone life. Enter antibiotics, the watershed miracle born along with the baby boomers. Since then, a near avalanche of medical advances has added an extra generation of time to life, but it has also transformed dying into a long-term affair. Today's major killers—cancer, heart disease, stroke—are all illnesses with which we can live for many years, but these are years filled with difficult symptoms and choices.

No longer at issue is whether doctors are "doing everything possible," but when and how treatment should wind down, questions none of our religious, family, or medical institutions are prepared for. Research confirms what the public already knows:

70 to 90 percent of us now die when some decision is made either to withhold or withdraw treatment such as drugs, respirators, or feeding tubes. Yet, the questions remain: Who decides? And how?

Hospitals, once places to treat pneumonia or appendicitis or to go to die, are now just short stops in the turnstile of modern dying. This new path involves roller-coaster crises that take us in and out of medical centers, with long gaps in between. We stay home, grow weaker, and ultimately need more and more care.

Physicians are not fully trained to address the staggering symptoms of lengthy declines. In 1995, the sorry findings began to appear of an eight-year, $28 million study, dubbed Support, of 10,000 seriously ill patients—5,000 of whom eventually died—in five teaching hospitals across the United States. To researchers' shock, 50 percent of the dying suffered moderate to severe pain, 31 percent had signed documents saying they preferred that CPR be withheld, yet 53 percent of their doctors didn't know that.

Other studies have come up with similar findings. A world-renowned pain research team at the University of Wisconsin found in studies of cancer patients that more than 40 percent of them suffered long-term and undertreated pain. A study at Memorial Sloan-Kettering Cancer Center in New York City found undertreated pain in nearly 85 percent of AIDS patients. Almost half of this pain might have been alleviated with stronger drugs. And pain wasn't the only symptom. Other Sloan-Kettering research showed that hospitalized cancer patients suffered an average of thirteen intolerable symptoms; AIDS patients averaged eighteen. Doctors weren't trained to address many of these symptoms.

These findings have since shaken the medical community into retraining doctors and nurses in better care for the dying and inspired state legislatures into initiatives on better pain management and improved ways of thinking about advanced directives.

Yet, a little-reported part of the Support study may be even more devastating to patients and families. More than half of the families studied suffered a major crisis in caring for a loved one. Thirty-four percent of the patients needed large amounts of family caregiving, causing 31 percent of the families to lose most of their savings, 29 percent to lose a major source of income, and 29 percent to require a major life change for another family member. In 12 percent, another family member became seriously ill from the stress the intensive caregiving required.

Surprisingly, all these patients had health insurance, yet the impact of their illness on families was extreme. It should come as no shock to anyone that most of these caregivers were women who are now struggling to care for ill relatives, while at the same time bringing in much-needed family income, caring often for children at the same time they are now caring not just for one, but—as we live longer—for *two* generations of aging family members. This is a major women's issue of our time. It will peak into the next century as more boomers themselves age and become chronically ill and, as their numbers mount, it becomes woefully obvious how inadequate the American health care system now is to address the quality of life in long-term, modern dying.

Illness and dying are far more complicated than ever before, yet this is a generation that has already lived through the transformations of natural childbirth and the ongoing abortion wars. It believes in autonomy and choice. At the same time, the dying and their loved ones are beginning to look for answers beyond the clinic and the hospital, sometimes, in the bargain, landing in the international news.

In 1990, Jack Kevorkian, MD, the notorious Michigan pathologist, helped Alzheimer's patient Janet Adkins die in the back of his rusty Volkswagen van. After he started a saline solution going, she activated his famous suicide machine, which first sent a sedative and then deadly potassium chloride to her heart. Since then and even after Dr. Kevorkian's medical license was taken away, after he resorted to using carbon monoxide for some of his patients, and finally after he landed in jail in 1999 for directly injecting lethal medications into Lou Gehrig's disease patient Thomas Youk on CBS's *60 Minutes,* polls have consistently shown that between 65 and 75 percent of the public supports physician-assisted suicide.

Those who oppose legalization of assisted suicide argue on ethical, religious, or legal grounds, and say they fear it may lead to patient abuse. Some see redemption in suffering, or fear abuse should their care be compromised by the oppressive weight of medical cost-cutting. And of course there are others who believe the reverse: that it is a matter of choice, that abuse, like back alley abortion, will come from keeping assisted suicide illegal, or that legalization will prevent Lone Ranger tactics like Kevorkian's and create fail-safe guidelines for states and medical institutions to use to guard patients against private suffering.

Yet, those national studies cited above give clues as to why there is strong public support for legalization. Government policy and the prickly atmosphere surrounding the practice of medicine have only compounded the problem. Drug laws in a "Just Say No" culture can prevent pain medications from reaching the dying. Doctors, fearing retaliation from medical licensing boards and federal agencies, tend to underprescribe. Medical insurance covers acute hospital care but not the very long-term care many ill people now require. Managed care has all too often taken medical decision-making away, not only from patients and families, but also from doctors. Doctors, patients, and families are all suffering under the ironic burdens of medicine's great success.

CONSUMERS TAKE CHARGE

In Denver in May 1998, I attended a statewide meeting of the Colorado Collaboration on End-of-Life Care, a coalition of doctors, nurses, hospice volunteers, AIDS workers, clergy, and everyday people brought together by their common desire to change how Colorado cares for its dying.

This group is just one of many that has now begun organizing to address the critical state of end-of-life care. At their meeting I heard talk about the issues that are troubling many, many people across the country: how to improve hospitals and nursing homes, how to make living wills carry more weight in health care institutions, how to make hospice care, with its focus on pain management, comfort, and spiritual closure, available to more people.

Members of the clergy mused about how to address psycho-spiritual concerns, especially in an era of near-death-experience spirituality. Everyone wanted to change state drug laws that inhibit doctors' prescribing pain medications.

There were also private concerns. A member of the generation whose men never changed their children's diapers wept quietly, remembering how he changed his dying wife's bedding, how long this went on, how humiliated she was and how terribly lonely they both felt. A man who had AIDS said prisons are filled with men and women with AIDS and that hospices there are sorely needed. Both men wanted policies changed, as did the majority of women in attendance at that meeting, but they also wanted to create support groups that would provide the everyday help they wished had been given to them when they needed it.

One major reason such groups as the Colorado Collaboration are cropping up across the country is that their ideas have been funded over the past few years by a handful of generous charitable foundations, which share their vision of reshaping the American culture of dying. Since the late 1980s, when it gave $28 million to fund the Support study, the Robert Wood Johnson Foundation (RWJF), catalyzed by that national study's dismal findings, has spent nearly $50 million on changing end-of-life medical care, from education on proper pain management to raising public awareness through dialogue groups and media projects.

Beginning in 1999, another multi-million-dollar RWJF-funded initiative poured money into community-state partnership grantee coalitions in each state, adding to its Last Acts Campaign to mobilize American health care organizations nationally. A four-part, RWJF-funded Bill Moyers special on dying is scheduled for fall of the year 2000.

Philanthropist George Soros' Open Society Institute inaugurated the Project on Death in America in New York in 1994, and since then has given some $15 million to help transform the experience of dying through research, scholarship, the arts and humanities, and education.

The thousands of community projects now emerging will, in the end, have the most profound effect. Some are new consumer advocacy organizations such as Americans for Better Care of the Dying and the Partnership for Caring. Others are volunteer efforts, begun by people who brushed shoulders with grief and came away with a vision of change.

THE NEXT STEPS

If we can learn anything from the abortion wars, it will be that choice and diversity matter. We are a diverse nation with as many different cultural and religious views of dying as we have of living—and all of it matters! If we divide over this issue, fighting each other, we risk failing to alter a medical care system that has outlived its capacity to care for the ill under today's conditions for modern dying. Medicine has now given us the gift of time. It's how we make use of it that counts. Not to honor, legalize, support, or address the diverse ways each of us wants to make use of this time will only leave us flailing in battle, no one getting desperately needed care.

Dying is a sacred, not just a medical event. But medicine has so complicated our life at the end of life that we do not address or understand the complexities involved until we are in the midst of personal and family chaos. It behooves us all to think and plan ahead. Since the publication of *The Good Death*—and inspired by the voices and stories I have heard on my travels—I've helped begin a nonprofit organization, The Good Death Initiative Inc., to build an educational campaign to change

how each of us understand and care for our own dying in the very villages and cities where we live.

We plan to hold public events called Town Meetings Across America on Death and Dying. My partners are Barbara Maltby, a movie producer, who helped make *Ordinary People,* and Paul Brenner, a New York hospice director, as well as other doctors, media people, attorneys, ethicists, and entertainers. We intend to go city to city, town to town, to explore what it means to make choices at the end of life, to empower communities to expand support to patients and families, to talk about the visionary programs we have heard about.

The following groups suggest a range of the enlightened resources now available. I hope that in addition to the political efforts now taking place to change state and national law, in addition to the retraining medical personnel are now receiving to reshape the way they give care, that these groups will inspire similar efforts in more communities around the country. If nothing else, what they are showing us is that a massive grassroots effort to change our healthcare system and how we all care for the dying is already here. Not surprisingly, much of it is being led and/or inspired by women, often the same women who transformed American culture and healthcare once before.

LIVES RECORDED FOR POSTERITY

In the small university town of Missoula, Montana, the Missoula Demonstration Project's Life Story Task Force has instituted a pilot effort to focus the town's citizens on what might dramatically improve the care of the dying. Among its most welcomed programs is Gathering Life Stories, whose aim is to help those who are dying to leave a family legacy.

Volunteers are trained to sit down with people in hospitals, hospices, nursing homes, senior centers, and housing projects and interview them there, recording and writing their life stories. Preliminary studies show that these sessions not only engender a sense of meaning in the lives elders have led, but also reduce their sadness and stress.

LAUNDRY HELPERS

Auntie Helen's Fluff 'n' Fold in San Diego, a free volunteer-run laundry service for men, women, and children who are ill with AIDS, was inspired by the simple idea that everyone should be able to die in a clean, dry bed. The service was named after the great-aunt of its founder, the late Gary Cheatham. "Gary had a friend named Ronnie," says executive director Bob Stanley, "who was so ill his laundry had piled up in a corner of his room. Gary picked it up, washed it, and brought it back. After that he got a washing machine for his garage and began doing laundry for other people who were sick with AIDS."

That was in 1988. Now the nonprofit organization has eight commercial washers and nine dryers and does 1,500 loads of laundry a month for approximately 350 clients, with a twenty-four-hour pickup and return time. "We have volunteers from every sector," Stanley says. "Senior citizens, people affected by HIV, the physically or emotionally challenged, college students. It makes everyone feel better to help others feel good. You know how a nice fresh pair of pajamas or clean sheets feel? Well, when you're so sick, they feel *really* great!"

PET VISITATION

I remember the day Maverick, a golden retriever, paid a visit to Hospice House, the residential unit of Hope Hospice in Fort Myers, Florida. He walked through the halls as though he owned them, greeting everyone as he wagged his tail. Then he lifted his leg and peed on the nurses' station. "Oh well," said the nurse to the dog's embarrassed human companion, "that's what hospice is all about." Maverick went on licking and nuzzling the dying, room by room, a working dog on a Wednesday afternoon.

Hope Hospice has six dog teams and one cat team. Some of these "therapy dogs" work in nursing homes; some visit in patients' homes. "There are studies that show that people who have pets live longer lives," says Melissa Mehlum, the volunteer coordinator. "It helps our patients, the touch, the smell, the company, the petting, the caregivers, and our staff."

Deaths take a toll on the animals as well as the people they comfort, according to Deni Elliott, who runs S.T.A.R. Dogs, a similar program of volunteers in hospices, hospitals, and nursing homes in Missoula, Montana. "Dogs understand death a lot better than people do," says Elliott. "We think dogs should be given a chance to see the person as dead, to go to the funeral so the dog understands that the person has died. There should be continuity with the hospice team so the dog does not feel a sense of continual loss."

Hope Hospice's dog and cat teams—all pets and their owners who want to volunteer by visiting at the hospice—are trained and certified locally. A national registration program is offered by Delta Society.

ASSISTED-SUICIDE SUPPORT

The terminally ill can buy Derek Humphry's best seller, *Final Exit*, to find out what drugs to take to end life, but unless physician-assisted suicide is legalized in the state where they live, they, and any loved ones who help them, run the risk of criminal charges. Sadly, they and many others who suffer, whether or not they take such steps, are left to die alone.

Enter Compassion in Dying, founded in Seattle in 1993 by minister Ralph Mero, but now led by Barbara Coombs Lee, a former hospice nurse and now an attorney, and staffed by health care workers, volunteers, and clergy. Its philosophy: No one should have to die alone, no matter what she is dying of or how.

Compassion in Dying is best known for having brought the suits to legalize assisted suicide to the Supreme Court and for helping to pass the nation's first assisted-suicide law, in Oregon. The court battle was led by dynamo attorney Kathryn Tucker, and the Oregon law's most visible craftsman and public champion was Barbara Coombs Lee.

The group started as a nonprofit service organization to provide non-judgmental information and emotional support to the terminally ill, making house visits, bringing in professionals to assess whether additional pain medications or hospice support might be needed, and, if it is a patient's final choice, to give advice about lethal medications and sit with those who ultimately decide to take them.

Paradoxically, the strict guidelines covering assessment of need that Compassion helped draft for the Oregon assisted-suicide law have resulted in improved care of the dying throughout the state's health care system. Some 30 percent of all Oregonians now die with the help of a hospice, as opposed to 14 to 21 percent in the rest of the country; more die at home than in hospitals; and Oregon's medical use of morphine has increased by 70 percent, making it one of the states with the highest morphine use for treating the terminally ill.

For those who believe in assisted suicide as a rational choice for the terminally ill or when all other palliative care measures do not work, or for those who only want to help with assessment and service support groups, Compassion in Dying can provide start-up materials.

GOURMET DINNER FOR CAREGIVERS

Suzanne Mintz, president of the National Family Caregivers Association, says that 80 to 90 percent of all at-home caring for the chronically ill and disabled in the US is provided by family members. This caregiving includes helping a loved one with cooking, cleaning, shopping, health care tasks, legal and financial matters, and giving huge amounts of emotional support. Studies show that the altruistic daughters, mothers, husbands, and partners of the dying who provide virtually around-the-clock care tend to suffer high levels of depression, frustration, and anxiety. When someone is dying, caregivers also grieve day by day. They need small respites. They need help.

The First Presbyterian Church in Annapolis, Maryland, like many churches and synagogues, has created a year-round caregivers program for its members, capped by an annual Caregivers Night Out. Often-isolated caregivers around town are invited to a gourmet dinner served by tuxedoed waiters. Someone is found to stay with the person who is ill, another to drive the caregiver to and from the event.

Church volunteers have also prepared a local resource guide for caregiver help, formed a support committee, and set up a squad of drivers to run errands for caregivers. All it takes is a car and a little time to help out a caregiver who might like to go out for a manicure or a long walk.

Good Mourning, America

AMY PAGNOZZI

Amy Pagnozzi, "Good Mourning, America," *MAMM*, October/November, 1998. Reprinted by permission.

When Betty Rollin's breast cancer recurred fourteen years ago, she never seriously considered the possibility she might die. Oh, she was scared, all right. But it was a generalized terror, not one that manifested itself in the living wills, powers of attorney, or advanced directives she advocates now as the vice president of Death with Dignity National Center, a San Mateo, California-based educational organization working to improve care for terminally ill patients and to decriminalize a patient's choice to die with a physician's aid. "I . . . never for myself," Rollin stammers, flummoxed, when asked if she considered it herself. "I mean, who wants to think about death unless they absolutely have to?" While recovering from each of her two bouts with cancer, her fears were usurped by a pure joy, unalloyed by mortal intimations. "I'm alive and I feel great and aren't I lucky and on with life," is how Rollin, newswoman for NBC for more than twenty-five years, describes this feeling.

But her utter lack of morbidity does set her apart,

given that she's one of this country's leading physician aid-in-dying advocates. Imagine the welcome Death with Dignity's executives must have given the much-respected and poised Rollin in 1994, knowing what wonders her authoritative and pleasant persona could bring to a debate that's veered toward the hysterical since Jack Kevorkian took center stage. Bear in mind, even Derek Humphry's landmark right-to-die manual *Final Exit* was too much for some (chapter 19: "Self-Deliverance Via the Plastic Bag"). Death is a delicate subject, something that Rollin hadn't really considered before being forced to, fifteen years ago, when her mother Ida was dying of ovarian cancer.

Her activism began accidentally. She was asked to help her mother and she did: It was no volunteer effort. "I've had a wonderful life, but now it's over," Ida Rollin told her daughter. Two and a half years after her diagnosis, she couldn't keep food down, walk, control her bladder or bowels. She'd been game enough to fight when there was hope—enduring eight months of punishing chemotherapy, then more, after a recurrence. Rather than wither away after her husband had died and her daughter was grown, she'd learned piano, joined a theater, made new friends, even taken a lover. "I'm not saying it couldn't be worse," she told Betty. "I know how some people suffer. But to me . . . life is taking a walk, visiting my children, eating! If I had life, I'd want it. I don't want this."

Betty and her mathematician husband, Harold M. Edwards ("Ed"), felt lost. It was 1983 and information about assisted dying was scarce. Humphry's *Final Exit* and its lethal dosage charts were not yet available; there was no Internet to browse for cyanide recipes; and legislation suggesting doctors should help people die wasn't even pending.

Misinformation, on the other hand, was rampant. A doctor in New York City hinted, before hanging up abruptly, that Dalmane (flurazepam), a hypnotic agent used for insomnia, alone could be fatal—which was unlikely. A nurse had offered to show Betty's mother how to use a hypodermic, so she could create an air embolism—which might

kill her or might merely blow out some brain cells. The Netherlands was one of the few places where assisted dying was permitted, and that's where they found the sole doctor who offered them accurate advice—an American-born friend-of-a-friend who provided drug information.

Luckily for Ida, Betty and Ed were only vaguely aware of the Kafkaesque scenarios that could befall her if they "botched" it, otherwise they might have put off acting until the matter was out of their hands. "People ask us, 'What was going through your mind?' But until the end, there was nothing," Betty says. "We were too afraid to be emotional, because if we got emotional it might upset her stomach, and then she wouldn't be able to keep the pills down and she'd wind up suffering more."

Wearing full makeup and a new flowered nightie, Ida Rollin downed two anti-anxiety drugs: one Compazine (prochlorperazine), prescribed for nausea, and then twenty Nembutal (pentobarbital sodium), the lethal part of the prescription cocktail. Then came five Dalmane. "I want you to know that I am a happy woman," she said before getting sleepy. "I made a man happy for forty years, and I gave birth to the most wonderful child, and later in life I had another child [Ed] whom I love as if I had given birth to him too. No one has been more blessed than I. I've had a wonderful life, and this is my wish." She fell unconscious almost immediately, and hours later, Ida died peacefully in her own bed.

And her daughter Betty has "never had a bad moment" about what she did because "we pulled it off, we made this thing happen, she escaped from life." She thought she would write a book as a tribute to her mother and forget about it. But that's not how things turned out. Although death was neither a fascination nor her life's work, before and after the book, *Last Wish*, was published in 1985, she was up to her neck in it. (Public Affairs is reissuing the book in paperback this September.)

Rollin, you probably already know, was breast cancer's first-ever "It" girl, a title she's held since her breast cancer memoir, *First, You Cry*, was published in 1976. But even documenting her battle with breast cancer, her mastectomy, her leaving her first husband for a new love, and her unsuccessful search for the perfect prosthetic breast (she ended up cruising a drapery store with a pair of scissors, snipping off kitchen curtain pom-poms for nipples), didn't make Rollin flinch, even afterward. She's a boldly honest, resolute optimist. She gives a stock lecture on the "bright side" of breast cancer, which was not altered a whit by a recurrence and second mastectomy more than a decade ago. Rollin's attitude is rooted in an extraordinary sense of perspective that never lets her lose sight of others' misery. It would not be oversimplifying to state that *Last Wish*, similarly, is about the bright side of death, since it is the story of Rollin's mother's triumph over pain and suffering. However, not everyone sees it from that angle.

In some minds, the publication of *Last Wish* transformed Rollin overnight from a shining icon for survivors into "that woman who killed her mother." She even got disinvited from several hospitals where she'd been scheduled to do her cheery breast cancer lecture, after a board member or some such figure realized Rollin had written *Last Wish*. Nonetheless, the book shot up the best seller lists, outdoing even *First, You Cry*. Ida Rollin the entrepreneur would have liked that. But as for the notoriety, Ida Rollin the mother would have told her daughter that it wasn't worth it.

Betty expected a minor fuss over the fact that she'd researched guns, carbon monoxide, and poison on Ida's behalf—but not the storm she was facing, which has never completely settled. A review of her book on the front page of the *Washington Post* suggested she might soon be indicted for murder. It wasn't true—the most she could be charged with in New York was criminally assisting a suicide— but it was interesting enough for Barbara Walters to come calling. Magazines put her on their covers, and the book became a network TV movie.

But it was only after letters began pouring in by the thousands that Rollin realized she had hit a nerve and accomplished more than simply sharing

"a powerful story about someone who happened to be my mother."

"Oh, I didn't think anyone else felt this way," or "I didn't think anyone went through this," wrote the daughters and sons, sisters and brothers, husbands and lovers. Their sense of relief that Rollin had again broken the silence on a taboo subject, as she had done with breast cancer, was palpable. "Me, too," said the letters. "My mother in County Clare is just like your mother." "My mother in Kyoto is just like your mother." Usually when they told their stories, Rollin says, "it didn't seem to me to be like my story at all," but she knew she had struck a chord. The writers, most of them anguished over what they had or had not done, wanted desperately to share their experience, and Rollin had been chosen.

An activist was born, reluctantly. "Assisting my mother to die really worked for my family, but I now know that this is absolutely not something families should be doing," Betty, still startlingly youthful at sixty-two, said recently in her sunny, Park Avenue penthouse. "You need a professional to help you, you need [to go to] a doctor. It's eminently sensible and merciful." Rollin continues to talk about death these days because "there are a lot of people in this country who think physician aid-in-dying is a bad idea, so I feel I am needed." Most of the people who feel that way "just don't get it," because it's never happened to them.

Her expectations for the movement are modest, and even if they weren't, this isn't exactly the sort of cause you wrap a ribbon around ("A nice noose-shaped twist of twine for that lapel, ma'am?"). Rollin reckons that it will be a long time before any kind of physician-assisted death is legal throughout the entire country, given that the US Supreme Court has tossed the debate back to the state courts. She suspects California could be next to allow doctors to prescribe lethal prescriptions and Michigan might conceivably follow. So far, Oregon is still the only state where the dying can be helped by their doctors. Since November 4, 1997, ten people have received lethal prescriptions, nine of whom were cancer patients. Eight used these prescriptions for self-deliverance and the other two died naturally of their diseases. Rollin wishes the act, basically limited to a prescription—"a piece of paper"—was a bit wider in scope so that it included some kind of provision for people who cannot swallow pills. But given that there wasn't even a Death With Dignity organization until 1994, the movement has come a long way. The public's consciousness has been raised.

"People don't have to go around thinking about death all the time to understand this issue," Rollin says. "I do think when they are called upon to vote on this issue, they might think how they would feel if they were at the end of life and suffering greatly and wanting to escape and not being able to." She's no zealot. Unlike some colleagues, she's "often thought that people who are against legal aid-in-dying are less cruel than inexperienced." As she wrote in a new introduction to *Last Wish*, "Many people, luckier than they know, have never had their bodies turned into torture chambers. Many people believe the myth that pain can (always) be stopped by drugs. Drugs are amazing, but they don't work equally well for everybody."

Before Ida Rollin actually asked her daughter for assistance in her death, she used this metaphor: "I'm locked in a room and I don't know where the key is." And Betty thinks that legislation addressing assisted suicide is "insurance" more than anything. "Look, intellectually, if I am ever in this situation, I want a choice," Rollin declares. "I just don't particularly expect to be in this situation."

Dying into Grace: Mother and Daughter . . . a Dance of Healing

ARTEMIS MARCH

Artemis March, PhD, excerpt from *Dying Into Grace*, Quantum Lens Press, 2007. Reprinted by permission.

There are all kinds of ties in one's life, all kinds of friendship, loves, complexities, but there is only one person whom one needs for dying. To have such a person is a great good fortune. To be that person, to have been such a person, is a heavy and blessed experience. . . . Once at least, in each lifetime, we are meant to be a blessing to each other.
—*Gerda Lerner,* A Death of One's Own

I had no choice but to write this book. What compelled its creation was the most extraordinary, grueling, exhausting, surprising, disruptive, rewarding, and transformative experience of my life: midwifing my mother's death.

The idea that I, who live four hours away, would ever move in and become her primary caregiver was about the last thing I could have imagined in my "normal" life, and no one could have predicted where her/our journey would take us. That journey uprooted my life and threatened my dreams while Olwen struggled with why, in her view, it was taking so long to die, once she—a pragmatic doer who did not know the meaning of procrastination—had decided it was time. Our dance was imprinted with stunning surprises and deep connections, yet it also exacted terrible demands to surrender what each of us held most dear: "How do I let go of my life?"

Ultimately, my mother and I transcended ancient patterns, kept her out of a nursing home nightmare, and healed our wounds and losses, the deepest of which long predated my birth. Shedding her inessentials, Olwen came home to herself, took immense risks, and broke through a lifetime of cautiousness. She was able to complete her relational and spiritual work with me and for herself in a profound and joyous way that was permanently transformative for each of us. Our intimate Dance of Death led to the hard-won and unexpected gift of mutual healing.

Olwen's death and dying were continuous and discontinuous with who she was in life. She looked life and death in the face, never backing away from hard things. A self-starter sustained by durable energy, she had a robust constitution, bones and joints which never broke or ached, and tremendous strength of will. Following life-shattering losses, she rebirthed herself three times, weaving a rich life as an independent woman in the prefeminist, prepsychological era. She was sustained by the steel in her backbone, her capacity for friendship, and her in-the-bones knowledge that every relationship is part of a larger fabric. A life is as strong as the fabric it weaves, and hers was strong indeed. But she had outlived all her lifelong friends, most of her small family, and most of her community networks.

Olwen's willpower, resilience, backbone, and the life she had woven were integral to how she dealt with her last years of subtle decline and her months of dying. Yet, in other respects, her dying was also discontinuous with the path she had been on since before I, her only child, was born to her late in her childbearing years.

Getting on with her life meant closing off the back rooms of her mind and living life in the front room. A friend recalls meeting my mother when Olwen was in her mid-eighties: "I met her once at the Cape and remember her vividly. She was nice— and she was precisely carved out of rock. A definite presence, formidable, not animated. I liked her." It was the closed rooms, the shadows, and the silences that I absorbed in my bones, that shaped so much of my life and our relationship. They were the underside of her survival and triumph over loss.

In those final weeks, however, everything shifted. The rooms that had been closed now opened and the real Olwen shone through more brilliantly than ever. She found again her whole self whom she had locked away before I was born.

I was to discover her letting go was inseparable from my own. While it had seemed her dying was about *her* letting go of *her* life, it was *I* who also had to let her go by truly surrendering to the process in order for her life journey to complete itself in a mutually transformative way.

"Transformation" has been overused for trivial purposes, but I must claim it as the only word that properly names the outcome of our journey. Transformation is altogether different from incremental change along a continuous path—a concept modeled after billiard ball trajectories. Transformation is a living process that represents discontinuity with the past, a catapulting into an After which feels altogether different than the Before— so different that you can't get yourself back to that old place.

Whereas "change" happens over time, transformation happens in a moment, after which life is never the same going forward, and our relationship to the past is forever altered. We see everything from a larger vantage point and through a new lens. Yet transformative moments are also intimately bound to the past, for they do not emerge from fallow ground. Like the order that self-structures from a rich chaos, or the birthing that emerges from months of gestation in the dark, transformation has a mysterious quality, arising as if from "nowhere."

I now look back at all the struggles, complexity, and ambivalence of the Before, and the fundamental fact that Olwen and I never gave up on each other as being the rich ground from which our After sprang. What if we had never gotten there? Having gone through this enduringly transformative process, it is unthinkable that we might have missed it. I discovered that:

> ➤ Dying can be the most powerful and transformative experience in life, not only for the dying, but also for those of us who enter deeply into their process.

> ➤ Yet most of us cheat ourselves and the dying.

> ➤ We can do something about that. We aren't in control, but we aren't powerless. We can empower ourselves to dance with our beloved dying.

You will find in our caregiving/dying story a new, relational paradigm—represented as a dance between the dying partner and her caregiving partner—for enhancing the probabilities that the dying process will open to *mutual* growth and healing. ("Healing" means movement toward greater wholeness, through which old wounds and losses become extinct.)

While the focal pair in my exposition of the dance is intergenerational and pertains especially to mother and daughter, it can be applied to any significant relationship in which one person—or animal companion—is dying.

My dance with Olwen was based on intuition and attunement, grounded through a lifetime's experience of who she was and what was important to her. I had read nothing about "dying well" or its deeper dimensions. As I was finalizing this book, I began to read books by professionals experienced in end-of-life care to help locate our story while clarifying its distinctiveness. Yes, it does happen that dying people become their whole and essential self. Yes, learning and growth do happen near the end of life. Yes, the dying do come to grace. And, most intriguing of all, the amazing things that sometimes happen between the dying and loved ones can be permanently transformative for both.

But, none of these things happen routinely. Indeed, their relative scarcity appears to have been the motivating impetus behind several books. The physical and medical foundations for supporting these emotional-spiritual openings are not even in place: people die badly, whether in pain, alone, abandoned, without witness, without presence, subjected to unwanted treatments and interventions, in alien environments, or at the least, without having made the best use of their precious time with loved ones.

And, these mysterious discontinuities near the end of life are not solo events. They arise in a context of presence and witnessing, and in relationships informed by authentic engagement. This truth is implicit in accounts illustrating what is possible emotionally, relationally, and spiritually at the end of life. The well-timed question, the consistent presence of compassionate witnessing, the ability to listen through symbolic language and engage with what the dying are really saying—all bespeak relational processes that triggered, enabled, or enhanced the more profound dimensions of "dying well."

But, the chroniclers and advocates for realizing full end-of-life potential lack a relational framework for presenting their experiences and observations. Informed by standard personal and transpersonal psychologies, expansion of the dying self is presented as a solo process, even when supported to varying degrees by the living.

The Dance of Death, by contrast, shifts primacy to *movement in and through relationship*. Movement is fostered by the emphatic attunement of the caregiving partner who is herself learning and growing while creating a safe, responsive space in which her beloved dying is more likely to open and grow. The Dance of Death is about each dance partner's opening more fully to themselves and each other, and, through their mutually responsive process, helping to heal both the self and the other.

We, as family caregivers—past, present, or future—who will ourselves be dying one day, can stop cheating ourselves and our elders, and enhance the possibilities for jointly experiencing growth, healing, and even transformation by doing three things:

➤ Reframing and living the dying process as a dance full of growth opportunities for everyone.

➤ Empowering ourselves to dance as well as possible, even if it is our first time up close and personal with dying.

➤ Becoming a political force that demands end-of-life environments, care, practices, policies, and programs that support rather than violate the dying and their family caregivers.

These three things are linked: When we understand in our bones what is possible in and through a dying process and that we can make a difference in whether and how those possibilities are realized, we are motivated to build the social-political-medical foundation that enables their realization to become typical rather than exceptional.

These principles are not intended to add more layers to the burden of caregiving, or ratchet up the standard so we feel we have never done enough—as has happened with parents who turn themselves into pretzels around their kids. Rather, they are directed to internally reconfiguring our intention and our priorities—and, when necessary, jolting our mental and emotional default settings—so that the urgent does not crowd out the important. These guiding principles are not about spending *more* time and energy, but paying attention to what we are doing with the time and energy available to us, so that we are doing what truly matters.

As my mother and I were living our story, however, we had no idea how things would turn out. How would the last phases of her life unfold? Over what period of time? Would it be possible not only to get her home again, but also to keep her there? Could I find the right help and would it be enough? Would we run out of money before she ran out of life? Might suddenly escalating care needs use up her money, forcing her out of her lovely apartment and onto Medicaid at some dreadful, fragile moment? Would I use up my small savings intended to launch my "real work" around which my own identity and life are formed? Would I, as I desperately hoped, be with her at the end, or would I have chosen the "wrong time" to go home?

ORIENTING CAREGIVERS

The ongoing trepidation kindled by these unknowns, the emotional roller coaster and totality of exhaustion endemic to caring for our beloved dying, and the necessity of riding multiple learning curves, initially inspired me to think about writing a book to provide orientation for those who un-

dertake to live it. As I became consumed by the process of caring for my mother, I was learning on the job, in the moment, with virtually no guidance. Like most of us thrust into this situation, I had no prior experience for the most important job of my life, and I had read but one book. Trying to get it right the first time with no rehearsals, no retakes, and a level of sleep deprivation that was previously unimaginable led me to realize I was accumulating knowledge and wisdom that was wasted if it never went beyond me.

All around me, friends and acquaintances are going through some stage of this process with one or both parents, or have just been through it, or are holding their breath about what the future will bring. There are millions of us in our forties, fifties, and sixties who are facing the end of our parents' lives, and, I daresay, have little preparation, foreknowledge, or grasp of what may lie ahead. Although the unique journey we each undertake with a dying parent is fraught with uncertainty and replete with surprises, there are markers that can keep us better oriented, and learning that can be pulled out of the journeys of those who have gone before us.

I felt a growing urge to share what I was learning in this process with people who may become, or are right now, or have been the primary caregiver for a declining/dying parent or elder. I did not want to write *about* the process after the fact from an expert point of view or cull and arrange material for topical consultation, but to capture the process itself.

What is it like to careen in and out of multiple mind-sets while experiencing a kaleidoscope of emotions telescoping in on each other? How do you cope with all the facets and levels of a mother's dying yet stop on a dime to be emotionally present to profound moments which often come out of "nowhere" and catch you by surprise? I wanted to get hold of the dying/caregiving/healing process I call the Dance of Death from the inside and in real time when you don't know how anything will turn out and are drowning in unbearable uncertainties. I wanted to tell a story that is at once my mother's story, my caregiving story, and the last phases of our journey together, yet simultaneously serves as a teaching/learning vehicle.

Only a narrative told in the first person and the unfolding present tense could weave together these stories and themes, and my expanding intentions. Because more and more of my professional work is directed toward improving the quality, safety, and patient-centeredness of health care delivery systems, what I chose to include in my narrative silently speaks from familiarity with the fragmented structure and misaligned incentives of our badly designed health care system. Particular encounters with that system are integral to our story and illustrate the devastating human consequences of that system even when it is not operating at its worst, but "merely" in its routinely mediocre ways.

VALIDATING AND WITNESSING CAREGIVERS

While my initial intent was to help orient caregivers, it expanded to validating that experience, whether past, present, or future. To the extent that this book can bear witness to your experience, it will also have done its job.

If you have already been through the caregiving process, your experience may or may not have received validation from people around you but certainly it is not recognized by our society. Most of us are lucky to get a day off from work for the funeral. Those who quit their jobs, draw down their savings, and put the rest of their life on hold to undertake this journey may jeopardize their own financial viability, job and/or career, other relationships, and even their own health. For most of us, neither caregiving nor grieving warrant a leave of absence, let alone with pay. No communal structures recognize, honor, and support the full, healthy cycle of grief and reconstruction of identity and meaning. By contrast, indigenous peoples accumulate enormous experience with the dying

and the dead; create community structures and rituals that witness, hold, and support the processes of dying, caregiving, and grieving; and integrate the living, the dead, the unborn, and the ancestors into a single sociocosmic fabric.

Despite social invisibility and lack of cultural valuation, family caregivers themselves instinctively recognize their value. Andrea Sankar, a medical anthropologist and gerontologist, has found that:

> Those family and friends who care for the dying experience their efforts as one of, if not *the*, most important accomplishments of their lives—their "finest hour" . . . People end their care of the dying frequently judging it to have been the "best and worst time" of their lives, and yet they have no one with whom to share it.[1]

Having long valued myself by the originality of my "real work," it was a surprise when I felt as Sankar's interviewees did.

In telling our story, part of my intention is to value and validate all those who take this journey with their beloved dying. Knowing how pushed and pulled caregivers are in daunting territory which health care professionals claim as their province, I have also extracted a model of the inherent structure obscured by the chaos of our unique situations. Located in the present moment from the perspective of the caregiver who is in the thick of things, it is intended as an orienting device for those going through it and validation for those who have completed such a journey. Its purpose is to give visibility, shape, and dignity to caregiving and make it seem a little less overwhelming, because you can see your situation as a whole from the outside, even while you are going through it.

COUNTERACTING A DEATH-DENYING CULTURE

By illuminating what is possible, this book also aims to counteract the consequences of our death-denying culture. It empowers caregivers and our elders by illustrating and explaining ways of navigating and dancing which may help give both partners greater closure and peace of mind than they ever imagined possible. If you can draw from my experiences so as to enhance the dying process in which you are a partner and reduce your potential regrets, this book will have also served its purpose.

Because cultural and medical phobia about death keeps us away from dying, most of us don't accumulate firsthand experience to draw on when we become decision-makers for someone close to us. We have to rely on others to fill us in. Too few of us get honest, reliable information about the dying and the death process even if we ask for it, and most of us don't have independent, informed sources to ask. As a result, we may cheat the dying and ourselves of the potentially most powerful, meaningful, and transformative experience of their or our lives.

I first crashed into this cultural reality in a shattering way a decade ago in the days following the stroke of my mother's friend, Elizabeth. Elizabeth was not just one of Mother's friends. She was the oldest and dearest of these relationships, the two having first connected in high school when Elizabeth admired Olwen's knitting and asked her to teach her how. It was to Elizabeth's family's home that Olwen repaired after each of the three great losses of her life, the losses that forever changed her life.

I was present for the third of these when we moved in with Elizabeth and her family for three years after the divorce, back in the days when no one was divorced. During those years of great bitterness between my parents, Elizabeth had the profound emotional intelligence to be able to be my mother's best friend, continue working for my father, and be the only adult who saw me in all this. As I told her many times over many years, I don't know how I would have survived emotionally, or where I would be or how I would be, if it had not been for her. At what level she took in the pro-

fundity of her gift I do not know, because on the surface she tossed it off, saying gracious things about how difficult it was in those days for each of my parents.

I persisted in telling her, however, because it was the primary way I could acknowledge the essence of who she really was, the largeness and wisdom of her being. I often thought I was the only one who truly saw her, and, since childhood, had gotten angry with each and every member of my family who at one time or another said diminishing things about her. From the day I was born, Elizabeth and I never did not see each other, never argued, never had any "stuff" between us. It was always a soul-to-soul, essence-to-essence relationship that never went off-course. Our ability to see each other even when no one else did was the gift we gave each other.

Although one side of Elizabeth's body was severely affected and her swallowing was impaired, her caretakers maintained she could go on for weeks. They talked about getting her well, got her up and dressed her every day, wheeled her down to the dining table at appointed times, and made a big to-do about the "swallow therapist" who, they made it seem, was going to perform a small miracle. Her big moment was to call for a differently shaped spoon to facilitate swallowing ice cream and such!

My head was spinning in this surreal environment. I felt like I was bouncing off rubber walls in a fun house. There was nothing to hang my hat on except my own intuition which was being validated by no one at the nursing home. No one seemed to be in charge of Elizabeth's case, and there was no one willing or able to explore my questions from a clear-eyed perspective independent of the party line that will not look death in the face, and insists on pushing the body to be here even if it and the being it houses are ready to move on.

My intuition said: How can our dear little Elizabeth go on like this? If one side of her body is barely working, how can her whole-body systems function?

How long before everything collapses? Aren't we talking about days or a week here? They would not address my common-sense questions about her clinical reality. Weeks, they said, or even longer, is quite possible, and they kept treating her as if she were recovering from a surgery or illness, and as if they could get her well or get some improvement.

I had dashed home to see Elizabeth unprepared for a lengthy visit and under the impression that her stroke, although serious, was not necessarily life-threatening. Now I had to make an agonizing decision: should I stay on longer, or leave (as I had originally planned) and come back for Christmas in a couple of weeks (or sooner if her situation were deteriorating) when I would be prepared for a longer visit? Having a realistic timetable was crucial for me.

I did not follow my intuition, however, and reluctantly drove back on a Thursday. I got daily reports from my mother, and on Sunday, she and the caretakers all thought Elizabeth was stronger. (Knowing what I have since learned, I think they were misled by what is called an "awakening" that often precedes death.) But Monday morning the nursing home called my mother to come over. On Monday afternoon, Elizabeth died.

I, who knew "nothing" about dying, turned out to be right. I wanted to be there and should have been there and could have been there. Because I did not follow my intuition, I failed one of the two people who had always been there for me and mattered most to me in the world.

A core principle emerged for me that I would follow in my Dance of Death with Olwen: be deeply attuned with my beloved dying, always respect and follow my intuition irrespective of what experienced providers or other people say. Intuition was my primary guide, and scary as the dance was, my intuition did not fail me.

MUTUAL GROWTH AND HEALING

As my journey with Olwen evolved, my reasons for writing this book not only expanded, but also found their center. I wanted to illuminate ways of being with a dying parent that can enhance the potential for mutually satisfying, emotional, relational, and spiritual outcomes. (A "parent" can be one's actual parent, or any elder who played that role and carries that meaning.)

If you haven't been through the death of a parent, it is almost impossible to imagine your way into the mercurial kaleidoscope of emotions generated by the ever-shifting situation, the impending loss and its finality while, amidst all the high-stake uncertainties, constantly having to make all kinds of decisions which can't be undone or redone.

You may discover you cannot make predictions about your choices or behavior or feelings based on linear extrapolations from the rest of your life experience or from your relationship up to this point, because the death of a parent is not like other losses, and the death of the mother is in a league all its own. You may surprise yourself because the Dance of Death is nonlinear:

➤ It may elicit behavior and feelings from both of you that is discontinuous with who you thought you were, who you thought she was, and the patterns that have shaped your relationship for a lifetime.

➤ Being open to the surprises and immediately flowing with them is possibly the most important, most healing, most transformative thing you will ever do.

➤ If the narrative of this book and the themes it highlights can help you to do that, then its central intention will be realized.

TELLING HER STORY

In the last weeks of Olwen's life, I felt a growing urge to "tell her story" and promised her she would not be forgotten. That need became more powerful as I became immersed in creating a collage and writing a eulogy for her memorial service, and found that one mirrored the other. I found myself focusing on her formative years, her resilience, and her capacity for picking up the pieces of her life each time it was shredded. Her "overstory" of triumph over loss was the right part of her story for that occasion.

The Olwen of her formative and prime years is not our focus here, yet they and her stunning willpower are essential backstory to who she was in those last months, weeks, and days of her life. The central narrative of this book intertwines the story of Olwen and her journey Home with my caregiving story about how I navigated a path through our Dance of Death and how we were each transformed by the process.

Our journey was precipitated by Olwen's hospitalization for pneumonia and a weakening heart. Olwen gave herself and me the gift of clarity: getting home, never ending up in a nursing home, and not "going on and on" while the quality of her life went down and down. Our journey unfolded from my efforts to translate my mother's wishes into reality, while our situations kept evolving and we encountered obstacles we each had to overcome as Olwen moved closer to death.

Working as a team, we emerged triumphant in the early rounds. She mustered her last reservoirs of strength and will, and I negotiated with all the stakeholders to get her home after her hospital and rehab incarcerations. Yet the question loomed: will she be able to *stay* there?

When Olwen started going downhill, the only way to avoid her nightmare of pointless cycling between hospitals and nursing homes was to get her off the endless treatment treadmill, bring in hospice, and shift the paradigm to palliative care. By fully vanquishing the first set of antagonists— the medical paradigm, providers, programs, and pharmaceuticals at cross-purposes with her needs and desires—and bringing in hospice, I unavoidably set up the next round of challenges.

I had to move in as Olwen's primary caregiver four hours from my own home and life. The mere existential fact of two people, each with her own needs, generated tensions between "my life or hers?" This tension between two subjectivities, between caring for the other and caring for oneself, is of course the fundamental tension in any family caregiving relationship. In addition, I had to struggle with our old patterns (always exacerbated by our coexisting in her space), try to stay outside of them, and not map old stuff onto her. Grappling with these internal challenges was much harder than rearranging the landscape to meet her ever-emerging needs.

Ultimately, we were struggling with the deepest and most intractable barrier to Olwen's dying well: her self-negating paradigm. Would it—even after all we had been through together and all we had each tried to do—would it defeat us both in the end? Winning this one was not about working together and being on the same side. It required something profound to surrender in each of us so there were no longer any sides to be on. Through the paradoxical mysteries of love and grace, we finally moved past all that had separated us. The grace through which transformation emerged lay beyond anything either of us had ever imagined.

NOTE

1. Andrea Sankar, *Dying at Home: A Family Guide for Caregiving*, Baltimore: Johns Hopkins University Press, 1999.

CHAPTER 23

Women's Health, Moving Forward

Changing Concepts of Women's Health: Advocating for Change

JULIA SCOTT

Julia Scott, excerpt from a speech given at the Canada-US Women's Health Forum, August 8, 1996, Ottawa, Canada. Reprinted by permission.

I want to reflect on the growth of the women's movement in the United States and its prospects for the future. I look at our current challenge as twofold. One is to get the word out about women's health status globally and not just in our own countries. The second, which is much harder, is getting past simply having the rhetoric and language about inclusiveness and diversity, and really getting down to the hard work for each of us and seeing how we hinder the expression and existence of that inclusiveness and diversity. It's very difficult to talk about these issues. Those of us who do are seen by the establishment as wild-eyed radicals, always bringing up things that might perhaps divide us. We want to be together in solidarity around gender issues. But we have to acknowledge that there are differences among us that impact our health. So if we raise these issues, it's not to be contentious or argumentative, although for some people that may be part of the reason, but to say that if we really believe in equality, we have to discuss what our differences are and not see them as ways that somehow make our effort less.

I always feel particularly challenged, particularly as a woman of color, to get up and speak on these issues. For the United States, I think we'll really be able to say that we have made progress in our movement when women other than women of color or poor women speak and work on these issues with the same fervor that they do on the issues of the so-called majority women.

Let's be clear that the women's health movement in the United States did not begin in the 1990s. The gains of the 1990s are directly related to and benefited from the organized women's movement of the 1970s and 1980s. The advances that we have been able to make in the 1990s, with the greater influx of women into positions of power, in legislation and administration, from the NIH to FDA, have been because of the hard work of women in the 1970s and 1980s. These women were not necessarily in the medical establishment, but they were activists and everyday women, who got sick and tired of not having answers and having all of our health problems labeled as hysterical or the results of our having our periods.

The woman's health movement also benefited from the struggles and the strategies of the civil rights movement. Many of the gains that the women's health movement has been able to make in the United States have been borne on the back of black men and women who struggled for racial equality in the United States.

What we know from the many gains we have made is that, in spite of the valiant efforts of so many women, including President Clinton's appointment of many women throughout this administration and the influx of women, especially women of color, into our own legislatures, they still have not afforded us the kind of access to health and health care that women so richly deserve. It's not enough simply to have women in place. We do have to question the philosophy of women who are appointed to these commissions and decision-making bodies, because very often some women who are not progressive have been some of our own worse enemies.

So, while it would not be possible to talk in detail about all the women's groups and organizations who have pioneered this work in the United States, I can still say that it is recognized that the group of women who came together to prepare publication of *Our Bodies, Ourselves* gave us the first work that paved the way to confronting some of women's anger and frustration about the lack of information and control we had concerning our bodies and the lack of access to health care treatment modalities. Also, the National Women's Health Network was and is the women's premier feminist health organization in the United States.

The National Black Woman's Health Project came out of that movement. Our founder, Byllye Avery, was on the board of that organization and became horrified when looking at the statistics and seeing the paucity of information available about black women's health. She was struck, especially, in 1979, by the National Health and Nutrition Examination Survey, conducted by the National Center for Health Statistics, Centers for Disease Control and Prevention (NCHS/CDC), which showed that black women, in a self-administered survey where they rated themselves, were in more psychological stress than white women who were institutionalized. It seemed to her—something that we have to acknowledge—even the best organizations that have the right kind of analyses in terms of race and class and their impact on our health status will never take the place of women of color having their own organizations and doing their own work. So, while we support and need the support of the broader white women's health movement, in our country and globally, we insist that work on these issues, especially issues that are critical to our health, are led by the women who are affected by them.

At the heart of our focus today is the fundamental question of how women can fully access good health and the best care that the United States, international leader in medical research, has to offer. We seek access for women who are poor or wealthy, married or single, migrant workers, office workers, homeless, differently abled, professionals, homemakers, heterosexual, bisexual, or lesbian. This perspective was not in the mix when the women's health movement first began agitating. The first inkling of a women's health movement was the 1960s campaign where a few isolated women were fighting for natural childbirth. They wanted to decrease the use of anesthetics women were being given during delivery. And they started to banish from the delivery room practices which had developed, not to improve the overall well being of mother and infant, but to increase the convenience for doctors. In raising these issues, the small group began to insert a new dynamic into the doctor-patient relationship.

Let me take a moment to talk about some of the differences in health concerns, fully aware that sometimes such discussions will be seen as a way of dividing us. However, it's really important for us to acknowledge that there are differences.

I will give just a few examples of those differences. While breast cancer doesn't affect black women at the same rates that it affects white women, it does affect us differently. We tend to get it at an earlier age, and the regulations which give an age at which women should get their first mammography is really problematic for us. That's why we have been fighting so valiantly to get those regulations changed. We would like it to be acknowledged that for black women, getting our first mammography at age forty or fifty is simply not good enough. We have also been fighting for more research on breast cancer to look at those differences. For instance, only last year a study came out suggesting that not only do we get it earlier but that we get a more virulent form of it. We, basically, have been told that the reason we die from breast cancer more frequently than other women is because of lack of access to such things as mammographies. While I'm sure that does have an impact on the situation, we have been struggling to make sure that we pay as much attention in our research agenda to the issues of the environment and of diet and how that relates to the different women of color communities.

The issue of AIDS is another area we have to look at differently. It's an issue that has been dealt with as a white male disease. But as the majority of the women who are being affected by this are minority women, mainly black, latino, and Native American women, we now find the money is start-

ing to dry up. Also we find a lot of punitive legislation being aimed at women who are HIV-infected. Instead of funding treatment programs and research programs that would look at how women are differently affected by HIV, we find that legislatures and judges want to mandate that women take medications like AZT against their judgments and that there be mandatory HIV testing. These are all things that we have to be concerned about.

The area of reproductive technologies is a huge issue for all women, but especially for women of color in the US. These are the same women who have been targeted for unsafe contraception, for sterilization abuse—and this is not something that has simply happened in the past. This is something that is happening right now.

Let's also think about the work on identifying the breast cancer gene. This is something we have to be very concerned about. Now insurance companies have or will have the ability to get at information that identifies certain people as being at risk for chronic and debilitating diseases. Then those people are going to be excluded from getting health care. So, while we cannot minimize the opportunities that allow more choice to women, we have to look at the downside, and pay attention to it.

The women of color movement has been very forceful in the US in looking at the use of long-acting contraceptives. We agree that this is something that is much needed in the very meager menu of choices that are available to women, but there are also serious problems with the discriminatory use of these methods aimed and targeted at poor women and women of color. We think it was the dragging of the feet of women and men in the health community, and the women's health community itself not joining us in that struggle, that has brought us to a place now where we have a method that could be valuable for some women, but is now in jeopardy in our country. We cannot continue to hide our heads in the sand over this issue.

I think the women's health movement has grown

to a place where it is starting to acknowledge, at least in rhetoric, that race, ethnicity, and class affect and impact the quality of health care for women; but I also think we have not gone that next step of working on how we can all very seriously talk together and address the racist practices in our institutions that keep us from working together. I hope we will spend more time talking about the issues and how we can address them. I hope we will come to a time when the broader women's community will be able to accept the leadership of women different from themselves, accept that we may have to change our strategies. Maybe we won't be able to get there the way everybody is used to getting there, but we will get there.

The Whole Woman

GERMAINE GREER

Germaine Greer, excerpt from *The Whole Woman,* New York: Knopf, 1999, with an introduction by Jennifer Baumgardner. Reprinted by permission.

Germaine Greer's new book *The Whole Woman,* her thirty-years-later follow-up to *The Female Eunuch,* is thoroughly disliked by everyone from the staid stylists at the *New York Times* to the chatty philosophers at salon.com. The consensus is that the book is shrill and disorganized, the work of a past-her-prime second-waver: bitter, batty, and male-bashing.

The fact that her critics, former fans all, find her to be so sour and incompetent points to the central difference between her audience then and now. *The Female Eunuch* spoke to women on the brink of a tumultuous shift in status and consciousness. *The Whole Woman* is written for feminists, women for whom finding the political roots of what appear to be personal problems is a matter of course. Instead of being happy with whatever progress has been made, Greer wants women to be insulted and angry by the scraps now offered us as "feminist emancipation," be it the "privilege" of abortion or "flex" time for overworked mothers.

With *Eunuch,* Greer said that women were castrated, cut off from their sexuality, and tried to get women to assert cunt power when most feminists were focusing on political power. Now that the pro-sex, get-on-top, use-toys, he-better-make-you-come aspect of feminism is ascendant (see *Bust, Minx, Susie Bright,* etc.), Greer is again fighting for the neglected side, turning her attention to politics . . . analyzing everything from deadbeat dads to transsexualism to girlie culture to female mutilation. And some of Greer's strongest inquiries concern women's health.

"Revolution," the final chapter of *The Female Eunuch,* concludes with the challenge, "What will you do?"; in *The Whole Woman,* Greer renews her question, asking not only what we will do, but what, during a three-decade interim, we actually have done.

I hope that despite the bad reviews, serious students of feminism will still read *The Whole Woman.* So much about what makes an ambitious book become big is timing. Yet the fact that the thirty-four heavy-hitting essayettes of *The Whole Woman* could be dismissed so easily is evidence that, despite the fragments of feminists' rhetoric in every atom of our culture, the whole of women's liberation that Greer envisions is still as hard for us to picture as the round earth was for Columbus's shipmates. To think that Greer is recanting on her free-your-ass credo from 1970 is to see just half the picture. Greer didn't think women could fuck themselves into liberty, but that we needed to be free to fuck as well as to do anything else. Her definition of *whole* means for women to be sexual and confident at the same time as they are political and conscious, and that's my definition, too.

—Jennifer Baumgardner

This sequel to *The Female Eunuch* is the book I said I would never write. I believed that each generation should produce its own statement of problems and priorities, and that I had no special authority or vocation to speak on behalf of women of any but my own age, class, background, and education. For thirty years I have done my best to champion all the styles of feminism that came to public attention because I wanted it to be clear that lipstick lesbianism and the prostitutes' union and La Leche and the Women's League for Peace and Freedom and pressure for the ordination of women were aspects of the same struggle toward awareness of oppression and triumph over it. Though I disagreed with some of the strategies and was as troubled as I should have been by some of the more fundamental conflicts, it was not until feminists of my own generation began to assert with apparent seriousness that feminism had gone too far that the fire flared up in my belly. When the lifestyle feminists chimed in that feminism had gone just far enough in giving them the right to "have it all," i.e., money, sex, and fashion, it would have been inexcusable to remain silent.

In 1970 the movement was called "women's liberation" or, contemptuously, "women's lib." When the name "libbers" was dropped for "feminists" we were all relieved. What none of us noticed was that the ideal of liberation was fading out with the word. We were settling for equality. Liberation struggles are not about assimilation but about asserting difference, endowing that difference with dignity and prestige, and insisting on it as a condition of self-definition and self-determination. The aim of women's liberation is to do as much for female people as has been done for colonized nations. Women's liberation did not see the female's potential in terms of the male's actual; the visionary feminists of the late sixties and early seventies knew that women could never find freedom by agreeing to live the lives of unfree men. Seekers after equality clamored to be admitted to smoke-filled male haunts. Liberationists sought the world over for clues to what women's lives could be if they were free to define their own values, order their own priorities, and decide their own fate.

The Female Eunuch was one feminist text that did not argue for equality. At a debate in Oxford one William J. Clinton heard me arguing that equality legislation could not give me the right to have broad hips or hairy thighs, to be at ease in my woman's body. Thirty years on, femininity is still compulsory for women and has become an option for men, while genuine femaleness remains grotesque to the point of obscenity. Meanwhile the price of the small advances we have made toward sexual equality has been the denial of femaleness as any kind of a distinguishing character. If femaleness is not to be interpreted as inferiority, it is not to signify anything at all. Even the distinction between the vagina, which only women have, and the rectum, which everybody has, has been declared, as it were, unconstitutional. Nonconsensual buggery, which can be inflicted on both sexes, has been nonsensically renamed "male rape." In June 1998 an overwhelming vote of the British House of Commons recognized the right of sixteen-year-old homosexual men "to have sex," by which they meant, apparently, for it was never explained, the right to penetrate and be penetrated anally. This the MPs saw as granting homosexual men the same rights as heterosexuals. For them at least, rectum and vagina were equivalent; in many cultures (and increasingly our own) the most desirable vagina is as tight and narrow as a rectum. Postmodernists are proud and pleased that gender now justifies fewer suppositions about an individual than ever before, but for women still wrestling with the same physical realities this new silence about their visceral experiences is the same old rapist's hand clamped across their mouths. Real women are being phased out; the first step, persuading them to deny their own existence, is almost complete.

In the last thirty years women have come a long, long way; our lives are nobler and richer than they were, but they are also fiendishly difficult. From the beginning feminists have been aware that the causes of female suffering can be grouped under the heading "contradictory expectations." The contradictions women face have never been more bruising than they are now. The career woman does not know if she is to do her job like a man or like herself. Is she supposed to change the organization or knuckle under to it? Is she supposed to endure harassment or kick ass and take names? Is motherhood a privilege or a punishment? Even if it had been real, equality would have been a poor substitute for liberation; fake equality is leading women into double jeopardy. The rhetoric of equality is being used in the name of political correctness to mask the hammering that women are taking. When *The Female Eunuch* was written our daughters were not cutting or starving themselves. On every side speechless women endure endless hardship, grief, and pain in a world system that creates billions of losers for every handful of winners.

It's time to get angry again.

The womb rudely awakens the growing girl to its presence by causing her to shed blood through her vagina. The more difficult the process, the more bloated and bilious she feels, the more dragging the pain, the more negative the ideas of a womb will seem to her. As she has heard the womb spoken of as a space inside her, like a room she did not know she had, her menstruation appears like a troublesome tenant after whom she has to clean up. . . . Though feminists have argued that we should celebrate the menarche as a young woman's coming of age, with a visible rise in status to compensate her for the inconvenience of menstruation and ward off any attempt on her part to cancel the whole process by remaining a skinny child, nothing has happened to endow the cycle with glamour or respect. We call the napkins used to soak up menstrual discharge "sanitary protection" as if the blood was both dirty and dangerous. Sanitary protection may now be advertised on television, not because women's functions are no longer considered shameful or disgusting but because the potential earnings are enormous. High profit margins on napkins that women have no choice but to buy are used to subsidize marketing campaigns for luxury products.

Neither women nor men have a positive attitude to menstruation. . . . The questions of the exorbitant cost of napkins and tampons has been raised regularly by feminists; feminists were the first to point out the dangers of asbestos in tampons and of toxic shock syndrome. . . . If women regard their own menstrual fluid as "googoomuck" we are a long way from taking the pride in our femaleness that is a necessary condition of liberation. Hundreds of feminists have tried all kinds of strategies for filling the idea of menstruation with positive significance, but it remains a kind of excretion, the liquefaction of abjection. Advertising of sanitary protection can no more mention blood than advertising of toilet paper can mention shit. When we come to recognize the taste of our menstrual blood on the lips or fingers or penis of a lover, perhaps then we will realize that it is not putrid, not dangerous, not in the least disgusting. One of the latest explanations of the real function of the uniquely human process of menstruation holds that the shedding of the blood is not an excretion but protection of the sloughing womb from infection.

For 30 years feminists have struggled to develop a positive imagery of the womb and ovaries. Feminist artists have painted, modeled, woven, potted, photographed, filmed, videoed, and embroidered sumptuous images of the female genitalia to absolutely no purpose. As far as mainstream culture was concerned, cunt art was no more than a subbranch of gynecology. Though much of the most influential art of the 1990s was focused upon the body as the locus of gender and the modality of socialization, no girl drifted off to sleep at night and dreamed of her mysterious innards under any shape she could recognize. Though women artists devised myriad fabulous boxes, purses lined with satin or fur, and glimmering bottomless caves, ordinary women derived little comfort from a new awareness of themselves as buried treasure. It would take more than a trip through the vagina of sculptor Niki de St. Phalle's ninety-foot-long female figure "Hon" to awaken the consciousness of the womb. More memorable perhaps were the artistic experiences of the womb dramatized as bruising encounters with obstetric technology.

Perhaps womb pride was too much to expect. The word "womb" originally meant any hollow space and by extension came to mean "belly" or "abdomen." The use of the word in modern times exclusively to signify the organ of gestation demonstrates our inability to think of the womb as anything but a passive receptacle, a pocket inside a person rather than the person herself. The ideal body is imperforate; the wombed body is grotesque and gaping, like Luna Park. Women's "inner space" implies a negative, an unsoundness, a hollowness, a harbor for otherness. But the term is misleading; there is no more a void inside a woman than there is inside a man. The unpregnant womb is not a space, but closed upon itself. The womb is not a sinus or a sac. The image of the uterus as a void waiting to be filled is an artifact derived from billions of lying diagrams that represent the fabulous baroque biochemistry of the womb as if it were the pocket of a billiard table. Women artists have done their best to counteract this by introducing fiber-optics into their own bodies, to show the quivering liveliness of the cervix's puppy-muzzle and the surging pulse of the fallopian tube amid its dancing fimbriae. Very few are watching, and for those who are there can be no shock of recognition. Consciousness is made of language, and we have no language for this. Cock and balls have a thousand names but uterus and ovaries have only their medical labels.

To justify the dragooning and torturing of women the public health establishment uses the rhetoric of feminism. Screening for cervical cancer was hailed as a woman's right; the taxpayer willingly stumped up for it, convinced that if women just had this itty-bitty test every now and then they would stop dying of cervical cancer. But they didn't. Deaths from cervical cancer, which were already falling, continued to fall, at a rate of about 7 percent a year. Meanwhile the one in six tested women called for retesting suffered agonies of fear and bewilderment, as well as all kinds of surgical interventions from colposcopy to hysterec-

tomy. Women were practiced on with an inefficient diagnostic tool because they were not the point; control was the point. The rest was oversold as an insurance against developing cervical and uterine cancer when it was no such thing. In case this sounds incredible, let me explain.

The current state of our understanding of cervical cancer is that it is in whole or in part a sexually transmitted disease, caused by the human papilloma virus (HVP), which causes genital warts and is carried by males and females. . . . Between 1960 and 1980 the incidence of cervical cancer in women under the age of thirty-five trebled and the number of deaths from the disease in this age group rose by 72 percent. In the nineties 15 percent of cases occur in this age group. The disease appears to progress slowly, taking about ten years to become manifest, but in general its career is not well understood.

The national cervical cancer screening program is based on the Papanicolaou smear, which has a false-negative rate estimated in 1979 as anywhere between 25 and 40 percent; where invasive cervical cancer is concerned, the rate may be as high as 50 percent. Abnormal Pap smears will also result from common infections. The remains of blood, or sperm, or contraceptive creams and jellies, vaginal douches, and deodorants in the vagina will affect the quality of the sample. Contraceptive pills and medications of other kinds can also distort the cell profile. If the test is not taken twelve to sixteen days after a period, and forty-eight hours or more after the last intercourse, its reliability may be compromised. As the supposedly premalignant changes in cell conformation are quite subtle, the job of evaluating cervical smears is both immensely boring and unremittingly stressful, even without the constant pressure for greater productivity. The *Wall Street Journal* reported in 1988 that a large proportion of US smear tests were read in high-volume cut-rate laboratories where technicians were sometimes given financial incentives to up the number of slides they read in a day to as many as 300, four times the maximum recommended if the human error rate was to be kept to a minimum. Some laboratories paid screeners on a piecework basis, sometimes as little as forty-five cents a slide. . . .

The adoption of a simple positive-negative classification conceals seven categories, from minor and almost certainly insignificant changes in the cell structure to changes considered definitely precancerous to actual in situ carcinoma. The difficulty in assessing smears correctly is clearly illustrated by the wide variations in practice between one region and another. . . . In Britain 5.5. million women a year are given smear tests; an average of 7 in every 100 of their smears will be considered positive, giving a total of 385,000 smears. In fact no more than 4,500 women will develop cervical cancer in any year, so 380,500 will have been frightened needlessly. . . . In June 1995 an article in the *Lancet* reported that "staff live in fear of being blamed for failing to prevent invasive cases of cancer. The desire to avoid overdiagnosis, which in the past kept the detection rates low, has now been outweighed by the need to avoid any possibility of being held responsible for missing a case." The result is an epidemic of terror. . . .

To be recalled for a second Pap smear is to catch the disease of fear. The test having been oversold in the first place, the woman is sure that there is something terribly wrong. After all, if it is true that atypical cells usually clear up spontaneously, what was the point of going through all the humiliating palaver of the test in the first place? The woman who is recalled may be given the all-clear after another sampling or two, but will she quite believe it? If she keeps being called back, every three months, or every month, she is very likely to make sure that she hasn't got cervical cancer by opting for and actively seeking a hysterectomy. A hysterectomy is a major operation with a long recovery period. The hysterectomized woman will need hormone replacement therapy and be "under the doctor" for a very long time, perhaps the rest of her life. . . .

Every time the newspapers report that a health authority has had to recall-screen women because

a second examination of their slides has led to different conclusions about their status, fear stalks the land. Public health consultant Dr. Angela Raffle dared to tell the truth, that cervical screening is "actually expensive, complicated, and relatively ineffective. Only about 50 percent of cases are picked up and there is huge and escalating overdetection and overtreatment." Raffle went on: "Screening has become something of a feminist icon and it is very hard to explain that cervical cancer was a rare and diminishing cause of death before we even began screening." Male-dominated governments are remarkably unaware of "feminist icons" and don't often, if ever, invest huge amounts of money in them. If the American government now spends $4.5 billion on Pap smears every year, it is not because they are being pushed around by a bunch of noisy feminists but because of the power and priorities of the medical establishment. . . .

No pressure group within the medical profession is lobbying for the right to save men's lives by regularly examining the prostate. Occasionally we hear that clinicians regret men's unwillingness to be routinely poked and prodded and X-rayed, but the temptation to set up a screening service for men has so far been successfully resisted, on the same sorts of considerations that should have prevented the setting up of women's screening programs. There is a strong impression that men are no more likely to submit their testicles to official care and attention than they are to wear their muffler when it is cold and keep their feet dry. The service exists for them to avail themselves of if they want to, and that is deemed to be sufficient. Men have the right to take care of themselves or not, as they see fit, but women are to be taken care of whether they like it or not. Screening is many times more likely to destroy a woman's peace of mind than it is to save her life. Women are driven through the health system like sheep through a dip. The disease they are being treated for is womanhood.

You and I need all the mothers we can get. Governments rely on taxes on current earnings for the funds that run our societies; the people now in work pay for the care and support of the people who are not in work. As the work force shrinks and life expectancy increases it becomes harder and harder to pay the social security bill. We all need the children being born now and we need them to grow up as well-educated, useful people, not circling aimlessly round the poverty trap. In *The Female Eunuch* I argued that motherhood should not be treated as a substitute career; now I would argue that motherhood should be regarded as a genuine career option, that is to say, as paid work and as such an alternative to other paid work. What this would mean is that every woman who decides to have a child would be paid enough money to raise that child in decent circumstances. The choice, whether to continue in her employment outside the home and use the money to pay for professional help in raising her child, or stay at home and devote her time to doing it herself, should be hers. By investing in motherhood we would inject more money into child care, which is the only way to improve a system that at present relies on the contribution of disenfranchised, low-paid, unresourced, and unqualified women. The sooner we decide that mothers are entitled to state support to use as they wish, the less it will cost us in the long run. We will be told on all sides that we can't afford it. If we weren't paying to send aircraft carriers to the Gulf and any other place Bill Clinton thinks a saber should be rattled, we could afford it. It is a question of priorities. Dignified motherhood is a feminist priority. A permanent seat on the UN Security Council is not.

In *The Female Eunuch* I argued that feminism would have to address the problem of male violence both spontaneous and institutionalized, but I could suggest no way of doing this beyond refusing to act as the warrior's reward. Even then radical women were demanding the right to aggression as a basic human right and women's groups were training in self-defense and martial arts. The assumption seemed to be that all human beings were violent unless they were deprived of the right to aggression by an oppressor. Freedom had to include the right to beat your enemies up. The outcome of a free-for-all seemed to me obvious: if violence is a right the strongest and the cruelest will always tyrannize over the gentle and the loving. Only those women who were strong and cruel enough could join in the butchery. The rest would be butchered.

That was not an outcome that I could tolerate, so I argued feebly that women should devalue violence by refusing to be attracted to it or to reward the victors. . . . In the years that followed aggression was carefully studied and we began to understand rather more about it. The role of women in for-menting male aggression is, I now believe, marginal, even irrelevant. . . . Our culture now depicts much more elaborate violence in more media more often than it did thirty years ago. Regardless of official ideologies our culture is therefore, by my judgment, less feminist than it was thirty years ago. Brutality, like other forms of pornography, damages everyone exposed to it. Violence disenfranchises all weaklings, including children, old people—and women.

Children, old people, and women are all short of testosterone. Even 10 years ago, testosterone was a word not often heard; nowadays the presence of testosterone in the environment is often remarked on. When the stands at the football ground are packed with vociferating fans it is described as a testosterone storm. When a driver kills another driver who cut him off at a corner, he does it in a "blind testosterone rage." . . . By invoking testosterone a man can abdicate responsibility for his own behavior.

Testosterone does seem to be powerful. Women who have been dosed with pharmaceutical testosterone as part of hormone replacement therapy report distinct and unnerving changes in personality, which are, as one might expect, increased tension and irritability, and clitoral sensitivity raised to the point of discomfort. When women began to complain of personality changes as well as irreversible changes in voice and distribution of body hair, HRT preparations containing testosterone were deleted. It would seem that testosterone is the hormone of dominance; a survey from Mount Sinai School of Medicine in New York found that, the higher up the career ladder women had risen, the higher their testosterone levels. . . .

Violent sex offenders have been found, again not consistently, to have the highest testosterone levels of all. The effect of alcohol and drugs is variable; habitual use suppresses testosterone but occasional use can stimulate secretion, possibly as a feedback effect of disinhibition. This raises a further possibility that violent men are not violent because they have more testosterone to cope with, but that they have more testosterone because they are more violent. . . .

Taking courage, then, from the notion of biology as alterable, we can entertain the possibility that ours is a culture in which elevated testosterone levels are sought, prized, and rewarded, no matter how destructive the consequence. . . . Testosterone converts fear into hostility; fear stimulates secretions of testosterone along with other body chemicals associated with aggression, and off float the pheromones into the surrounding air. Could it be that we enjoy being scared and angry more than we enjoy serenity? . . .

Pluggers of the "future is female" line like to tell us that women's management skills are different, because women are nonconfrontational and more interested in compromise and settlement than in imposing their will. If aggression is fun and if the biochemistry of aggression can be stimulated by cultural demand, we cannot rule out the possibility that women will gradually become as dangerous to themselves and others as men are. If the nonviolent woman is simply a subservient creature, too repressed to acknowledge her own murderous propensities, war will continue to be the human condition. War will not be rendered obsolete unless feminism and pacifism agree to persist in their historical cohabitation and build a culture of nonviolence.

The propaganda machine that is now aimed at our daughters is more powerful than any form of indoctrination that has ever existed before. Pop is followed by print is followed by video and film, and nothing that a parent generation can do will have any effect other than to increase the desirability of the girlpower way of life. Nobody observing the incitement of little girls to initiate sexual contact with boys can remain unconcerned. Regardless of the dutiful pushing of condoms in the girls' press, the exposure of baby vaginas and cervixes to the penis is more likely to result in pregnancy and infection than orgasm. We know that some of today's young women regard oral sex as little more than a courtesy routinely offered by cool girls to demanding boys, the girls themselves having no expectation that any man would ever do as much for them. The girls' press does not question this iniquity; rather it reinforces the idea that boys are nabobs who can get any kind of sex anywhere and mostly cannot be bothered. To deny a woman's sexuality is certainly to oppress her, but to portray her as nothing but a sexual being is equally to oppress her. No one doubts that teenage boys have peremptory sexual urges, but they are never depicted as prepared to accept any humiliation, endure any indignity, just to get close to some, any, girl. Nor are they pushed to spend money on their appearance or to dress revealingly or drink too much in order to attract the attention of the opposite sex. In every color spread the British girls' press trumpets the triumph of misogyny and the hopelessness of the cause of female pride.

The trouble is not that sisterhood is powerful, as the title of Robin Morgan's book has it, but that it isn't. Sisterhood does not rule and will never rule, OK? The principle of sisterhood is power-sharing, which is another name for powerlessness. In a society constructed of self-perpetuating elites, a grassroots movement exists to be walked on. Elites tumble down but the grass survives to spring again through the thickest pavement. All studies of gender difference agree on one thing, that females are less variable than males. If men and women were poppies, both the tallest and shortest poppies would be men. The women would cluster around the median, the norm. If we look at intelligence or mathematical ability we can see the same phenomenon. Men are, as it were, built for competition, already separated out into winners and losers, while women are built to understand each other, to cooperate, to pull shoulder to shoulder. Indeed, we could see the historic pattern of binding a woman to a man and forcibly separating her from her female peers as a precaution against the development of a female tendency to agglomerate. Men are afraid of women in groups.

One of the advances in the last thirty years has been that women's friendship is now a serious topic, and an entrenched value in women's lives. Girls' magazines treat the vicissitudes of friendship with more seriousness than the endless flummery about boys. Women's "being there for each other" features in soap operas. Women students consider themselves bound to accept each other's word without question, flying in the face of the prejudice that women are incapable of loyalty or trust. Only when sisterhood is real can sisterhood become powerful. We are on the way.

Women's Health and Government Regulation: 1950–1980

SUZANNE WHITE JUNOD

©1999 by Suzanne White Junod. Reprinted by permission.

Many of the medical discoveries that were made in the first half of the twentieth century came to fruition in the second half. New techniques for detecting cancer and fetal abnormalities were developed. A number of new products were introduced into the market—not always with happy results. And women's struggle to make informed decisions about their own bodies often led to clashes with both the government and private industry. Some of these clashes took place in the courts; others, in the streets.

By 1955, four different research groups were credited with discovering that the sex of the fetus could be predicted through analysis of fetal cells in amniotic fluid. This information was important in cases of genetically transmitted sex-linked diseases.

In 1959, French cytogeneticist Jerome LeJeune discovered that one form of Down's syndrome was caused by trisomy of the twenty-first chromosome; this paved the way for a wider use of amniocentesis in diagnosing fetal genetic abnormalities. By 1966, the problems in culturing fetal cells obtained through amniocentesis were solved, and two years later, the first abortions after midtrimester amniocentesis and karyotyping were performed.

A cooperative registry was set up in 1971 to ascertain the safety of amniocentesis. By 1976, amniocentesis was shown to have favorable results in clinical trials. By the late 1970s, there were a number of successful lawsuits against obstetricians who had failed to refer a patient over the age of 35 for amniocentesis. As a result, amniocentesis came in to greatly expanded use.

Ultrasound, which Lars Leksell had used successfully in 1953 to diagnose a hematoma in an infant's brain, became a routine part of obstetrical practice after 1975, when improvements in gray-scale and real-time imaging made it commercially successful.

IN VITRO FERTILIZATION

The first successful use of follicle-stimulating hormone for ovulation induction was reported in 1958. The first pregnancy after treatment with human pituitary gonadotropin was reported in 1960; this led to studies of the hypothalamic-releasing factors that enable or block ovulation.

In 1969, Patrick Steptoe and Robert Edwards began collaboration on the human IVF project. Steptoe had improved the laparoscopy instrument in the 1950s and used it to operate on the fallopian tubes and to extract ova.

In 1973, Landrum Settles of Columbia University extracted an ovum from a patient with dysfunctional fallopian tubes, fertilized it with her husband's sperm, and incubated it in his lab in preparation for implantation in her womb. Horrified, the chairman of the Department of Obstetrics and Gynecology deliberately destroyed Settles' experiment, claiming that it was both unethical and a risk to the woman's health.

On July 25, 1978, Steptoe and Edwards reported the birth of the first "test-tube" (IVF) baby in England.

CANCER DETECTION AND TREATMENT

PAP SMEAR During the 1950s, cytology laboratories were established in the United States, signifying the medical community's growing acceptance of the Pap smear as a means of detecting cervical cancer, as well women's increasing demand for the test. The American Cancer Society was instrumental in educating physicians on its use. By the 1960s, the Pap smear was part of regular gynecology practice. Pap Check, a do-it-yourself test that had never received FDA approval, was finally recalled in 1973.

MAMMOGRAPHY In 1960, Robert Egan at M. D. Anderson Hospital in Houston revolutionized breast imaging when he adapted a high-resolution industrial film to a mammographic technique. In 1962, Egan reported the discovery of unsuspected "occult carcinomas."

In 1963, Health Insurance Plan of New York tested Egan's breast-imaging technique and, in 1964, organized the first randomized controlled study to evaluate the effect of screening on mortality. Women who were screened were a third less likely to die from breast cancer than those who received physical examination only. This study served as a model for a national study sponsored by the American Cancer Society and the National Cancer Institute that included 250,000

women. In 1965, the American College of Radiology held its first conference on mammography.

Throughout the 1970s, however, there was concern about the side effects from mammography, especially in women who had undergone radiation treatment. Xerox Corporation replaced the film of the traditional X-ray with a selenium-coated aluminum plate prepared for exposure after being electrically charged. Xeroradiology reduced exposure and produced better quality images. Magnification mammography, which allowed better analysis of suspicious areas, was also introduced.

TAMOXIFEN Paclitaxel (Taxol) was first isolated from the Pacific yew in 1966. Dr. Craig Jordan, professor of cancer pharmacology and director of the breast cancer research program at the Lurie Comprehensive Cancer Center at Northwestern University Medical School in Chicago, began studying tamoxifen as a graduate student in 1969. "It was the age of making love and not war, and everybody was looking for more contraceptives." Tamoxifen was a great postcoital contraceptive in rats, but it proved totally ineffective in women, so it went back on the shelf, at least temporarily.

But then Dr. Jordan found that tamoxifen could prevent breast cancer in animals, so in 1974 he began testing it on American women with breast cancer. In 1977, Tamoxifen was approved for patients with advanced breast cancer, and in June 1990, it was approved for node-negative patients.

NEW TREATMENTS, NEW PRODUCTS, NEW THREATS

DES In 1940, Charles Huggins first reported the value of a potent hormone, diethylstilbestrol (DES), in the treatment of prostate tumors. Over the next three decades, DES was prescribed to pregnant women, supposedly to improve the chances of a healthy delivery. A generation later physicians found that it caused adenosis (abnormal gland development) and vaginal adenocarcinoma (a form of cancer) in the daughters of women who took the drug. Genitourinary defects have also been found in sons, and more recent lawsuits allege harm to grandchildren as well. Since the 1970s, several thousand DES victims have sued pharmaceutical companies nationwide.

ENOVID In 1959, the FDA approved Enovid (produced by G. D. Searle) as an oral contraceptive. This profoundly altered the scope of the FDA's authority and established what evolved into a long-term interest in women's health issues. As FDA commissioner George Larrick pointed out, pregnancy was not a "disease." The agency had no experience in either approving or regulating a drug for such a purpose, and although the efficacy of the pill was not in doubt, its safety was soon rendered suspect when reports of associated thromboemolic problems began to surface. In 1967, British epidemiological studies confirmed the statistical link between thromboembolism and oral contraceptives. In 1968, the FDA instituted an Adverse Reaction Data Reporting Program on oral contraceptive drugs.

SILICONE IMPLANTS The first breast implant was in 1962. In 1963, Dow Corning launched a national advertising campaign for Dow Corning Medical Fluid 360, a liquid silicone preparation that could be injected into the body "for removing facial wrinkles, recontouring women's breasts, and reshaping other parts of the body." FDA agents seized some of the product in the office of an osteopath and in the offices of two California cosmetic surgeons. The agents discovered that the California physicians had not only used the Dow silicone "360" in their medical practice, but also a laboratory-grade silicone and an industrial-grade silicone, which the physicians had ordered through a furniture dealer.

In 1968, Dow defendants moved to dismiss the government's criminal indictment against them, arguing that the product that they had shipped, silicone fluid, was not a "drug" or a "new drug" under the law. The court ruled that it could not make such a determination until the evidence was heard at trial. The defendants also charged that the statutory definitions of "drug," "device," "cosmetic," and "new drug" were unconstitutionally vague in regard to their product. The court also rejected this argument, saying "the choice of the proper classification is not as difficult as defendants make it out to be. With the guidance of the avowed Congressional policy of protecting the public health, when an item is capable of coming within two definitions, there is really only one answer, namely, that which affords the public the greater protection."

In 1971, Dow Corning and S. W. Rhode, former director of Dow's Medical Products Division, entered pleas of no contest to charges that they had sold a silicone product for rejuvenating middle-aged women in violation of the federal Food, Drug, and Cosmetic Act. The company acknowledged that it had failed to obtain premarket clearance for their product as a drug. Rhodes and Dow were subject to maximum fines of $8,000 and eight years in prison.

Four years later Dow Corning modified its original breast implant product. The FDA responded in a Talk Paper that it had "never approved injectable liquid silicone for breast augmentation or enlargement. Serious injury and at least four known deaths have been attributed to this procedure," and warned against medical use of nonsterile industrial-grade silicone. The FDA further noted that "there is another method of breast augmentation which is performed in the United States. It involves the use of silicone in a pliable plastic bag placed over the chest muscles. None of the problems connected with liquid silicone have been reported for this procedure."

On March 24, and July 6, 1978, the General and Plastic Surgery Devices Panel recommended that the silicone inflatable breast prosthesis be given a class II designation, but identified certain risks to health presented by the device.

DALKON SHIELD The Dalkon Shield, marketed by A. H. Robbins Pharmaceutical Company, was developed before passage of the 1976 Medical Devices Amendment and therefore did not go through a premarketing screening. Regulators had concerns about the device from the beginning, however, and it was targeted for investigation when reports of injury began to emerge.

Litigation began in 1974 and ultimately involved hundreds of thousands of claimants from among the 2.2 million women who had had the Shield implanted. By 1980, clear evidence of corporate wrongdoing and fraud had emerged, and juries routinely began awarding multimillion-dollar punitive damages. As a result, Robins entered bankruptcy court voluntarily in 1985, and in 1989 a plan was implemented to permit injured women to choose an administrative compensation scheme instead of litigation.

TOXIC SHOCK SYNDROME Toxic shock syndrome (TSS) was first identified in 1989. The earliest reported cases occurred among seven children; all were linked to the presence of *staphylococcus aureus*. Symptoms of the disease include vomiting, diarrhea, high fever, and a sunburnlike rash.

Before 1977 all tampon products were made of rayon or a rayon-cotton blend. Since 1977, 40 percent of tampon products have contained more absorbent synthetic material. In 1979, the FDA listed tampons as a class II device under the 1976 Medical Device Amendments and ruled that they must not contain drugs or antimicrobial agents. Today, 70 percent of menstruating women used vaginal tampons.

In 1978, TSS was identified as a distinct disease. A dramatic upsurge in cases reported to CDC occurred in 1980, when 890 cases were reported, 812 among women whose illness coincided with the start of their menstrual periods. The fatality rate among early TSS patients was around 8 percent. This striking association of TSS with menstruating women stimulated careful epidemiological analysis. When information collected by the Utah Department of Health suggested that a particular tampon brand, Rely, had been sued by many women with TSS, a detailed study was devised by the Centers for Disease Control in September 1980 to examine tampon brand use. This study found that 71 percent of a recent group of women with TSS had used Rely tampons.

On September 22, 1980, Procter and Gamble recalled all Rely tampons on the market, and all tampon manufacturers subsequently lowered the absorbency of their tampons. The FDA began requiring that all tampon packages carry information on TSS and advise women to use tampons with the minimum absorbency needed to control menstrual flow.

In 1980, the American Society for Testing and Materials organized a task force to develop uniform absorbency testing and labeling at the FDA's request.

Although cases of menstrually related TSS fell off dramatically after 1984, the overall number of cases is suspected to have risen as the staphylococcal bacteria that produces the deadly toxin has spread to more people. Today, only about half of the cases of staphylococcal toxic shock syndrome are connected with menstruating women. TSS has been reported in men, children, and older women, and in conjunction with surgery, a wound, influenza, sinusitis, childbirth, use of a contraceptive sponge, cervical cap, or diaphragm, intravenous drug abuse, an abscess, boil, cut, or even an insect bite.

THE WOMEN'S HEALTH MOVEMENT TAKES OFF

➤ 1969: Journalist Barbara Seaman publishes *The Doctors' Case Against the Pill,* charging that women were not being adequately informed about dangerous side effects from the pill, including stroke, heart disease, diabetes, depression, and other ailments.

➤ 1970: Senate hearings on the pill; activist Alice Wolfson demanded to know why no women were being allowed to testify. TV cameras recorded the disruption as Seaman and other women joined the protest. The dissent helped to launch a political movement focusing on women's health.

➤ 1975: Seaman, Wolfson, and three other women activists went on to found the National Women's Health Network as an umbrella institution for nearly 2,000 women's self-help medical projects. The movement centered on the overuse of medical technology, insufficiently rigorous drug testing, and refusal to listen to patients (paternalism).

➤ 1970: Alice Wolfson took the first critical steps to open a dialogue between the FDA Obstetrics and Gynecology Advisory Committee and the FDA. The meetings were closed to the public, but Wolfson and several colleagues persisted in attending anyway. "What are you discussing that women shouldn't hear?" she asked. This was the occasion of the first sit-in at the FDA.

➤ 1970: The AMA House of Delegates passed a resolution opposing the product package insert (PPI) on the grounds that it would "confuse and alarm many patients." A compromise was reached wherein a modified version was mailed to physicians to hand out with every pill prescription. Over the next five years, the AMA distributed only 4 million copies, although an estimated 10 million US women per annum were taking the pill. In time, the FDA went back to its original concept—distributing the PPI in the pill packet through pharmacists. Again there was opposition from doctors and the drug industry. This time the consumer groups were more successful. It is likely that the PPI has contributed to the subsequent decline in pill use.

➤ 1971: Self-help gynecology helped transform women's health and body issues into a separate social movement. The movement was born on April 7, 1971, at the Everywoman's Bookstore in Los Angeles. For some time feminists had met there to discuss health and abortion issues. After exhausting "book learning," Carol Downer, a member of the group, suggested empirical observation. After inserting a speculum in her own vagina, she invited other women present to observe her cervix.

➤ 1972: Police officers arrested Carol Downer and Colleen Wilson on charges of practicing medicine without a license. Margaret Mead observed that "men began taking over obstetrics and they invented a tool that allowed them to look inside women. You could call this progress—except that when women tried to look inside themselves, this was called 'practicing medicine without a license.'" (*Los Angeles Times,* February 5, 1974). Several months later, Downer was acquitted after two days of deliberation by the jury.

➤ 1972: Boston women organized Speakoutrage, a public hearing for women to testify about their experiences with abortion, forced sterilization, unnecessary surgery, and other forms of exploitation and mistreatment. Conditions at the Boston City Hospital ob-gyn clinic were especially decried. As evidence of medical abuse came to light in city after city and hospital after hospital, it generated a broader-based women's health movement.

Carol Downer, the "mother" of self-help gynecology, was arrested for using yogurt to treat yeast infections and for using a device called the Del-Em for menstrual extraction, also called "self-abortion." Her defense was eloquent and long-quoted as a cornerstone of the concerns of the women's health movement:

> In what has been described as "rape of the pelvis," our uteri and ovaries are removed, often needlessly. Our breasts and all supporting muscular tissue are carved out brutally in radical mastectomy. Abortion and preventive birth control methods are denied us unless we are a certain age, or married, or perhaps they are denied us completely. Hospital committees decide whether or not we can have our tubes tied. Unless our uterus has "done its duty," we're often denied. We give birth in hospitals run for the convenience of the staff. We're drugged, strapped, cut, ignored, enemaed, probed, shaved—all in the name of "superior care." How can we rescue ourselves from the dilemma that male supremacy has landed

us in? The answer is simple. We women must taken women's medicine back into our own capable hands.

MEN, WOMEN, WHAT'S THE DIFFERENCE?

In 1961, news that the hypnotic drug thalidomide had been linked with an epidemic of malformed infants in Europe focused attention on women and pregnancy. Worldwide concern about thalidomide led to the passage of drug reform legislation in the United States which shut women out of the early phases of clinical drug testing and virtually orphaned clinical studies of pediatric drug efficacy and safety.

In the 1970s it was discovered that women taking the prescription drug Premarin to treat menopausal symptoms showed a lower risk of cardiovascular illness. As a result, in 1975 Rush-Cook County undertook a hormone therapy study—on *men* —to see what effects estrogen drugs had on heart disease. This study remains the only randomized, controlled scientific study about estrogen therapy and heart disease.

In 1977, the FDA published research guidelines that officially excluded women of reproductive age from early phases of clinical drug trials. As a result, drugs were routinely approved for general use that had not been tested on women. "Nobody was thinking much about how drugs might act differently in men and women," said Dr. Lainie Friedman Ross, assistant director of the MacLean Center for Clinical Medical Ethics at the University of Chicago. "Men are steady-state subjects. The problem is, about half of the people eventually taking the tested drugs were women with monthly hormonal changes."

The scratch-your-head logic of using men to test women's treatments helped garnish important support for the Women's Health Initiative in the 1980s.

Map of the Women's Health Movement

SHERYL BURT RUZEK

Sheryl Burt Ruzek, excerpt from "The Map of the Women's Health Movement," paper presented at the Seminar on the History and Future of Women's Health, Washington DC, June 11, 1998; Sheryl Burt Ruzek and Julie Becker, "The Women's Health Movement in the United States: From Grass-Roots Activism to Professional Agendas," *Journal of the American Medical Women's Association*, Winter 1999. Reprinted by permission.

Women's health activists have generated public debate and spearheaded social action in a number of waves throughout US history, waves that University of Michigan Sociologist Carol Weisman views as part of a women's health "megamovement" that has spanned two centuries. The US women's health movement grew rapidly through the 1970s; broadened its base with women of color and others in the early 1980s; and contracted, was co-opted, and became institutionalized during the late 1980s and 1990s. The general feminist movement of the 1960s and 1970s spawned dozens of specific movements and hundreds of movement organizations, shaping public consciousness.

RISE AND DEVELOPMENT OF THE WOMEN'S HEALTH MOVEMENT

Looking back now at the early days of the women's health movement in the late 1960s, it seems almost incredible how hard it was to get access to medical information unless you were a doctor—and most doctors were men. Few books on women's health could be found in bookstores, except for books on childbirth. The assumption was simply that physicians were the experts and women were to do as instructed. Breaking open this closed system, laywomen asserted that personal, subjective knowledge of one's own body was a valid source of information and deserved recognition, not scorn. The idea of women creating "observational" data out of their own health and body experiences was truly "revolutionary."

From demonstrations during the Senate hearings on the pill to gynecological self-help groups in homes, the women's health movement grew rapidly through the early 1970s. This activism didn't emerge in a vacuum, but out of a social environment in which a wide array of social movements was re-shaping the landscape.

The women's health movement grew rapidly through the leadership of several grassroots groups with strong ties to other social change movements, particularly the abortion rights, prepared childbirth, and consumer health movements. As the general feminist movement of the 1960s and 1970s sought equal rights and the full participation of women in all public spheres, many believed that without control over reproduction, all other rights were in jeopardy. Thus in the early years, reproductive issues defined many branches of the movement and shaped group consciousness and social action. Reproductive rights remain central to feminist health agendas worldwide.

Feminist health writers such as Barbara Seaman, Barbara Ehrenreich, Deirdre English, Ellen Frankfort, Gena Corea, Claudia Dreifus, and columnists for prominent feminist newspapers galvanized women to explore their own health, providing critical mo-mentum for the emerging grassroots movement. The Boston Women's Health Book Collective pro-duced the enormously popular *Our Bodies, Ourselves,* which has had numerous US and foreign language printings. The Federation of Feminist Women's Health Centers "invented" and championed gyne-cological self-help and woman-centered reproduc-tive health services. The National Women's Health Network (NWHN) linked a wide array of local groups to provide a voice for women in Washington. Monitoring legislation, Food and Drug Adminis-tration actions, and informing the public about women's health issues continue to be central to this organization's mission. A few nationally promi-nent groups focused on specific diseases or condition (e.g., DES Action, the Endometriosis Association).

Members of pivotal groups and other health activists traveled, spoke, and published widely, and used contacts with the media effectively, becoming spokespeople for the rapidly growing movement.

Movement activists also sought a number of reforms: regulation of drugs and devices; out of hospital birthing centers and midwifery; alternative and complementary therapies; lay access to medical information; and better communication between patients and health providers. Activists have also questioned medical orthodoxies—particularly birth practices, hormone replacement therapies, and cancer prevention and treatment.

An important achievement of the women's health movement was transferring women's health from the domain of largely male experts to women themselves. Developing in parallel with self-help medical care movements, consciousness-raising and gynecological self-help became strategies for empowering women to define their own health and create alternative services. Local movement groups in all fifty states were providing gynecol-ogical self-help, women-controlled reproductive health clinics, clearinghouses for health information and referral services, and producing their own health educational materials. Advocacy ranged from accompanying individual women seeking medical care to advising and influencing state and local health departments.

By the mid-1970s, more than 250 formally iden-tifiable groups provided education, advocacy, and direct service in the United States. Nearly 2,000 informal self-help groups and projects provided additional momentum to the movement. Although ideologically committed to being inclusive, the leadership of the women's health movement re-mained largely white and middle class in North America during the early years. Sterilization abuse mobilized women of color to seek government protection during the 1970s, and groups such as the Committee to End Sterilization Abuse (CESA) were founded.

The women's health movement grew visibly global, with groups such as ISIS in Geneva creating opportunities for worldwide feminist health activism. By the mid-1970s, there were more than seventy feminist health groups in Canada, Europe, and Australia. Today, there are growing efforts to make connections with feminist health activists, both in industrialized and developing countries.

As the women's health movement evolved in the United States, the distinct health needs of diverse women emerged, and women of color formed their own movement organizations such as the National Black Women's Health Project, the National Latina Women's Health Organization, the Native American Women's Health Education and Research Center, and the National Asian Women's Health Organization. Women of color health organizations gained national recognition and developed agendas to protect women against racist sterilization and contraceptive practices; to widen access to medical care for lower income women, including abortions no longer covered by Medicaid; and to focus on diseases and conditions affecting women of color such as lupus, fetal alcohol syndrome, hypertension, obesity, drug addiction, and stress related to racism and poverty that were ignored or misunderstood by largely white movement groups. By the late 1980s, the National Black Women's Health Project had established local chapters with more than 150 self-help groups for African-American women. Women's health agendas also grew within organizations that addressed a broad range of issues for both men and women of color.

Other women added distinct health agendas in the 1970s and 1980s. Lesbians (the Lesbian Health Agenda), rural women, and women with disabilities (the Dis-Abled Women's Network) joined older women's groups (the Older Women's League) and women with specific health concerns to broaden constituencies and issues. With the rise of environmental health concerns, groups such as the Women's Environmental Development Organization (WEDO) built bridges between feminist health activism and other movements for social change.

Of course social movements never retain their peak levels of participation, and like other movements, grassroots feminist health organizations declined in the 1980s, apparently as a result of changes in movement adherents and the social context in which movement groups operated. For example, many founders of movement organizations returned to school, began families, or entered the paid labor force, as have the next generation of women who increasingly juggle careers and families, thus reducing the traditional volunteer labor pool. Much of organized feminism, as it evolved both in media imagery and academe, came to be seen as distant or disconnected from ordinary women's lives.

The success of single-issue groups, particularly acquired immune deficiency syndrome (AIDS) organizations, to secure funding for direct services, education, and research presented new models for health activism. And the discovery of mainstream health institutions that "marketing to women" could increase profits led to the designation of a wide array of clinical services as "women's health clinics." By the 1990s, women's health services were widespread, although most were now part of larger medical institutions. In her recent national survey of women's health services, Weisman found that most centers founded in the 1960s and 1970s claimed a commitment to a feminist ideology; those founded later or sponsored by hospitals were significantly less likely to report this commitment. Within the movement, concerns emerged over whether new interest in women's health reflected co-optation or institutionalization. One price of "success" is that it is increasingly difficult for women to know whether particular "women's health centers" are truly woman-centered or simply marketed as such.

By the end of the 1980s, most alternative feminist health clinics had ceased to exist, and the survivors had broadened their range of services and affiliated with larger health systems. Gynecological self-help has virtually disappeared. The surviving grassroots movement advocacy and education groups such as the NWHN must work hard to retain support from both individuals and foundations as they compete with newer organizations for members and resources. Thus, grassroots groups contracted internally as they were diluted externally by the growing prominence of both mainstream women's support groups (on a wide array of health issues ranging form alcohol problems to breast cancer) and disease-focused health advocacy groups whose efforts supported the growing federal initiatives for greater equity in women's health research.

FROM GRASSROOTS IDEOLOGIES TO PROFESSIONAL INSTITUTIONAL AGENDAS

The success of the women's health movement is reflected in the extent to which mainstream organizations and institutions, particularly federal agencies, have incorporated or adopted core ideas and created new opportunities for women's health advocates. By 1990, the reform wings of feminism had made significant claims for gender equity in all social institutions and federal equity agendas emerged. With a growing number of women in Congress, in the biomedical professions, and in health advocacy communities, organizations that had pursued very different paths to improving women's health coalesced around the 1989 General Accounting Office (GAO) report. This report, showing that the National Institutes of Health (NIH) had failed to implement its policy of including women in study populations, proved to be a catalyst for pressuring Congress and the NIH to take action, and by the end of 1990 the Women's Health Equity Act was passed, and the NIH established the Office of Research on Women's Health. In 1991, the NIH undertook the Women's Health Initiative, the largest project of its kind, seeking data on prevention and treatment of cancer, cardiovascular disease, and osteoporosis. Scientific and professional interest in women's health burgeoned. Spurred by growing federal investment in women's health and by the "Cold War dividend" funding of women's research

through the Department of Defense, health activists saw opportunities to collaborate with scientists and professionals who were eager to take advantage of these new research priorities.

Although grassroots women's health groups have criticized many aspects of federally funded research, and have attempted to rectify perceived problems in consent procedures and inclusion criteria, they have largely supported greater federal funding of biomedical and psychosocial research on women's health. Thus after two decades of activism, the health movement's critique of biomedicine and the call for de-medicalizing women's health care was largely reframed into a bipartisan agenda for parity in funding for women's and men's health-related research.

The 1990s became a period of heightened activism. To maximize the likelihood of obtaining federal funding for research on women's health, scientists and their consumer allies focused on specific diseases—from AIDS to breast cancer. This narrowing of focus was critical for navigating federal funding streams that are tied to specific diseases and organ systems. The new "disease-oriented" organizations reflect the interests of women who expect a high level of professionalism. Facing dual roles as workers outside the home and traditional caretakers inside the home, the highly educated women who support the new single-issue groups may find that their interests lie in organizations that dispense professionally endorsed information, solicit donations, and carry out advocacy efforts on behalf of women. Thus the success of women's entry into the labor force, changes in cultural ethos, and women's own commitment to specialization and professionalism may explain why the narrower, highly professionalized women's health organizations that emphasize parity for women's health research attract women who do not identify either with broader movements for social change or with feminism per se.

AIDS advocacy groups also raised a new standard of effectiveness for health activists. They not only successfully increased funding for education and research, but gained a voice in how these added appropriations from government and foundations would be spent. Julie Becker, a public health advocate, observes that thereafter, breast cancer advocates and others (ovarian cancer advocates, Parkinson's patients and their families, etc.) adopted many of the AIDS organizations' strategies, albeit with a more professional and less confrontational style. A growing willingness to own illness and become "poster people" for cancer, as people with AIDS had done effectively, put a face on diseases that women privately and pervasively feared. Creating strong alliances between consumers, medical professionals, and researchers, breast cancer advocates rallied behind a specific cause that affected many of them directly or through family and friends. Many activists who threw their energy into propelling the such as the national breast cancer coalition into national prominence left behind older-style support groups and feminist health organizations with broader agendas.

Using well-established letter-writing and advocacy strategies, breast cancer activists testified at hearings, held press conferences, and took their case to the NIH. In collaboration with growing bipartisan support in Congress and the scientific community, advocates succeeded in increasing federal funding for breast cancer research from $84 million to more than $400 million in 1993. Breast cancer advocates also insisted that survivors be involved in shaping research agendas and educational efforts and aligned themselves more consistently and collaboratively with scientists than had some AIDS activists or earlier grassroots movement leaders.

The success of breast cancer advocacy quickly created a "disease *du jour*" climate, where professionals rallied people directly or indirectly affected by particular diseases to lobby for increased funding. Ovarian cancer was the next women's disease to achieve national prominence. While this approach secures more resources or particular groups in the short run, it pits diseases against each other, turning research funding into a "popularity contest" or war

of each against all—to be won by the group that can make the most noise or wield the greatest political pressure. A result may be overfunding some diseases without regard for their prevalence, contribution to overall population health, or likelihood of scientific value. In this environment, orphan diseases will join orphan drugs as unfortunate, but probably unavoidable downsides of market-driven research and medicine.

A question that both Ruzek and Weissman have pondered together is the extent to which these newer groups are part of the women's health movement—or represent, at least in part, a separate and distinct, although overlapping, wave of activism.

DIFFERENCES BETWEEN GRASSROOTS AND PROFESSIONALIZED WOMEN'S HEALTH ORGANIZATIONS

Many grassroots women's health movement groups see themselves as different from what they perceive to be more professional mainstream organizations, although these differences are not always clearly articulated. After observing a wide range of groups for three decades, Ruzek argues that surviving grassroots advocacy groups can be differentiated from most professionalized, disease-focused groups in the following six ways:

➤ *Social movement orientation.* The founders of many grassroots feminist groups had ties to progressive or radical social movements that emphasized social justice and social change, to which many remain committed. In contrast, the newer professionalized support and advocacy organizations are typically more narrowly focused on a single disease or health issue, and except for environmentally focused groups such as WEDO, few are integral to broader social movements for social change (although some individual members may have such commitments).

➤ *Leadership.* Although some women physicians who were critical of medical education, training, and practice were leaders of the grassroots women's health movement, lay leadership was the norm. The role of physicians relative to others remains a point of contention among some feminist groups. In contrast, the professionalized support and advocacy groups formed in the 1990s had a growing pool of women physicians, scientists, and other highly trained professionals to turn to for leadership.

➤ *Attitude toward biomedicine.* A recurring theme in the grassroots women's health movement has been the demand for "evidence-based medicine," long before this term came into vogue. Major feminist advocacy groups aligned themselves with scientists and physicians who sought to put medical practice on a more scientific basis at a time when it was resisted by many clinicians. Grassroots health activists were critical of the side effects of inadequately tested drugs and devices, particularly early high-dose oral contraceptives, diethylstilbestrol, and intrauterine devices. They also questioned the number of unnecessary hysterectomies and radical mastectomies performed. In short, consumer groups sought to protect women from unsafe or unnecessary biomedical interventions. The professionalized advocacy groups founded in the 1990s focus more on ensuring women an "equal" share of biopsychosocial science and treatment—a stance that concerns many grassroots activists who fear overmedicalization and overtreatment of both men and women. The growing number of women physicians and scientists also facilitates alliances with women consumers because perceived interests in safety and effectiveness make these relationships seem mutually beneficial to many women.

➤ *Relationships with corporate sponsors.* Older grassroots advocacy groups remain deeply concerned about the effects of drug and device manufacturers sponsoring journals and organizational activities. In fact, this issue is a pivotal source of strain between grassroots groups and highly professional women's health organizations. While organizations of women physicians and professional advocacy groups rely heavily on corporate sponsorships, older grassroots groups avoid such relationships on grounds that financial ties affect the willingness of groups to criticize sponsors, promote competitors' products, or address alternative or complementary therapies that might undermine conventional prescribing patterns. Research confirms that sponsorship has this effect. Refusing support from corporate sponsors remains a hallmark of grassroots movement groups, but they struggle financially as a result. Because professional groups accept corporate support from drug and device manufacturers, they have more resources for education and advocacy.

➤ *Goals of education.* Both older and newer women's health organizations share the goal of educating women to improve their own health and make decisions about their own care. Grassroots feminist groups, particularly through the 1970s, focused on demystifying medicine and encouraging women to trust their subjective experience of their own health. Having access to larger number of women physicians may have reduced the perceived need to demystify medicine, and professional organizations appear largely concerned with making their highly educated constituencies aware of medical and scientific information.

➤ *Lay versus professional authority.* Grassroots health groups remain committed to substantial lay control over health and healing and to expanding the roles of such nonphysician healers as midwives, nurses, and counseling professionals. They would involve consumers in all aspects of health policy making, not simply transfer legitimate authority from male to female physicians. In largely professional organizations, women physicians are viewed as the primary societal experts on women's health matters.

The grassroots women's health movement organizations leave a legacy of making health an important social concern and educating women to take responsibility for their own health and health care decision making. The movement as a whole has made substantial efforts to influence powerful social institutions—organized medicine, the pharmaceutical industry, and regulatory agencies. In partnership with newer, professionalized equity organizations, health movement activists have taken up mainstream reform efforts that will become increasingly important as medical care is dominated by market forces. Thus the current episode of women's health activism overlaps with, but is, in many ways, different from the activism of the 1960s and 1970s. These distinct episodes of women's health activism need to be differentiated and understood in the specific historical contexts in which they emerged, recognizing the distinct roles that their history may lead them to play in the future. Because of the complexity of assessing the safety, effectiveness, and cost effectiveness of medical technologies worldwide, social justice demands ways to include women's health advocates who are committed to good science that is free from conflict of interest in patient education and health system coverage decisions. Finding ways to ensure women access to such information needs to be a priority for both grassroots and professionalized advocacy organizations.

The next challenge: who will speak for women in the electronic age? The electronic communication technologies foster a climate in which researchers and consumers expect to find information instantaneously and effortlessly. The reliability of information in electronic media is often questionable, however. Until data can be transformed into usable knowledge that can shape human action, the information age will not fulfill its promise. Neither grassroots women's health movement organizations nor newer professionalized disease agenda groups have adequately grappled with how to communicate with their constituencies effectively. Both types of groups as well as government and mainstream health organizations need to assess, manage, and distribute what each sees as "reliable" health information. Organizational survival may depend increasingly on teaching both "customers" and staff how to use reliable information effectively.

Because of the role of advocacy groups in health policy making in the United States, it is important how they present themselves and are perceived. As electronic media provide all comers the opportunity to claim organizational status in an increasingly "virtual" world, and the number of groups claiming to speak for women increases, how will the public differentiate among them? As we navigate the uncharted "information age," the ability of the grassroots women's health movement to remain nationally recognized as critical spokespersons may become problematic because the technology allows anyone with a computer and minimal skill to "create" an organization with worldwide visibly. Most movement organizations are just beginning to move from hard copy resource centers and clearinghouses to electronic purveyors of information. Newer professional advocacy groups that are better funded and more attuned to technological advancements are likely to gain because those who position themselves in electronic media will be perceived as speaking for women. In an effort to address the complexity of electronic media, the boston women's health book collective included a section on how to assess the adequacy of electronic sources of information in the 1998 edition of *Our Bodies, Ourselves.*

Who speaks for women's health in the electronic age very much depends on where one looks—Yahoo, for instance, or Healthfinders, the electronic database the Department of Health and Human Services unveiled for public use in May 1999—and how willing one is to sift through hundreds of self-characterized "women's health organizations." Becker, who is researching how Web sites present reliable information, emphasizes that women need to be vigilant in assessing information gleaned from the Internet, because it is so "easy" to log on and "find something."

Both grassroots and professionalized women's health advocates need new strategies for remaining key information brokers in an increasingly complex sea of women's health information. Grassroots health movement groups remain important forces for increasing awareness of women's health issues and are viewed as trustworthy sources of information by feminist groups in the United States and worldwide. But the cacophony of often contradictory and conflicting medical advice—from all sorts of journals, newsletters, Internet "chat rooms," and government and private health organizations—is likely to strain the individual's ability to sort out fact from fiction, established scientific evidence from snake oil, and hypotheses from hype. As it becomes more complex to be a well-informed consumer, the divide between information "haves" and "have nots" will widen. However, professionalized equity organizations, too, face competition from a growing array of institutions that claim expertise in matters of women's health. The challenge for both types of women's health groups will be to differentiate themselves for others whose interests lie more in marketing than in meeting diverse women's health needs.

As we enter the new millennium we must address growing disparities in wealth and access to health insurance among women. Women's health advocates need to find ways to widen access and equity to care for all women.

Cindy Pearson

INTERVIEW BY TANIA KETENJIAN

Cindy Pearson is the executive director of the National Women's Health Network. This interview was conducted in May 1999.

TK: What is the central belief of the National Women's Health Network?

CP: We believe that women need a watchdog organization to look out for their health interests because too many women have received health care based either on someone's unproven opinion about what works, or on someone's interest in making a profit. We try to provide information to women who don't have a source they can trust and, because we don't take any money from drug companies or companies that manufacture medical devices, we believe we can present an independent voice that isn't influenced by anything other than what women would consider in making decisions for themselves.

TK: How are women at a disadvantage when they enter the doctor's office?

CP: Women interact with the health care system much more often than men do. We go when we're young and healthy for reproductive health services and, because we live longer than men, we're more likely to have chronic health conditions. So whatever is wrong with the health care system, women experience it more. Over the years that's led to all kinds of abuses and unnecessary and inappropriate treatment. Because of the lingering effects of sexism in the health care system, women's true needs are ignored by their health care providers. Women are given the brush-off or are thought of as "just another complaining woman," so women are at a real disadvantage when it comes to the health care system.

TK: I've realized in talking to leaders in the women's health movement that doctors intervene too much. Can you talk about that a bit?

CP: American life is overmedicalized, especially for women, although also for men. My hope is that our women's health movement, to the extent that it succeeds in improving health care and making it more humane for women, will apply to men as well. Basically, we have paid a price in this country for making great technological improvements. Personally, I'm delighted that if my body is broken in a car crash there is high-tech medical care available to put me back together. Similarly, acute, raging infections can be treated by wonderful antibiotics. But what I don't like, and what I'm part of a movement to oppose, is the complete medicalization of the normal aspects of life. For example, we schedule our children to be seen by pediatricians in the first couple years of life more than they're seen by their grandparents. Those pediatricians prescribe unnecessary drugs, maybe as often as every third or fourth visit, leading these kids, some would say, to more health problems in their future than they would have had in the first place and making those drugs less effective when you really need them. I'm also part of a movement working against turning pregnancy and childbirth into a medical procedure, which happened decades ago in this country. It doesn't need to happen, and if it weren't that way, if there were a midwife instead of an obstetrician for every woman, we would have healthier women and babies in the United States. I certainly don't like it that there's an entire profession telling women that menopause is the beginning of an estrogen deficiency disease that lasts the rest of their lives and will cause them all kinds of ill health if they don't take drugs to stop it. Menopause, which is the reverse side of the coin of puberty, is a time of hormonal transition, turmoil, and turbulence; but it's no more the beginning of ill health than puberty is the beginning of ill health. Each of the examples that I could give you about the medicalization of women's lives is not supported by scientific medicine, but by a veneration of physicians that, in some instances, is appropriate, but not in this instance. If we can challenge that which I think we have started to do in this country and take back our health from the medical realm altogether, we're going to be much better off.

TK: What do you think of the current state of medical practice as a whole?

CP: A lot of women think that finding a nice woman doctor is the answer to their problems with health care, but you know what? Women doctors are more doctor than they are woman. Now, I don't mean to be insulting at all because there are plenty of wonderful women physicians who I respect and love, but the fact is that going through training as a physician in the United States is so intensive and so weighted toward a certain viewpoint, that most people, whether male or female, can only come out with that viewpoint. For the most part our advice to women is to bring

knowledge and a questioning attitude to their doctors. You can't just search for the right kind of doctor or a woman doctor and think that guarantees you the right kind of treatment. One thing that's particularly frustrating to women who don't like the medicalization of normal life processes like childbirth and menopause, is how incredibly medicalized most female ob-gyns are. They're just as likely to do cesarean sections as men; they're just as likely to intervene in slow labors; they're just as likely to push hormone replacement therapy to women going through the menopause; and, even though there may be an empathy factor, they may take a little more time, they may listen a little more, they're—for the most part—still going to offer you the same tried and true techniques that though tried and true, aren't actually good for our health.

TK: So what changes would you like to see in women's health care?

CP: When I think of the world as I would like it to be for women's health, I think of a world in which women start to learn about their health at home: they learn about their bodies; they're familiar with self-examination techniques; they know home remedies that have been passed down through their family; and they really have a sense of, "I'm the one who knows my body best." They go on from there to get well-woman care whenever possible from either lay health workers, peer education counselors, nurse practitioners, certified nurse midwives, allied health professionals who are like the people they care for, and who work from an holistic perspective. I would like to see a world in which profit and patentability driving what gets approved by the FDA no longer causes problems. Then the long-standing remedies that we now call "alternative," but that have been used in many cultures for millennia, the ones that actually work, can be marketed. This would differ from today when no one will invest in these products because they can't get the return they get from manufacturing a brand name prescription drug. I would like to see the use of physician specialists for primary care fade away so that when women are seeing physicians for primary care, they are seeing someone who supports the healthy-person approach, rather than supporting this test and that procedure, the let's-dive-in-and-intervene approach. Then we'd certainly have a less expensive, all-around healthier approach to women's health.

TK: What are some issues that need to be addressed but aren't always recognized?

CP: Some of the issues that don't get recognized as women's health issues have a big impact on younger women who should expect the best of health. One, for example, is the effect of domestic violence on health. It's only in recent years that domestic violence has been pushed out of the closet that violent men would like to keep it in, and brought out, not only as a social problem, or a problem of violence, but also as a problem that effects women's health. Domestic violence is one of the leading reasons women go to the emergency room. Another issue, for example, is women's work in reducing the rate of deaths and injuries caused by drunk drivers through Mothers Against Drunk Drivers. You wouldn't think of drunk driving as a women's health issue, but the fact that women got active and came up with an effective prevention strategy of tighter rules for blood alcohol levels has lowered the rate of these accidents and led to better health and longer lives. So you can look at important women's health issues from a general, public health perspective and find a very broad approach to women's health.

TK: What do you think of demystifying patients' health issues?

CP: Thirty years ago if anyone talked about a bad experience they had with the health care system, if they found a friendly ear, the response would usually be, "You need a better doctor, let me give you my doctor's number," or "Let me tell you about the person I heard speak." The response was "Find a better professional" not "Take charge

yourself." The movements—the feminist health movement, the patient's rights movement, the AIDS movement, and the emphasis on alternative health have all started to shift that to, instead of finding a better professional or a good doctor, educating yourself, taking charge, and being the decision-maker for yourself as much as possible. It's interesting to me that, in this time when many individual consumers and patients are trying to have more power, we're seeing more groups focused on health care that are really just trying to change practitioners to different or better professionals, like nicer doctors or more female doctors and researchers. In reality, the core of being in charge of your own health is taking control yourself. There's a subtle but important difference between groups that say, "We need better, nicer doctors, more female doctors, doctors that know more about alternative medicine," and groups or movements that say, "Patients and consumers need to be in control." That's where the women's health movement started. People talked about finding a good doctor, but then realized, good doctors aren't the answer, informed patients are the answer.

TK: So what do you think can be done to give patients a stronger voice and more power when dealing with their doctors?

CP: If you believe in a health care movement with the goal of putting power in the hands of patients, you have to believe in information being freely available to everybody, and the source of information being visible, identified. This means no hidden, sneaky drug company information that masquerades as an educational effort by a nonprofit group, and no fake web sites named as if they're nonprofit and represent the patient's perspective, but in fact are financed by drug companies. You know, to really make a movement that changes things around so that people are in control of their own health, people must have information from a trustworthy source.

TK: How does one judge whether or not the information provided by an expert physician or scientist in a medical journal is biased? In other words, how can a lay person be sure that the information from these prominent people isn't tainted by outside influences from politics or drug manufacturers?

CP: One of the things we always advise consumers is to watch for the source of the information they're getting, and to see if there's any potential bias that might be subtly influencing its recommendations. You can hear an eminent researcher or scientist on a morning talk show, or on the nightly news, or you can read a newspaper account of an article that's been published in a prestigious journal; what you may not hear is that that researcher's results have been funded by the manufacturer whose product they're talking about. It's starting to be possible to occasionally find that information in written disclosures in medical journals. If you have access to a medical journal, you can see who funds the work. It's very rare to get that kind of disclosure in average, mainstream, broadcast media. The morning talk shows put people on all the time giving their opinion about certain health issues; we activists know just how tightly connected these people are to the companies that make the products they're talking about. There's no way you would know that from watching the TV shows. Similarly, the people who are turned to to give their ten seconds of august opinion in broadcast news almost never disclose their connections. We encourage anyone who sees experts with connections to drug or medical or insurance companies acting as if they're a neutral source to report them, to just call back the media source that's featured this person and say, "Look, I know that X, Y, and Z companies support this person's research, and I think you should have put that into your coverage." The National Women's Health Network is trying to get a campaign going for a data bank journalists could use to check the financial ties of medical spokespeople that are often in the media. But it's a challenge because uncovering that information is hard going.

TK: Is overprescription of drugs common?

CP: Years ago we used to complain that the only drugs women could get out of their doctors were tranquilizers; that if women came in with anything from arthritis to back trouble to endometriosis they would get a literal or verbal pat on the head, and a prescription for tranquilizers. I think that's changed somewhat, although there are still lots of prescriptions written for mood-altering drugs. Drug companies have realized that women are a fabulous market for prescription drugs: women are concerned about their health; they're used to seeing the doctor frequently; they like to stay informed; and now they're being targeted in the same way that Nike targets young adults for their shoe ads. Women are being targeted with drug ads to convince them that it would be a good idea to take any number of drugs on an ongoing basis.

TK: So what are the main consequences of that targeting by pharmaceutical companies?

CP: "There's no drug safe enough to be worth taking if you don't need it." That axiom comes from Dr. Philip Corfman, a Food and Drug Administration medical officer with a lot of years of experience in women's health. The basic point is that if you're in dire straits, and a drug has been shown to work, it's probably worth taking, even if it has some pretty serious side effects. But if you're healthy to start with, and what you need from the medical system is a way in which to manage your reproduction, or a way to go through the menopausal transition more comfortably, you don't want to deal with any extra risks.

TK: What are the effects of pharmaceutical industries advertising directly to the public?

CP: Unless you're a hermit, you know that the rules have changed about advertising brand name prescription drugs. There are ads on TV that name drugs, and there are ads that don't have any of the long list of warnings and details that used to be in tiny fine print in the back of magazine ads. For consumer groups, that means a mixed blessing. Thirty years ago, we were fighting desperately for people to get information about the drugs they were taking. How can we say that it's bad to get information about drugs through an ad? Shouldn't we be for information? But what is information that's in an ad; is it actually informative, or is it really a sales technique? Our experience so far with direct-to-consumer ads on television is that it's much more of a sales technique than it is informative or educational in any way. Ads naming the drug have been allowed on television for a little less than two years now. In that time, the FDA has found that over half of the pharmaceutical companies that advertise their drugs on television have been breaking the rules: they exaggerate the benefits; they minimize or don't mention the risks; they try to claim that the drug works for groups of people in whom it hasn't been studied; and they try to mislead the public in other ways. The trouble is that the FDA has no power to preview these ads before they're on the air. They don't have nearly the staff or resources they need to watch all these ads. Many times they take action after receiving a complaint from a group like ours; all they can do is tell the company to pull the ad. Maybe the drug company was likely to change that ad anyway to get a fresh image out before people's minds. But the damage has already been done when a consumer sees a misleading ad on television, even if it's later pulled by the FDA. We're concerned that in the long run, something needs to change in terms of laws and regulations so that at a minimum, the FDA has the power and the resources to review ads before they go on TV. In the short term, patients and consmers need to insist that if they even have the faintest glimmer of talking to their doctor about a drug because of direct advertising, they need to insist that they get written medication guides produced by the government, or by an independent consumer group, before they swallow their first pill. It's vitally important that people see the contraindications to taking a drug in writing. The women's health movement that in the 1970s held a memorial service in front of the FDA proved that if women could get their hands on information,

they could make the use of a drug safer by ruling themselves out if it was too risky for them, or quickly getting off it if they had any complications. If patients and consumers would insist on that kind of written information now, we could counterbalance the hard sell that's going on with television ads for brand name drugs.

TK: The Network has had some major successes in the past few years involving the National Institutes of Health, the FDA, the National Cancer Institute, to give some examples. Can you discuss some of these?

CP: Some of the things the network has tried to accomplish in the last few years have really been about the misuse of research that puts healthy women at much higher risks than necessary. We've been concerned that too many research trials have been designed by short-sighted doctors used to dealing with dangerous medications, day in and day out. They don't seem to realize that, in designing a prevention study with healthy volunteer subjects, they should be starting with the safest approach possible. We have complained bitterly about the design of the tamoxifen trial for healthy women. We got the consent forms changed and women really listened to us; many that were at low risk actually stayed out of that trial. Another accomplishment was that we told the National Institutes of Health that they were making a mistake in the design of their estrogen replacement therapy study in healthy women. They originally wanted to ask women to volunteer to take estrogen, which is known to cause cancer of the uterus. We told them, "This is wrong, this is ethically wrong; even in a research environment, you shouldn't be asking women to put themselves at risk with a known cancer-causing agent." They finally listened to us, although not until two years later, and after much cost and bureaucratic hassle. But they did change the way they organized that trial. So I think those are some of the accomplishments that have really made a difference in the last few years: protecting healthy people from unnecessary risks in government-funded research.

TK: There are many controversies surrounding breast cancer; can you tell me what some of the most prominent ones are?

CP: Breast cancer has been controversial since the first courageous women started talking to each other about it. Even now that it's a big, justice-based social movement that has mobilized millions of women to agitate for more funding for research, for better treatment, for more respect for survivors, all those things; so many issues related to breast cancer are controversial. One example is that even a good ten years after it's been accepted by leading researchers and policy makers that removing the cancer itself, in a lumpectomy, is as likely to lead to the woman's survival as removing her whole breast, many doctors still routinely do mastectomies. Many hundreds of thousands of women are having mastectomies, having their breasts removed, who don't need that procedure. That's one area that's still controversial. Another area is how to treat advanced disease, because in contrast to women who are diagnosed with their breast cancer early and have good odds of surviving as long as women have been followed so far (about fifteen or twenty years), women whose cancer is diagnosed in an advanced state, or whose cancer recurs in another part of their body, don't have any treatment that's been shown to work for any considerable length of time. A few women do survive for many years; but most women who have advanced breast cancer face continued progression of the disease to the point where it kills them. These women want to live, and their doctors want to help them find a way to live. And all they've been able to offer so far is more of the same: literally, more chemotherapy. If some chemotherapy can't stop advanced cancer, well maybe lots of chemotherapy could. The trouble is that lots of chemotherapy by itself can kill you because it kills the cells in the bone marrow which produce new blood cells and new infec-tion-fighting cells. A very expensive, elaborate procedure designed several years ago has been shown to be effective in cancers based in the blood: high-dose chemotherapy followed by a bone marrow transplant. Very soon after that was shown to be effective in cancers based in the blood, it was offered to women with breast cancer, mostly out of a feeling of "We've got nothing else, so let's give it a try." It became very controversial: it's extremely expensive (in the realm of $100,000), it has fatal side effects itself. Even in the best centers that do it frequently, a percentage of women die within the following couple of weeks as a result of this treatment. Yet women were told, "This is your only chance; this has a twenty-five percent chance of creating a complete remission as opposed to a three percent chance if you just have regular chemotherapy." So women fought for it: sued their insurance companies, lobbied Congress, got state laws passed to mandate that this be covered. In the last several years, about twelve thousand women in the United States have had this procedure, but sadly, only about a thousand of them received it in a clinical trial, so it's taken all this time and all this fighting to find out that it's not a better treatment. We now have five studies that, with the exception of one, have found the high-dose chemotherapy approach is no better than regular chemotherapy. So we're really left back where we were eight, nine, or ten years ago. It's a sad commentary on the way our medical system approaches diseases like cancer. They keep trying the same approaches even when they haven't worked. We've wasted a lot of time that could have been spent looking for approaches that do work.

TK: In the magazine *MAMM*, you were quoted as saying, "What makes it harder for the breast cancer movement than for other movements (such as the AIDS movement) is women's issues about putting themselves first." Can you comment on this?

CP: You know, over the years, there have been so many different kinds of health movements, and when people ask me to comment on the women's health movement, or women-specific disease movements like the breast cancer movement, I'm always struck by how much harder it is for women to sustain the kind of energy that men feel so free to give to the causes that affect them. The AIDS movement, for example, liberated tremendous amounts of energy from individuals who gave several nights a week to be part of Act Up or other AIDS projects. On the other hand, the breast cancer movement sparked the same kind of fire in women, but so many women found themselves paying a terrible cost in terms of their families. There were the judgments about them not spending time with their kids because they were gone every night at these meetings; they weren't with their boyfriends or husbands. Women are so much less free to put themselves first, even when their own lives depend on it. So it's really been impressive to me that, fighting against such odds, the breast cancer movement has strongly sustained itself throughout this decade. Because it's not easy to be a woman feminist health activist, let me tell you.

TK: To what do you attribute the success of the National Women's Health Network?

CP: The National Women's Health Network is small, poor, and beleaguered. We're often in a David-versus-Goliath situation; the only reason we have existed for nearly twenty-five years is because we represent the heartfelt wishes of a strong constituency of individual women (and some of the men who support them) who want a more humane health care system for both women who receive healthcare and women who provide it. They keep us alive with their support and their input, and we go out and try to take their words and make them heard by the people in power. We do a good enough job for our members to keep us alive.

On Young Feminism

SUNNY DALY

Sunny Daly, "On Young Feminism," 2008. Original for this publication.

At twenty-six I am fortunate to have had diverse experiences with movements for women's empowerment in the global West. As a girl, my mother encouraged my use of the word "feminist," and made it clear that I could literally be anything I wanted to be. In academics, I thought it silly to focus on women because aren't women a part of regular history and regular literature anyway? It took me until my senior year of college to realize that I had learned far too little about us through this strategy, so I focused my year-long research project on women to see how it felt. Suddenly, I knew what I wanted to do with myself—I had direction in life! My thesis, a history of the first birth control pill in America, brought me more contacts and insight into this world of feminism than I imagined possible, and for the first time I found my attention span lengthening. I left school with a goal: to make a living helping to empower women. This was not easy, but after enough dues-paying to drain the waitressing income and a few transcontinental moves, I landed a full-time position in a national women's organization.

Too quickly, I became frustrated. Unwieldy organizational structures fraught with inefficiency, wayward and unfocused agendas for progress, stunted respect, and the lack of substantive work available for my level were revealed. Though many individual mentors inspire me time and again, I worry about how I will maintain my "professionalized feminism" without losing faith in the movement. What I see is a lot of time spent reinventing the wheel, competition for funding, and brushing off of new ideas. The serious lack of diversity and rare collaboration is alarming. Many projects do not feel relevant to me and I feel slighted considering my profound commitment to the organization (and for a salary that limits life outside of work).

This job is a first step, I realize, and I am not about to quit. My generation will untangle the problems and address our frustrations in many ways. Personally, I've decided to look abroad to learn about other potential paths for the movement. There are many ways of achieving empowerment and many definitions of feminism, power, and success. I wish to understand this heterogeneity and learn best practices, if you will, from within women's own contexts in other parts of the globe. I believe that learning about the rest of the world will not only help me to find my own fulfillment in this field, but it will help me to make real contributions by highlighting the true urgencies and successful (and unsuccessful) ways to tackle them. Others, I see, will absorb institutional memory to keep today's feminist organizations running and they will be candidates for succession when that day inevitably comes. Still others will lose patience and take their talents to other sectors, to be waitresses or executives, but, not having lost their faith, they will instill our feminist values in bosses, coworkers, mentees, and children.

Some feminists of the second wave fret about the lack of younger women in the movement and our weak dedication. Really, there are many, many women my age committed to building upon the progress we've so fortunately inherited (and yes, we know we're lucky). Many of the questions and solutions have changed, however, and the integration of new, often more global, perspectives is a very real priority to us. It is inevitable that we will lead in time but this should not be taken as a threat. Rather, it is an opportunity to expand and texturize the meaning of feminism and the goals we pursue under its banner.

Our Bodies, Our Voices, Our Choices

NATIONAL BLACK WOMEN'S HEALTH PROJECT

National Black Women's Health Project, excerpt from *Our Bodies, Our Voices, Our Choices: A Black Woman's Primer on Reproductive Health and Rights*, Washington, DC: National Black Women's Health Project, 1998. Reprinted by permission.

Since its inception in 1981, the National Black Women's Health Project (NBWHP) has worked to bring together women to talk about our experiences, hopes, and dreams—and to share information that will enhance our lives and health. This primer is designed for black women to use as an introductory policy reference on reproductive health issues. It contains historical background, the contemporary context, and NBWHP policy statements. We hope it will stimulate greater interest and understanding of reproductive health issues as well as encourage women to take positive action for themselves, their families, and their communities. There is much to learn and much to do.

The principle of self-help guides our fundamental belief that every woman—whether heterosexual, bisexual, or lesbian—may substantially increase her chances of achieving overall health and well-being if:

➤ She is knowledgeable about her body
➤ She is aware of her rights and empowered to ask necessary questions
➤ She knows that she is entitled to information and services that are delivered with dignity and respect

We also believe that when women appreciate how history and contemporary events combine to impact our ability to make decisions and to have choices, they will want to get politically involved on matters close to home, across the nation, or around the world.

Historically, all women in the United States have struggled to achieve reproductive health and reproductive rights. While this struggle has been most challenging for poor women and women of color, the fact that blacks were brought to this country in chains, sold as slaves, and held in bondage for generations has had a deep and enduring impact on our lives.

For 244 years, black women in America suffered the harsh realities of slave labor, forced breeding, and the wrenching separation of children from mothers and other loved ones. Since emancipation, we have been burdened by a racist mythology that distorts our sexuality and paints us as loose, immoral, and unfit to be mothers. Over time, we have borne the brunt of a dizzying array of racist policies and programs aimed at controlling our reproduction. In the past 30 years alone, we have dealt with forced or involuntary sterilization, court-ordered insertion of long-acting contraceptives, deadly illegal abortions, punitive welfare policies, and arrest and prosecution instead of treatment and compassion for using drugs while pregnant . . . the list goes on.

Out of this dismal experience, black women have grasped a fundamental truth: unless and until we are free to control our own fertility, we will never be able to take care of ourselves or our families, or take full advantage of opportunities in education, employment, and society at large.

Spurred on by this truth, black women have been involved in the movement for "voluntary motherhood" and reproductive rights since the turn of the century. Racism and discrimination meant that our efforts were largely within our own community, although over time, a number of black women have played prominent roles in the national reproductive rights movement.

Today, most people think of the phrase "reproductive rights" as the right to choose an abortion. Black women have always understood that the correct phrase is "reproductive *health* and rights"—that our struggle goes beyond our ability to decide whether, when, and how to have a child.

Black women understand that genuine reproductive health and rights are possible *only* when society allows healthy mothers and healthy babies to flourish. Genuine reproductive *health* will be achieved when society ensures that young girls and women have access to all necessary information and basic services, from health care and housing to education and employment. Genuine reproductive *rights* will be achieved when women can make decisions about their sexuality and re-

production that are free from coercion, actual or threatened violence, soul-crushing addictions, and despair—and when society ensures that the resources necessary to support those decisions are readily available.

There are many compelling ways to bring this expansive view of reproductive health and rights into reality. Black women put creative energy and volunteer time into the prevention of violence and homelessness, the promotion of prenatal care and mammography screening, and much more.

Those of us who have been active in the reproductive rights movement have been vital partners in the effort to expand these rights and broaden women's choices. But we have also been vocal critics of options that present problems for many women, such as technologies that have negative side effects or do not provide protection against sexually transmitted diseases, as well as programs that do not offer an ongoing support system for women.

Our historical experience has taught us to examine any new reproductive technology or social program through our triple screen: race, class, and gender. As a result, our view often diverges from the mainstream. Unless we are convinced that a new technology or program will genuinely add to a woman's choices and enhance her health and well-being, we voice our opposition and urge all black women to consider seriously the facts before accepting that technology or program.

As women of the African diaspora, we have traveled great distances, literally and figuratively. We have survived and often thrived. Let us celebrate our lives as black women—vital, vibrant, and strong—and move forward to secure genuine reproductive health and rights for ourselves, our daughters, and all our sisters.

Julia R. Scott, RN
President and CEO,
National Black Women's Health Project

SEXUAL HEALTH AND EDUCATION

HISTORICAL EXPERIENCE: RACIST MYTHOLOGY

Racist mythology has defined African-American sexuality and childbearing since slavery. Both African-American women and men were labeled "naturally immoral" and considered sexually irresponsible. After slavery, African-American women were referred to as "Jezebels" and portrayed as promiscuous, "bad" mothers who, unrestrained in their childbearing, passed these same traits on to their children. At the same time, African-American women were involved extensively in child care and rearing of white children as wet nurses and nannies.

For centuries, black women were caught in a vicious catch-22. First, whites claimed we were sexually "loose" and therefore fair game for white rapists and sexual predators. Then, our sexuality was blamed for helping to "cause" black men to rape white women, an alleged act which led to brutal, often fatal consequences for many of our men.

CONTEMPORARY CONTEXT: SEXUALITY, SHAME, AND SILENCE

One consequence of our legacy from slavery and the continuing public mythologies about African-American sexuality is that many of us have deeply buried the interconnectedness of our emotional, sexual, and reproductive experiences. Our sexuality is often associated with feelings of shame. Problems related to our reproductive health—from unwanted pregnancies or infertility to cancers of the breast or reproductive organs—are usually kept private.

In addition, mainstream cultural taboos tend to prevent discussion of healthy sexuality among all women. Attacks on public school, family life, and sex education programs by some conservative and religious fundamentalists have severely limited opportunities to help adolescent girls (and boys) at a crucial time in their sexual development to understand and practice decision-making and negotiation skills. Oftentimes, the premises of these attacks are accepted without in-depth examination of cause and effect.

This "conspiracy of silence" has an invisible yet potent impact on the overall health and well-being of black women. When we are discouraged from asking questions and when we cannot discuss important issues related to our reproductive health and sexuality, our health and that of future generations is jeopardized. Lack of knowledge about sexuality and reproduction is often cited as a major reason that young women engage in irresponsible sexual practices, resulting in high rates of unintended pregnancies and sexually transmitted infections. However, knowledge alone is not the answer either. Confidence, self-respect, and awareness of the benefits of delayed gratification are essential elements as well.

NBWHP POLICY STATEMENT: HEALTHY SEXUALITY BEGINS WITH EDUCATION

A vital component of sexual health is access to age-appropriate family life and sex education programs. All humans are sexual beings from the moment of birth, so it makes sense that attention to our sexual health should begin at the earliest possible age.

African-American girls and adolescents have a critical need for adequate knowledge and understanding of sexuality for two reasons: they are vulnerable to internalizing the negative stereotypes about black female sexuality; and they are likely to be subjected to sexual abuse or violence. In fact, one in three black women report sexual abuse at some point in their lives.

Programs for boys are equally important for factual knowledge and understanding about responsible sexuality, respect for self, and others. We must teach all children appropriate ways to show love and affection and encourage them to disclose and negative incidents in order to reduce their potential for sexual abuse.

NBWHP supports age-appropriate sex education in multiple settings, including public and private schools, as well as efforts to help families and caregivers to provide accurate information regarding sex and sexuality to their children. Sex education and family life skills should be taught in schools, churches, community centers—as well as in the home—by caring adults. This is the first challenge, and often the most critical one, for achieving a life of good health.

African-American women must take the lead in fostering sexual health for today's young girls and for the generations to come. As adults, we can play an essential role in helping young girls and adolescents to develop healthy attitudes and feelings about their bodies and their sexuality. We can do this by willingly and openly discussing any or all topics related to sexuality, by modeling respectful and loving relationships with others, and by demonstrating love for ourselves through healthy behaviors.

PREGNANCY AND PRENATAL CARE

HISTORICAL EXPERIENCE: FORCED BREEDING

During slavery, black women in America had no control over their reproductive lives. We were subjected to forced breeding, rape and sexual abuse, and our families were torn apart on the auction block. As slaves, we were valuable for our field labor and as reproducers. Our babies were the "new stock" for slave owners who depended on a continual supply of infants after the import of new slaves was banned in 1808.

Centuries before modern medicine was able to define and treat the fetus separately from the mother, slave owners saw the fetus as a distinct piece of property with great potential value. When a slave owner would punish a pregnant slave, he had to balance his interest in disciplining his worker with his interest in gaining a healthy new infant. The solution became a common practice throughout the South: the pregnant slave was forced to lie down in a depression in the ground so that her fetus would not be injured while she was bullwhipped.

Babies are our hopes and wishes for the future,

symbolizing love for our partner, for our families—for life itself. Having a baby that you want is one of life's most glorious gifts. There is a delicious excitement and sense of wonder.

The most powerful act of "resistance" by slave women was ensuring the survival of their children. An enduring legacy from our days in slavery is the strong African-American tradition of forging communal bonds among nonrelated individuals, of taking in children without parents, of caring for one another in the face of extreme odds. This spirit of life-affirming "resistance" continues in our community today.

CONTEMPORARY CONTEXT: HEALTHY MOTHERS = HEALTHY BABIES

The intergenerational cycle of poverty and near poverty makes it difficult for many African-American families to build and maintain preventive health care habits. An estimated 25–30 percent of inner-city African-American women receive little or no prenatal care during their pregnancies. This is oftentimes due to lack of access to health care services, inadequate care when health care is delivered, language barriers, and/or a lack of information, especially among pregnant adolescents.

Prenatal care is essential for a safe pregnancy and a healthy, full-term infant. In addition to monitoring the pregnant woman's diet and encouraging her to quit smoking, prenatal care includes screening for sexually transmitted diseases, high blood pressure, gestational diabetes, abuse of alcohol and illegal drugs, and domestic violence. When the health care needs of childbearing African-American women are not met, there are grave consequences.

Scientists at the Centers for Disease Control and Prevention (CDC) report that African-American women are four times more likely to die from pregnancy-related causes than white women. On average, an African-American woman dies every two and a half days in the United States from pregnancy-related causes. Many of them could be saved by regular checkups during pregnancy.

Infant mortality rates in African-American communities resemble those in developing nations. Black babies die at the rate of 6,000 more per year than white babies in the same geographical area.

The primary contributing factor to infant mortality is low birth weight. Surprisingly, the frequency of low-birthweight babies is not limited just to poor women in medically underserved areas. Middle-class black women have more low-birthweight babies than white women of the same socioeconomic class. And, approximately one-quarter of all pregnancies in women of every socioeconomic class and race end in miscarriage.

The fact that high rates of infant morbidity and mortality span all economic classes suggests that elements other than poverty are to blame. Women who are happy to be pregnant are more likely to seek and get medical care before their baby is born (prenatal care). But when our pregnancies are unplanned or unwanted, we often experience mixed feelings and denial—both of which can cause a delay in seeking appropriate medical care for ourselves and the developing child.

NBWHP POLICY STATEMENT: UNIVERSAL PRENATAL CARE IS ESSENTIAL

It is a simple formula: Healthy mothers have healthy babies. Prenatal care truly begins with the health of the mother when she is a child. NBWHP supports lifelong access to adequate medical care, decent housing, and educational opportunities, as well as efforts to promote good nutrition and exercise and opportunities to develop healthy behaviors.

NBWHP opposes mandatory drug testing of pregnant women. Such testing is not an appropriate component of maternal care. However, voluntary drug screening, when accompanied by appropriate counseling and referral to professional treatment, is critical for the health of mother and infant. For women who are willing to seek treatment, there must be adequate access to treatment programs and facilities for pregnant women and women with children.

HISTORICAL EXPERIENCE: "VOLUNTARY MOTHERHOOD" PROMOTED

Black people have always recognized the value of spaced and well-timed births as a way to reduce high maternal and infant mortality rates and strengthen family life. At the turn of the century, black women were controlling their own fertility, chiefly by marrying late, having fewer children, and using contraception and abortion. The black women's club movement had emerged as a dominant force in promoting new social and family values among African-American women. The clubs supported "voluntary motherhood" and shared information about contraceptives.

Historically, babies in this country were delivered at home. The vast majority of babies born in the United States were delivered by midwives during home births. The "granny" midwife was a respected figure in the black community, especially in rural Southern states where she was the only person who could help mothers—black and white—to deliver their babies. Grannies would often stay for several days with a mother, helping to care for other children and the house until the mother regained her strength. Many grannies were illiterate; their traditions and knowledge of herbal remedies and medicines were shared and passed along to the next generation through oral stories and apprenticeships. However, by the middle of this century, doctors succeeded in taking control of childbirth by banning midwives and prohibiting women from attending medical school.

CONTEMPORARY CONTEXT: BIRTHS TO OLDER WOMEN INCREASE, TEEN PREGNANCIES DECLINE

Between 1980 and 1994, the birth rates for all women remained fairly stable, at an average of 21 per 1,000 for black women, and 15 per 1,000 white women. However, increasing numbers of black women are choosing to give birth at later ages. The number of births for African-American women ages thirty to forty-four increased from 1980 to

1996, while births to African-American women ages twenty-nine and younger decreased. The percentage of intended births increases with the age of the mother. In 1995, only 23.4 percent of births to black women under twenty were intended, compared to 51.8 percent for women ages twenty to twenty-nine, and 70.2 percent for women ages thirty to forty-four.

Teenage pregnancy rates—although declining during the 1990s—still remain high, especially for young black women. Half a million adolescents give birth each year. In 1996, births among girls aged fifteen through seventeen were more than twice as likely among African-American teenage girls than white teenage girls. Birth rates among African-American girls younger than fifteen were 4.5 times higher than for white girls.

Among black teenagers, 75 percent of pregnancies are "unwanted" or "mis-timed." This is a major concern because of the potential social and economic consequences as well as the health effects. Indirectly, patterns of poverty and low educational attainment often become solidified as a result of early childbearing.

NBWHP POLICY STATEMENT: WOMEN HAVE THE RIGHT TO GIVE BIRTH

NBWHP supports the availability of wide options for childbirth, as well as the education of women about these options in advance. In some areas, women have a choice of settings for delivery, ranging from hospital operating rooms or birthing centers to their own homes. Many women are asking nurse-midwives to help them prepare for childbirth and to assist during labor and delivery. Some women prepare for natural childbirth by taking birthing classes where they learn breathing and relaxation exercises; at the time of delivery, some women choose to have little or no pain medication. Others opt for a stronger pain reliever. Pregnant women have a right to participate in the decision about where and how they will have their babies.

In the United States, one in four babies is delivered by cesarean section. It is the most frequently performed major surgical procedure among reproductive-age women. There are several medical conditions that lead to C-sections; however, nonmedical factors also influence the decision. Women who have private medical insurance, who are patients at private (rather than public) clinics, and who are married, older, and/or in a higher socioeconomic bracket are more likely to have c-sections. Nonmedical reasons include the avoidance of pain, convenience, financial incentives for providers (C-sections cost nearly twice as much as vaginal births), and fear of being sued for delivering an infant with a poor outcome after prolonged labor.

A C-section is major surgery and can result in infections, hemorrhage, injury to other organs, and other physical and psychological complications. The maternal mortality rate for C-sections is two to four times greater than that for vaginal deliveries. C-sections not necessitated by medical reasons increase the risk to the infant of premature birth and breathing problems. C-sections can also interfere with breast-feeding and the establishment of the mother-child bond. For all of there reasons, NBWHP opposes the use of C-sections for nonmedical purposes.

NBWHP also opposes efforts to limit reproductive choice, such as recently passed welfare reform legislation that includes "child exclusion" provisions to discourage women receiving welfare from having children. Instead of providing the necessary services, job-training opportunities, education, child support enforcement, and transitional benefits to poor families, the "child exclusion" provisions deny increases in benefits that are needed to raise an additional child. This punishes welfare recipients for choosing childbirth. Ironically, Medicaid covers pregnancy, childbirth, and sterilization but does not provide funds for abortion.

Not only are fertility rates of welfare recipients lower than those of the general population, but the longer a woman remains on welfare, the less likely she is to give birth. Furthermore, the great majority of pregnancies among women on welfare are unintended.

There is no evidence to support the assumption that poor people's childbearing decisions are motivated by minimal grant increases or incentives. There is evidence, however, that teens are more likely to have children when other life options—such as education and jobs—are unavailable.

As the discussion of welfare reform inevitably turns to "individual responsibility," NBWHP insists that the federal, state, and local governments also act "responsibly" and be held accountable for their failures in providing the economic and social conditions that allow all citizens to have a decent standard of living.

CONTRACEPTION AND DISEASE PREVENTION

HISTORICAL EXPERIENCE: SUPPORT OF BIRTH CONTROL, DISTRUST OF MEDICAL COMMUNITY

By the end of the nineteenth century, black fertility rates had plummeted by one-third. This was often blamed on racial discrimination, inadequate wages, poor nutrition, substandard housing, and lack of medical care for most African Americans. While these circumstances did in fact exist, ample evidence also indicates that many African Americans were using "folk" contraceptives and abortion.

The fledgling birth control movement of the early twentieth century drew initial interest and support among black women and men. As Margaret Sanger's birth control movement grew, many black women insisted on expanding birth control services in their communities; they were enthusiastic users of the few clinics across the country that were available to them. Because most clinics were operated by whites, some blacks were suspicious that birth control would be used for genocide or that blacks would be subject to reproductive medical experiments. Despite such opposition and fear, black women generally supported family planning and organized to promote it in their communities throughout the first half of the twentieth century.

As part of the 1960s "war on poverty," the federal government began to establish family planning clinics in predominantly black urban areas. Black nationalists (mostly men) attacked these programs as genocide-suicide—but black women once more affirmed their right to make their own reproductive choices and resisted efforts to shut down these clinics.

The most notable historical event with regard to African Americans and sexually transmitted diseases is the notorious Tuskegee study. In 1972, the US Public Health Service admitted that for the prior forty years, it had been studying the course of untreated latent syphilis in hundreds of poor black sharecroppers in Tuskegee, Alabama. The physicians conducting the study deceived the men about their condition and deliberately withheld effective treatment for the disease, even after penicillin became available.

Published medical reports estimate that twenty-eight out of one hundred men died as a result of their syphilis. The wives and families of these men also were affected. Studies later showed that twenty-seven out of fifty wives tested positive for syphilis. As a consequence of the research study in Tuskegee, many African Americans continue to distrust the medical and public health authorities.

CONTEMPORARY CONTEXT: UNINTENDED PREGNANCIES, STDS, AND HIV/AIDS AFFECT BLACK WOMEN DISPROPORTIONATELY

High rates of unintended pregnancy, abortion, and teenage childbearing among black women speak to the great need for better access to and use of effective contraceptives. In addition, with skyrocketing rates of HIV/AIDS and other infections, it is urgent that black women protect themselves from unwanted pregnancy and *sexually transmitted diseases* (STDs) at the same time.

In 1996, African Americans accounted for 78 percent of all reported cases of *gonorrhea.* African-American teenagers aged fifteen to nineteen have infection rates that are twenty-four times higher than whites. Among young black adults aged twenty to twenty-four, the rate is thirty times higher than whites.

The highest rates of *chlamydia* infection are found in individuals aged fifteen to nineteen and twenty to twenty-four for all racial and ethnic groups. Blacks are infected at much higher rates than whites.

Up to 20–30 percent of sexually active Americans of all races are thought to be infected with *human papillomavirus* (HPV), which causes genital warts.

It is estimated that 45–60 million Americans are infected with *herpes genitalis*. About 80 percent of African-American women and 60 percent of African-American men will be infected with herpes at some time in their lives.

Rates of *syphilis* infection are 62 percent higher for African Americans than whites. Between 1985 and 1990, this disease increased by 230 percent among African-American women.

In 1995, 10.6 percent of all black women were treated for *pelvic inflammatory disease* (*PID*), compared to 7.2 percent of white women.

The fastest-growing group of persons infected by HIV—the virus that causes AIDS (*acquired immune deficiency syndrome*)—are heterosexual women. In 1996, African-American women comprised 56 percent of AIDS cases among women in the United States. In the majority of cases, they were infected as adolescents or young girls.

Women are at greater risk than men of contracting sexually transmitted diseases and HIV/AIDS because of our anatomical differences. The risks are even higher for adolescent women due to age-related physiological changes in the cervix. Lesbian and bisexual women are also at risk of spreading STDs and HIV/AIDS through the exchange of bodily fluids.

STDs are more difficult to diagnose and less likely to be treated in women. If undiagnosed and untreated, STDs can do great long-term damage to a woman's health, causing premature delivery, stillbirth, infertility, and genital cancers. The presence of an STD—whether it has open, visible sores or is invisible and asymptomatic—will increase a woman's risk of contracting HIV/AIDS.

A wide range of contraceptive methods are available that can greatly reduce the risk of pregnancy; however, few also protect against STDs.

Barrier methods—including the *male condom, female condom, diaphragm,* and *cervical cap*—prevent sperm from reaching the egg and protect against STDs. Used correctly, latex male condoms (not those made from animal tissue) offer the best protection against STDs and HIV/AIDS and are most effective when used with a spermicide containing nonoxynol-9. Unfortunately, spermicides may irritate the vaginal lining of some sensitive women, making them more susceptible to HIV/AIDS infection through the broken skin.

Hormonal contraceptives—including the *pill, intrauterine device* (IUD), *Depo-Provera* ("the shot"), and *Norplant*—are an effective way to prevent pregnancy. However, they may not be appropriate for women with certain health conditions, such as high blood pressure or a history of cancer or diabetes—and they do not protect against STDs or HIV/AIDS.

"Emergency" contraception (ECP, or the "morning-after pill") is used in the event of unprotected sex, contraceptive failure, rape, or incest. The Food and Drug Administration (FDA) has approved a product for emergency contraception called Preven. The Preven contraceptive kit is currently available by prescription from doctors and other health care professionals.

The only 100 percent guarantee a women has against unwanted pregnancy and STDs is celibacy (no sexual activity), a practice often encouraged by religious groups for unmarried people.

NBWHP POLICY STATEMENT: CHOOSE BIRTH CONTROL, DISEASE PREVENTION, AND HEALTH CARE

NBWHP supports universal access to health care and family planning services for all women. Black women should insist on full and accurate information from their health care providers about all contraceptive options, including side effects, health risks and benefits, costs to obtain the method, procedures, and costs necessary to have a method removed.

Much attention has recently been placed on new hormonal contraceptive technologies that provide long-term protection from pregnancy without the need to "think about it." It has been argued that these methods are "liberating" for women. NBWHP believes that if ever there was a time for women to think carefully about sexual activity, it is now. Women need to own the fact that sexuality is a natural and normal part of adult life. We need to think carefully—and ahead of time—about whether and when we will engage in sex and how we will prevent unwanted pregnancies and the spread of infections. All women must become comfortable with their bodies and their sexuality so that we can take control of our decision making around the issues of sexual health and reproduction.

NBWHP believes that barrier methods—used properly and every time—should be considered as the first choice for contraception as well as disease prevention. Barrier methods can be integrated into sexual foreplay, and the rewards include increased intimacy with one's sex partner and greater comfort and familiarity with one's own body and sexuality. Family planning programs and health care providers must invest necessary time and resources to ensure that women are encouraged to use barrier methods to reduce their risk of STDs and HIV/AIDS.

Sexually active African-American women of all ages—whether heterosexual, bisexual, or lesbian—need a strong foundation of accurate information as well as support for practicing safer sex if we are going to win the battle against HIV/AIDS and STDs. NBWHP supports HIV/AIDS education and STD prevention programs as the best weapons against the continuing spread of STDs and HIV/AIDS throughout all segments of the population.

NBWHP is also a strong advocate of efforts to ensure that AIDS diagnosis and treatment services are available for early HIV detection within geographic and fiscal reach of at-risk populations such as low-income women and their families, rural dwellers, and the homeless. Outpatient care must entitle patients to receive services appropriate to their needs, including mental health care, housing assistance, and family services, as well as clinical and hospice care.

Early detection and medical intervention are now providing many HIV-infected women a greater life expectancy. Unfortunately, women and adolescent girls infected with HIV receive fewer medical services, such as medication, hospital admissions, and outpatient visits, than similarly diagnosed men. An asymptomatic, HIV-infected female is 20 percent less likely to receive azidothymidine (AZT) than an asymptomatic, HIV-infected male. A female with AIDS is also 20 percent less likely than a male injection drug user to be hospitalized for AIDS-related conditions.

Statistics demonstrate that African Americans do not receive enough early, routine, and preventative health care. Hospital emergency rooms and clinics are a much more common source of medical care for African Americans than for whites, and 20 percent of African Americans (compared to 13 percent of whites) report no usual source of medical care. NBWHP calls for improvements in the health care delivery system to ensure that women of color have access to quality, affordable preventative services, early detection and treatment, and appropriate follow-up care and counseling.

There is currently a debate about making the pill—which is now a prescription drug—available as an over-the-counter drug. NBWHP supports keeping oral contraceptives as prescription drugs because the annual health care visit for birth control pills is the only time many black women have access to medical services. Furthermore, the side effects of nausea, weight gain, and depression may cause a woman on the pill to need more frequent checkups. Black women have high rates of obesity, diabetes, and high blood pressure and therefore require adequate screening before using the pill. NBWHP is not confident that pharmacists are sufficiently trained to screen customers who would buy the pill over the counter. In addition, pharmacists may not have the time to thoroughly counsel customers.

A seminal issue for the reproductive health and rights of African-American women has been the marketing of long-acting contraceptives. Norplant and Depo-Provera function as short-term or temporary sterilizations, and their potential for abuse was quickly realized. Prior to its approval for use as a contraceptive (in addition to its use as cancer therapy), Depo-Provera had been regularly administered as birth control to women in developing countries, and to black and Native American women in clinical trials.

In 1982, the National Women's Health Network and its new program, the Black Women's Health Project, announced a class action suit against the Upjohn Pharmaceutical Company. The media focused on the use of the drug at Grady Hospital in Atlanta, where women were not fully informed of the adverse effects of the drug. While the use of Depo-Provera caused many problems, the suit was dropped because the drug did not cause any deaths.

NBWHP and other advocacy groups still oppose the use of Depo-Provera due to the possible increased risk of breast cancer in women under age thirty-five. This may be especially dangerous for black women, who are more likely to develop this cancer at younger ages. Weight gain of up to twenty to seventy pounds is not unusual, and this poses a threat to the health of many black women—50 percent of whom are already overweight and may suffer from diabetes or hypertension. Loss of bone density is another serious risk, especially to adolescent girls whose bones are still growing, and to women who may be susceptible to osteoporosis. Depression is a side effect with a greater negative impact on the health of poor and black women, many of whom have high levels of psychological stress in their daily lives due to racism, sexism, and economic struggles.

NBWHP also opposes any "incentives" for poor women and women of color to use Norplant or any other long-acting contraceptive, as well as any efforts to restrict choice among forms of contraception. In 1990, Norplant was on the market for just one month when judges began to order it inserted in women. An editorial in a major newspaper suggested that welfare recipients should be given financial incentives to take the drug and reduce their childbearing. Black activists were outraged that legislators would propose laws that would effectively sterilize women for years, simply because they were poor. Furthermore, there was mounting evidence that women having trouble with the drug's side effects were having difficulty obtaining necessary medical assistance to remove the capsules from their arms.

NBWHP supports efforts to develop female-controlled barrier methods of prevention, such as an inexpensive microbicide or virucide. Microbicides and virucides are chemical compounds that women could put in their vaginas before intercourse to block HIV. A women could protect herself against STDs and HIV/AIDS without having to negotiate condom use with her partner. Ideally, microbicides would be made with and without spermicides so that women who want to get pregnant could do so without worrying about contracting a disease.

Scientists are also pursuing several other options, including hormone-releasing vaginal rings that would be placed in the vagina for several weeks or months, skin patches, and vaccines/anti-fertility drugs that generate a temporary immune system reaction against eggs or sperm. Researchers are examining two options for a "male contraceptive," an implant and a vaccine.

The single most urgent concern of all health advocates regarding vaccines is how to prevent their abuse, on both individual and mass scales. An agent that could be secretly combined with other vaccinations or injections, or added to food and water supplies, poses a chilling threat to reproductive rights of women around the world. NBWHP urges the public, press, and legislators to demand answers to critical questions surrounding how these drugs will be used in studies and then used with the public.

HISTORICAL EXPERIENCE: STERILIZATION WITHOUT CONSENT

At the turn of the twentieth century, the so-called science of eugenics emerged, teaching that intelligence and other traits were "genetically determined" and if society were to improve, control over reproduction must be exercised. Proponents of eugenics played to white race suicide fears by encouraging "positive eugenics" (more births by white women) and the practice of "negative eugenics" (preventing births by "inferior" people). Compulsory sterilization was advocated by eugenicists to eliminate the "socially inadequate" members of society: the mentally retarded, the mentally ill, epileptics, criminals, prostitutes, and the poor.

Between 1907 and 1913, a dozen states passed involuntary sterilization laws, but constitutional challenges kept them on hold. However, in 1927, the US Supreme Court upheld the sterilization of a "feeble-minded" white girl in Virginia, and the floodgates opened. In short order, thirty states enacted compulsory sterilization laws. State governments initially focused on sterilizing institutionalized young women who were deemed unfit to be mothers. Women who were deemed promiscuous or who had children out of wedlock were often declared "feeble-minded" and institutionalized simply to be sterilized. The economic crisis in the 1930s prompted sterilization proponents to turn their attention to poor southern blacks. As the Depression deepened, whites were concerned that a larger number of black children would require more public funding.

When Nazi atrocities and their systematic destruction of "undesirable" people came to light in the 1940s, eugenics was discredited as a science, and mandatory sterilization laws were repealed. But the "population bomb" theory of the 1950s triggered racist fears of black and brown people overwhelming the white world. White fears were particularly sparked by images of a growing "welfare class" in U.S. cities.

By World War II, more sterilizations were being performed on institutionalized blacks than whites. In 1973, a legal case involving two teenaged sisters uncovered the widespread practice of government-funded sterilization of women without their knowledge or consent. The case of the Relf sisters revealed the fact that 100,000 to 150,000 poor women—one-half of them black—were being sterilized each year under the auspices of the US Department of Health, Education, and Welfare.

The scope of the abuse was terrifying. Women of color with no choice among health care providers often had to submit to "voluntary" sterilization to have their babies delivered. Many women were sterilized without their knowledge or permission: they would undergo gynecological procedures only to later discover that they had been sterilized. This was so widespread in the South that these operations came to be known as "Mississippi appendectomies." Physicians routinely performed more complicated surgical hysterectomies rather than simpler tubal ligations because their reimbursement fee was higher, and teaching hospitals permitted unnecessary hysterectomies as "practice" for their medical residents.

CONTEMPORARY CONTEXT: VOLUNTARY STERILIZATION IS AN OPTION, INVOLUNTARY STERILIZATION REMAINS A PROBLEM

Current research suggests that women, by and large, desire to control their family size. Most low-income black women want and have a small number of children, and spend most of their reproductive lives trying to avoid pregnancy. Although black women do outweigh their white counterparts in rates of unintended pregnancy, black women with higher educational and income levels have fewer children. Overall birth trends in the United States exemplify this, with family sizes decreasing from an average of six children in the 1960s to approximately three in 1995.

Sterilization as a means of contraception can be the right choice for individuals who are certain that they do not wish to have any (or any more) children. Today, women are usually sterilized by open (mini-laparotomy) tubal ligation or laparoscopic tubal cauterization, or clip placement. These are operations in which the fallopian tubes are cut, blocked, or clipped to prevent the egg from joining the sperm. Men are sterilized by vasectomy, an operation in which the vas deferens (the tubes that carry sperm) are cut or blocked.

For women over the age of thirty, voluntary sterilization via tubal ligation is more commonly used than any other method of birth control. There is usually a high one-time cost for tubal ligation or vasectomy, and these operations are considered permanent, although reversal is sometimes possible. When one partner is sterilized, there is a rate of 99 percent effectiveness in preventing pregnancy. However, *sterilization does not protect against STDs and HIV/AIDS.*

Involuntary sterilization, primarily via hysterectomy to treat gynecological problems, remains a problem today. Hysterectomy—the removal of the uterus—is the second most frequently performed major surgical procedure among reproductive-age women. More than one-fourth of women in the United States will undergo a hysterectomy before their sixtieth birthday. The Centers for Disease Control and Prevention (CDC) report that the number of hysterectomies has stabilized at 600,000 per year with no difference in the rate of hysterectomies based on race.

Although most hysterectomies involve the removal of only the uterus and the cervix, there has been an increase in hysterectomies in which the ovaries are also removed. Surgical removal of the ovaries can result in a need for hormonal treatment for some women.

The most frequent reason for black women having hysterectomies is fibroid tumors, a condition that disproportionately affects African-American women. However, treatments that provide alternatives to hysterectomies have always been available to certain women. These include laser and other ablative therapies, surgical excision (myomectomy),

and medications that, at least, temporarily shrink fibroid tumors.

NBWHP POLICY STATEMENT: BALANCE ISSUES OF ACCESS WITH SAFEGUARDS AGAINST ABUSE

The historical use of involuntary sterilization reflects a societal misconception that black women have too many children, and this is the cause of our social problems. This belief disregards issues of equity with respect to education and employment, and essentially overshadows the political, social, and economic issues that impact women's quality of life. These ideas are actually contrary to the beliefs that women hold about their won reproductive goals.

NBWHP believes that reproductive freedom is a right of all women regardless of race or socioeconomic status. Current data illustrates that when knowledge and access are increased, women can and do make reproductive decisions that will ultimately have a positive impact on their sexual status. NBWHP supports all voluntary and informed decisions about sterilization. Further, these decisions must be made without coercion. The focus of intervention should not be dictated by stereotypes and inaccurate beliefs, but rather an acknowledgment and effort to address the disparities in education, health care, and opportunities facing black women.

Because black women and other women of color were sterilized against their will or without their knowledge through federally supported programs as recently as twenty-five years ago, safeguards have been put in place to prevent such abuse. NBWHP believes it is possible to balance safeguards against sterilization abuse with a woman's right to choose sterilization without undue bureaucratic red tape or delays.

Involuntary sterilization presents another set of issues. NBWHP believes that hysterectomy should not be considered as the first and only option for the treatment of fibroids. Only after alternatives have been explored—and it has been determined that this procedure is medically warranted—should a hysterectomy be considered. Black women must be presented with options and opportunities to make educated choices about this and all procedures affecting their reproductive abilities. Through appropriate education and exploration of options, a woman can decide, in conjunction with her physician, which choice is best for her. Always seek a second opinion when a hysterectomy is recommended.

NBWHP also advocates for the continued research on alternatives to hysterectomies in the treatment of gynecological problems. Because there is no universally adopted medical standard for hysterectomy, a vast opportunity is created for non-medical factors such as race, age, religion, and socioeconomic status to become part of the decision-making process. Further research into the appropriateness and impact of this and other treatments as they relate to black women is needed.

Black women must also become savvy self-advocates when exploring options of care. We need to exercise our patient rights and feel empowered to question and/or challenge the medical community in order to make decisions that are right for us.

ABORTION

HISTORICAL EXPERIENCE: A LONGSTANDING PRACTICE

There is evidence that some black women refused to bear children as slaves—and therefore used contraceptives and abortion, in addition to outright refusing to be mated or raped. It is impossible to determine what percentage of the recorded instances of miscarriage and stillbirth among slave women were self-induced or the result of harsh living conditions and forced labor. The same is true with recorded cases of infanticide.

When "modern" contraceptives first became available at the turn of the century, African-American women were quick to understand the clear need to have access to contraception: Illegal abortion was a major method of controlling fertility for African-American women desperate to limit their childbear-

ing. The high rates of illegal abortion translated into tragically high rates of septic abortion and death.

In the 1950s, the medical establishment began to crack down on illegal abortion providers. African-American women who were underground providers were targeted more often than their white counterparts. As access to these generally safe but illegal providers decreased, more and more black women suffered the deadly consequences of self-induced abortion.

An "underground railroad" offered women access to illegal abortion providers throughout the 1960s. Groups of women learned how to perform abortions and then offered their services at low cost to poor women of color. Black women played important roles in these efforts across the country.

The 1973 Supreme Court decision to legalize abortion was critically important for all women and widely welcomed by the many black women who had struggled for this basic right. In 1976, Congress passed the Hyde Amendment which eliminated Medicaid funding of abortions for poor women, the majority of whom are African American. Many black activists were troubled by the failure of the predominantly white, middle-class abortion rights movement to fight harder to prevent passage of the Hyde Amendment.

CONTEMPORARY CONTEXT: ABORTION RIGHTS THREATENED

Abortion is a highly politicized medical procedure in the United States. In 1998, more restrictions on abortions exist than at any time in the past twenty-five years. Legislation ranging from parental consent/notification and waiting periods to "informed consent" and "gag rules" has virtually succeeded in limiting poor women and adolescents to either have a child or submit to temporary and/or permanent sterilization. The requirement in some states that a teenager obtain the consent and/or notify both parents is a serious impediment to many more African-American teens whose fathers are not available or whose pregnancy is a result of incest.

There is well-organized opposition to women

making their own choices about abortion. Opponents' tactics range from fake abortion clinics to "sidewalk counseling" and spreading false information—such as a link between breast cancer and abortion, a claim that has been scientifically debunked. Fanatics have killed health care providers at clinics; even their homes are no longer safe! Many of the targeted clinics are private, nonprofit clinics that provide low-cost services to black women and adolescents; this threatens young women's access to health care as well as places their lives in jeopardy.

According to estimates based on the National Survey of Family Growth, contraceptive failure is responsible for about half of the 3.5 million unintended pregnancies—approximately 1.7 million. Many women become pregnant even while using contraception because no method is 100 percent effective. Additionally, some women have limited power in negotiations with their partners about whether and when to have children or about the use of a specific contraceptive method.

When faced with an unintended pregnancy, the ratio of black women who choose abortion is about equal to that of white women. However, black women experience unintended pregnancies 2.5 times more often than white women, so we are twice as likely to have abortions.

Having an abortion is oftentimes a painful choice for women, but it may be the right choice at the particular time. Many women struggle with the decision to have an abortion and see it only as a last resort. Too often, they delay their decisions and thus require abortions later in their pregnancies.

Currently, there are two forms of abortion: *surgical* and *medical*.

The majority of *surgical abortions* are performed in the first trimester (three months of pregnancy). Early surgical abortion is a low-risk and relatively simple procedure. Surgical abortions in the second trimester are more complex and require two days.

Late-term abortions (twenty-four to twenty-six weeks) are complicated surgical procedures usually requiring general anesthesia. Most late-term abortions are performed to save the life or health of the mother, but they are subject to intense legal controversy. Opponents of the procedure have been succeeding in their attempts to limit or ban the procedure.

Medical abortion is a two-step procedure in which a woman takes one drug and then returns two days later to take another drug, which brings on uterine contractions. This regimen must be undertaken within the first seven weeks of pregnancy to be effective. Two drugs currently being used for medical abortions are mifepristone (the abortion pill RU-486) and methotrexate.

The advantages of medical abortion include the privacy of taking the drugs in one's own home and lower risks of infection or damage. Some women have said that they feel "in charge" of the medical abortion process, but women should be forewarned that heavy bleeding and cramping—similar to that experienced with a miscarriage—will occur.

NBWHP POLICY STATEMENT: KEEP ABORTION SAFE AND LEGAL

NBWHP unequivocally supports:

➤ The right of all women—regardless of age, income, or education—to make their own decisions regarding whether, when, and under what conditions she will bear children. We firmly believe that each woman, in consultation with her health care provider, is capable of deciding whether or not to carry a pregnancy to term.

➤ Access to complete information and safe, legal, and accessible abortion services for all women, including young and poor women. We encourage young women to consult with parents or other responsible adults in making this decision.

➤ Mandatory requirements that all medical school curricula include surgical abortion procedure training.

➤ The speedy regulation and release process of drugs for medical abortion, and increased training of health care professionals in their use.

➤ Demand for research to determine what, if any, specific side effects there are for black women undergoing medical abortion.

NBWHP opposes:

➤ Mandatory parental consent or notification laws and regulations.

➤ Restrictive or prohibitive laws or regulations that limit access to abortion services or information, such as the Hyde Amendment and child exclusion policies.

➤ Policies that limit or ban certain medical procedures determined necessary by health professionals. We believe that every woman in consultation with her health care provider can determine which abortion procedure is best for her.

DISEASES AND CONDITIONS OF THE REPRODUCTIVE SYSTEM

HISTORICAL EXPERIENCE

Historically, tension has existed between the medical community and the African-American community. One hundred years before Nazi atrocities led to the adoption of ethical guidelines for human medical experimentation, black women were used as medical subjects in studies of reproductive health. Surgical techniques in gynecology were developed in the nineteenth century through countless operations performed without anesthesia on black women purchased expressly for these experiments.

Based on these and other violations of trust by the medical community, many African Americans remain apprehensive about professional medical care. This problem is particularly disturbing because black women continue to face conditions that result in poor health and increase the need for competent medical care.

CONTEMPORARY CONTEXT: AFRICAN-AMERICAN WOMEN AT GREATER RISK.

All women face health risks related to their reproductive system, but certain diseases and conditions tend to be either more prevalent or more deadly in the African-American community. These include cancer, fibroids, pelvic inflammatory disease (PID), and infertility.

CANCER is defined by the American Cancer Society as "a group of diseases characterized by uncontrolled growth and spread of abnormal cells." Advanced cancer, the condition in which the disease has spread throughout the body, usually results in death. Cancers of the reproductive organs are a serious health concern for African-American women.

Breast cancer is the leading cause of cancer deaths among African-American women between the ages of thirty and fifty-four. Compared to white women, African-American women have a lower incidence but higher death rate from breast cancer. Detection at an early stage strongly influences the success of treatment. Some health professionals believe that black women should have a baseline mammogram at age thirty (rather than at age forty) because breast cancer strikes many black women at earlier ages.

Cancer of the uterus, which includes cervical cancer, is the second largest cause of cancer deaths among African-American women ages fifteen to thirty-four. African-American women are 2.5 times more likely to have cervical cancer than white women. Risk factors for cervical cancer include multiple sexual partners, early age at first intercourse, a history of STDs (particularly the human papillomavirus), and oral contraception use.

Little is known about the causes of ovarian cancer. Age is listed as the highest risk factor especially for women over sixty, yet ovarian cancer appears as one of the five leading cancer sites for African-American females ages thirty-five to fifty-four. Furthermore, for women with breast cancer, the chance of developing ovarian cancer doubles. Incidence rates for ovarian cancer are slightly lower for African-American women than for white women, but as with breast cancer, our survival rates are also slightly lower.

If detected early enough, there is an almost

100 percent survival rate for all three of these cancers. However, because a disproportionate number of African-American women live in poverty, have inadequate or no health education, and encounter obstacles to quality health care, most are diagnosed too late to save their lives.

FIBROIDS are benign (noncancerous) tumors that occur in the uterine wall. Fibroids often go undetected because they do not always produce symptoms. More than 50 percent of black women have fibroids, and fibroids are three to five times more prevalent among African-American women than white women. Most fibroids are small and harmless. However, if fibroids grow unchecked, health problems may result, including heavy or prolonged menstrual bleeding, abdominal bloating, lower-back pain, fatigue due to iron deficiency, painful sexual intercourse, difficulty becoming pregnant, and recurrent miscarriage.

There are several treatments for fibroids. Injections of hormone (GnRH) Lupron shrinks fibroids temporarily. Also available in a nasal spray, these medications induce a menopausal state in a woman's body, causing the ovaries to cease hormone (estrogen/progesterone/testosterone) production. Small fibroids can also be removed surgically by burning away with a laser or by being scraped off. For larger tumors, a small incision is made in the abdomen for removal by laser or other medical instruments. Another procedure involves cutting off the estrogen and blood supply to the fibroid, which causes it to wither and die. Women who choose removal of fibroids must be made aware of a 30 to 50 percent recurrence rate when multiple tumors are present (within five years). Hysterectomy—complete removal of uterus—is still the most common treatment for fibroids, but it is often unnecessary.

INFERTILITY affects African Americans at a rate up to one and a half times higher than for whites. The causes most often cited include untreated sexually transmitted infections (particularly chlamydia and gonorrhea) which cause pelvic inflammatory disease (PID); endometriosis (the growth of intrauterine [endometrial] tissue outside of the uterus); nutritional deficiencies; complications from childbirth and abortion; and environmental and workplace hazards.

NBWHP POLICY STATEMENT: GREATER ACCESS TO HEALTH CARE IS NEEDED

Stronger preventive health care and early detection are important steps to protect our health from cancer. Cancer survival hinges on early detection. The sooner the disease is diagnosed and treatment begun, the higher the chances are that the spread of abnormal cells will be stopped before invading other areas of the body. Therefore, women of color must have access to quality, affordable preventive screening (including regular gynecological checkups, breast exams, Pap smears, and mammograms), education regarding prevention as well as warning signals, and follow-up counseling for all types of cancer. Our efforts at prevention must include knowing the importance of nutrition, exercise, regular stress reduction techniques, and the importance of controlling modifiable habits, such as smoking, alcohol, and/or drug use.

There is evidence that many African-American women do not participate in cancer screening programs because they do not know about them. In one study, nearly 60 percent of women of color stated that their reason for not complying with screening guidelines was a lack of appreciation of the importance of screening. Another reason for the continued higher cancer death rate among African-American women may be a less complete follow-up of positive tests, particularly if they do not have a regular source of care.

NBWHP also supports the development of new tests to detect breast cancer in its early stages. Mammograms are not effective in detecting breast cancer in women under thirty-five years of age because of denser breast tissue. Only 25 percent of early cases are caught by mammograms in this age group. However, mammography remains a very important tool in breast cancer detection, as improved technology is devised.

NBWHP calls for an end to the barriers faced by African Americans seeking treatment for infertility. These barriers include the high cost of infertility treatment; advertising by infertility treatment centers that feature only white infants and fuel the unspoken assumption that white babies are more highly valued by society; and the continued portrayal of black women as overly fertile, which generates a lesser sense of urgency for treatment of our infertility. Attention must be focused on improving the basic conditions that contribute to infertility, and on improving access to preventive health care and prompt diagnosis and treatment of STDs. Taking these steps might reduce the infertility rate and allow black women to achieve greater overall health.

Both private and public health care programs have looked at managed care as a way to improve the quality and control the costs of health care. Although managed-care programs have the potential for providing high-quality health care, they have been largely used as vehicle to control costs among the insured, particularly with federal health programs. Managed care programs have been widely criticized for limiting patient choice of physicians and for lack of quality assurance mechanisms.

NBWHP believes that comprehensive health care reform is crucial to provide all Americans with equal access to quality health care.

MENOPAUSE

HISTORICAL EXPERIENCE: A TABOO TOPIC

Before the turn of the century, any discussion of menopause was considered taboo. In fact, women whose childbearing years were over were widely looked upon as old and sexually unattractive. Menopause itself was viewed as an unpleasant condition to be dreaded and feared, much like a disease.

These attitudes can be attributed, in part, to the fact that until the early 1900s, most women did not live to see menopause. Due to disease, physical labor, and complications related to childbirth, the average life span for a woman was about forty-five years. Those who lived into their fifties were considered elderly.

Fortunately, things are changing. Approximately 40 million female "baby boomers" will reach menopause around the decade of the 1990s. As a result of this demographic trend as well as dramatically increasing life expectancies, menopause has become much more of a topic for study and discussion.

CURRENT CONTEXT: THE MEDICALIZATION OF MENOPAUSE

Menopause is the process in which ovarian hormone levels diminish, signaling the end of a woman's reproductive years and cessation of menstrual periods (or flow). Menopause has three phases: premenopause (active menstruation), perimenopause (noticeable changes), and postmenopause (after periods have ended). A woman will know she has reached menopause when she has completed one year without menstruation. A health care provider can confirm this by measuring hormone levels.

Perimenopause is the two- to ten-year period before the end of menstrual periods, occurring between the ages of about thirty-five to forty-eight. During this phase, the length, amount, and frequency of menstrual flow may change. Pregnancy and the spread of sexually transmitted diseases can still occur at this time, so precautions must be taken.

Many women pass through menopause with few discomforting signs. Other women who experience a sharp decline in hormone levels may suffer more discomfort. The most common discomforts associated with menopause are hot flashes, insomnia, mood swings, vaginal dryness leading to painful intercourse, weight gain, forgetfulness, waning libido, and irregular vaginal bleeding.

Heavy periods are common during this time, but often subside as estrogen levels drop. Prolonged menstrual bleeding, especially after periods have begun to diminish, may be a sign of abnormal growths in the uterus or an overgrowth of the uterine lining. These problems may lead to cancer. Thus, regular gynecological checkups are important for early detection and obtaining treatment as early as possible.

There are few scientific data regarding how menopause affects African-American women differently than other women. However, anecdotal information indicates that black women may view this change of life more positively than white women. Many African-American women see menopause as a natural part of life and look forward to the end of their childbearing years. Those who suffer discomforts may turn to home remedies, natural herbs, vitamins, and spirituality rather than, or in addition to, Western medicine for relief.

As a result of widespread media campaigns by pharmaceutical companies that urge women to combat the signs of menopause and aging, many midlife women utilize hormone replacement therapy (HRT). Premarin (a brand of estrogen) has become one of the largest-selling prescription drugs in the United States. However, this drug is primarily used by middle-class women, while poorer women—including those who need the drug after a hysterectomy—are unable to obtain it.

Any decision about using HRT should be made individually, based on complete and accurate information regarding the risks and benefits. HRT is generally inadvisable for women who have had a stroke or heart attack; have had breast or uterine cancer; suffer from impairment of liver function; have unexplained vaginal bleeding; are pregnant; or face a variety of other health conditions. HRT is known to increase the risk of breast cancer after long-term use; increase the risk of endometrial cancer (if estrogen is used alone); and cause (in some women) nausea, weight gain, breast tenderness, uterine bleeding, fluid retention, and/or depression. However, estrogen may reduce the risk of heart disease and osteoporosis.

NBWHP POLICY STATEMENT: MENOPAUSE SHOULD BE TREATED AS A NATURAL CONDITION

NBWHP opposes the medicalization of menopause. It is not a disease, but a natural stage in a woman's life. Because pharmaceutical companies have promoted the medical treatment of "estrogen deficiency disease," many women have been cut off from seeking the advice and wisdom of elder women who have dealt already with this life transition. Furthermore, the ad campaign has contributed to the problem of some in the medical community mistakenly attributing health concerns reported by midlife women to menopause when the actual cause may be serious conditions such as gallbladder disease, hypertension, or clinical depression.

NBWHP supports the management of any uncomfortable signs of menopause with natural, self-help methods, including a diet rich in fresh fruits and vegetables, soy products, plenty of exercise, and stress-reduction activities. However, when signs are severe or women desire a medical approach, access to appropriate medical treatment of menopause must be available. Furthermore, all African-American women approaching menopause must have access to annual medical exams that include a mammogram, Pap smear, and bone density test.

EMPOWERMENT THROUGH SELF-HELP

NBWHP is firmly committed to the conviction that self-help—on both personal and community levels—is the foundation on which African-American women will shape the future for themselves and their families.

Black women simultaneously face racism, sexism, classism, and heterosexism. This umbrella of oppression affects us in all areas of our lives, even when we believe ourselves to be surviving and thriving. By better understanding the ways in which these interlocking oppressions affect our health status, we can examine our wellness within the broader social/political/economic context that is our reality. In this way, efforts to promote our health are clearly political in nature as we take control of our lives and support each other to do the same.

Through self-help, many of us have been able to achieve personal empowerment and make changes in our lives to make ourselves healthier. However, those of us who promote self-help and practice it daily recognize that such activities alone cannot secure democratic rights and freedom. No one can "self-help" her way to employment, housing, education, or health care when basic access is blocked by the discriminatory practices of employers, lenders, service providers, and governments.

We must make the connection between personal empowerment and community empowerment in order to advocate collectively for the public policy changes necessary to improve the quality of life for black women, our children, families, and community.

THE PROCESS OF SELF-HELP

Self-help begins when we are willing to confront our reluctance to discuss our sexual and reproductive health issues, and when we commit to breaking the "conspiracy of silence" and to taking good care of ourselves.

Self-help continues when we remember that a woman's sexual and reproductive health cannot be separated from the political, social, and economic context in which she lives.

Self-help is strengthened when we understand that true choice is possible only when women have adequate nutrition, health care, education, employment, and housing—and enjoy full and equal access to economic and political power.

Self-help grows when we challenge discrimination in the form of racism, sexism, or heterosexism—all of which kill African-American women—and when we are willing to face our own classism that divides African-American women into "haves" and "have-nots."

Self-help is rooted in our awareness that if the rights of one women are limited, then the rights of all women are threatened—and a commitment to

positive action to ensure that women achieve genuine reproductive health and rights.

SELF-HELP: PERSONAL EMPOWERMENT

The effects of racism and internalized oppression—combined with the effects of poverty and violence—cause much of the stress in our lives and contribute to our poor physical, emotional, and economic health. NBWHP urges you to adopt the following self-help activities that lead to good health and personal empowerment.

➤ *Take positive steps toward your own good health.* Seek appropriate, competent, thorough medical care on a regular basis. Learn about self-examination and become familiar and comfortable with your own body.

➤ *Discover what works to lift your spirits and cheer your mind* —music, meditation, talking with friends, bubble baths, reading, yoga, laughing with children—and then nourish yourself everyday in at least one special way.

➤ *Share information.* Ask the women in your life—mother, aunts, grandmothers, sisters, cousins, close family friends—to talk about their sexual and reproductive health experiences. Uncover secrets. Get to know your personal history.

➤ *Learn about principles of sexual responsibility.* Apply them to your own life, and help friends and family to do the same. Have the courage to ask for and receive accurate information about sex and sexuality.

➤ *Protect yourself and others from sexual abuse or exploitation.* Value your ability to control your decision making around sex. Create respectful, mutually satisfying relationships that may or may not include sex.

➤ *Commit to achieving a healthy weight,* to selecting and eating more nutritious foods, and to engaging in regular exercise such as Walking for Wellness, the fitness component of NBWHP's self-help groups that involves sisters walking individually and in groups.

> *If you choose to drink alcohol, do so in moderation.* Avoid illegal drugs and do not abuse over-the-counter or prescription medications.

> *Do your homework on the women's issues in your community.* Decide to become personally involved in community groups or volunteer organizations.

> *Exercise your rights!* Register to vote, and be sure to vote in all elections.

SELF-HELP: COMMUNITY EMPOWERMENT

Once you have started to empower yourself, you can help others to do the same. Whether your community is a small town, an inner-city housing project, or a college campus, there are many opportunities to help African-American women achieve better health for themselves and their families. Wherever people are, you can get involved:

> Join the local chapter of NBWHP. If there isn't one, start one!

> Encourage all women in your life to schedule medical checkups and any necessary screenings. Offer to accompany them and hold their hands for mammograms or medical appointments. Make this part of birthday gifts: after the appointments, take them to lunch!

> Volunteer in reproductive health clinics that serve women of color.

> Volunteer in schools. Get involved in the PTA, and work for effective sex education for students from the elementary grades through high school.

> Volunteer with church groups that are serving the homeless and hungry.

> Sponsor walkathons or other health-promoting events for black women.

> Support nonprofit advocacy organizations working on reproductive health and rights issues with either your money, your time, or both.

> Join local civic or social organizations and put reproductive health and rights on their agenda. Volunteer to get speakers.

> Encourage your family and friends to register and vote. Help get people to the polls on election day.

> Write or call elected officials to express your views on political issues affecting the lives and health of African-American women.

> Become familiar and involved with local and state politics on reproductive health and rights issues. Organize voter registration drives, circulate, petitions, sponsor educational forums, and promote reproductive health care services.

> Let us know what community self-help actions you are undertaking. And remember, NBWHP is available to help with information and assistance.

Patsy Mink on Health Issues for Asian Women

INTERVIEW BY TANIA KETENJIAN

Congresswoman Patsy Mink (D-HI) served in the House of Representatives from 1990 until her death in 2002. This interview was conducted in June 1999.

TK: What would you say are some of the most prominent health issues facing Asian women?

PM: The statistics with reference to Asian health are shocking and startling in terms of lack of access to typical health facilities. We have to do a lot more to get our health care system to be more aware of the difficulties of getting health information to Asian women. They're not going for mammograms in many cases until they're very, very terminally ill. They're not accustomed to the typical invasive methodologies of the regular health care system and, as a consequence, they withdraw from it. The system doesn't allow things that are culturally comfortable for the Asian population, for example, acupuncture and herbal medicines are not covered services. The two systems do not come together, but diverge, and the quality of life for Asian communities is therefore greatly diminished. President Clinton recently established the President's Advisory Commission on Asian American Health and other concerns. The National Institutes of Health is supposed to make studies and recommendations and to see how these discrepancies can be resolved. The President and the departments of government recognize that the quality of life for Asian Americans is being severely impacted by the failure of the regular health care system.

Breast cancer rates increase dramatically for Japanese women when they move to the United States. This can be attributed to diet or other circumstances of their changed life, but those statistics are really quite alarming. There is a large incidence of cancer and heart disease among all Asian population categories—male and female—as they move to the United States and become second- and third-generation Americans.

TK: What would you like to see changed or developed in health care for Asian women?

PM: Asian women are not very receptive to the calls that traditionally are made to the rest of the population to have annual mammograms, and Pap tests, and so forth. One study showed that only 18 percent of Vietnamese women have ever had a Pap smear. A random sample of 157 Chinese-American women in California showed that 68 percent did not know what a Pap smear was; they had never heard of it! Hepatitis B is thirteen times more common in the Asian population than in other American populations. Native Hawaiian women have the highest incidence of breast cancer of all minority women. This is the population group within our country that is suffering and we need to pay attention. We need to find out what it is that we aren't doing right.

TK: Why do you think this situation exists?

PM: If I knew, I would already have begun to implement the solution. We're trying to figure out what we can do to reach out to this population and get them health care services—whether it's the regular variety or alternative medicine—whatever can bring them up to normal health levels.

TK: In *The Conversation Begins,* you say that the women's movement still focuses on middle-class white women. What do you think can be done to change that?

PM: Very little. I don't think that there are enough minority Asian women who participate, who think it's worthwhile to express themselves on behalf of the minority population. As a result, years go by with people paying no attention to anything other than what the middle-class white population is concerned about. There is even less attention to minority women's issues now than there was ten or twenty years ago.

I think it's mainly that there's no exposure, there's no sensitivity training, there's no one there to keep poking at the white majority when they make a mistake, or forget a certain population, or gear their message to white populations while leaving out the minorities. The absence of even black women in these groups is quite astounding, so I don't know how we can get Asian women to participate. It's very tough. When we all started the efforts to organize the National Organization for Women and the Women's Caucus, I tried very hard to bring in Asian communities, but they wouldn't participate. Even in my state of Hawaii, neither organization is in existence. I can't even say that in my own circumstances I've been able to create an awareness of the importance of political participation.

TK: Because of the absence of black women in health organizations, Byllye Avery founded the National Black Women's Health Project. Are there corresponding Asian groups?

PM: We have a lot of Asian health groups. But that doesn't make up for the absence of attention or insensitivity toward our concerns from groups like NOW and the Women's Caucus. They will acknowledge each other as groups, but that's very different from having the population sitting right there in your executive committee and at your conventions, pounding away about exclusions.

TK: What should be done to increase participation?

PM: I don't know how you can get populations to *want* to participate. Even in our own exclusively Asian groups, there are not large numbers participating. A few people in leadership positions have to speak for the many that are silent.

TK: Would you call yourself one of those people?

PM: Yes.

TK: Would you call yourself an activist?

PM: Of course, always.

TK: And how did you get involved in activism?

PM: I think it's just in my nature to run into a problem and to fix it rather than to simply say, "Well, that's a problem; that's the way things are and always will be." I have a personality that says, "Let's go see if we can fix it."

TK: So that's what activism is?

PM: Yes; that's all it is. It is to believe that things can be better, that you don't have to accept the status quo.

TK: How did you decide to become a lawyer?

PM: Well, that was quite accidental. Actually, I was trying to become a medical doctor, but I couldn't get into medical school because women were excluded. I wrote to a dozen or more medical schools and each wrote back saying, "I'm sorry, but we don't take women." So I was very disenchanted. I got my bachelor's degree and I started working as a clerk out in the private, nonprofit sector. One of the women I ran into who was the director of a program said, "Well, why don't you try for just any professional school; it doesn't have to be medicine; if you have the talent, you can direct your professional education

into doing other things." She persuaded me to write an application to law school. By some great magic, I got into law school the first time I tried without knowing what the study of law really was. I went as an experiment, and I found it fascinating, very engrossing. So I stuck with it for three years, got my law degree, came home, and really felt better equipped to challenge the status quo because I had that fantastic educational background.

TK: What do you feel is lacking in the political sector; what needs more focus regarding women?

PM: More women need to be part of the process. I think we could make much greater headway if more women were active instead of just sort of background participants—making coffee, serving whatever, not engaging in the stream of political ideas and immediate change. We need women to get to the forefront and become part of policy making.

TK: How can that happen?

PM: One by one. One by one.

TK: What issues would you like to work on in the future?

PM: We are working very hard on education right now. We want to find ways to improve education because that is the source of the strength of our country and our ability to keep up with global scientific and technological advances. If our educational prowess falls, we're going to diminish our ability to be competitive; so I think that education is terribly important. While it is important for the individual, it is even more important for the nation as a whole; so that's my number one issue. My number two issue is all the health issues: the ability to maintain Medicare, for instance, to provide enough for families to take care of the medical needs of their elderly and sick. And finally, I am concerned about Social Security and the needs of the Asian population. I would say that those three are at the top of my list.

Charon Asetoyer

INTERVIEW BY TANIA KETENJIAN

Charon Asetoyer is the founder of the Native American Women's Health Education Resource Center. This interview was conducted in June 1999.

TK: What do you think are some of the most prominent reproductive health issues for indigenous women?

CA: The lack of delivery services within communities—women have to travel long distances to deliver their babies and get prenatal care. And reproductive tract infections are at an all-time high. The Indian Health Service doesn't offer education in prevention and that causes these problems. Too many non-barrier contraceptives are promoted.

We have people who are working on issues of boarding school survivors, people who were going to boarding schools where there was sexual abuse committed against our children by the Catholic Church. People are just now starting to talk about it. This information is surfacing, and it has had a devastating effect on our reproductive health and will continue to do so until these issues are addressed.

The social problems in our community create situations in which our young women feel that starting their families at an early age is the right thing. In reality, a fourteen-year-old should still be in school, should be looking at how she can have fun and be a fourteen-year-old and not at how to be a mother. We need to look at why this is happening to our young people, why they feel that their options are so limited that they start a family. We need to look at what can go on within our communities that will support our young people in staying in school. They need to realize that they have a future and choices. There are very few services that look at improving the status of our young women and that would have a very profound, integrating effect on our reproductive health and rights.

Development, any kind of development, affects the status of health and our families. We need to look at why we haven't made the same forward moves in community development as other people. When you start uncovering all of these issues, you are going to come up with the same answer. We're talking about 500 years of contact—we call it "AC" instead of "AD"—500 years after contact, that's how we look at things, 500 years after Columbus. For us, that has had a very profound impact on our current existence and people seem to forget that. People whose culture is completely devoid of origins want us to assimilate into the mainstream. They do not respect cultural differences. There are light-years of difference between that and a people who still feels proud of its culture. I think it is very important that people stop to think, that people respect differences, even if they have lost their knowledge of their traditional ways because they are no longer in their homeland, no longer in Europe. They are here in this country where we lived and flourished long before they came. They need to stop trying to take away very important fundamental human rights that make cultures cultures, and to acknowledge our autonomy, our sovereignty. When that happens, then you will see an increase in the status of health of indigenous patients. We're just so busy trying to fight off corporate America and trying to maintain who we are and to fight the assimilation and fight the mainstreaming. It's very difficult to have time in your day to pay attention to your health like other people do. We don't have the same access as other people and it is fundamentally important to recognize that.

TK: Can you tell me some specific pros and cons of the Indian Health Service?

CA: The Indian Health Service is our primary health care provider, and we have to do everything we can to make it a good provider, to improve its services. The Indian Health Service needs to look at community response in order to improve its services. It needs to make more information about sexually transmitted diseases and reproductive tract infections accessible and available to the community. It needs to improve on its preventive services; it needs to establish better informed consent. The Indian Health Service headquarters has established informed consent, but it's amazing that it is not uniformly mandated. This means that every Indian Health Service clinic does not have to use the same informed consent procedures. In some instances, when you walk in the door, that's considered consent; that's not acceptable. So they have to have more continuity and consistency within their services. They also need to have more culturally sensitive practitioners who are aware of our traditional practices. They need to respect them so that both approaches can work together. There may be patients who are using both—the biomedical approach as well as the traditional, spiritual approaches—for treating their problems. So the physicians need to realize that they are on a reservation, that they are functioning within a different culture, and that it is unacceptable to force a person into complying with all of their procedures. Practitioners need to become more familiar with indigenous practices and, through that, will achieve much better outcomes.

TK: Do issues of self-worth play a role in the difficulties indigenous women have in seeking health care?

CA: I don't think that we don't feel worthy enough to seek health care. The problem is more one of fear. Because of our history, we're dealing with fear of the Western health care provider. There is not a lot of trust within the community for the Indian Health Service. Too many of our women have been sterilized, too many of our babies have died, our midwifery practices have almost been lost because of our being forced to use IHS services, so there is a mistrust of the services the government provides. A lot of people don't want to go to IHS clinics, and will turn to our traditional spirituality and medical practices, or to what remains of them after they were outlawed. For us, it has to do with trust, or lack of it.

TK: What kind of involvement does the Native American Women's Health Education Resource Center have with other women's groups and minority groups?

CA: We try very hard to do as much networking as we can, to network with other indigenous organizations, to network and work with other women of color, and to also work with mainstream women's organizations because, when it comes right down to it, we have to if we're all to survive. Many of us are victims of the same perpetrator: pharmaceutical companies and capitalism—multinational corporations trying to turn a buck on our gender. So it's very important that we work together and respect each others' philosophies, communities, and cultures. Together we can make changes; fragmented and working against each other, we can't.

TK: What changes would you like most to see in the next few years?

CA: I would like to see more indigenous women and more women of color sitting on boards of mainstream organizations. I would like to see more foundations and philanthropic efforts directed at women of color and indigenous women so that we can address the kinds of issues in our communities that need to be addressed. We need to develop programs that assist our young women in being able to have better reproductive health and that provide services to improve the status of young women. I'm sure that would create a turnaround in childbearing. I'd like to see healthier women; I'd like to see a reduction in diabetes within our community. I'd like to see respect for indigenous women from the biomedical community; and I would like to see the government back off from so much control and acknowledge the policies that we would like to see implemented in our health care system.

TK: Can you tell me a little bit about your experiences in the National Women's Health Network [NWHN]?

CA: I still feel that the National Women's Health Network is a very important organization and that it's a voice in Washington for all women. They have been incredible advocates, and have impacted policy in Washington for women's reproductive health. I think that the organization needs to continue its existence. I served on the board of directors of the National Women's Health Network for eight years, and I support the organization wholeheartedly. In fact, the NWHN, and the National Latina Health Project and the National Black Women's Health Project, helped us to develop the Native American Women's Health Education and Resource Center fourteen years ago. So I have very high respect for the National Women's Health Network.

TK: Let's say an indigenous woman wanted to turn to someone or someplace for superior care, better care than what is normally available to them, where would you send them?

CA: Well, I would send them to a woman's clinic in Sioux Falls. That is 150 miles away from us. We are in the Yankton Sioux Reservation in Lake Andes, South Dakota. If a woman does not have an automobile, or does not have money to buy gas or hire someone to take her 300 miles round trip, she's out of luck. Most indigenous women on reservations in this country live in very rural, isolated communities. We not only lack access to services within our own community, but we also lack resources that could provide us with other kinds of services.

TK: I know you did some reports on Norplant. Why did you do them and what did you discover?

CA: We did reports on the impact of Depo-Provera and the impact of Norplant in the Native American communities because they seemed to be the Indian Health Service's contraceptives of choice as opposed to the contraceptives of choice of the women in the community. Women were not getting all of the information about these contraceptives, or about the impact they would have on their health, both in the long- and short-term. On the surface, Depo or Norplant look like the best things since sliced bread; but that couldn't be more wrong. So it was important that we examine the situation and publish documented reports that

would bring all of these issues to the fore. We found that in the case of Norplant, when women realized, "This isn't the right kind of contraceptive for me because I'm having some kind of side effect; I want to have it removed," their request was being denied. Women were being forced to lose their reproductive health, and their reproductive rights were being violated. Women no longer had choice or control. They were at the mercy of the health care provider. In terms of Depo-Provera, it was and still is the form of contraception women are being encouraged to use. After they use it for a while and realize the side effects related to the drug, it's too late to do something about it. Again, it's a provider-controlled contraceptive.

TK: What can indigenous women do to overcome and change all the obstacles they face?

CA: It's not a matter of overcoming these kinds of reproductive health problems; it is one, rather, of being able to organize ourselves in order to move policies forward to prevent these kinds of things from continuing to happen. We have been organizing women for over ten years now. We have seen some changes, positive changes, because of the work that we're doing, both at local and national levels in the form of policy changes and service improvements. I really think that a lot of that is because women are organizing and getting more involved and bringing our day-to-day reality into the policy arena. It's important for indigenous women, for *all* women for that matter, to continue to organize and work on issues of reproductive health.

IN CONCLUSION, IN MEMORIAM, IN HOPE

IN FEBRUARY 2008, the women's health movement lost one of its mothers, and I lost one of mine. Barbara Seaman, the coauthor of this book and a tireless activist on behalf of women's rights, died of lung cancer at her home in Manhattan. After her diagnosis in April 2007, Barbara was determined to write her memoirs, to put to paper her various experiences working to reform women's health care, to offer advice and tales of victory and caution for young women who would fight the next generation of battles for better, safer lives. She never got the chance.

During the summer of 2007 I conducted a series of interviews with Barbara, asking her to talk about different points in her great career. She never could decide which moment or experience first put her on the path to a life of health advocacy. Was it the death of her Aunt Sally from hormone treatment (HT)–induced cancer, or the time a doctor ignored her stated intentions to breast feed and gave her postpartum drugs that leeched into her breast milk and poisoned her infant son? I like to think that, at least subconsciously, it was the moment when Barbara was seventeen and a doctor, in response to her queries on how to lose weight, put a free sample pack of cigarettes in her hand and told her to have one or two after dinner instead of dessert.

She was similarly undecided when asked about her greatest accomplishments. Some days she would say that her best contribution was her book *Women and the Crisis in Sex Hormones*, which predicted the HT debacle following the resolutions of the Women's Health Initiative in 2002. In other moments, the *Doctors' Case Against the Pill* and the resulting hearings, protests, and the world's first patient packet insert occupied her thoughts. In the end she decided it was a tie between her grandchildren (including two feminist granddaughters) and the creation of the National Women's Health Network.

On her greatest regret, she was decided. It was her inability to stop women from suffering the unnecessary side effects and even irreparable harm of bad drugs. She saw it as a recurring pattern: undertested drugs were pushed by irresponsible profit-hungry pharmaceutical companies on a population of women, and the damage was done before the truth could emerge. She saw it happen with the birth control pill, and again with DES, HT, Norplant, and fertility drugs. In recent years she worried about menstrual suppression drugs, bisphosphonates, statins, and the HPV vaccine Gardisil. Barbara saw the connections between these situations and was frustrated and discouraged that others couldn't. Each time we read or heard a story about a woman with a tragic outcome or an avoidable cancer or simply a serious life disruption, Barbara despaired that she had failed. She wondered how, after decades of activism and reporting, she was unable to prevent the same sorts of health tragedies that inspired her to begin her immense work. This was ironic to me, because Barbara was someone who refused to accept individual credit for her successes, preferring instead to spread the accomplishments around to other activists, writers, doctors, and feminists, yet she wanted to bear the responsibility for the movement's failures herself.

Barbara Seaman's greatest legacy, as dozens of people like myself rushed to eulogize, was her tireless work to mentor, educate, and encourage young women toward their own great works. I met her during my junior years of college when I was a directionless, restless young woman desperately searching for opportunities to work for positive change in the world. Barbara taught me to be passionate about health care and feminism. She gave me the skills and opportunity to write about these subjects, and introduced me to great thinkers and activists with whom I could work, organize, improvise, and theorize about how to continue the projects of the women's health movement. This book shows what Barbara always believed—that there is continuity between the generations, and that even as a young woman answers the questions of those who came before, she poses a new set that those who follow her will have to work to address.

Barbara originally imagined *Voices of the Women's Health Movement* as a comprehensive women's health manual organized around parts of the body. This sort of organizational scheme appealed to her. The book's unique structure is like the body—fluid, complicated, and gloriously disorganized. The process of grieving and letting go of Barbara is much the same. I think it is interesting that since she has died, I, and others who love her, have tried to reassemble a portrait of her, to recall each detail or preference, to try and build a more complete whole. We tell stories that capture her unique sense of humor, or recite poems she liked, or ruminate on new health problems that had started to occupy her thoughts. For all of these reasons, I am glad the book has taken the form it has. In a way, it is the memoir my dear friend never found the time to write.

Barbara's joy in her work was contextual—it always came from seeing her personal accomplishments alongside the work of others. Talk to her about her groundbreaking book on birth control, and she would start to describe Alice Wolfson's protests of the Senate pill hearings. Compliment her book *Women and the Crisis in Sex Hormones*, and she would detail the courageous scientists who helped underline the dangers of HT, or the work of a brave lawyer like Sybil Shainwald who helped get legal justice for DES victims. Barbara was never looking for individual attention, which is another reason I think this book constitutes a fitting biography of its author. Barbara's private stories appear alongside the great writings of her "heroic antecedents," peers, and intellectual and political daughters and granddaughters.

The heart of it all, while often personal and anecdotal, is fundamentally communal, instructional, and political.

There are so many health battles facing young women today. In the United States, our crumbling health system has created a world where very few, regardless of sex or gender, can receive adequate health care, and the drug companies have worked hard to see that those who do are full of dubious long-term drugs. Hysterectomies are still performed too frequently, despite strong evidence that unnecessary gynecological surgery shortens the lifespan. The right to a safe abortion, of course, continues to suffer constant assault. The rights of lesbian, gay, bisexual, and transgender people continue to be abused and curtailed. The political challenges of childbirth and motherhood continue unresolved, and even as younger women reap the expanded educational and career opportunities earned by second-wave feminism, they struggle to navigate a society that treats women and men, mothers and fathers differently, and always asks women to make fantastically difficult choices and suffer in a vocational world that is, sadly, still rife with sexism. Teenage and preteen women must contemplate a society where drug makers insist that periods are unnecessary and that the burden of STD prevention is still a predominantly female enterprise. More troubling still is the erosion of comprehensive sexual education programs and their replacement with "abstinence only" curricula that prevent young women from receiving basic information about their bodies and sexual health. In this world we must define and fight the new health care battles of the twenty-first century and carry forth the women's health movement. My hope and my belief is that the example, memory, and inspiration of women who have come before us, including Barbara, will help us to keep fighting.

—Laura Eldridge, November 2011

ABOUT THE CONTRIBUTORS

MARGOT ADLER is a correspondent for National Public Radio (NPR) and the author of *Drawing Down the Moon*, the classic study of contemporary paganism, *Goddess Spirituality*, and *Heretic's Heart*, a memoir of the 1960s. Since September 11, 2001, she has focused much of her work on stories exploring the human factors in New York City, from the loss of loved ones, homes, and jobs, to work in the relief effort. She is presently the host of *Justice Talking* and she is a regular voice on *Morning Edition* and *All Things Considered* on NPR.

AMY ALLINA is on the board of directors and the executive committee of the Guttmacher Institute, an organization that advances sexual and reproductive health through research, policy analysis, and public education. Prior to joining the National Women's Health Network (HNWHN) in 1999, Allina worked for the Reproductive Health Technologies Project and on other women's health policy issues at the consulting firm of Bass and Howes. She was also a political organizer for the Maryland affiliate of National Abortion and Reproductive Rights Action League (NARAL) and an associate editor at *Multinational Monitor*, a monthly magazine founded by Ralph Nader.

CHARON ASETOYER is currently the executive director and founder of the Native American Women's Health Education Resource Center and the Native American Community Board. Asetoyer has served on the board of directors for the Indigenous Women's Network, the Honor the Earth Campaign, and the National Women's Health Network.

BYLLYE Y. AVERY co-founded the Gainsville Women's Health Center and co-founded Birthplace, an alternative birthing center in Gainsville, Florida. She moved to Atlanta in 1981 to begin the NBWHP, a nonprofit organization committed to defining, promoting, and maintaining the physical, mental, and emotional well-being of African-American women. Avery has received the MacArthur Foundation Fellowship for Social Contribution, the Essence Award for community service, and many other awards and honors. She was honored by *Women eNews* as one of "21 Leaders for the 21st Century."

LORI BARER, originally from New Jersey, is a graduate of the University of Michigan and a PhD candidate for public health at the University of Michigan.

PAULINE B. BART is professor emerita of sociology and women's studies in the department of psychiatry at the University of Illinois. Her most recent books are *Stopping Rape: Successful Survival Strategies,* coauthored with Patricia O'Brien, and *Violence Against Women: The Bloody Footprints,* coauthored with Eileen Moran. As an activist in issues of violence against women and women's health, fields which have recently substantially converged, she considers her task to demystify the world for women.

CYNTHIA BASEMAN, born and raised in Los Angeles, California, began her career as a motion picture and television development executive selling stories to studios and networks including TNT, ABC, and NBC. In 1995 she suffered the loss of her daughter, who was stillborn. Devastated, Baseman struggled to find meaning in life again. In *Love, Mom,* Baseman gives a first hand account of her experiences in order to help others find the tools to search for happiness in the wake of misfortune.

SHARON BATT is a breast cancer survivor and the founder of Breast Cancer Action Montreal. She has been a journalist, author, professor, advocate, and university chair. She lives and works in Canada.

JENNIFER BAUMGARDNER is a New York–based writer and activist. Once an editor at *Ms.,* she has written for *Bust,* the *Nation, Jane, Out, HUES, Glamour, Marie Claire, Z,* and *Ms.,* among other magazines. She is the coauthor of two books on the state of feminism and activism, *Manifesta: Young Women, Feminism, and the Future* and *Grassroots: A Field Guide for Feminist Activism* with Amy Richards. In 2007, Baumgardner published *Look Both Ways: Bisexual Politics.*

KAREN BEKKER studied Judaic studies and art at Oberlin College. She served on the board of New York National Organization for Women (NOW), and has been actively involved in the feminist movement for several years. Her writing includes several articles in *Lilith.* She received a JD degree, magna cum laude, from the Benjamin N. Cardozo School of Law, where she served as senior editor on the Law Review Editorial Board. Bekker is an associate at Satterlee Stephens Burke & Burke LLP, where her practice focuses on commercial and first amendment litigation.

SUSAN BROWNMILLER is the author of *Against Our Will, Femininity, Waverly Place,* and *Seeing Vietnam.* Her most recent book is *In Our Time: Memoir of a Revloution.* She is an adjunct professor of women's and gender studies at Pace University in New York City.

MEGAN BUCKLEY interned with Barbara Seaman in 2006. She graduated from Gettysburg College in May 2008, and is currently working at Special Ops Media, a full service interactive marketing agency.

CAEDMON MAGBOO is a graduate of Barnard College and the University of Washington Law School. She currently works as a public defender in Seattle and has been active on the issue of military tour lengths.

PAULA J. CAPLAN was named an "eminent woman psychologist" by the American Psychiatric Association. She the author of several books including *Don't Blame Mother* and the best-selling *The Myth of Women's Masochism.* She is a clinical and research psychologist.

CARRIE CARMICHAEL is a writer and performer living in New York City. She is the author of the classic *Non-Sexist Childraising, How to Relieve Menstrual Cramps and Other Menstrual Problems* with Marcia L. Storch, MD, and three other books. Carmichael won broadcast awards for her work on the NBC Radio Network and has contributed to numerous magazines and broadcasts.

ELEANOR CASEY is the author and editor of two anthologies, *An Uncertain Inheritance: Writers on Caring for Family* and *Unholy Ghost: Writers on Depression.* Her writing has appeared in the *New York Times, Slate, Salon,* the *Guardian, Self, Fitness, Cookie,* and *Elle.* She is a mental health journalism fellow at the Carter Center. She lives in Brooklyn with her husband and son.

MICHAEL CASTLEMAN is "one of the nation's top health writers" (*Library Journal*). He is the author of over fifteen books, most recently *Great Sex: A Man's Guide to the Secrets of Total-Body Sensuality, There's Still a Person in There,* and *Blended Medicine.* Castleman has also written for dozens of magazines. He has taught medical writing at the University of California, Berkeley, Graduate School of Journalism. He is the husband of a breast cancer survivor.

VERONICA CHAMBERS is the author of several books including *Having it All?*, *Mama's Girl*, *The Joy of Doing Things Badly*, and *Kickboxing Geishas*. She is a former culture writer for *Newsweek* and has written for *Premiere*, *Savoy*, *Glamour*, *O, The Oprah Magazine*, and the *New York Times*. She lives in Philadelphia.

DEBORAH CHASE is the author of seven books, including *Terms of Adornment* and *The Extend Your Life Diet*. She is an alumnus of Bronx High School of Science, a winner of the Westinghouse Science Talent Search, and graduated from New York University with a dual degree in science and journalism. She has done research at the National Cancer Institute and the New York University School of Medicine.

ARIEL CHESLER is a lawyer living in Manhattan.

PHYLLIS CHESLER, PHD, is an emerita professor of psychology and women's studies at City University of New York. She has lectured and organized political, legal, religious, and human rights campaigns in the United States and in Canada, Europe, the Middle East, and the Far East. Dr. Chesler is co-founder of the still-ongoing Association for Women in Psychology (1969) and the National Women's Health Network (1974), and is a charter member of the Women's Forum (1973–74). Dr. Chesler's thirteen books and thousands of articles and speeches have inspired people on many diverse issues.

SUZANNE CLORES is the author of a children's book, *Native American Women*, and the books *Memoirs of a Spiritual Outsider* and *The Wisdom of the Saints*. She is a professor of writing at DePaul University.

MARCIA COHEN is an editor and writer whose work has appeared in the *New York Times Magazine* as well as many other national newspapers and magazines. She is the author of *The Sisterhood*, a Book of the Month Club Featured Alternate. She is also coauthor, with Dr. Gilbert Simon, of *The Parents' Pediatric Companion* and the author of *Gender and Groupwork*.

VICTOR COHN was a former science editor of the *Washington Post* whose long-time coverage of science and medicine won him many of journalism's highest honors. His contribution here is drawn from his book *News & Numbers: A Guide to Reporting Statistical Claims and Controversies in Health and Other Fields*, now in an eighth printing and in use at many journalism schools. Cohn died in 2000.

GENA COREA is a writer, dancer, co-founder of the Feminist International Network of Resistance to Reproductive and Genetic Engineering (FINRRAGE), and a certified focusing trainer. She gives workshops on creating a first person science of reproduction and also on developing a relationship with body symptoms. Her books include *The Hidden Malpractice, The Mother Machine*, and *The Invisible Epidemic*.

PHILIP CORFMAN, MD, a graduate of Oberlin College, Harvard Medical School, and obstetrics and gynecology residencies at Harvard Hospital, practiced his specialty at one of the first HMOs in the county, the Rip Van Winkle Clinic in upstate New York. In 1968 he became the first Director of the Center for Population Research. During this period, he was at the World Health Organization (WHO) and served on several of its advisory committees. In 1984, he was detailed full time by the National Institutes of Health (NIH) to the Human Reproduction Programme to reorganize and direct its research and development activities. In 1987, at the end of his WHO assignment, Dr. Corfman moved to the FDA to be in charge of the medical review of drugs for contraception, fertility, obstetrics, and gynecology. He retired from the FDA in late 1997 and is now doing consulting work.

BELITA COWAN is president of the Lymphoma Foundation of America, Inc. She is the author of *Health Care Shoppers Guide: 59 Ways to Save Money, Nursing Homes: What You Need to Know*, and *Women's Health Care: Resources, Writings, and Bibliographies*. She has testified before the US Senate, the US House of Representatives, the US Food and Drug Administration, and the District of Columbia City Council.

SUNNY DALY is a student with a committed interest in international women's movements, activism, and reproductive health. She has a bachelor's degree in history from Reed College, where she wrote her thesis, "Changing Images of the Birth Control Pill, 1960–1973." She is currently pursuing master's degrees in both political science and gender and women's studies at the American University in Cairo.

ANGELA Y. DAVIS is a radical black activist, feminist, organizer, and author. Her advocacy on behalf of political prisoners led to three capital charges, sixteen months in jail awaiting trial, and a highly publicized campaign, then acquittal, in 1972. During this period, an international Free Angela Davis movement grew, and Davis used the momentum to found the National Alliance Against Racist and Political Repression, an organization that remains active today. Davis has taught in all fifty states, as well as throughout Europe, Africa, the Caribbean, Russia, and the Pacific. Through her teaching and writing she remains a powerful role model and inspiration for social movements, as well as a prominent figure in the struggle against the death penalty in California.

ANSELMA DELL'OLIO is a writer, lecturer, founder and director of the New Feminist Theater, and associate producer of *Woman* on WCBS-TV in New York. She currently lives and works as a journalist in Italy.

JOAN DITZION is a founder of the Boston Women's Health Book Collective and a coauthor of all editions of *Our Bodies, Ourselves* and *Ourselves and Our Children*. She also contributed to *Ourselves, Growing Older*.

BETTY DODSON, PHD, artist, author, and sex educator, is an international authority on women's sexuality. In 1974, Betty Dodson wrote, illustrated, and self-published her first book, *Liberating Masturbation: a Meditation on Selflove*, which by the eighties had become a feminist classic. Her bold, innovative teaching methods have been documented in a series of videos. Her latest book, *Orgasms for Two*, was published in 2002. Dodson has a private practice in New York City.

CAROL DOWNER has become a legendary figure in the women's health movement. In the early seventies she pioneered the concept of vaginal and cervical self-examination as a key to self-empowerment. A lawyer, she is the founding executive director of the Federation of Feminist Women's Health Centers. She has served on the Board of Directors for the National Abortion Federation.

MARTA DRURY is a donor-activist with a focus on women and children of color. Her activism led her to a nomination for the Nobel Peace Prize as part of the project entitled, "1,000 Women," an effort to recognize the efforts of 1,000 women all over the world working for peace and equality.

ANDREA EAGAN was the author of the first feminist advice book for girls, *Why Am I So Miserable If These Are The Best Years Of My Life?*, and the author of *The Newborn Mother: Stages of Her Growth*. She was the editor of the National Women's Health Network series for Pantheon Books and president of HealthRights, a nonprofit organization. She was the founding president of the National Writer Union and a founding board member of the Writers Room in New York City. She died in 1993.

BARBARA EHRENREICH is the author of fourteen books, including *Nickel and Dimed: On (Not) Getting By in America* and *Bait and Switch*. Most recently she published *Dancing in the Streets: A History of Collective Joy*. Ehrenreich has contributed to *Harper's* and the *Nation* and was a columnist for the *New York Times* and *Time Magazine*.

MARVIN S. EIGER, MD is a nationally known pediatrician who practiced in New York City for thirty years. Educated at Harvard University, Dr. Eiger received medical training at New York University School of Medicine and served his residency in pediatrics at Bellevue Hospital. Dr. Eiger is the father of two children and lives in Manhattan with his wife, Carol.

ARLENE EISENBERG was the author of several best-selling books, including *What to Expect When You're Expecting*, *What to Eat When You're Expecting*, *What to Expect the First Year*, and *What to Expect the Toddler Years*. Updated every six weeks, the "expect" books are in their seventy-fifth printing. Together they have sold nearly 17 million copies and have been translated into twenty-one different languages. Arlene Eisenberg died in 2001.

VICTORIA ENG lives and works in New York City. She earned an MFA in creative nonfiction from Columbia University.

DEIRDRE ENGLISH is the coauthor (with Barbara Ehrenreich) of the classic feminist work *Witches, Midwives and Nurses: A History of Women Healers*. She is a former editor in chief of *Mother Jones* and has been a public affairs commentator for San Francisco Public Radio.

SAMUEL S. EPSTEIN, M.D. is professor emeritus of Environmental and Occupational Medicine at the University of Illinois School of Public Health, and Chairman of the Cancer Prevention Coalition. He has published some 260 peer reviewed articles, and authored or co-authored 11 books including: the prize-winning *The Politics of Cancer* (1978); *The Safe Shopper's Bible* (1995); and *GOT (Genetically Engineered) MILK! The Monsanto rBGH/BST Milk Wars Handbook* (2001).

BARBARA FINDLEN was an editor-at-large for *Ms.*, and is the editor of the anthology *Listen Up: Voices From the Next Feminist Generation*, and coauthor, with Kristen Golden, of *Remarkable Women of the Twentieth Century: 100 Portraits of Achievement*.

PHYLLIS L. FINE is a psychotherapist in private practice and the co-founder of Midwest Support, an organization formed specifically to work with victims of professional abuse. She is also a founder of Families Against Sexually Abusive Therapists and Other Professionals (FAST).

SHULAMITH FIRESTONE was a founder of the Women's Liberation Movement in the late sixties and author of the classic *The Dialectic of Sex: The Case for Feminist Revolution*. More recently she has been writing fiction, notably *Airless Spaces*.

AUDREY FLACK is one of the world's leading photorealist painters. Her work is in museums around the globe. In recent decades she has turned to sculpture, where, in particular, she has been "searching for the Goddess." Flack has been called the feminist conscience of the College Art Association.

ANNE ROCHON FORD has worked in Canada as a writer and activist on women's health issues for the past twenty-four years. She co-founded several national, provincial, and local women's health groups, including the Canadian Women's Health Network and DES Action Toronto. A particular focus of her work has remained the issue of women and pharmaceuticals.

JANE P. FOWLER was diagnosed with HIV at the age of fifty-five. Recognizing a need for awareness and support for older women affected by HIV, Jane formed HIV Wisdom for Older Women in 2002. She has spoken hundreds of times since 1995 and has been a guest on *Oprah* and a contributor to *Our Bodies, Ourselves: Menopause*.

ELLEN FRANKFORT was the health columnist for the *Village Voice* and the author of several books. She was one of the key journalists who popularized the women's health movement. In the early 1970s, she served as a trustee at the Women's Medical Center on Irving Place in New York City, the first freestanding legal abortion clinic in the Western world. She died in 1987.

LUCINDA FRANKS is a winner of the Pulitzer Prize for National Reporting (1972) and many other awards. She has written for the *New York Times*, the *New Yorker*, and *Talk* magazine. Franks is the author of *My Father's Secret War, Waiting Out a War*, and *Wild Apples*.

SARA GERMAIN has a Bachelor of Arts degree in English and women's studies from the State University of New York College at Geneseo. She is one of many young women who have been mentored and influenced by Barbara Seaman, and she looks forward to many more years of study in women's health. An avid reader and writer, Germain hopes to make an influence, as her mentor did, with her pen.

JENNIFER GONNERMAN has been a staff writer for the *Village Voice* since 1997. She covers the criminal justice beat and has reported on prisons, drugs, gangs, domestic violence, and the courts. Her stories have also appeared in *Vibe, Ms., Glamour, The Source*, the *New York Observer*, and the *Nation*. She earned a 2004 National Book Award nomination for *Life on the Outside*.

LOIS GOULD has written eight novels, two works of nonfiction, two satires posing as children's fables, and a collection of personal essays. A frequent contributor of articles and reviews to the *New York Times*, she created the personal column "HERS." Her memoir about her mother, the fashion designer Jo Copeland, titled *Mommy Dressing: A Love Story*, was published in 1998. Gould died in 2002.

MADELINE GRAY published one of the first patient-to-patient menopause manuals, *The Changing Years*, in 1951. Gray was a writer and editor who lived and worked in New York for decades.

TARA GREENWAY is a mind/body practitioner with a private practice in Brooklyn Heights, New York City. Tara was trained in Theta Healing by Eric Brumett and by Vianna Stibal, the founder of the Theta technique. She is a member of MBS Connect, an organization which brings wellness speakers and practitioners into Fortune 500 companies. With collaborator/director Ariane Brandt, Tara has written and performed *Missionary Position*, a play about one woman's fight for sexual and spiritual freedom, which premiered off-Broadway at the Grove Street Playhouse in New York City after its original workshop production at the HERE Arts Center.

GERMAINE GREER is a journalist and scholar of early modern English literature, widely regarded as one of the most significant feminist voices of the later twentieth century. Greer's ideas have created controversy ever since her groundbreaking book *The Female Eunuch* became an international best seller in 1970, turning her overnight into a household name and bringing her both adulation and criticism. She is also the author of *Sex and Destiny: The Politics of Human Fertility*, *The Change: Women, Ageing and the Menopause*, and most recently *Shakespeare's Wife*.

RUTH GRUBER is an American journalist, photographer, writer, humanitarian, and a former United States government official. At age twenty, she received a PhD in one year, becoming the youngest person in the world to receive a doctorate. In 1935, the *New York Herald Tribune* asked her to write a feature series about women under Fascism and Communism. In 1944, she was assigned a secret mission to Europe to bring one thousand Jewish refugees and wounded American soldiers from Italy to the US. Gruber has received many awards for her writing and humanitarian acts, and she has published two autobiographies, *Ahead of Time: My Early Years as a Foreign Correspondent* and *Inside of Time: My Journey From Alaska to Israel*.

CATHERINE GUND is a film/videomaker, writer, teacher, and activist. Her media work—which focuses on the radical right, art and culture, HIV/AIDS, and gay and lesbian issues—has screened around the world in festivals, on public and cable television, at community-based organizations, universities, and museums. She was the founding director of BENT TV, the video workshop at the Hetrick-Martin Institute for gay, lesbian, bisexual, and transgender youth.

DORIS B. HAIRE is best known for *The Cultural Warping of Childbirth*, a well-referenced analysis of worldwide obstetric practices published by the International Childbirth Education Association in 1972, while she was the president. Haire, a consumer activist and pioneer in the area of informed consent, has also authored *The Pregnant Patient's Bill of Rights*, *How the FDA Determined the "Safety" of Drugs: Just How Safe is Safe*, and *Drugs in Labor and Birth*. She has observed obstetric care in seventy-two countries and continues to lecture worldwide.

MICHELLE HARRISON, MD, is a physician, writer, teacher, and leader in women's health. She consults and lectures internationally about women's health and other related health policy issues. Harrison is the author of *A Woman in Residence*, *The Pre-teen's First Book About Love, Sex, and AIDS*, *Self-Help for Premenstrual Syndrome*, and *A Safe Place to Live, A Story for Children Who Have Experienced Domestic Violence*.

FLORENCE HASELTINE is currently the director of the Center for Population Research. Dr. Haseltine has served as the director of the Center for Population Research since 1985. She is an obstetrician and gynecologist (OB-GYN) trained in reproductive endocrinology and genetics. Dr. Haseltine received a medical degree from the Albert Einstein College of Medicine. She did a residency at Boston Hospital for Women, and was on the faculty at the Yale University School of Medicine before assuming her current position.

MOLLY HASKELL is a film critic and has written for the *New York Times*, the *New York Times Book Review*, the *Nation*, and *Film Comment*, among other publications. She lectures on film at numerous universities and is a member of the New York Film Critics Circle and the National Society of Film Critics.

JUDITH LEWIS HERMAN, MD, is associate clinical professor of psychiatry at the Harvard Medical School and director of training at the Victims of Violence Program at Cambridge Hospital. She is the author of several books including *Trauma of Recovery* and *Father-Daughter Incest*.

SHERE HITE's groundbreaking Hite Reports have had a profound and lasting influence on generations of readers—countless millions all over the world. The four Hite Reports have been translated into fifteen languages and published in thirty-five countries, receiving numerous academic and professional awards and honors. The initial Hite Report was named as one of the one hundred key books of the twentieth century by the *Times* in 1998. In 2006, Hite published *The Shere Hite Reader*, a collection of some of her most notable writings.

MARY HOWELL, also known as MARGARET CAMPBELL, was a co-founder of the National Women's Health Network and a contributor to the Boston Women's Health Book Collective. She had a law degree as well as a medical degree, and a PhD in child development, besides being the author of many books. In 1973 she was the first woman ever hired as a dean at Harvard Medical School.

RUTH HUBBARD is a professor of biology at Harvard University. Ruth Hubbard is best known for her challenges to colleagues who promote sociobiology and her criticisms of those who justify discrimination against women on the basis of genetics. She is the author of several books, including *Exploding the Gene Myth.*

JANE WEGSCHEIDER HYMAN, PHD, is a researcher and writer on women's health and contributed to both *Ourselves, Growing Older* and *The New Our Bodies, Ourselves.* She is author of several books, including *I Am More Than One.* During her graduate studies in psychology, she specialized in mental health problems that primarily afflicted women.

ERICA JONG is the author of eight novels, including the international best seller *Fear of Flying.* In print in twenty-seven languages, this modern classic has sold eight million copies in the US alone. Jong's latest book is *Seducing the Demon: Writing for My Life.* Jong lives in New York City and Weston, Connecticut.

SUSAN JORDAN is a former partner of Dresner, Sykes, Jordan, and Townsend, a nationally known political and commercial research consulting firm. A lifelong feminist, she worked on a successful seven-year campaign to legalize the cervical cap in the US. She cur-

rently defends all types of criminal cases in State and Federal Court. Jordan was recently honored by being sworn in as the first tribal judge for the Hopland Band of Pomo Indians. She is listed in *The Best Lawyers in America.*

SUZANNE WHITE JUNOD is a medical historian with a PhD from Emory University, and she is employed by the US Food and Drug Administration. She has a special interest in women's health issues and is currently working on a published history in the field.

PAULA KAMEN is the author of what is widely noted as the first and still the only journalistic book on young women and feminism, *Feminist Fatale: Voices from the "Twentysomething" Generation Explore the Future of the "Women's Movement."* Her writing has appeared in about a dozen anthologies, the *New York Times, Washington Post, Chicago Tribune, Salon,* and many other publications. Her new book, *All in My Head,* addresses the idea of framing chronic pain as a "woman's issue."

DR. STEPHEN KANDALL retired in 1998 as chief of neonatology at Beth Israel Medical Center in New York and professor of pediatrics at the Albert Einstein College of Medicine. During his professional career he lectured widely nationally and internationally and published more than ninety articles and book chapters. His book, *Substance and Shadow,* grew from his advocacy efforts on behalf of women prosecuted for drug use during pregnancy.

ANNE S. KASPER, PHD, is a founding member of the US women's health movement, and has been an advocate, sociologist, researcher, and public policy expert on women's health for more than twenty years. Anne was health editor for *New Directions for Women* for five years and on the editorial board of *Women and Health* and the author of its health and public policy column for five years. She has also written for a number of other women's publications. Her new book, *Breast Cancer: Society Shapes an Epidemic,* examines the transition of breast cancer from a medical to a societal issue.

TANIA KETENJIAN is a journalist, documentarian, and sound artist. She has contributed nationally to PRI's *Studio 360,* APM's *Weekend America,* NPR's *Day to Day* and PRI's and BBC's *The World.* She has contributed internationally to the BBC and the BBC World Service in England, CBC in Canada, ABC in Australia, and RTE in Ireland. Tania hosts and produces a half-hour weekly program on the arts called *Sight Unseen* which airs in the San Francisco Bay Area and London. She has spoken with artists and thinkers as wide ranging as John Waters, Charlie Kaufman, and His Holiness the Dalai Lama. She has produced several long format audio documentaries including *The Pursuit of Happiness*, *Birth*, and *Born*. She has written for *Paper Magazine*, *Dazed and Confused*, *The Times* (UK) and *Icon Magazine*. Tania is a member of an artist's collective, Quorum, where she contributes sound pieces for exhibitions, and she shares a studio space with artists collectively called Compound 21. Tania lives in San Francisco with her husband, Philip Wood, with whom she co-founded *The [Un]Observed: A Radio Magazine*.

FRANCINE KLAGSBURN is the author of more than a dozen books and often writes and lectures on feminist issues. Her most recent book, *The Fourth Commandment: Remember the Sabbath Day,* was a National Jewish Book Award Finalist. Her column, "Thinking Aloud," appears monthly in the *Jewish Week*.

ROSE KUSHNER was a pioneer in the field of breast cancer activism. She first gained national recognition in 1975, when she wrote about her battle with breast cancer in the book *Why Me? What Every Woman Should Know About Breast Cancer to Save Her Life*. She was the founder and director of the Breast Cancer Advisory Center in Kensington, a member of the National Breast Cancer Advisory Board from 1980 to 1986, and was appointed to the American Cancer Society's Breast Cancer Task Force. At the time of her death in 1990, Kushner was lobbying to encourage the Federal Government to require that health insurance companies cover mammograms.

VIVIEN LABATON was the founding director of the Third Wave Foundation. She is curently a fellow at Atlantic Philanthropies. A graduate of Barnard College, Labaton earned her JD at NYU Law School. She is the coeditor, with Dawn Lundy Martin (a Third Wave co-founder), of *The Fire This Time*, a collection of essays by young activists on the future of feminism.

SONIA LANDER is a midwife and nurse living in New York City. She graduated from Barnard College and earned an MS in nursing from Yale.

BERNARD LEFKOWITZ is the author of *Our Guys: The Glen Ridge Rape and the Secret Life of the Perfect Suburb*. He has written three previous books on social issues. He died in 2004.

BARRON H. LERNER, MD, PHD, is a medical historian and internist at the College of Physicians and Surgeons of Columbia University. Dr. Lerner, who is the Angelica Berrie Gold Foundation assistant professor of medicine and public health, is the author of *Contagion and Confinement: Controlling Tuberculosis Along the Skid Road* and *The Breast Cancer Wars: Hope, Fear, and the Pursuit of a Cure in Twentieth Century America*.

NICOLE LEVITZ is a recent graduate of Boston University, where she co-founded the Coalition for Consensual Sex, a student group which brought sexual assault survivor services to the Boston University campus. She is currently the program associate for the Lawyers Alliance for New York and has worked at the Center for Reproductive Rights and the Boston Area Rape Crisis Center.

CHARLOTTE LIBOV is an award-winning author and professional speaker specializing in women's health issues. She is the author of *Beat Your Risk Factors: A Woman's Guide to Reducing Her Risk for Cancer, Heart Disease, Stroke, Diabetes and Osteoporosis* and *The Woman's Heart Book*, and lives in Bethlehem, Connecticut.

BETTY JEAN LIFTON, PHD, is an author and psychologist, and has an adoption counseling practice in New York City. Her adoption books include: *Twice Born: Memoirs of An Adopted Daughter; Lost and Found: The Adoption Experience; Journey of the Adopted Self: A Quest For Wholeness;* and the picture book *Tell Me A Real Adoption Story*.

MEIKA LOE is an assistant professor of sociology and anthropology and women's studies at Colgate University. She is the author of *The Rise of Viagra: How the Little Blue Pill Changed Sex in America*.

BARBARA LOVE is an editor, writer, and journalist. She is the author of *Foremost Women in Communications* and the co-author of *Sappho Was a Right-On*

Woman (with Sidney Abbott). She is on the board of the Veteran Feminists of America and co-authored the book *Feminists Who Changed America, 1963–1975* (with Nancy F. Cott).

SUSAN LOVE, MD, is an author, teacher, surgeon, lecturer, researcher, and activist. *Dr. Susan Love's Breast Book* has been termed the bible for women with breast cancer; released in 1997, *Dr. Susan Love's Hormone Book* (updated and re-published in 2003 as *Dr. Susan Love's Menopause and Hormone Book)* provides an equally authoritative range of information about menopause.

MICHAEL LOWENTHAL is the author of the novels *Charity Girl, Avoidance* and *The Same Embrace*. His short stories have appeared in *Tin House*, the *Southern Review*, the *Kenyon Review*, and *Esquire.com*. He has also written nonfiction for the *New York Times Magazine, Boston Magazine*, the *Washington Post*, the *Boston Globe, Out*, and many other publications. Lowenthal teaches creative writing in the low-residency MFA program at Lesley University.

HELEN LOWERY is a twenty-four-year-old law student at the American University Washington College of Law in Washington, DC. She is interested in women's advocacy and has worked on issues of women's health, sexual assault, and reproductive justice. In her free time, Lowery is a baking enthusiast and likes to dance. She expects to receive her JD in May 2009.

KIRSTEN LUKER, PHD, is professor of sociology and a professor in the Jurisprudence and Social Policy Program (Boalt Hall School of Law) at the University of California, Berkeley. She is the author of many scholarly articles, as well as three books: *Taking Chances: Abortion and the Decision Not to Contracept, Abortion and the Politics of Motherhood*, and *Dubious Conceptions: The Politics of Teenage Pregnancy*. She is currently at work on her fourth book, tentatively entitled *Bodies and Politics*.

HARRIET LYONS was an original editor of *Ms*. She was a recipient of the Women in Communications' Clarion Award for "The Decade of Women: A *Ms*. History of the '70s in Words & Pictures." As a *McCall's* and *Redbook* senior editor from 1993 to 1997, she edited cover profiles, articles concerning social issues, and

human interest stories. She is currently Special Sections editor at the *Daily News*.

CAROLYN MACKLER is a young adult novelist living and working in New York City. Her books include: *The Earth, My Butt, and Other Big Round Things, Vegan Virgin Valentine, Love and Other Four Letter Words*, and *Guyaholic*. Mackler was a contributing editor at *Ms*., and her articles and essays have also appeared in publications including the *Los Angeles Times, HUES*, and *New Moon*.

ARTEMIS MARCH, PHD, has been evolving her own brand of narrative nonfiction for twenty years without realizing it was preparing her to write *Dying Into Grace*, a book about caregiving relationships and her mother's death. A sociologist by training, she first got into the storytelling business at the Harvard Business School where she designed dozens of teaching case studies, many of them bestsellers, for students and executives. Her consulting practice focuses on patient-centered care at every stage of life.

MARJORIE MARGOLIES served one term as a Democratic member of the US House of Representatives from Pennsylvania. She graduated from the University of Pennsylvania in 1963 and was in broadcast journalism for over twenty-four years, winning five Emmy Awards for her work. She currently serves as the founder and chair of Women's Campaign International (WCI), a group that provides advocacy training for women throughout the world. She is also a professor at the Fels Institute of Government at the University of Pennsylvania.

HELEN I. MARIESKIND has been active in women's health issues since the early 1970s. She is author of the landmark *Evaluation of Caesarean Section in the United States, Women in the Health System: Patients, Providers and Programs*, and the founder and editor for six years of *Women & Health*. She lives in Washington, DC and works as a writer and editor for the Office of Juvenile Justice and Delinquency Prevention, Office of Justice Programs, US Department of Justice.

NORMA FOX MAZER is the author of over thirty novels for children and young adults, plus two collections of short stories. She has edited an anthology of women's poetry and contributed articles, essays, and short stories to numerous journals and anthologies. Among her awards are a Newbery Honor, the California Young Readers Medal, a Christopher Medal, and an Edgar.

NORMA MCCORVEY has worked as a crisis counselor in a Dallas women's clinic. She is a frequent speaker on abortion rights and women's issues. She lives in Dallas, Texas.

JEAN BAKER MILLER is a clinical professor of psychiatry at Boston University School of Medicine and director of the Jean Baker Miller Training Institute at the Stone Center, Wellesley College. She has written *Toward a New Psychology of Women*; coauthored *The Healing Connection: How Women Form Relationships in Therapy and in Life; Women's Growth in Connection;* and edited *Psychoanalysis and Women*.

MARCIA MILLMAN is a professor of sociology at the University of California, Santa Cruz and a social psychologist. She is the author of several books including *Such a Pretty Face: On Being Fat in America, Kind Hearts and Cold Cash, The Unkindest Cut: Life in the Backrooms of Medicine*, and *The Perfect Sister: What Draws Us Together, What Drives Us Apart*. She lives in the San Francisco Bay area.

PATSY T. MINK was a third generation Japanese-American graduate of University of Chicago Law School (1951). Her lawsuit, *Mink vs. EPA et al.,* established the core principles of the Freedom of Information Act. An environmentalist, advocate of consumer rights, individual rights, and civil rights, Mink made her mark first as an opponent of the Vietnam War. She died in 2002.

THE NATIONAL WOMEN'S HEALTH NETWORK is an independent, member-supported organization dedicated to safeguarding women's health rights and interests by providing accurate, unbiased health information to women and advocating for national health policies that address women's health needs. The director of the Network is Cynthia Pearson, and the founders are Barbara Seaman, Belita Cowan, Phylis Chesler, Mary Howell, and Alice Wolfson.

MARYANN NAPOLI is a co-founder and the associate director of the Center for Medical Consumers in New York City. She writes *Health Facts,* the Center's monthly newsletter.

HEDDA NUSSBAUM was abruptly thrown into the public spotlight in November 1987 after her long-time partner, Joel Steinberg, assaulted and killed their daughter, Lisa. She went on to become an advocate for other battered women. A former senior editor at Random House and the author of children's books, Ms. Nussbaum has written a memoir about her experiences, *Surviving Intimate Terrorism*, which was published in the fall of 2005.

SALLY WENDKOS OLDS has written extensively about relationships, health, and personal growth, and has won national awards for both her book and magazine writing. Her college textbooks on child and adult development, *A Child's World* and *Human Development*, coauthored with psychologist Diane E. Papalia, PhD, have been read by more than two million students and are the leading texts in their fields.

SUSIE ORBACH has written extensively about women's psychology and the construction of femininity, gender, the making of the body, psychoanalysis and social policy, eating difficulties, obesity to anorexia, women and brands, globalism and body image, and emotional literacy in business, education, and government. She has been consultant to The World Bank and is currently consultant to the National Health Service (NHS) and to Dove®. She is the author of several books, including *Fat is a Feminist Issue.*

LESYLE E. ORLOFF founded Ayuda's unique domestic violence program, dedicated to serving the interrelated legal and social service needs of battered latina and immigrant women and children. Ms. Orloff was a cofounder of the National Network on Behalf of Battered Immigrant Women and is the Washington, DC spokesperson for that organization. In 1999, Ms. Orloff joined NOW Legal Defense and Education Fund's Washington, DC office as the director of the Immigrant Women Program and senior staff attorney.

AMY PAGNOZZI writes for *New York, Vanity Fair, Glamour,* and *Penthouse.*

CINDY PEARSON is executive director of the National Women's Health Network. She has worked at NWHN since 1987 and has coordinated the internship program, managed the information clearinghouse, and directed NWHN's program and policy work. Cindy became NWHN's executive director in May 1996.

She is currently the president of the board of directors of Women's Health Specialists in Northern California and is the treasurer of the National Breast Cancer Coalition.

JOANNA PERLMAN is a marketing and public relations specialist at the law firm Skadden, Arps, Slate, Meagher and Flom. She is a former press secretary for the New York City Department of Finance. She is a graduate of Barnard College and has also worked for NOW and the television station New York One.

REBECCA PLANTE is an assistant professor of sociology at Ithaca College. She is the author of *Sexualities, Identities, Behaviors and Societies* and *Sexualities in Context: A Social Perspective*. She has also worked as an evaluator of various state level HIV/AIDS education programs.

LETTY COTTIN POGREBIN is a writer and lecturer. Among her books are *Growing Up Free, Stories for Free Children*, and *Getting Over Getting Older: An Intimate Journey*. She was a founding editor of *Ms.*, and a former president of the Author's Guild. Most recently she has written her first novel, titled *Three Daughters*.

LAUREN PORSCH is the founder of the New York Abortion Access Fund, a nonprofit organization that provides financial assistance to low-income women who cannot afford the cost of an abortion, as well as being actively involved in health promotion and access to care campaigns for Lesbian, Gay, Bisexual, and Transgender communities.

AMY RICHARDS is a writer, researcher, organizer, and fundraising consultant. A co-founder and executive committee member of the Third Wave Foundation, Richards was profiled by *Ms.* in 1997 in "21 for the 21st: Leaders for the Next Century." She is the coauthor of *Manifesta: Young Women, Feminism and the Future* and *Grassroots: A Field Guide for Feminist Activism*. Richards's most recent book is *Opting In: Having a Child Without Losing Yourself*.

HELEN RODRIGUEZ-TRIAS was a founding member of both the Committee to End Sterilization Abuse and the Committee for Abortion Rights and Against Sterilization Abuse. In the 1980s she served as medical director of the New York State Department of Health AIDS Institute, where she worked on behalf of women

with HIV. In the 1990s, she focused on reproductive health as co-director of the Pacific Institute for Women's Health, a nonprofit research and advocacy group dedicated to improving women's well being worldwide.

ESTHER (SIEDMAN) ROME was a founding member of the Boston Women's Health Book Collective and coauthor of its best-selling book *Our Bodies, Ourselves*. For most of the 1980s she served as a consumer representative to a task force of the American Society for Testing Materials, which after many years of meetings, and due largely to Esther's persistence, finally enacted a uniform standard for tampon labeling. When confronted with breast cancer, Esther persistently and energetically researched treatment options and shared what she had learned with all who were interested.

JUDITH ROSSNER is the author of such best-selling novels as *Looking for Mr. Goodbar, August*, and *Emmeline*, on which the opera by Tobias Picker is based. She died in August 2005.

BETTY ROTHBART, MSW, is a health columnist for *Hadassah* magazine and the author of a number of books on health and parenting. She is the author of four curricula on HIV/AIDS and abuse prevention for the New York City Board of Education, where she conducts teacher trainings on health and sexuality education. She coauthored her most recent book, *Healthy Teens, Body and Soul: A Parent's Complete Guide*, with Andrea Marks.

BARBARA KATZ ROTHMAN is a professor of sociology at the City University of New York. She has served as president of Sociologists for the Study of Social Problems and Sociologists for Women in Society. Her books include *Weaving a Family: Untangling Race and Adoption, The Book of Life, Recreating Motherhood, The Tentative Pregnancy*, and *In Labor*. She lives in Brooklyn, New York.

SHERYL BURT RUZEK, PHD, is professor of health studies at Temple University. She is currently working on a second edition of her 1978 book, *The Women's Health Movement, Feminist Alternatives to Medicine Control* and is a consultant to numerous public health organizations. Her recent publications include *Women's Health: Complexities and Differences* (with

Virginia Olesen and Adele Clarke) and articles on the future of health reform.

GILLIAN SANSON is a women's health educator, researcher, and author. Her book *Mid-Life Energy and Happiness* was published in 1999, followed by *The Osteoporosis 'Epidemic': Well Women and the Marketing of Fear*. Her work has received international recognition and endorsement and was the subject of a *20/20* documentary in New Zealand in 2001. Gill lives in Auckland, New Zealand.

MEI HWEI ASTELLA SAW graduated from Northwestern University and worked as an associate editor at Seven Stories Press. A daughter of two fine doctors, she doesn't think members of the medical profession are gods.

HAGAR SCHER is a journalist and writer living in New York City. Her articles about politics, feminism, sex, women's health, fitness, sports, and first-person experiences have appeared in *Ms., Glamour, New Woman, Fitness, Ladies' Home Journal,* and *Latina* magazines. A woman of the world, Hagar was raised in Israel and Canada, and has resided in Italy and England.

LYNNE SHARON SCHWARTZ has written many books since the start of her career in the 1970s, including *Rough Strife* (nominated for a National Book Award), a collection of stories called *Referred Pain*, the novel *The Writing on the Wall*, and *The Emergence of Memory: Conversations with W.B. Sebald*, a book of interviews with the late German author. Lynne Sharon Schwartz's reviews and criticism have appeared in many leading magazines and papers. She has received grants from the Guggenheim Foundation, the National Endowment for the Arts, and the New York State Foundation for the Arts, and has taught in many writing programs here and abroad.

JULIA R. SCOTT is president of the National Black Woman's Health Project, and has a long history as a leader and activist in preventive health and in the struggle for the advancement of people of color. She has held a variety of other posts, including director of training for the Boston Family Planning Project, and reproductive rights field coordinator and executive director of the Foundation of Women. She has received the Gloria Steinem Women of Vision award.

SYBIL SHAINWALD'S legal career has focused almost exclusively on women's health issues. She was co-counsel in the nation's first DES daughter victory, *Bichler v. Lilly*, and she litigated thousands of cases involving drugs and devices harmful to women and their children. She co-founded Health Action International and is deeply involved with the National Women's Health Network. Shainwald was one of the first and most vocal opponents of the use of Norplant, especially its widespread use in developing nations. Her writings, lectures, and appearances before congressional subcommittees have raised the national consciousness on crucial women's health issues.

CASSANDRA SHAYLOR is an attorney and activist based in Oakland, California. She is the co-founder and co-director of Justice Now, a prison organization and training center focused on people in women's prisons in the United States. Shaylor speaks regularly to academic and activist audiences on issues of women in prison, prison abolition, and the intersections of race and sexuality in the prison-industrial complex.

SARAH J. SHEY received her MFA in nonfiction writing from Columbia University in October 1999. She has been published in such publications as the *Christian Science Monitor*, the *Philadelphia Inquirer*, and *This Old House Magazine*. She is the author of the children's books *Blue Lake Days* and *Sky All Around*.

ALIX KATES SHULMAN's twelve books include two books on the anarchist Emma Goldman, three books for children, four novels, and three memoirs (the award winning *Drinking the Rain* and *A Good Enough Daughter*). Hailed by the *New York Times* as "the voice that has for three decades provided a lyrical narrative of the changing position of women in American society," her works have been translated into eleven languages. Her most recent memoir, *To Love What Is*, will be published in September of 2008.

KATIE SINGER is certified to teach Fertility Awareness by the Ovulation Method Teachers' Association. She teaches at Women's Health Services in Santa Fe, New Mexico. Her first novel, *The Wholeness of a Broken Heart*, has recently been published by Riverhead Books. Her other writings include *The Garden of Fertility, Honoring Our Cycles: A Natural Family Planning Workbook*, and articles about Fertility Awareness.

Katie is currently working on a new novel and essays about fertility and ecology.

MARGOT SLADE is deputy editor, special sections, of the *New York Times* and the mother of twins, Emma and Jacob.

ELIZABETH CADY STANTON, the boldest and most brilliant of the nineteenth-century American feminists, was born in 1815 in upstate New York. For more than fifty years, there seemed to be no impediment to women's full equality that Elizabeth did not notice and attempt to route: besides suffrage, she campaigned for birth control, property rights for wives, custody rights for mothers, equal wages, cooperative nurseries, coeducation, and "deliverance from the tyranny of self-styled medical, religious, and legal authorities." Through it all Elizabeth was a doting, hands-on mother of five sons and two daughters.

EDITH STEIN was a German philosopher, a Carmelite nun, martyr, and saint of the Catholic Church who died at Auschwitz. In 1922, she converted to Christianity, was baptized into the Roman Catholic Church, and was received into the Discalced Carmelite Order in 1934. She was canonized as Saint Teresa Benedicta of the Cross (her Carmelite monastic name) by Pope John Paul II in 1998.

GLORIA STEINEM is one of the most influential writers, editors, and activists of our time. She travels worldwide as a lecturer and feminist organizer, and is a frequent media spokeswoman on issues of equality. In the words of her biographer, Carolyn Heilbrun, "She is most honored and most cherished by people throughout the country who remember her speaking, her helping to start their rape crisis center, her timely support for their various burgeoning organizations." Gloria co-founded *Ms.* in 1971 and was one of its editors for fifteen years. She continues to write and lecture on various political and feminist issues.

KOFI TAHA is a writer, activist, entrepreneur, and renowned philanthropist. His poems, essays, and articles have been published in various forms, ranging from academic journals to newspapers to hip-hop tabloids. He is the author of a book of poetry entitled *Postdiluvian America: Drought of Humility*.

LEORA TANENBAUM is the author of *Slut! Growing Up Female with a Bad Reputation*. Her writing has appeared in *Newsday, Seventeen, Ms.*, and other newspapers and magazines. She lives in New York City. Her most recent books are *Catfight: Rivalries Among Women—from Diets to Dating, from the Boardroom to the Delivery Room* and *Bad Shoes & the Women Who Love Them*.

NOY THRUPKAEW is a senior correspondent for the *American Prospect*. Previously she was the news editor of *Sojourner: The Women's Forum*, a national feminist newspaper based in Boston. She has lived in Japan and Thailand, and frequently writes on international women's human rights, welfare policy, and Southeast and East Asian literature and film.

LEONORE TIEFER, PHD, is an author, educator, researcher, therapist, and activist who has specialized in many areas of sexuality. Dr. Tiefer has written widely about the medicalization of men's and women's sexuality. She has been interviewed by news media around the world and appeared on many news shows as the foremost critic of "disease-mongering" trends in the medical management of women's sexual problems. The website of her educational anti-medicalization campaign, newviewcampaign.org, is a major resource on this topic for journalists, colleagues, and the public. Dr. Tiefer has written over 150 scientific and professional publications.

ANDREA TONE is a professor of history at McGill University. She is the author of several books and edited volumes, including *Devices and Desires: A History of Contraceptives in America*, which was named one of the best books of the year by the *Washington Post* and, most recently, *Medicating Modern America: Prescription Drugs in History*, with Elizabeth Siegel Watkins. Her work has been featured on ABC News, PBS, National Public Radio, the Canadian Broadcasting Corporation (CBC), the History Channel, and in the *New York Times.*

SOJOURNER TRUTH was born into slavery in New York State. She won her freedom in 1827, when that state emancipated its slaves. Sojourner Truth consistently and actively identified herself with the cause of women's rights. She was the only black woman present at the First National Woman's Rights Convention in Worcester, Massachusetts, in 1850.

SARI TUDIVER, PHD, is the resource coordinator at the Women's Health Clinic, a community health center in Winnipeg, Manitoba and an editor of *A Friend Indeed*, an international newsletter for women on menopause and midlife. An anthropologist by training, she has been involved in research, writing, education, and advocacy on many aspects of women's health, including reproductive technologies and the international pharmaceutical industry. She is a founding member of the Canadian Women's Health Network.

LILA A. WALLIS, MD, is clinical professor of medicine at Cornell University Medical College and an attending physician at the New York Hospital in New York City. Dr. Wallis is an internationally recognized expert on estrogen replacement therapy, menopause, and osteoporosis. She is also celebrated for her contributions to women's health and medical education through her organizational activities, lectures, and publications. Dr. Wallis is senior author of *The Whole Woman— Take Charge of Your Health in Every Phase of Your Life*, published in May 1999.

ELIZABETH SIEGAL WATKINS has a PhD in the history of science from Harvard University, from which her book *On the Pill* is derived. She is a historian with the Historical Society of Western Pennsylvania in Pittsburgh, and writes, teaches, and consults in Pennsylvania. Her most recent books are *The Estrogen Elixir: A History of Hormone Replacement Therapy in America* and *Medicating Modern America: Prescription Drugs in History* with Andrea Tone. Both were published in 2007.

ERICA WARREN is a freelance writer living in Brooklyn, New York.

KATHRYN WATTERSON, who teaches writing at the University of Pennsylvania, has written several prize-winning nonfiction books, including, most recently, *Not by the Sword*, which won the 1996 Christopher Award. Her first book, *Women in Prison*, is considered a classic on the subject and was the basis for the ABC documentary *Women In Prison*.

MARILYN WEBB is one of the early founders of the Second Wave of the women's movement. An organizer, speaker, and writer, she also began *Off Our Backs*, one of the first feminist newspapers, the nation's

first college-based women's studies program, and Sagaris, a feminist think-tank. Most recently she has become a leader of a new movement to improve the care of the dying. She is the author of the influential book, *The Good Death: The New American Search to Reshape the End of Life*.

ELAINE WEISS has conducted dozens of domestic violence training sessions around the country. Her writings about domestic abuse have appeared in local and national publications and are used as teaching resources in a number of battered women's shelters. Dr. Weiss is an adjunct professor at the University of Utah School of Medicine, in the Department of Family and Preventive Medicine. There, she teaches medical students and faculty how to recognize and support patients who are victims of domestic violence.

Author and neuroscientist NAOMI WEISSTEIN, known for her powerful oratory, is a Professor of Psychology at SUNY, Buffalo. A Guggenheim Fellow and a Fellow of the American Association for the Advancement of Science and the American Psychological Society, she has written over sixty articles on science, feminism, culture, and politics, including her famous "Kinder, Kirche, Kuche," credited for starting the discipline of the psychology of women.

EDITH WHITE, the author of *Breastfeeding and HIV/AIDS: The Research, the Politics, the Women's Responses*, spent more than twenty-five years teaching breast-feeding management to health professionals, and was one of the founders of the International Board of Lactation Consultants. She is now executive director of the South Shore AIDS Project, Inc. in Plymouth, Massachusetts.

FRANCES CERRA WHITTELSEY is an award-winning journalist, magazine editor, and author who teaches journalism part-time at Hofstra University.

NAOMI WOLF was born in San Francisco in 1962. Her essays have appeared in various publications including: *The New Republic, Wall Street Journal, Glamour, Ms., Esquire*, the *Washington Post*, and the *New York Times*. Her books include *The Beauty Myth, Fire With Fire: The New Female Power And How It Will Change The 21st Century, Promiscuities: The Secret Struggle for Womanhood*, and *Misconceptions*, a book on the politics of motherhood in America. Wolf's most recent book is *The End Of America: A Letter of Warning to a Young Patriot.*

ALICE WOLFSON is an attorney specializing in defending the rights of insurance policy holders for the firm Bourhis, Wolfson, and Schlichtmann in San Francisco, California. She is one of the founders of the National Women's Health Network.

SUSAN WOOD is a research professor in the Department of Environmental and Occupational Health at George Washington University. A long-time champion of women's health, Dr. Wood previously served as Director for Policy and Program Development at the US Department of Health and Human Services in the Office on Women's Health. Professor Wood has been honored with the FDA Commissioner's Special Citation (2004), the DHHS Secretary's Distinguished Service Award (2003), and the Keystone Award in Women's Health Research (2000), among other awards.

IRENE XANTHOUDAKIS works with the New York Abortion Access Fund and the Haven Coalition as well as other agencies committed to ending homelessness and providing services to formerly incarcerated individuals. Irene graduated with a Masters of Public Administration from the School of International and Public Affairs at Columbia University in February 2007.

LAURA YEAGER has published fiction in such magazines as *Paris Review, Missouri Review, North American Review, Ohio Short Fiction,* and *Kaleidoscope.* She has taught at Kent State University, Walsh University, Malone College, and Rhode Island School of Design. Laura holds a BA from Oberlin College, an MA in English from Iowa State University, and an MFA in English from the University of Iowa.

ABOUT THE EDITORS

BARBARA SEAMAN was a founding member of the women's health movement. In 1969, her landmark book on hormonal contraceptives, *The Doctors' Case Against the Pill*, sparked Congressional hearings into the safety of birth control pills and catapulted women's health issues into the national spotlight. Her work led to the creation of the world's first patient packet insert (now included in most pharmaceutical products) as well as other innovations for patient safety. In 1975 she co-founded the National Women's Health Network, an advocacy and watchdog group in Washington DC that worked to eliminate quotas for women in medical schools and give women the right to information about medical treatments and alternatives. The organization remains one of the few women's advocacy groups that refuses all money from drug and device makers. In her book, *The Greatest Experiment Ever Performed on Women*, she demonstrated the failure of the FDA and the medical establishment to demand rigorous testing of hormone therapy before mass prescribing took place and castigated the pharmaceutical industry for putting profits above women's lives. Since 2003 she has written passionately on the dangers of fertility drugs and unnecessary gynecological procedures. She is the author of seven books on women's health. She died in February 2008 at the age of seventy-two.

LAURA ELDRIDGE is Barbara Seaman's longtime collaborator and associate. She has been researching and writing about women's health topics for nearly ten years. She contributed to Seaman's *The Greatest Experiment Ever Performed on Women: Exploding the Estrogen Myth* and coauthored *The No-Nonsense Guide to Menopause*. She is the author of the book *In Our Control: The Complete Guide to Contraceptive Choices for Women*. Eldridge has degrees from Barnard College and New York University and lives and writes in Brooklyn, New York.

Index

abortions, 29. *See also*
menstrual extraction
clinics, 49, 57
illegal, 49
laws, 49
legal, 335–36
as longstanding practice,
334
with rape, 48
rights, 334–35
self-, 48, 51, 54, 307
women's death rate, 54
Abrams, Elliott, 217
abuse. *See also specific forms of
abuse*
Amytal, 74, 79, 80–81, 83
child, 82, 89–90, 134–39,
155–56
lineal victims of, 83–84
of mental patients, 77, 78–
83
physical, 134
sexual, 90, 134
with sterilization, 333–34
with trauma and recovery,
130–39
ACE. *See* AIDS Counseling and
Education Program
acquaintance rape, 88–89, 119
activists
becoming, 34–36
legacy of, 37–38, 234
New View as outlet for older
and younger, 6
activities
approved female, 70–71
dominants with domain of
valued, 75
excessive athletic, 163–64
addiction
alcohol, 106–13
tranquilizers, 100–104

women and drug, 100–113
Adkins, Janet, 277
Adler, Margot, 256–57
adolescent, clitoral orgasm as,
10, 23
advertisements
prescription drugs, 271–72
vibrators, 7, 8
advocacy, 77–78, 142
domestic violence victims,
143–44
for end of life issues, 281–84
Africa, 55. *See also specific
countries in Africa*
age
female sexuality and, 26–27
with makeup, 183–85
rapists and average, 119
sunscreen and, 181
ageism, HIV/AIDS and, 219
aggression, indirect, 90–92
"Aging" (Jong), 179–80
AIDS Counseling and
Education (ACE) Program,
219–20
AIDS/HIV. *See* HIV/AIDS
alcoholism, 106–13
American Cancer Society, as
wealthiest nonprofit, 272–
73
American Psychiatric
Association (APA), 7, 27,
77–78. *See also Diagnostic
and Statistical Manual of
Disorders*
apology issued by, 79
Amytal
abuse, 74, 79, 80–81, 83
use during pregnancy, 82
anatomy, 30, 32. *See also*
bodies, female; bodies,
intersex; bodies, male

The Ancient Gorgon
(sculpture), 126, *128*
Angier, Natalie, 91
animal fat, 182
anorexia nervosa, 177
APA. *See* American Psychiatric
Association
Apollo and Daphne
(sculpture), *125*, 126
appearance, makeup and, 183–
85
areola, 196
Argaw, Seble W., 202–3, 204–6
art, rape depictions
The Ancient Gorgon, 126,
128
Apollo and Daphne, *125*,
126
Colossal Head of Medusa,
126, *128*
*The Expulsion of Adam and
Eve from the Garden*, 123,
124
Iris, Messenger of the Gods,
126, *127*
Leda and the Swan, *124*, 125
Luncheon on the Grass, 126,
127
in paintings and sculpture,
122–28
*Perseus with the Head of
Medusa*, 126, *127*
*Rape of the Daughters of
Leucippus*, 126
Rape of the Sabine Woman,
125, 126
The Rape of Europa, *125*,
126
Venus of Willendorf, 122,
123
Asetoyer, Charon, 344–46
Asia, MR in, 55

Asians, health issues for, 341–43
aspirin, 240, 261
assisted suicide, 277–78, 280–81, 283–84
asylums
    female experience in families akin to experiences in, 73
    lineal victims and, 83–84
    mental patients abused in, 77, 78–83
    as patriarchal institutions, 94
    pregnancy in, 74
    rape in, 73–74, 78
    as sanctuary for wealthy whites, 72
    sexism in, 72
    sexual repression in, 73
    shock therapy in, 73–74
    women's experiences in, 70–75
athletes, women. See sports, women in
athletic triad, 163–64
attitudes, of doctors toward patients, 57–58
Avery, Byllye, 294, 342

babies
    with breast milk, 196–98, 214–17
    drug, 105
    gender assigned to, 32
    HIV/AIDS deaths, 216–17
    HIV and breast milk infecting, 214–17
    intersex, 31–32
    midwives catching, 56
Badri, Rana, 202, 203–5, 206
Baker, 216
barbiturates, 81–82, 83
Barlow, J. J., 254
Barr, Pat, 229
Barrett-Connor, Elizabeth, 229
Bart, Pauline, 103, 118–22
Bashir, Layli Miller, 204
batterers, 144. See also domestic violence victims
    cycle of abuse for, 157–58
    domestic violence victims killing, 152–55
    statistics, 140–41, 152
Baumgardner, Jennifer, 296
Beach, Frank, 35–36
beauty
    cultural ideals, 176
    facial appearance and makeup, 183–85
    facial cleansing, 180–83

hair associated with, 187
learning about looks and food, 176
    in media, 85
    myth, 175
Beck, Max, 33
Becker, Julie, 312, 314
Bedford Hills Correctional Facility, 219
    ACE staff, *220*
Bégin, Monique, 233
Bellamy, Carol, 203, 205
Bergin, Eugene, 154, 155
Bergman, Ingrid, 145
Berman, Jennifer, 62
Berman, Laura, 62
Bernini, Gian Lorenzo, 125–26
Bethune, David R., 273
Bettelheim, Bruno, 66
bias, 259, 263–64
Bigelow, Billy, 145
Binder, Gordon, 273
binge eating, 177. See also eating disorders
biofeedback, 213–14
birth control pill, 22, 64. See also contraceptives
    on college campuses, 212
    DES as morning-after, 250, 255–56
    for men, 12
blacks
    hair and dreadlocks, 193–95
    negative stereotypes of, 87
    women with HIV/AIDS, 328–29
blood pressure, high, 228, 240
bodies, female
    aerobic power of, 162
    with asylum experiences, 70–75
    beauty myth and, 175
    body fat's role with, 176–77
    breasts, 195–201
    eating disorders and, 176–77
    face, 179–85
    fat as antisocial figure with, 171–75
    fat as feminist issue with, 168–71
    hair, 185–95
    image and, 167–77
    laws and, 56–57
    under male control, 39, 41
    milk production, 196–98, 214–17
    parts of, 179–206

as pathological, 2, 39
    psychology with minds and, 65–113
    self-help gynecology as liberation of, 49
    in sports, 159–65
    vagina, 201–6
bodies, intersex, 31–34
bodies, male, 2
Bodies Like Ours, 31
body fat, role of, 176–77
body hair, 186
    shaving, 185, 189–91
body parts. See breasts; face; hair; vagina
Bologna, Giovanni, 125–26
bone density, 245. See also osteoporosis
borderline personality disorder, 135–37, 138
Boston Forum
    expert-ownership at, 41–42
    FSD and, 39–40
    players, 40–41
Boston Women's Health Book Collective (BWHBC), 2
Boyer, Charles, 145
Boynton, Grace, 185
boys
    intellectual differences between girls and, 69
    sexual double standard with, 44–45
    variables of experience in, 30–34
Brady law, 164
Brahen, Leonard S., 102
bras, 197, 198–200
breast cancer, 223
    activist legacy, 234
    in Asians, 342
    control regained, 233–34
    fundraising, 232
    information and support, 233
    oral history, 224–25
    privacy with, 233
    as property, 230–31
    research, 231–32
    treatment, 231
breast-feeding
    babies infected with HIV/AIDS through, 214–17
    breast milk and, 196–98, 214–17
    UNICEF and WHO's negligence with HIV/AIDS and, 214–15

breasts
    anatomy of, 195–98
    areola and nipple, 196
    bras and, 197, 198–200
    let-down reflex and, 197–98
    milk production, 196–98, 214–17
    reduction, 201
    silicone implants, 305
    size, 196
    supporting structure, 197
Brenner, Barbara, 224
Brenner, Paul, 279
Briere, John, 134
Briquet, Paul, 137
broken genetic recipe, 31
Broverman, Inge K., 71
Brownmiller, Susan, 2, 115
    interview, 183–85, 188–89
Brundidge, Archie (brother-in-law), 155
Brundidge, Charline, 152–55
Brundidge, Marvin (husband), 152–55
Bryer, Jeffrey, 134
bulimia nervosa, 177
Burkina Faso, FC/FGM ban in, 201
Burnett, W. S., 254
Burney, Fanny, 223
Bush, George, 227
BWHBC. *See* Boston Women's Health Book Collective

Cambridge Hospital Victims of Violence (VOV) Program, 97
cancer, 256–57. *See also* breast cancer
    cervical, 299
    DES connected to, 237
    detection and treatment, 304
    reproductive system and, 336–37
    uterine, 54
captivity, trauma of, 130–32
caregivers
    dying partner's relationship to, 284–91
    gourmet dinners for, 281
    orienting, 287–88
    validating and witnessing, 288
Carmichael, Carrie, 183–85, 188–89
Carroll, Diahann, 194
Carter, Jimmy, 224
Casey, Nell, 98–100
celiac disease, 244–45

Cellini, Benvenuto, 126–27
Central African Republic, FC/FGM ban in, 201
cervical cancer, 299
cervical caps, 47–48
Chalker, Rebecca, 48, 49, 54
chamomile, 104
Charcot, Jean-Martin, 137
Charity Girl (Lowenthal), 207, 208–11
Chase, Cheryl, 30
Cheatham, Gary, 280
Chesler, Phyllis, 66, 86, 92–98
childbirth
    increase among older women, 326–27
    voluntary motherhood promoted with, 326
    women's right with, 327–28
children. *See also* babies; boys; girls
    abuse of, 82, 89–90, 134–39, 155–56
    gender assigned to, 32–34
    HIV/AIDS in breast milk infecting, 214–17
    as lineal victims of abuse, 83–84
    molestation, 82
    as survivors of trauma, 134–39
    trauma's influence on, 133
Childs, E. Kitch, 97
Chile, 51
Chodorow, Nancy, 86, 89
cholesterol, high, 240–41
Christie, Ed, 192
chronic illness, 223–24, 315. *See also* breast cancer; heart disease; osteoporosis
circumcision. *See* female circumcision/female genital mutilation
classism, in asylums, 72
cleansing cream, 182
clinical trials, Gardasil, 208
clinics. *See also* Feminist Women's Health Center
    abortion, 49, 57
    self-help, 50, 52
Clinton, Bill, 42–43, 294, 297, 301, 342
Clinton, Chelsea, 43
Clinton, Hillary, 43, 188–89
clitoral orgasm, 15, 62
    as adolescent, 10, 23
    with clitoral removal, 17

Masters and Johnson on, 14, 16, 17, 18
clitoris
    hood, 16
    "normal" and medically acceptable size, 32
Coalition for Consensual Sex, 129
college campuses
    birth control pills on, 212
    DES on, 255
    rape on, 115–16
    sexual violence prevention on, 128–29
    STDs on, 211–12
Colossal Head of Medusa (sculpture), 126, *128*
community empowerment, 341
competitiveness
    indirect aggression and, 90–92
    resentment with, 88–89
    with women, 85–92
    women's essential natures and, 89–90
complex post-traumatic stress disorder (PTSD), 133–34, 139
conflict, dominants avoiding, 76
conflict of interest
    dirty money and, 267–68
    pharmaceutical companies with informed consent and, 247–74
    prescriptions and, 265–70
Congress, U.S., 164, 254–55
consciousness, PTSD and, 139
contraceptives, 22. *See also* *specific types of contraceptives*
    birth control pills, 12, 22, 64, 212, 250
    DES as morning-after, 250, 255–56
    in developing countries, 54
    disease prevention and, 328–31
Cooperstock, Ruth, 103
Corea, Gena, 309
Corfman, Philip, 251, 318
cosmetics. *See also* facial cleansing; makeup
    labels, 181
Costich, Jim, 33–34
countries. *See* developing countries; *specific countries*
Cowan, Belita, 255
Cowan study, 255–56
craziness, 70–75, 95. *See also* asylums

crimes, violent, 89–90. *See also* rape
criminals, minority men deemed as, 72
culture
 beauty ideals in, 176
 death denied in, 288–90
 with expectations, 91
 FC/FGM embedded in, 206

Dalkon Shield, 305–6
Daly, Michael, 17
date rape drugs, 211
Dawidowicz, Lucy, 131
deaths
 cervical cancer, 299
 child abuse ending in, 155–56
 counteracting culture's denial of, 288–90
 DES, 249–50
 domestic violence with silence and, 144
 end of life issues and, 275–92
 heart disease, 239
 HIV/AIDS in babies, 216–17
 pain and anger with, 276–81
 in prison from HIV/AIDS, 219
 spousal abuse ending in, 152–55
 in women from abortions, 54
Defending Our Lives (documentary film), 116
Delaney, Janice, 49
Del Em (DLM), 48, 49, 307
 with menstrual extraction, 50, 52–54
Depo-Provera, 346
depression, 93, 241
 manic, 98–100
 in women and men, 66
DES. *See* diethylstilbestrol
Dessert, George, 273
destiny, anatomy as, 32
Deutsch, Helene, 117–18
developing countries. *See also* *specific developing countries*
 contraceptives in, 54
 double standard for infant feeding in, 216
 MR in, 54–55
Dewar, Elaine, 245
diagnosis
 diagnostic mislabeling with, 131–32
 doctors disguising, 257
 heart disease, 242–43
 PTSD, 133

 with survivors of childhood abuse, 134–36
 trauma, recovery and new, 130–31
Diagnostic and Statistical Manual of Disorders (DSM) (APA), 27, 28
diaphragm, 56, 64
Diaware, Demba, 203
Dieckmann, William J., 252
diethylstilbestrol (DES), 304–5
 cancer connected to, 237
 on college campuses, 255
 congressional hearings on, 254–55
 deaths, 249–50
 failure to test, 250
 in food, 250
 Greenwald report on, 253–54
 Herbst report on, 252–53
 as morning-after contraceptive, 250, 255–56
 origins of, 250–51
 pharmaceutical companies and, 250–51, 256
 as poison, 252, 255
 pregnancy and, 237, 249–53
 studies, 251–52, 255–56
 testing, 250, 252
diets, 177, 244–45. *See also* eating disorders
DiFranco, Ani, 191
dildos, 62, 63. *See also* vibrators
Diouf, Abdou, 203
dirty money, 267–68
disease, 2, 7. *See also* heart disease; sexually transmitted diseases; *specific types of disease*
 prevention with contraceptives, 328–31
 reproductive system and, 336–38
Disney, Walt, 273
DLM. *See* Del Em
doctors
 abortion and harassment of, 57
 diagnosis disguised by, 257
 domestic violence victims and role of, 140–43
 genital massage performed by, 6, 7–8, 9
 against menstrual extraction, 55–56
 midwives and, 56

 patients and attitudes of, 57–58, 65
 pelvic exams and dialogue with, 59
 psychological manipulation in, 65
 vibrators as medical instrument for, 8
Dodd, Charles (Sir), 250
Dodson, Betty, 60–64
Dohrenrend, Barbara, 72
Dohrenrend, Bruce, 72
domestic violence decision tree
 identifying victims, 142
 encourage open discussion, 142
 listening without judgment, 142
 validating experiences, 142
 documenting, 142
 assessing danger, 142–43
 treatment, referral and support, 143
 clinical findings to support abuse, 143
 specific questioning, 143
 with patient denial, 143
 judging success of intervention, 143
domestic violence intervention strategy
 identifying questions, 141
 validating experiences, 142
 advocating for safety and offering help, 142
 supporting choices, 142
domestic violence victims, 116, 139
 advocacy for, 143–44
 batterers killed by, 152–55
 doctor's role in, 140–43
 medical response measured in, 140
 neighbor's role with, 144–45
 police with, 140, 153–54
 pregnancy and, 141
 in prison, 154–55
 recognizing and treating, 142–43
 regulations and intervention strategy with, 141–42
 with silence and death, 144
 spouse abuse and, 145–47
 statistics, 140–41
 time frame with, 140–41
dominants
 conflict avoided by, 76

subordinates with, 75–76
donor insemination, 51
double-orgasm theory,
    debunked, 10–11, 67
double standard
    infant feeding in developing
        countries, 216
    of mental health, 71
    sexual, 44–45
Downer, Carol, 47–49, 54, 56, 307.
    See also self-help gynecology
dreadlocks, 193–95
Dreifus, Claudia, 309
driving drunk, 108
drugs, 94. *See also* homeopathic
    remedies; *specific types of
    drugs*
    abuse, 74, 79, 80–81
    addiction to, 100–113
    alcoholism, 106–13
    babies, 105
    date rape, 211
    habit-forming, 81–82, 83
    labels, 256
    prescription, 265–72
drunk driving, 108
DSM. *See Diagnostic and
    Statistical Manual of
    Disorders*
Dworkin, Andrea, 48

Eagleton, Thomas, 181
Earhart, Amelia, 187
eating disorders, 70–71, 97, 165
    anorexia and bulimia nervosa,
        177
    body fat's role and, 176–77
    cultural ideals and, 176
    fighting, 177
    learning about looks and food,
        176
    starvation with, 176, 177
Eberstadt, Nicholas, 217
economic factors, sexual
    problems and, 29
ED. *See* erectile dysfunction
education, 219–20
    rape prevention, 97
    sexual health and, 324–25
Edwards, Charles, 254
Edwards, Harold M. "Ed," 282
Edwards, Robert, 303
Egan, Robert, 304
Egypt, FC/FGM and, 201, 202,
    204
Ehrenreich, Barbara, 309
Einstein, Albert, 192

ejaculation, 10
    female, 63
Eldridge, Laura, 115, 275, 349
Eli Lilly, 256
Elliott, Deni, 280
empowerment
    community, 341
    personal, 340–41
    self-help and, 339–41
end of life issues. *See also* deaths
    advocacy for, 281–84
    assisted-suicide support, 280–
        81
    with caregivers and dying
        partners, 284–91
    clergy with, 278
    consumers taking charge of,
        278–79
    counteracting death-denying
        culture with, 288–90
    cultural conversations about,
        275
    gourmet dinners for
        caregivers, 281
    growth and healing with, 290
    laundry helpers and, 280
    lives recorded for posterity,
        279, 290–91
    next steps, 279
    with pain and anger in death,
        276–81
    pet visitation with, 280
English, Deirdre, 309
Enovid, 305
Equanil, 101
erectile dysfunction (ED), 39, 40
Erikson, Erik, 66–67
estrogen, 240, 242. *See also*
    diethylstilbestrol
    studies, 251–52
    synthetic, 250
ethics, slave, 89
Ethiopia, FC/FGM in, 202, 205,
    206
European Collaborative Study,
    216
Ewing, Charles, 154
exams. *See also* pelvic exams
    bimanual rectovaginal, 59
    bimanual vaginoabdominal,
        58–59
    speculum, 58
exercise, 242
experience, variables of
    in boys, girls, men and
        women, 30–34
    sex variations with, 31–34

*The Expulsion of Adam and Eve
    from the Garden* (painting),
    123, *124*
eyebrows, 192–93
Eyerly, Stacia, 44

face
    aging, 179–80
    appearance and makeup, 183–
        85
    cleansing routines, 180–83
facial cleansing, 180
    with cream and lotion
        cleansers, 182
    oil-balance control with, 182
    soaps and, 181–82
    sunscreens and, 181
    toning and, 182–83
faking, orgasms, 12–13, 22
families. *See also* domestic
    violence victims
    alcoholism in, 106–13
    asylum experiences akin to
        female experiences in, 73
    heart disease and medical
        history of, 240–41
    manic depression in, 98–100
    mental illness and, 98–100
    violence, 93
Fanon, Frantz, 87
fantasies, 21
    rape, 116–18
fat. *See also* overweight
    animal, 182
    as antisocial figure, 171–75
    as feminist issue, 168–71
    in foods, 241–42
    role of body, 176–77
FC/FGM. *See* female
    circumcision/female genital
    mutilation
FDA. *See* Food and Drug
    Administration, U.S.
female circumcision/female
    genital mutilation (FC/FGM)
    breakthroughs against, 201–6
    history and practice, 205–6
    with human rights and
        holistic approaches, 205
    laws, 201–2, 203
    literature, 204, 205
    media and, 203
    new models and old problems
        with, 203–4
    statistics, 202
    Tostan's grassroots efforts and,
        202–3

Western awareness of, 204–5
WHO and, 202, 205–6
female ejaculation, 63
females. *See also* bodies, female
    activities approved for, 70–71
    as assigned gender, 32–33
    frigidity, 10, 12, 39
    love's importance to, 11
    myths about interest in sex, 25
    Viagra, 5–6, 38–40
female sexual dysfunction (FSD)
    in media, 41
    pharmaceutical companies
        promoting, 5–6, 40–42
    rise of, 39–40
female sexuality
    age and, 26–27
    outdated attitudes about, 8–9
femininity, hair and, 188–89
feminists
    fat as issue of, 168–71
    first-wave, 1–2 (*See also
        specific feminists*)
    legacy of boomer, 45–46
    mental health and influence
        of, 96
    second-wave, 47
    on trial, 56–57
    young, 321–22
Feminist Women's Health Center
    (FWHC), 48
    evolution of, 49–50
    information-sharing and
        literature of, 51–52
    police raid on, 56
    with women's health
        movement, 50–51
Ferguson, John Henry, 252
Ferlise, Donald V., 204–5
fetal studies, 303
fibroids, 337
films. *See also specific film titles*
    about rape, 116
    lesbians in, 43–44
    sluts in, 44
Fitzgerald, Scott, 71
Fitzgerald, Zelda, asylum
    experience of, 70–71
Flack, Audrey, 122, 126, 128
fluid-bonded, 64
Folley, S. J., 198
Food, Drug and Cosmetic Act,
    305
Food and Drug Administration,
    U.S. (FDA), 6, 39, 254, 263
foods, 176. *See also* eating
    disorders

DES in, 250
fats in, 241–42
gluten-free, 244–45
Fountain, L. H., 254, 255
Fowler, Jane, 207
Frankfort, Ellen, 49, 55–56, 309
Freedman, 81
freedom
    of expression for
        subordinates, 76
    mental health and influence
        of, 98
Freud, Sigmund, 8, 10, 16, 213
    Hite's debunking of vaginal
        orgasm and, 23–27
Frisch, Rose, 159
FSD. *See* female sexual
    dysfunction
fundraising, breast cancer, 232
FWHC. *See* Feminist Women's
    Health Center

Gage, Suzann, 51
Galen, 7
gang rape, 119
Gardasil, 208
Gelinas, Denise, 134
Geloo, 217
gender, 29
    assigning, 32–34
    bias with heart disease, 240
    language bias and, 12
    roles, 70–71, 87
    studies on stereotypes with,
        93
genital massage, 6–9
genital mutilation, 32–34, 205.
    See also female
    circumcision/female genital
    mutilation
Gevertzen, Alan, 273
Gies, Miep, 145
Gilbert, David, 270
Gilligan, Carol, 89
Gilman, Charlotte Perkins, 65, 87
girls. *See also* eating disorders;
    female circumcision/female
    genital mutilation
    athletic triad in young, 164
    Gardasil clinical trials on, 208
    good, 44–45
    indirect aggression in, 90–92
    intellectual differences
        between boys and, 69
    learning about looks and food,
        176
    in Little League, 162–63

role models and hair models
    for, 186–88
sexual double standard with,
    44–45
variables of experience in, 30–
    34
Glenn, Jules, 18
Glen Ridge rape, 150–51
gluten-free diets, 244–45
Goetsch, Martha, 213
Goffman, Erving, 73
Goldstein, Irwin, 39, 40, 41
good girls, 44–45
Goodwin, Jean, 133
government regulations,
    women's health and, 303–8
Grady, Hugh C., 252
Grant, James, 216
Gray, Ross, 233
Greenwald, Peter, 253–54
Greer, Germaine, 296–303
Gren, Deborah, 229
Grier, Pam, 195
Gross, Al, 157–58
guilt, 8, 22, 119
Gusfield, Joseph, 41
gynecology. *See* self-help
    gynecology

habit-forming drugs, 81–82, 83.
    *See also specific habit-
    forming drugs*
hair
    beauty associated with, 187
    body, 185–86, 189–91
    dreadlocks, 193–95
    eyebrows, 192–93
    femininity associated with,
        188–89
    flat, 189
    in media, 187
    pubic, 185
    role models as models for,
        186–88
    shaving body, 185, 189–91
Haring, Keith, 144
Harris, Dorothy V., 160
Harris Games, 160–61
Harvard University, 250–51. *See
    also* diethylstilbestrol
Harvey, Mary, 97
Haskell, Molly, 187
hatred, self-, 87, 95
health, women's, 7, 13. *See also*
    mental health; sexual health;
    women's health movement
    Asians, 341–43

cancer detection and
    treatment, 304
changing concepts of, 293–96
fetal studies, 303
government regulation and,
    303–8
Internet health information
    and, 274
IVF and, 303–4
men's health and, 308
MR and influence on, 54–55
new treatments, products and
    threats, 304–6
in prisons with HIV/AIDS,
    220–21
health insurance coverage, 218
health movements. *See* women's
    health movement
Hearst, Patricia, 130
heart attacks, 242
heart disease
    aspirin study with, 240
    deaths, 239
    diagnosing, 242–43
    explanation of coronary, 240
    family medical history and,
        240–41
    gender bias and, 240
    myths, 239–40
    prevention, 241–42
    risk factors, 241
    treatment, 243
    in women, 239–43
Hefner, Hugh, 14
Henderson, Craig, 232
Henie, Sonja, 187
herbal medicines, 341
Herbst, Arthur, 249, 251, 254
Herbst report, on DES, 252–53
Herman, Judith Lewis, 95–96, 97,
    116
hierarchy of studies, with
    science, 260
Himler, George, 254
hind milk, 197
Hippocrates, 6, 79
Hirsch, Lolly, 49
Hite, Shere
    Freud's vaginal orgasm
        debunked by, 23–27
    influence of, 5–6, 24
    *The Hite Report on Female
        Sexuality* (Hite), 5, 6
    age and female sexuality, 26–
        27
    influence of, 23

on orgasm via intercourse, 24–
    25
sexist definition of sex in, 25
women in control of female
    orgasms, 25–26
HIV/AIDS, 207, 212, 295
    ageism and, 219
    in black women, 328–29
    breast milk and babies
        infected with, 214–17
    in media, 218–19
    midlife and older women
        living with, 217–19
    prisons and women's health
        care with, 220–21
    women in prison with, 219–20
HIV Wisdom for Older Women,
    218
hoax, sexual revolution as, 10
Holck, Susan E., 215
Holocaust, 131, 133
homeopathic remedies, 1, 56,
    104, 214
hooks, bell, 97
hormone replacement therapy
    (HRT), 227–28, 242, 245–46,
    263
hospitals, in cases of rape, 122
Houston, Whitney, 193
Howell, Mary, 225–26
HPV. *See* Human Papilloma Virus
HRT. *See* hormone replacement
    therapy
Huggins, Charles, 304
Hughes, Sylvia Plath. *See* Plath,
    Sylvia
Human Papilloma Virus (HPV),
    208, 299
Humphry, Derek, 280, 282
husbands. *See* males; men;
    spousal rape; spouse abuse
hypertension. *See* blood
    pressure, high
hysteria, 6, 7–8, 39, 135

ideal weight, 165, 176
identity
    of rapists, 119, 120
    women and mixed messages
        about, 85–86
illegal abortions, 49
illness. *See* chronic illness;
    mental illness
impotence, 12, 37
incest, 93, 97
Indian Health Service, 344–45
Indonesia

FC/FGM in, 202
MR in, 55
infants. *See* babies
information-sharing
    breast cancer, 233
    FWHC's literature and, 51–52
informed consent
    with Indian Health Service,
        345
    pharmaceutical companies,
        conflict of interest and,
        247–74
Ingraham, Hollis S., 254
injuries, sports-related, 164
insemination, donor, 51
intercourse, 21, 24–25
international views, of sexual
    rights and sexual health, 28–
    29
Internet, evaluating health
    information, 274
intersex, 30–34
in vitro fertilization (IVF), 303–4
Iris, Messenger of the Gods
    (sculpture), 126, *127*
IVF. *See* in vitro fertilization

Jack, Dana Crowley, 91
Janus Report, on sexual double
    standard, 44
Jews, 145, 210. *See also* Holocaust
Johnson, Virginia E., 5, 9, 10, 23,
    117
    on orgasms, 14, 16, 17
    on sexual dysfunction, 27
    on sexual frustration, 19
Jong, Erica, 179–80
Jordan, Craig, 304
Jordan, Julie, 145

Kahlo, Frida, 192
Kaplan, Eugene, 18
Karman, Harvey, 52
Kasper, Ann S., 224–25, 236–39
Kassindja, Fauziya, 204–5
Kate, Carolyn, 88–89
Keenan, Richard, 155
Keniston, Kenneth, 18
Kennedy, Edward "Ted," 102, 103,
    255
Kessler, Suzanne, 31
Ketenjian, Tania
    Asetoyer interview, 344–46
    Kasper interview, 236–38
    Love interview, 225–30
    Mink interview, 164, 341–43
    Pearson interview, 315–21

Petitti interview, 261–65
Kevorkian, Jack, 277–78, 282
King, Billy Jean, 160
King, Don, 193
King, Martin Luther, Jr., 36
Kinsey, Alfred, 9–10, 18, 23, 117
Kline, Nathan, 101
Klinefelter syndrome, 30
knockout orgasms, 17
Koedt, Ann, 23, 25
Kohn, 87
Kolb, Lawrence, 133
Koop, Everett, 140
Kushner, Harvey, 239
Kushner, Rose, 224–25, 229, 236–39

labels
    for cosmetics, 181
    drug, 256
    subordinate and dominant, 75–76
    trauma, recover and mis-, 131–32
Lachaise, Gaston, 123
Lallemant, Marc, 215
language bias, gender and, 12
Larrick, George, 305
Lasker, Albert, 232
Lasker, Mary, 232
Lasser, J. K., 223
Lasser, Terese, 223–24
laundry helpers, 280
laws. *See also specific legislation*
    abortions, 49
    assisted-suicide, 281
    Brady, 164
    FC/FGM, 201–2, 203
    licensure, 56
    self-help gynecology and, 56–57
    Title IX, 159, 164
Lazarus, Margaret, 116
LDL. *See* low-density lipoprotein
Leary, Timothy, 102
Le Coeur, Sophie, 215
Leda and the Swan (painting), *124*, 125
Lee, Barbara Coombs, 280
Lee, Harper, 104
Lee, Spike, 44
legal abortions, 335–36
LeJeune, Jerome, 303
Leksell, Lars, 303
Lerner, Gerda, 284
lesbians, in film, 43–44
let-down reflex, 197–98

Levitz, Nicole, 116
Lewinsky, Monica, 42–43, 86
Lewis, John, 251
licensure laws, 56
life. *See* end of life issues
lineal victims, of abuse, 83–84
Lipton, Eunice, 185
literature
    FC/FGM, 204, 205
    FWHC's information-sharing and, 51–52
Little League, girls in, 162–63
locker-room talk, women's, 45–46
looks, 176, 183–85
Lorde, Audre, 233
Los Angeles Self-Help Clinic, 52
lotions, 182, 183
love, 11
Love, Susan, 224, 225–30
low-density lipoprotein (LDL), 240–41
Lowenthal, Michael, 207, 208–11
Lowery, Helen, 116
Luncheon on the Grass (painting), 126, *127*
Lupton, Mary Jane, 49
Lydon, Susan, 12
Lynch, Mary, 153, 154, 155
Lyons, Harriet, 192

Maccoby, Eleanor, 69
Madagascar, 216
madness, 71–73. *See also* asylums
    women and, 92–98
Maginnis, Cyndie, 100–101, 102
Maines, Rachel, 6–9
makeup, 183–85
Malaysia, FC/FGM in, 202
males. *See also* bodies, male; female circumcision/female genital mutilation
    as assigned gender, 32
    female bodies under control of, 39, 41
    female orgasm and ignorance of, 10
    female sexuality and outdated attitudes of, 8–9
    impotence, 12
    as sexual revolution winners, 9–13
    with women's liberation associated with sexual revolution, 9
    work's importance to, 11
Maltby, Barbara, 279
mammogram, 304

Manet, Édouard, 126–27
manic depression, 98–100
Marley, Bob, 195
Masaccio, 123–24
masks, facial, 183
masochistic personality disorder, 132
Masserman, Jules, 78–83
Masserman, Mrs., 79, 83
mastectomy, 223–24, 236–37
Masters, William H., 5, 9, 10, 23, 117
    on orgasms, 14, 16, 17
    on sexual dysfunction, 27
    on sexual frustration, 19
masturbation, 61
    as health hazard, 7
    in lieu of sexual relationships, 14
    orgasm during, 27, 63
    questionnaire, 21, 22
    as taboo, 10, 12
mature, vaginal orgasm as, 10, 23
Mayer-Rokitansky-Kuster-Hauser (MRKH) syndrome, 32
McCarthy, Joseph, 273
McCoach, David, 154
Mead, Margaret, 13, 307
media
    beauty images in, 85
    on drug addiction, 102–3
    FC/FGM and, 203
    FSD in, 41
    hair in, 187
    HIV/AIDS in, 218–19
    menstrual extraction in, 48
    prescription drugs in, 271–72
    sex misinformation in, 63
    vibrators in, 7–8
medical factors, sexual problems and, 30
medical history, heart disease and, 240–41
medicalization, of menopause, 338–39
medical model, of sexuality and beyond, 27–28
medical response, domestic violence and, 140
medical treatments
    genital massage viewed as, 6–9
    intersex, 31–34
    women with STDs and forced, 207, 208–11
medicine, licensure laws with, 56
Mehlum, Melissa, 280

Meir, Golda, 192–93
Melching, Molly, 202
men. *See also* female
    circumcision/female genital
    mutilation; males
    birth control pill for, 12
    craziness and, 71–72, 73
    depression in, 66
    hairiness in, 185–86
    minorities as medical test
        subjects, 39
    psychiatrists, 73
    rape and, 116–18
    as rape victims, 118
    sex differences theory of
        women and, 69
    social stress in, 72
    spouse abuse and, 145–47
    variables of experience in, 30–
        34
    violent crimes committed by,
        89
    women's health and health of,
        308
menopause
    as disease, 2
    medicalization of, 338–39
    as natural condition, 339
    as taboo, 338
menstrual extraction
    cultural history of, 53–54
    Del Em and, 50, 52–54
    in developing nations, 54–55
    FWHC's evolution with, 49–52
    materials and methods, 52–53
    media's mislabeling of, 48
    procedures, 52–53
    resistance against, 55–56
    results, 53
menstrual regulation, 54–55
menstruation, athletic triad and
    abnormal, 163–64
mental health
    airless space of, 84–85
    double standard of, 71
    families, mental illness and,
        98–100
    feminists influencing, 96
    freedom's influence on, 98
    of men, 66, 71–72
    of women in asylums, 70–75
    of women writers, 70–71
mental illness, 94, 98–100. *See
    also* asylums
Mero, Ralph, 280
Michelangelo, 124–25
midwives

    doctors and, 56
    with domestic violence
        victims, 143–44
    genital massage performed by,
        6, 7–8, 9
Milano, Carol, 14
Milford, Carol, 71
Milgram, Stanley, 68
milk production, breasts and,
    196–98, 214–17
Miller, Diane Disney, 273
Miller, Jean Baker, 66
Mills, Don Harper, 254–55
Miltown, 101, 103
minds
    with asylum experiences, 70–
        75
    MP-PAC as advocates for
        mental patients', 77–78
    psychology, women's bodies
        and, 65–113
Mink, Patsy T., 159, 164, 341–43
minorities
    as medical test subjects, 39
    men deemed criminal or
        psychotic, 72
    on prison, 221
Mintz, Suzanne, 281
mixed messages, 85–86, 91
molestation, 82
Morgan, Robin, 56, 302
Morganthau, Robert, 156
morning-after pill, 250, 255–56
Moyers, Bill, 279
MR. *See* menstrual regulation
MRKH. *See* Mayer-Rokitansky-
    Kuster-Hauser syndrome
multiple orgasms, 17
multiple personality disorder,
    135–36, 138–39
Musal, Karen, 204
myths, 25
    about women in sports, 161
    about women's nature, 69
    beauty, 175
    double-orgasm theory, 10–11,
        67
    heart disease, 239–40
    osteoporosis, 243–46
    race, 324
    of rape and violence, *124*, 125
    sexual, 64
    women as kinder and gentler,
        90

Nasca, P. C., 254

National Black Women's Health
    Project (NBWHP). *See also
    Our Bodies, Our Voices, Our
    Choices*
    origins, 322–23
National Institutes of Health
    (NIH), 37, 264
National Women's Health
    Network (NWHN), 3, 48, 294,
    307, 345–46
Native American Indians, 344–46
NBWHP. *See* National Black
    Women's Health Project
neighbors/witnesses, with
    domestic violence victims,
    144–45
Nelson, Jill, 87
Niederland, William, 133
Nietzsche, Friedrich, 88–89
NIH. *See* National Institutes of
    Health
nipples, 196
Nixon, Richard, 235
Noël, Barbara, 74, 79, 83. *See also*
    Masserman, Jules
nonstandard genitalia, 31
Norplant, 346
Norsigian, Judy, 2–3
Novello, Antonio, 140
Nussbaum, Hedda, 116, 155–58
NWHN. *See* National Women's
    Health Network

obedience experiments, 68–69
obesity, 241. *See also* overweight
OBOS. *See Our Bodies, Ourselves*
oils, categories of, 182
orgasmic platforms, 16
orgasms. *See also The Technology
    of Orgasm*
    with artificial vaginas and
        clitoris removal, 17
    clitoral, 10, 14–18, 62
    excitement, 16
    faking, 12–13, 22
    with female sex cycle, 16–17
    with intercourse, 24–25
    knockout, 17
    liberated, 13–19
    male ignorance of female, 10
    during masturbation, 27, 63
    multiple, 17
    myth of double-, 10–11, 67
    myths about female, 25
    penetration tied to, 7–8
    plateau, 16
    questionnaire, 20–21, 22

resolution, 17–19
speed-of-response differential with, 10
survey, 14
vaginal, 10, 14–15, 16, 18, 23–27
women in control of female, 25–26
orgasms, male. *See also* ejaculation
as health necessity, 13
The Origin of the Milky Way (painting), 198
osteoporosis, 243–46
Our Bodies, Ourselves (OBOS) (Boston Women's Health Book Collective), 2
Our Bodies, Our Voices, Our Choices (NBWHP)
abortion, 334–36
childbirth, 326–28
contraception and disease prevention, 328–31
diseases and conditions of reproductive system, 336–38
menopause, 338–39
NBWHP's origins, 322–23
pregnancy and prenatal care, 325–26
self-help and empowerment, 339–41
sexual health and education, 324–25
sterilization, 332–34
overweight, 241. *See also* weight loss
antisocial figure of being, 171–75
with fat as feminist issue, 168–71
Ovid, 13, 126
oxytocin, 197–98

paintings, 198. *See also* art, rape depictions
Pakistan, FC/FGM in, 202
Papinicaloau, George, 208
Pap smear, 208, 230, 299–300, 304
partner abuse. *See* domestic violence victims
partners
end of life issues with caregivers and dying, 284–91
sexual problems with, 29–30
with spousal abuse, 145–47

Pataki, George, 152, 155
Pataki, Libby, 152
pathology, of female bodies, 2, 39
patients. *See also* asylums
abuse of mental, 77, 78–83
airless space and, 84–85
breast cancer and control regained by, 233–34
doctors and attitudes toward, 57–58, 65
lineal victims and, 83–84
trauma survivors as psychiatric, 134–39
patriarchy, asylums as domain of, 94
PC muscle. *See* pubococcygeus muscle
Pearson, Cynthia, 3, 48, 229, 315–21
pelvic exams
bimanual rectovaginal exam with, 59
bimanual vaginoabdominal exam with, 58–59
collection of specimens in, 58–59
dialogue with doctors for, 59
explanation of, 58
external genitalia and, 58
questions, 57–58
speculum exam with, 58
women's attitudes toward, 59–60
penetration, orgasm tied to, 7–8
penis, 23
"normal" and medically acceptable size, 32
Pentothal, 81
period extraction. *See* menstrual extraction
perpetrator, PTSD and perception of, 139
Perseus with the Head of Medusa (sculpture), 126, *127*
personal empowerment, 340–41
Petitti, Diana, 261–65
pet visitation, 280
Pfrender, Ann, 256
pharmaceutical companies
DES and, 250–51, 256
drugs advertised by, 271–72
female Viagra and, 39
FSD promoted by, 5–6, 40–42
Gardasil promoted by, 208
informed consent and conflict of interest with, 247–74
resources for researching, 270

tranquilizers promoted by, 101–3
physical abuse, 134
physicians. *See* doctors
physiology
DSM's reduction of normal sexual function to, 28
with female sex cycle, 16–19
of women athletes, 160–63
Pincus, Gregory, 251
plateau, with female sex cycle, 16
Plath, Sylvia, asylum experience of, 70–71
poisons, 252, 255, 268. *See also* diethylstilbestrol
police
with domestic violence victims, 140, 153–54
FWHC raided by, 56
in rape cases, 120, 121–22
political factors, sexual problems and, 29
politics
sexology research with, 36–37
sluts in, 42–43
vaginal, 49, 55–56
Pollitt, Katha, 90
pornography, 21
Poskanzer, D. C., 253
posterity, end of life issues and, 279, 290–91
post-traumatic stress disorder (PTSD). *See also* trauma
characteristics, 139
diagnosis of, 133
renaming, 133–34
potency, 12, 13
power. *See also* empowerment
female aerobic, 162
potency as symbol for, 12, 13
rape as issue of, 118
in statistics, 259
pregnancy
Amytal use during, 82
in asylums, 74
DES and, 237, 249–53
domestic violence victims and, 141
forced breeding, 325
IVF, 303–4
prenatal care and, 325–26
in prisons, 220
teenagers, 211
prenatal care, 325–26. *See also* pregnancy
prescription drugs. *See also* drugs
advertisements, 271–72

pharmaceutical companies and conflict of interest with, 265–70
prevention, heart disease, 241–42
Preves, Sharon, 31
prisons, 51
    domestic violence victims in, 154–55
    FC/FGM and, 204–5
    population growth of women in, 221
    pregnancy in, 220
    trauma of captivity and, 130–32
    women's health care in, 220–21
    women with HIV/AIDS in, 219–20
privacy, with breast cancer, 233
probability, in science, 258–59
products, women's health and new, 304–6
property, breast cancer as, 230–31
Prozac, 104
psychiatrists
    mental patients abused by, 78–83
    MP-PAC and, 77–78
    percentage of men, 73
psychological factors, sexual problems and, 30
psychological manipulation, 65
psychologists, mental patients abused by, 78–79
psychology
    with asylum experiences, 70–75
    of competitiveness in women, 85–92
    of dominants and subordinates, 75–76
    lineal victims and, 83–84
    Masserman, Jules, interview and, 78–83
    MP-PAC and, 77–78
    obedience experiments in, 68–69
    women and madness with, 92–98
    women as constructs of, 66–70
    women's minds and bodies with, 65–113
psychotics, minority men deemed as, 72
PTSD. *See* post-traumatic stress disorder

pubic hair, 185
pubococcygeus (PC) muscle, 62
Putnam, Frank, 136

questionnaires
    research, 23
    sexuality, 19–23
questions
    domestic violence decision tree, 143
    domestic violence intervention strategy, 141
    pelvic exam, 57–58
    sex, 60–64
    women in sports, 165

race, heart disease and, 240
race, mythology of, 324
Rachel's Environment and Health Weekly, 270
Raffle, Angela, 300
randomized trials, 262
Rangel, Charles, 42
rape, 51, 94
    abortions with, 48
    acquaintance, 88–89, 119
    art and depictions of, 122–28
    in asylums, 73–74, 78
    on college campuses, 115–16
    date, 119, 211
    documentary films about, 116
    gang, 119
    Glen Ridge, 150–51
    hospitals in cases of, 122
    men as victims of, 118
    myths of violence and, *124*, 125
    police in cases of, 120, 121–22
    as power trip, 118
    prevention education, 97
    spousal, 153
    victims and setting, 116–18
    victims survey and statistics, 118–22
    with violence against women, 115–58
Rape of the Daughters of Leucippus (painting), 126
Rape of the Sabine Woman (sculpture), *125*, 126
The Rape of Europa (painting), *125*, 126
Raphael, Dana, 215
rapists
    age of, 119
    identity of, 119, 120

Rapunzel (fictional character), 194
recovery, trauma and, 130–39
rectal contact, 21
Redstone, Sumner M., 273
reduction, breast, 201
regulations
    with domestic violence cases, 141
    menstrual, 54–55
    PTSD and affect, 139
relationships, 11, 14
    caregivers and dying partners, 284–91
    PTSD and alterations in, 139
    sexual problems with, 29–30
repression, sexual, 73
reproductive system
    cancer and, 336–37
    diseases and conditions of, 336–38
    fibroids in, 337
    infertility and, 337
research
    breast cancer, 231–32
    politics and sexology, 36–37
research questionnaires, 23
resentment, 88–89
resolution, with female sex cycle, 16–17
Reubens, 126
Rheingold, Joseph, 67
Rheingold, Paul, 250
Rhode, S. W., 305
Richards, Amelia, 165
rights
    abortion, 334–35
    sexual, 28–29
risk factors, heart disease, 241
Rivera, Diego, 192
Robert Wood Johnson Foundation (RWJF), 278–79
Rodin, Auguste, 126–27
Roe v. Wade, 48
role models, as hair models, 186–88
Rollin, Betty, 281–84
Rollin, Ida, 282–83
romance, mixed messages, 85
Roosevelt, Eleanor, 225
Rose, Deborah, 56
Rosenblatt, Rebecca, 192
Ross, Lainie Friedman, 308
Rothman, Lorraine, 47–48, 49, 52. *See also* self-help gynecology
Ruddick, Sara, 89
RuPaul, 193

Russell, Cheryl, 79
Ruzek, Sheryl Burt, 308, 312
RWJF. *See* Robert Wood Johnson
    Foundation

Saddoff, 81
sado-masochism, 22
Sankar, Andrea, 288
Schacter, 69
Schiavo, Terri, 275
Schmidt, Alexander, 256
science, 257
    bias in, 259
    hierarchy of studies with, 260
    probability in, 258–59
    statistical power and, 259
    uncertainty and, 258
    variability in, 259–60
Scott, Julia R., 323
sculpture. *See* art, rape
    depictions
Seaman, Barbara, 23, 179, 225,
    275, 306–7, 309
    in memoriam, 347–49
Seconal, 81
second-wave feminists, 47
selective estrogen receptor
    modulators (SERMs), 242
self-abortions, 48, 51, 54, 307. *See
    also* menstrual extraction
self-defense techniques, 51
self-hatred, 87, 95
self-help
    empowerment through, 339–
    41
    process of, 340
self-help clinics, 50, 52
self-help gynecology, 307. *See
    also* menstrual extraction
    in developing countries, 54–55
    female bodies liberated with,
    49
    FWHC's evolution with, 49–52
    law and, 56–57
    menstrual extraction
        procedures, 52–53
    menstruation's cultural
        history and, 53–54
    origins, 47, 60–64
    pelvic exams, 57–59
    women's attitudes toward, 59–
    60
self-perception, PTSD and, 139
Sengegal, 201. *See also* female
    circumcision/female genital
    mutilation

SERMs. *See* selective estrogen
    receptor modulators
Settles, Landrum, 304
sex
    attitudes toward, 5–6
    genital massage as medical
        treatment unrelated to, 6–9
    liberated orgasm and, 13–19
    media and misinformation
        about, 63
    questions about, 60–64
    sexist definition of, 25, 27
    with sexuality questionnaire,
        19–23
    sexual revolution and, 9–13
    taboo and talking about, 12–
    13
sex aids, vibrators as, 8, 61, 64
sex assignment, 32–34
sex cycle, female, physiology of,
    16–19
"Sex in America" national survey,
    6
sexism
    in asylums, 72
    with definition of sex, 25
Sex Is Not a Natural Act (Tiefer)
    activist beginnings, 34–36
    activists' legacy, 37–38
    sexology, changes and
        influence of, 36–37
sexology, 36–37
sex skin reaction, 16
sexual abuse, 90, 134
sexual acts. *See also specific
    sexual acts*
    coitus as most frequent
        heterosexual, 6
sexual double standards, 44–45
sexual dysfunctions, 27–28
sexual frustration, 19
sexual function, 28
sexual health, 28–29
    education and, 324–25
sexuality, 27–28, 324
sexuality questionnaire
    explanation of, 19–20
    from January 1973, 20–23
sexually transmitted diseases
    (STDs). *See also specific STDs*
    biofeedback in treatment of,
        213–14
    breast-feeding and babies
        infected with HIV/AIDS,
        214–17
    on college campuses, 211–12

midlife and older women with
    HIV/AIDS, 217–19
vulvar vestibulitis support
    groups, 212–14
World War I and treatment
    forced upon women with,
    207, 208–11
sexual myths, 64
sexual practices, 6
sexual problems
    beyond medical model of
        sexuality, 27–28
    due to sociocultural, political
        or economic factors, 29
    four categories of, 27–28
    with international view on
        sexual health and sexual
        rights, 28–29
    with partners and
        relationships, 29–30
sexual relationships,
    masturbation in lieu of, 14
sexual repression, 73
sexual revolution
    as backward step for women,
    26
    as hoax, 10
    hypocrisy of, 9–13
    male association of women's
        liberation with, 9
    need and love in, 11
sexual rights, 28–29
sexual violence, 28, 128–29
sex variations, 30, 31–34
Shainess, Natalie, 18
Shainwald, Sybil, 348
shame, 29, 30, 47, 49–50, 324
shaving
    body hair, 185, 189–91
    customs, 185
Sherfey, Mary Jane, 23
Sherman Antitrust Act, 57
Shilts, Randy, 214
Shimkin, Michael B., 252
shock therapy, 73–74
Sianga, Mavis, 217
silence
    about HIV/AIDS and breast-
        feeding, 214–17
    domestic violence and, 144
    HIV/AIDS, women in prison
        and breaking, 219–20
    sexuality, shame and, 324
silicone implants, 305
Simpson, O. J., 145
Singer, 69
Siragusa, Charles, 154

size
    breasts, 196
    clitoris and penis, 32
slave ethics, 89
slavery, 325
sluts
    in film, 44
    in politics, 42–43
    sexual double standard with,
        44–45
Smith, Olive Watkins, 250–53
smoking, 241
snake pits, 94. *See also* asylums
Snodgrass, Sara, 90
Snyder, Myra, 271
soaps
    with fruit, vegetable or herb
        extracts, 182
    types of, 181–82
social stress, 72
sociocultural factors, sexual
    problems and, 29
Socrates, 82
Somalia, FC/FGM in, 202, 205
somatization disorder, 135, 137–
    38
Soranus, 7
Soros, George, 279
Speakoutrage, 307
specimens, in pelvic exams, 58–
    59
speed-of-response differential,
    between male and female
    orgasm, 10
Speranza, John, 141
Spiegel, David, 83
sponge, 63
sports, women in, 159
    athletic triad and, 163–64
    injuries, 164
    physiology of, 160–63
    questions and answers about,
        165
    Title IX and influence on, 164
spousal rape, 153
spouse abuse, 145–47, 152–55.
        See also domestic violence
        victims
St. John's wort, 104
Stamps, Timothy, 214
Stanley, Bob, 280
Stanton, Elizabeth Cady
    as first-wave feminist, 1–2
    influence of, 47
Stark, Eli, 254
Starr, Kenneth, 43

starvation, 176, 177. *See also*
    eating disorders
statistical significance, 260–61
statistics, 259
    domestic violence, 140–41,
        152
    FC/FGM, 202
    HIV/AIDS, 214–17
    rape, 118–22
    sports-related injuries, 164
    STDs, 211–12
status orgasmus, 17
STDs. *See* sexually transmitted
    diseases
Steinberg, Joel, 116, 155–58
Steinberg, Lisa, 116, 155–56
Stephanopoulos, George, 188
Steptoe, Patrick, 303
stereotypes
    blacks and negative, 87
    studies on gender, 93
sterilization
    abuse, 333–34
    without consent, 332
    voluntary, 332–33
stilbestrol. *See also*
        diethylstilbestrol
    failure to test, 250
Stoltenberg, John, 48
stress, 72, 241. *See also* post-
    traumatic stress disorder
studies
    DES, 251–52, 255–56
    fetal, 303
    gender-stereotyping, 93
    heart disease and aspirin, 240
    HIV/AIDS and breast-feeding,
        216
    truthful medical, 261–65
    "The Wife-Beater's Wife," 131–
        32
subordinates
    with dominants, 75–76
    freedom of expression
        blocked for, 76
Sudan, FC/FGM in, 202, 204, 205
Sugg, Nancy Kathleen, 141
suicide, 70, 71, 93, 103
    assisted, 277–78, 280–81, 283–
        84
sunscreens, 181
support
    assisted suicide, 280–81
    breast cancer, 233
    breast structure, 197
    with domestic violence, 142–
        43

groups for STDs, 212–14
surgeries, forced intersex, 31–34.
        See also specific surgeries
Surrey, Janet, 95
surveys. *See also* questionnaires
    orgasms, 14
    rape victims, 118–22
    "Sex in America," 6
Surviving Domestic Terrorism
    (Nussbaum), 116
Surviving Intimate Terrorism
    (Nussbaum)
    cycle of abuse, 157–58
    first time, 156–57
    introduction, 155–56
Survivor Project, 31
survivors
    Holocaust, 133
    of trauma as psychiatric
        patients, 134–39
systems of meaning, PTSD and,
    139

taboo
    masturbation as, 10, 12
    menopause as, 338
    talking about sex, 12–13
"Take Back the Night" march,
    115–16, 129
Tamoxifen, 304
Tanay, Emmanuel, 133
Tanenbaum, Leora, 66
Tavris, Carol, 90
Taylor, Elizabeth, 176
The Technology of Orgasm
    (Maines), review of, 6–9
teenagers
    pregnancy, 211
    violence in, 147–51
Terr, Lenore, 133
testing
    DES as poison, 252
    DES disseminated without,
        250
    women and minority men
        with medical, 39
testosterone, 301–2
thalidomide, 101–2
threats, women's health and new,
    304–6
Tiefer, Leonore, 6, 41
Tintoretto, Jacopo, 198
Tiresias, 13
Titian, 125–26
Title IX, 159, 164
Togo, FC/FGM ban in, 201
toning, for face, 182–83

Tostan, 202–3. *See also* female circumcision/female genital mutilation
Toth, Emily, 49
touching, 22
toxic shock syndrome (TSS), 306
tranquilizers, 74, 100–104. *See also specific types of tranquilizers*
transference, 83
Traore, Cheikh, 203
trauma
    of captivity, 130–32
    children and influence of, 133
    complex PTSD and, 133–34, 139
    diagnostic mislabeling with, 131–32
    masochistic personality disorder with, 132
    with need for new concept, 132–34
    new diagnosis with, 130–31
    recovery and, 130–39
    with survivors as psychiatric patients, 134–39
treatment. *See also* medical treatments
    breast cancer, 231
    cancer, 304
    domestic violence and, 143
    heart disease, 243
    new products, threats and, 304–6
    STD, 207, 208–11, 213–14
trials. *See also* clinical trials
    Brundidge, Charline, 152–55
    feminists on, 56–57
triglycerides, 240
Tripp, Linda, 86
trust, 64, 256–57
truth, 261–65
TSS. *See* toxic shock syndrome
Tucker, Kathryn, 280
Turner syndrome, 30
Twiggy, 176

Uganda, 217
Ulfelder, Howard, 253
uncertainty, truth and, 258
undernutrition, 176
UNICEF, 205
    HIV/AIDS, breast-feeding and silence of, 214–17
United States (U.S.), FC/FGM awareness in, 204–5
uterine cancer, 54

vaccinations, HPV, 208
vagina. *See also* pelvic exams
    with FC/FGM, 201–6
vaginal orgasm, 14–15, 16
    artificial vaginas and, 17
    debunked, 23–27
    as mature, 10, 23
    as proprioceptive, 17–18
vaginoplasty, 33
valerian, 104
validation, 142, 288
Valium, 104
Van Siclen Smith, George, 250–53
variability, in science, 259–60
vasectomy, 12
vasocongestion, 16, 17
vegetable oil, 182
Venus of Willendorf (sculpture), 122, *123*
Viagra
    expert-ownership and, 41–42
    players, 40–41
    rise of FSD, 39–40
    search for female, 5–6, 38–40
vibrators, 6
    advertisements, 7, 8
    as medical instrument, 8
    questionnaire, 21
    as sex aids, 8–9, 61, 64
victims. *See also* domestic violence victims
    blaming, 131–32
    men as rape, 118
    psychology and lineal, 83–84
    setting for rape, 116–18
    survey of rape, 118–22
violence. *See also* domestic violence victims; rape
    crime and, 89–90
    family, 93
    myths of rape and, *124*, 125
    sexual, 28, 128–29
    in teenagers, 147–51
    VOV and, 97
    women with rape and, 115–58
Visco, Fran, 229
Voltaire, 105
VOV. *See* Cambridge Hospital Victims of Violence Program
vulvar vestibulitis, 212–14

Walker, Alice, 194, 204
Wallace, Hanna, 44
Warren, Erica, 106–13
Watterson, Kathryn, 78–83
Webb, Marilyn, 275

weight, ideal, 165, 176
weight loss, 241
    athletic triad and, 163–64
    ideal weight and, 165
Weisstein, Naomi, 23, 27, 65–66
West, Ellen, 70–71
WHO. *See* World Health Organization
"The Wife-Beater's Wife" study, 131–32
Williams, Dar, 191
Williams, Esther, 187
Wilson, Colleen, 56, 307
Winnow, Jackie, 233
witches, 56
witnesses/neighbors, domestic violence victims and role of, 144–45
wives. *See* females; spousal rape; spouse abuse; women
Wolberg, Louis, 80, 81
Wolfson, Alice, 306–7, 348
women. *See also* health, women's
    with competitiveness, 85–92
    in control of female orgasms, 25–26
    craziness and asylum experiences of, 70–75
    depression in, 66
    drug addiction and, 100–113
    essential nature of, 89–90
    with expectations of other women, 86
    hairlessness in, 185–86
    health issues for Asian, 341–43
    heart disease in, 239–43
    HIV/AIDS in black, 328–29
    HIV/AIDS in midlife and older, 217–19
    identity and mixed messages for, 85–86
    imprisonment for Chilean, 51
    indirect aggression in, 90–92
    kinder, gentler myths about, 90
    with locker-room talk, 45–46
    madness and, 92–98
    as medical test subjects, 39
    mental health of writers, 70–71
    with mixed messages at work, 85
    myths about nature of, 69
    pelvic exams and attitudes of, 59–60
    population in prison, 221

in prison with HIV/AIDS, 219–20

psychology and constructs of, 66–70

psychology with minds and bodies of, 65–113

rape and violence against, 115–58

resentment and, 88–89

sex differences theory of men and, 69

sexual problems of, 29–30

sexual revolution as backward step for, 26

social stress in, 72

somatization disorder in, 135, 137–38

in sports, 159–65

variables of experience in, 30–34

Viagra for, 5–6, 38–40

violent crimes committed by, 89–90

World War I and STD treatment forced upon, 207, 208–11

women's health movement
flourishing of, 306–8

FWHC and, 50–51

grassroots and professionalized organizations, 312–15

ideologies and professional institutional agendas with, 311–12

legacy and influence of, 59–60

map of, 308–15

menstrual extraction and influence on, 55–56

moving forward with, 293–346

rise and development of, 308–11

work
male relationship to, 11

tranquilizers and connection to, 103

women and mixed messages at, 85

The Working Group on a New View of Women's Sexual Problems, 29

at Boston Forum, 40–41

World Association of Sexology, 29

World Health Organization (WHO), 28–29, 264–65

FC/FGM and, 202, 205–6

HIV/AIDS, breast-feeding and silence of, 214–17

World War I, forced STD treatment in, 207, 208–11

writers, mental health of women, 70–71

Yalom, Irvin, 135

Youk, Thomas, 278

Voices of the Women's Health Movement
VOLUME ONE

Contents

CHAPTER 1: IN THE BEGINNING

Witches, Midwives, and Nurses: A History of Women Healers by Barbara Ehrenreich
   and Deirdre English

Out of Conflict Comes Strength and Healing: Women's Health Movements by Helen I. Marieskind

Medicine and Morality in the Nineteenth Century by Kristin Luker

Ain't I a Woman? by Sojourner Truth

On Motherhood by Elizabeth Cady Stanton

Why Elizabeth Isn't on Your Silver Dollar by Barbara Seaman

Sylvia Bernstein Seaman (1900-95) by Karen Bekker

Fanny Burney's Letter to Her Sister, 1812, describing her mastectomy in December of 1811
   by Fanny Burney

Women's Health and Government Regulation: 1820-1949 by Suzanne White Junod

A My Name is Alice by Jennifer Baumgardner

CHAPTER 2: TAKING OUR BODIES BACK: THE WOMEN'S HEALTH MOVEMENT

The Role of Advocacy Groups in Research on Women's Health by Barbara Seaman and Susan F. Wood

Inside and Out: Two Stories of the Rumblings Beneath the Quiet compiled by Suzanne Clores

Women's Health and Government Regulation: 1950-1980 by Suzanne White Junod

Sisterhood by Gloria Steinem

Dear Injurious Physician by Barbara Seaman

The Ultimate Revolution by Shulamith Firestone

Our Bodies, Ourselves: Remembering the Dignity edited by Mei Hwei Astella Saw and Sarah J. Shey

Looking Back on Our Bodies, Ourselves edited by Joanna Perlman and Sarah J. Shey

The Boston Women's Health Book Collective and Our Bodies, Ourselves

Alice Wolfson interview by Tania Ketenjian

Belita Cowan interview by Tania Ketenjian

A Mother's Story by Helen Rodriguez-Trias

Helen Rodriguez-Trias interview by Tania Ketenjian

A Is for Activism by Byllye Avery

Byllye Avery interview by Tania Ketenjian

The Female Eunuch by Germaine Greer

The Hite Report on Shere Hite: Voice of a Daughter in Exile by Shere Hite

In Defense of Shere Hite by Sarah J. Shey

Susan Brownmiller: Memoir of a Revolutionary by Carrie Carmichael

A Mother's Story by Patsy Mink

DES Litigation by Sybil Shainwald

CHAPTER 3: BIRTH CONTROL

In the Matter of Rosemarie Lewis: Women and the Corporatization of Contraception by Andrea Tone

Racism, Birth Control, and Reproductive Rights by Angela Y. Davis
Informed Consent by Elizabeth Siegel Watkins
Julie Is Not a Statistic by Barbara Seaman
Philip Corfman interview by Tania Ketenjian
A Pill for Men by Barbara Seaman
Norplant: The Contraception You're Stuck With by Barbara Seaman
Cycles of Hot and Cold: Trying to Learn Fertility Awareness in North America by Katie Singer

CHAPTER 4: MENSTRUATION
If Men Could Menstruate by Gloria Steinem
The Selling of Premenstrual Syndrome by Andrea Eagan
No More T.O.M. by Sara Germain

CHAPTER 5: PREGNANCY AND BIRTHING
Childbirth in America edited by Victoria Eng and Sonia Lander
The Cultural Warping of Childbirth by Doris Haire
Motherhood by Letty Cottin Pogrebin
In Which a Sensible Woman Persuades Her Doctor, Her Family, and Her Friends to Help Her Give
    Birth at Home by Barbara Katz Rothman
How Late Can You Wait to Have a Baby? by Barbara Seaman
How Science is Redefining Parenthood by Barbara Katz Rothman
Having Anne by Laura Yeager
Preface to *With Child* by Ariel Chesler
Misconceptions by Gena Corea
Determination by Barbara Katz Rothman
Patenting Life: Are Genes Objects of Commerce? by Barbara Katz Rothman and Ruth Hubbard
Geriatric Obstetrics: Oh, Baby! by Carrie Carmichael
Bold Type: Childbirth Is Powerful by Barbara Findlen
Arlene Eisenberg interview by Tania Ketenjian
Lives: When One Is Enough by Amy Richards, as told to Amy Barrett
Hate Mail by Amy Richards
Love, Mom: A Mother's Journey from Loss to Hope by Cynthia Baseman
Is This Any Way to Have a Baby? by Barbara Seaman

CHAPTER 6: MOTHERHOOD
Yes, We Have No Bambinos by Molly Haskell
Dr. Spock's Advice to New Mothers by Alix Kates Shulman
Lovely Me by Barbara Seaman
My Mother's Death: Thoughts on Being a Separate Person by Judith Rossner
Take the Blame off Mother by Paula J. Caplan
The Madonna's Tears for a Crack in My Heart by Audrey Flack
Breastfeeding Revisited by Margot Slade
Moms in Dark about OTC Drugs, Survey Shows by Frances Cerra Whittelsey
The Baby Contract by Susan Jordan
Monster Mommies by Erica Jong
They Came to Stay by Marjorie Margolies and Ruth Gruber
An Adopted Daughter Meets Her Natural Mother by Betty Jean Lifton

What Do You Love about Being a Lesbian Mom? by Catherine Gund
On Becoming a Grandmother by Francine Klagsbrun

CHAPTER 7: MENOPAUSE AND AGING
Flashback: A History of Menopause by Laura Eldridge
The Changing Years by Madeline Gray
Promise Her Anything, but Give Her . . . Cancer: The Selling of ERT by Barbara Seaman
Exploding the Estrogen Myth by Barbara Seaman
The Bitter Pill by Leora Tanenbaum
A Friend Indeed: The Grandmother of Menopause Newsletters by Sari Tudiver
The Truth about Hormone Replacement Therapy: How to Break Free from the Medical Myths of
    Menopause by the National Women's Health Network
On Aging by Joan Ditzion

CHAPTER 8: GYNECOLOGICAL SURGERY
Needless Hysterectomies by Marcia Cohen
So, You're Going to Have a New Body! by Lynne Sharon Schwartz
Keeping All Your Eggs in One Basket by Barbara Seaman

CHAPTER 9: ABORTION
I Am Roe by Norma McCorvey
The Jane Collective by Pauline Bart
The Abortion by Alix Kates Shulman
Starting the New York Abortion Access Fund: Grassroots Activism on Abortion Rights, from Vision to
    Reality by Irene Xanthoudakis and Lauren Porsch

CHAPTER 10: LESBIAN, BISEXUAL AND TRANSGENDER HEALTH
Sappho Was a Right-On Woman by Sidney Abbott and Barbara Love
Putting Lesbian Health in Focus by Vivien Labaton
Lesbian Health Gains Long Due Attention from Institute of Medicine by Amy Allina
Look Both Ways by Jennifer Baumgardner
Women's Health/Transgender Health: Intersections by Lauren Porsch

CHAPTER 11: GENDER AND MEDICINE
Why Would a Girl Go into Medicine? by Margaret A. Campbell
A Woman in Residence by Michelle Harrison
Venus and the Doctor by Betty Rothbart
Woman Doctor by Florence Haseltine and Yvonne Yaw
Essays on Women by Edith Stein
Susan Wood interview by Meghan Buckley